T0384894

Hypnosis

The International Library of Psychology
Series Editor: David Canter

Titles in the Series

Human Perception
Marco Bertamini and Michael Kubovy

Environmental Psychology
David Canter, Terry Hartig and Mirilia Bonnes

Hypnosis
Michael Heap and Irving Kirsch

Counseling Psychology
Frederick Leong

Psychology and Law
Clinical Forensic Perspectives
Ronald Roesch

Psychology and Law
Criminal and Civil Perspectives
Ronald Roesch

Parapsychology
Richard Wiseman and Caroline Watt

History of Psychology Revisited
William Woodward and Sandy Lovie

Hypnosis

Theory, Research and Application

Edited by

Michael Heap

Wathwood Hospital, UK

and

Irving Kirsch

University of Connecticut, USA and University of Plymouth, UK

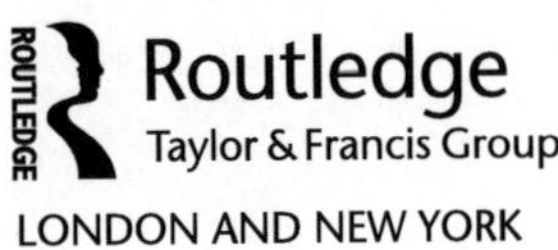

LONDON AND NEW YORK

First published 2006 by Ashgate Publishing

Published 2016 by Routledge
2 Park Square, Milton Park, Abingdon, Oxon OX14 4RN
605 Third Avenue, New York, NY 10017

Routledge is an imprint of the Taylor & Francis Group, an informa business

British Library Cataloguing in Publication Data
Hypnosis : theory, research and application. –
(International library of essays in psychology)
1. Hypnotism
I. Heap, Michael II. Kirsch, Irving, 1943
154.7

Library of Congress Cataloging-in-Publication Data
Hypnosis : theory, research, and application / edited by Michael Heap and Irving Kirsch.
p. cm. — (The international library of essays in psychology)
Includes bibliographical references.
ISBN 0-7546-2454-4 (alk. paper)
1. Hypnotism. I. Heap, Michael. II. Kirsch, Irving. III. Series.

BF1141.H89 2006
154.7—dc22

2005045341

ISBN 13: 978-0-7546-2454-7 (hbk)

DOI: 10.4324/9781315252858

Contents

PART IV INDIVIDUAL DIFFERENCES IN HYPNOTIC SUGGESTIBILITY

PART V INVESTIGATING HYPNOTIC PHENOMENA

PART VI NEUROPSYCHOLOGICAL AND NEUROPHYSIOLOGICAL RESEARCH AND THEORIES

PART VII CLINICAL APPLICATIONS

PART VIII PROFESSIONAL AND LEGAL ISSUES

Acknowledgements

The editors and publishers wish to thank the following for permission to use copyright material.

American Association for the Advancement of Science for the essay: Pierre Rainville, Gary H. Duncan, Donald D. Price, Benoît Carrier and M. Catherine Bushnell (1997), 'Pain Affect Encoded in Human Anterior Cingulate but not Somatosensory Cortex', *Science*, **277**, pp. 968–71. Copyright © 1997 AAAS.

American Medical Association for the essay: American Medical Association (1985), 'Scientific Status of Refreshing Recollection by the Use of Hypnosis', *Journal of the American Medical Association*, **253**, pp. 1918–23.

American Psychological Association for the essays: Irving Kirsch (1985), 'Response Expectancy as a Determinant of Experience and Behavior', *American Psychologist*, **40**, pp. 1189–202. Copyright © 1985 American Psychological Assocation; Arlene H. Morgan (1973), 'The Heritability of Hypnotic Susceptibility in Twins', *Journal of Abnormal Psychology*, **82**, pp. 55–61. Copyright © 1973 American Psychological Association; Auke Tellegen and Gilbert Atkinson (1974), 'Openness to Absorbing and Self-Altering Experiences ("Absorption"), a Trait Related to Hypnotic Susceptibility', *Journal of Abnormal Psychology*, **83**, pp. 268–77. Copyright © 1974 American Psychological Association; Donald R. Gorassini and Nicholas P. Spanos (1986), 'A Social-Cognitive Skills Approach to the Successful Modification of Hypnotic Susceptibility', *Journal of Personality and Social Psychology*, **50**, pp. 1004–12. Copyright © 1986 American Psychological Association; Steven Jay Lynn and Judith W. Rhue (1988), 'Fantasy-Proneness: Hypnosis, Developmental Antecedents, and Psychopathology', *American Psychologist*, **43**, pp. 35–44. Copyright © 1988 American Psychological Association; Carlo Piccione, Ernest R. Hilgard and Philip G. Zimbardo (1989), 'On the Degree of Stability of Measured Hypnotizability Over a 25-Year Period', *Journal of Personality and Social Psychology*, **56**, pp. 289–95. Copyright © 1989 American Psychological Association; Ernest R. Hilgard, Arlene H. Morgan and Hugh Macdonald (1975), 'Pain and Dissociation in the Cold Pressor Test: A Study of Hypnotic Analgesia with "Hidden Reports" Through Automatic Key Pressing and Automatic Talking', *Journal of Abnormal Psychology*, **84**, pp. 280–89. Copyright © 1975 American Psychological Association; William C. Coe and Anne S.E. Sluis (1989), 'Increasing Contextual Pressures to Breach Posthypnotic Amnesia', *Journal of Personality and Social Psychology*, **57**, pp. 885–94. Copyright © 1989 American Psychological Association; Irving Kirsch, Guy Montgomery and Guy Sapirstein (1995), 'Hypnosis as an Adjunct to Cognitive-Behavioral Psychotherapy: A Meta-Analysis', *Journal of Consulting and Clinical Psychology*, **63**, pp. 214–20. Copyright © 1995 American Psychological Association; David R. Patterson and Mark P. Jensen (2003), 'Hypnosis and Clinical Pain', *Psychological Bulletin*, **129**, pp. 495–521. Copyright © 2003 American Psychological Association; Alan Scoboria, Giuliana Mazzoni, Irving Kirsch and Leonard S. Milling (2002), 'Immediate and Persisting Effects of Misleading Questions and Hypnosis on Memory Reports', *Journal of Experimental Psychology: Applied*, **8**, pp. 26–32. Copyright © 2002 American Psychological Association. All reprinted with permission.

Blackwell Publishing for the essays: Ernest R. Hilgard (1974), 'Toward a Neo-Dissociation Theory: Multiple Cognitive Controls in Human Functioning', *Perspectives in Biology and Medicine*, **17**, pp. 301–16; Irving Kirsch, and Wayne Braffman (2001), 'Imaginative Suggestibility and Hypnotizability', *Current Directions in Psychological Science*, **10**, pp. 57–61; Steven Jay Lynn, Timothy G. Lock, Bryan Myers and David G. Payne (1997), 'Recalling the Unrecallable: Should Hypnosis be used to Recover Memories in Psychotherapy?', *Current Directions in Psychological Science*, **6**, pp. 79–83.

BMJ Publishing Group for the essay: W.M. Gonsalkorale, V. Miller, A. Afzal and P.J. Whorwell (2003), 'Long Term Benefits of Hypnotherapy for Irritable Bowel Syndrome', *Gut*, **52**, pp. 1623–29.

Contemporary Hypnosis for the essay: Nicholas P. Spanos, Deborah M. Flynn and Maxwell I. Gwynn (1988), 'Contextual Demands, Negative Hallucinations, and Hidden Observer Responding: Three Hidden Observers Observed', *British Journal of Experimental and Clinical Hypnosis*, **5**, pp. 5–10.

Guilford Publications, Inc. for the essay: Erik Z. Woody and Kenneth S. Bowers (1994), 'A Frontal Assault on Dissociated Control', in Steven Jay Lynn and Judith W. Rhue (eds), *Dissociation: Clinical and Theoretical Perspectives*, New York and London: The Guilford Press, pp. 52–79.

The International Library of Psychology for the essays: Amanda J. Barnier and Kevin M. McConkey (1999), 'Hypnotic and Posthypnotic Suggestion: Finding Meaning in the Message of the Hypnotist', *International Journal of Clinical and Experimental Hypnosis*, **47**, pp. 192–208; Helen J. Crawford (1994),'Brain Dynamics and Hypnosis: Attentional and Disattentional Processes', *International Journal of Clinical and Experimental Hypnosis*, **42**, pp. 204–32; Vilfredo De Pascalis (1999), 'Psychophysiological Correlates of Hypnosis and Hypnotic Susceptibility', *International Journal of Clinical and Experimental Hypnosis*, **47**, pp. 117–43.

John Wiley & Sons Ltd for the essays: John Gruzelier (1998), 'A Working Model of the Neuropsychophysiology of Hypnosis: A Review of Evidence', *Contemporary Hypnosis*, **15**, pp. 3–21; Michael Heap (2000), 'The Alleged Dangers of Stage Hypnosis', *Contemporary Hypnosis*, **17**, pp. 117–26.

Johns Hopkins University Press for the essay: Ernest R. Hilgard (1974), 'Toward a Neo-Dissociation Theory: Multiple Cognitive Controls in Human Functioning', *Perspectives in Biology and Medicine*, **17**, pp. 301–16. Copyright © 1974 The Johns Hopkins University Press. Reprinted with permission of The Johns Hopkins University Press.

Lippincott Williams and Wilkins for the essay: Ernest R. Hilgard (1969), 'Altered States of Awareness', *Journal of Nervous and Mental Disease*, **149**, pp. 68–79.

Rowman and Littlefield Publishing Group for the essay: Theodore X. Barber (1969/1995), 'Toward a Scientific Explanation of "Hypnotic" Behavior', in T.X. Barber, *Hypnosis: A Scientific Approach*, Northvale, NJ: Jason Aronson, pp. 221–42.

Every effort has been made to trace all the copyright holders, but if any have been inadvertently overlooked the publishers will be pleased to make the necessary arrangement at the first opportunity.

Series Preface

Psychology now touches every corner of our lives. No serious consideration of any newsworthy topic, from eating disorders to crime, from terrorism to new age beliefs, from trauma to happiness, is complete without some examination of what systematic, scientific psychology has to say on these matters. This means that psychology now runs the gamut from neuroscience to sociology, by way of medicine and anthropology, geography and molecular biology, connecting to virtually every area of scientific and professional life. This diversity produces a vibrant and rich discipline in which every area of activity finds outlets across a broad spectrum of publications.

Those who wish to gain an understanding of any area of psychology therefore either have to rely on secondary sources or, if they want to connect with the original contributions that define any domain of the discipline, must hunt through many areas of the library, often under diverse headings.

The volumes in this series obviate those difficulties by bringing together under one set of covers, carefully selected existing publications that are the definitive papers that characterize a specific topic in psychology.

The editors for each volume have been chosen because they are internationally recognized authorities. Therefore the selection of each editor, and the way in which it is organized into discrete sections, is an important statement about the field.

Each volume of the International Library of Psychology thus collects in one place the seminal and definitive journal articles that are creating current understanding of a specific aspect of present-day psychology. As a resource for study and research the volumes ensure that scholars and other professionals can gain ready access to original source material. As a statement of the essence of the topic covered they provide a benchmark for understanding and evaluating that aspect of psychology.

As this International Library emerges over the coming years it will help to specify what the nature of 21st century psychology is and what its contribution is to the future of humanity.

DAVID CANTER
Series Editor
Professor of Psychology
University of Liverpool, UK

Introduction

Definition and Description

According to Heap *et al.* (2001, p. 3):

> The term 'hypnosis' denotes an interaction between one person, the 'hypnotist', and another person or people, the 'subject' or 'subjects'. In this interaction the hypnotist attempts to influence the subjects' perceptions, feelings, thinking and behaviour by asking them to concentrate on ideas and images that may evoke the intended effects. The verbal communications that the hypnotist uses to achieve these effects are termed 'suggestions'. Suggestions differ from everyday kinds of instructions in that they imply that a 'successful' response is experienced by the subject as having a quality of involuntariness or effortlessness.

Occasionally, the hypnotist and subject are the same person. In this case, the person attempts to alter his or her experience by thinking of the suggestions without the aid of a hypnotist. This is termed 'self-hypnosis'. Many believe that all hypnosis can be thought of as self-hypnosis, because subjects must accept the suggestion if it is to have the intended effect.

Suggestion

There are a number of different kinds of suggestion that may be given during hypnosis. One common type of suggestion is 'ideomotor suggestion' in which the idea is conveyed of a simple, automatic movement of a part of the body, such as a finger or arm. This kind of suggestion often also includes the idea of some alteration in perceptual experience – for example, in the case of arm levitation, a feeling of lightness in the arm. Inhibition of a movement may be suggested, such as arm immobility or eye catalepsy. Suggestions of this sort are termed 'challenge suggestions'. Other changes in perceptions or cognitive function include suggested hallucinations, pain reduction, and memory inhibition (amnesia). These are generally termed 'cognitive suggestions'. Very often, suggestions are augmented by descriptions of appropriate imagery, such as a helium-filled balloon in the case of arm levitation, or immersion of the hand in icy water in the case of suggested hand numbness (glove anaesthesia).

The hypnotist may indicate that the response is to take place *after* the conclusion of hypnosis, in which case we use the term 'posthypnotic suggestion'. For example, the subjects may be told that, at some point after they have opened their eyes, the hypnotist will tap on the table and they will immediately touch their right ear, without remembering that they had been instructed to do so.

There is one important characteristic of a successful suggested response – namely that it entails a change in subjective experience, rather than merely a change in outward behaviour. With ideomotor responses, the essential component is the experience that the behaviour is occurring involuntarily or effortlessly. This characteristic is often called 'the classic suggestion effect'.

The Hypnotic Induction and the Concept of the 'Hypnotic Trance'

A session of hypnosis normally begins with a 'hypnotic induction'. Although the contents of hypnotic inductions vary widely, current inductions usually include suggestions that direct the subjects to relax and to become absorbed in inner processes, such as feelings, thoughts and imagery. During self-hypnosis, subjects go through this process under their own direction.

Traditionally, it has been considered that the hypnotic induction places the subject in a special altered state of consciousness or 'trance' in which he or she is particularly suggestible. Another presumed property of this trance state is that it facilitates access to unconscious processes. The validity of the concept of 'hypnotic trance' has been the subject of longstanding controversy and, in order to understand how this controversy developed, it is necessary to summarize the main historical milestones in the evolution of modern hypnosis. Before we do this, we conclude the present section with a brief examination of the measurement of suggestibility.

Hypnotic Suggestibility

A subject's response to any given suggestion can be measured in various ways, and the 1950s and 1960s saw the development of standard psychometric methods for the assessment of an individual's hypnotic suggestibility. These scales typically consist of a hypnotic induction followed by a series of suggestions. The subject's *hypnotizability* (or, more accurately, *hypnotic suggestibility*) is measured by the number of suggestions to which he or she successfully responds. Scores on these scales have a broad distribution with a clear central tendency.

The scales now in use have high internal consistency, with significant intercorrelations between responsiveness to different kinds of suggestion. However, it has also been reliably demonstrated that the proportion of subjects 'passing' declines from ideomotor, to challenge, to cognitive suggestions. Thus, some suggestions are more difficult than others to experience.

The most commonly used scales have high test–retest reliability. For example, Piccione, Hilgard and Zimbardo (Chapter 15, this volume), have demonstrated that hypnotizability, as measured by the Stanford Hypnotic Susceptibility Scales, Forms A and B, has high test–retest reliability (0.71) over a period of 25 years. Findings such as this support the contention that hypnotic susceptibility is a stable individual characteristic or trait, although not all authorities accept this. This topic will be discussed later.

The Historical Development of Modern Hypnosis

Although comparisons are sometimes drawn between procedures used in the 'sleep temples' of ancient Greece and Egypt, modern hypnosis itself can be traced directly back to the ideas and practices of the Austrian physician Franz Anton Mesmer (1734–1815). Mesmer proposed the existence of a universal force called 'animal magnetism' and claimed that disturbances in the natural flow of animal magnetism in the body were responsible for certain illnesses. He further claimed that he had the ability to restore this flow and thus heal the patient. For this purpose he initially used real magnets, but later he favoured slow passes of the hands over the patient's body. In response to these passes, patients would experience 'crises' (swooning, convulsing, crying, laughing hysterically and so on). They would then enter a stuporous state and thus they were healed.

The subsequent development of mesmerism was characterized by an emphasis on achieving a state of mental and physical relaxation in the patient and a narrow focus of attention. For example, Mesmer's student, the Marquis de Puységur (1751–1825), in preference to the mesmeric 'crises', encouraged in his patients a relaxed, calm state of mind that he termed 'artificial somnambulism'. The Abbé de Faria (1756–1819) used the term 'lucid sleep'; this was achieved by the subject concentrating on the idea of sleep rather than by mesmeric passes. Later, James Braid (1795–1860) described 'hypnosis' (the term he preferred) as a physiological state. This was characterized by a fixed stare, complete body relaxation, suppressed breathing and concentration on the words of the hypnotist. He later introduced the concept of 'monoideism', the idea that hypnosis is characterized by a state of heightened concentration on a single idea suggested by the hypnotist. Imagination, belief, and expectancy were thus intensified.

During this period mesmerism, as a clinical and therapeutic procedure, spread throughout Europe and North America. Of particular interest was its use in surgery and dentistry as an anaesthetic. This application had the support of some eminent physicians such as John Elliotson (1791–1868) and the surgeon James Esdaile (1808–1859).

After Braid, the terms 'mesmerism' and 'animal magnetism' were gradually replaced with the modern label, 'hypnosis'. The next important theoretical developments occurred in France with the ideas of Jean Martin Charcot (1835–1893) and Hippolyte Bernheim (1837–1919). Charcot was a leading neurologist and surgeon at the Salpêtrière Institute near Paris, and Bernheim was professor of medicine at Nancy. Charcot noted the similarity of hypnotic phenomena to symptoms exhibited by his hysterical patients such as involuntary catalepsy, anaesthesia, amnesia and hallucinations. He therefore insisted that hypnosis was an abnormal state of mind found in the mentally ill. He also put forward a three-stage theory of hypnosis, namely lethargy, then catalepsy, then somnambulism.

In contrast, Bernheim viewed hypnosis as a normal phenomenon based on the 'power of suggestion' rather than a special state. He demonstrated that the entire range of hypnotic phenomena could be elicited in 15 per cent of the normal population. He was also very critical of Charcot's three stages and demonstrated that they were not representative of the usual response of subjects to hypnosis. Thus, rather than a special state, we now have the emphasis on suggestibility – the idea that hypnosis has something to do with enhanced responsiveness to suggestion. In the end, Bernheim's arguments held sway and Charcot's were largely abandoned. However, Charcot's influence remains in the scales used to measure hypnotizability, as the suggestions included in those scales are requests to briefly experience the symptoms exhibited by his hysterical patients (for example, catalepsy, anaesthesia, amnesia and hallucinations).

From Braid onwards, we witness the increasing influence of psychiatrists and psychologists. Pierre Janet (1859–1947) was a French psychologist and psychotherapist who developed a theory of hypnosis based on Charcot's notion of dissociation (see Freud, 1856–1939). According to this theory, hypnosis produces a division of consciousness and eliminates conscious control of certain behaviours. Seventy years later, these ideas were revived by the American psychologist Ernest Hilgard, in his neodissociation theory, which will be considered later.

Hypnosis then appeared to go into decline. First, it became associated with popular practices, notably phrenology and spiritualism, that were eventually discredited by science. A second reason was the advent of psychoanalysis. In his formative years, Sigmund Freud (1856–1939) worked with Charcot and used hypnosis, but he eventually abandoned it in favour of methods such as free association, dream analysis, and interpretations based on transference. Third, there was the rise of behaviourism. Surprisingly, however, the behavioural psychologist Clark Hull *was* interested in hypnosis and in 1933, he wrote a book called *Hypnosis and Suggestibility* in which he described laboratory experiments on suggestion. He wished 'to divest hypnosis of its air of mystery, which surrounds it', but it was not for another 20 years or so that this goal was seriously pursued. From 1950 onwards, hypnosis began to be taken seriously again both as a subject for scientific study and as a treatment modality.

Modern Theories of Hypnosis

Modern theories of hypnosis endeavour to account for what Coe and Sarbin (1991) term the 'counter-expectational' nature of the subject's behaviour and experience. Why is it, for example, that a hypnotic subject forgets something when instructed to do so and remembers it again when the instruction is reversed? Similarly, why does he or she, when instructed, not feel pain, fail to see an object that is clearly in view, smell an odour that is clearly not present and so on? It is also necessary to account for individual differences in hypnotic suggestibility and its consistency over time.

'State' or 'Special Process' Theories of Hypnosis

The classic approach to explaining hypnotic experiences is to postulate that, as a result of the hypnotic induction, the subject is placed in an altered state of consciousness or 'trance' (for example, Shor, 1959, 1962). While in this trance state, special processes operate that account for the 'counter-expectational' nature of the subject's response to the hypnotist's suggestions. Some suggestions are harder to respond to than others because they require a deeper level of trance. For example, a suggestion of arm levitation is said to require only a 'light trance', whereas to respond to a suggestion of a negative hallucination or profound amnesia a 'deep trance' is required. People differ in the 'depth' of trance that they can attain and this is a stable characteristic, hence the wide range of hypnotic suggestibility found in the general population.

Ego-psychological theory

The ego-psychological model is a modern theoretical account of hypnosis developed by Fromm (1979, 1992) from the ideas proposed by Shor (1959, 1962). In the hypnotic trance, the 'general reality orientation' is diminished, and the deeper the trance, the less the subject is able to distinguish fantasy and reality. Another central feature of the model is the distinction between primary and secondary processes (Freud, 1923/1961). Primary processes are most evident in dreaming. They are emotional, holistic, illogical, unconscious and developmentally immature. Secondary processes are affect-free, analytic, logical, conscious and developmentally mature. Normal functioning relies mainly on secondary processes. During hypnosis there is an increased tendency in favour of primary mental processing, a kind of psychological 'regression' (Gill and Brenman, 1959), resulting in increased suggestibility and the apparent involuntariness of suggested phenomena.

This approach to understanding hypnosis has not been particularly influential amongst modern cognitive psychologists and there has been mixed support in the experimental literature (see Nash, 1991, for a review).

Neodissociation theory

Hilgard's neodissociation theory (for example, Hilgard, 1979, 1986) represents a revival of Janet's ideas summarized earlier. Hypnotic phenomena are brought about through a process of dissociation. However, for Hilgard, dissociation is a normal cognitive process, rather than a pathological one.

Neodissociation theory posits a hierarchical arrangement of 'cognitive control systems' responsible for learned cognitive and behavioural activities that are carried out in everyday life. Each of these structures has a certain autonomy of function; they are interactive, but they may also be isolated or dissociated from each other in certain circumstances (for example, in the case of automatic, overlearned activities). The idea of a hierarchical arrangement acknowledges the fact that, at any one time, some priority is needed as to what structure is to be dominant. Monitoring and controlling these structures is a superordinate mechanism, the executive ego, which may assign attentional priority to activities according to the demands of the situation. However, the executive ego is limited in this function: for example, driving a car is often done relatively automatically so that the driver is able to attend to a conversation with his or her passenger at the same time. However, should the driver encounter some severe weather on the journey, he or she may have to ignore the conversation and give full attention to driving. Thus, Hilgard refers to 'constraints on ego autonomy'.

Hypnosis and hypnotic suggestions are ways in which the hypnotist can influence the subject's executive ego in the assignment of attentional priority to various activities and experiences. More specifically, the hypnotic induction causes a 'fractionation' or dissociation within the executive system. Although part of the executive continues to function as normal during hypnosis, another, dissociated part is outside of awareness. This part can exert control in the usual manner, but such control is prevented from representing itself in consciousness by the formation of an 'amnesic barrier'. The hypnotist's suggestions direct the dissociated part of the executive to instigate actions or changes in cognitive processing. As the hypnotized subject is aware only of the resultant changes in behaviour and experience, and not the cognitive activity by which such changes are brought about, they experience their responses to hypnotic suggestion as involuntary. According to neodissociation theory, hypnotizability is a stable cognitive trait related to an individual's ability to experience dissociative phenomena in the manner described.

The most influential laboratory demonstrations of Hilgard's neodissociation theory concern the presumed accessing of the dissociated part of the executive by the 'hidden observer' paradigm. The classic demonstration of this involves the elicitation of profound analgesia in highly susceptible subjects (see Hilgard, Morgan and Macdonald, Chapter 17, this volume). In these experiments subjects immerse their hand in a bucket of ice and water and rate the pain experienced on a scale from 0 to 10. In response to suggestions of analgesia, these ratings may come down from the upper to the lower end of this scale. The experimenter then suggests that there is a hidden, 'unhypnotized' part of the person that continues to experience the pain as usual. This 'hidden observer' is instructed to rate the 'true' pain on the 0–10 scale by pressing keys with the free hand. Typically, these ratings correspond to the pain ratings given during hypnosis without the suggestion of analgesia. Similar experiments have been done using suggested deafness (Crawford, Macdonald and Hilgard 1979).

The concept of the hidden observer has been criticized by a number of writers (for example, Kirsch and Lynn, 1998; Spanos, 1986; Wagstaff, 1981), who consider it to be an artefact created by the experimenter, with the subject duly complying. For example, Spanos and his colleagues have shown that the hidden observer may be exquisitely sensitive to the wording of the instructions used to elicit it. In one study (Spanos and Hewitt, 1980) subjects were told that the hidden part was 'so deeply hidden' it would experience even less pain than the hypnotized part. As suggested, the hidden observers rated their pain as even less intense, rather than more intense.

Of relevance to neodissociation theory is the concept of 'trance logic' due to Martin Orne. Orne (Chapter 4, this volume, 1962, 1972) demonstrated that genuine hypnotic subjects, when asked to hallucinate a person sitting in a chair in front of them, would also describe objects that would normally be obscured by the person's body. Simulators tended to respond logically, denying being able to see the objects because these were behind the hallucinated person. Orne also reported that true hypnotic subjects would avoid colliding with a chair for which they had been given a negative hallucination suggestion, whereas, again, simulators tended to behave logically by bumping into the chair.

'Trance logic' is the ability to accept two contradictory beliefs or pieces of information without experiencing the usual sense of conflict, and this may be explained in terms of dissociation. However, other explanations are available (see Spanos, 1986; Wagstaff, 1981). For example, in the positive hallucination test, it may simply be that most hypnotic subjects fail to create a stable, opaque image. Instead, they 'see' what most of us see when asked to imagine something. Hence, when people who have not been hypnotized are instructed to imagine something, they often report the resultant image as being unstable and transparent.

Dissociated control theory

Dissociated control theory (see Woody and Bowers, Chapter 7, this volume) is a relative newcomer, but is proving influential, being based on modern neurocognitve concepts concerning the regulation of behaviour and on Hilgard's neodissociation theory. In particular, it draws on the model of the voluntary and involuntary regulation of behaviour put forward by Norman and Shallice (1986). This model describes two systems that regulate everyday behaviour. The lower-level, 'decentralized', system consists of units or schemas that govern particular actions, similar to Hilgard's cognitive control systems. When a schema is activated at a certain threshold, the associated action is executed. Schemas can be activated or inhibited by other schemas or by environmental triggers. This process is termed 'contention scheduling' and, for well-learned habits, this occurs automatically with little centralized control.

When complex or unfamiliar sequences of actions are required, or when strong habitual tendencies need to be inhibited, a higher-level mechanism comes into play, the 'supervisory attention system', not unlike Hilgard's executive ego. This controls the activation of the schemas, biasing the distribution of activation according to the requirements of the situation. This represents the basis of willed, as opposed to automatic, action.

Woody and Bowers (Chapter 7) propose that hypnosis disengages the supervisory attention system from its influence on the lower-level system. In other words, the fractionation is not *within* the high-level control system, as in the case of the neodissociation model, but between higher and lower levels of control. Accordingly, the behaviour and experiences of the hypnotized subject are automatically triggered by the hypnotist's suggestions.

According to Norman and Shallice (1986), the supervisory attention system is a function of the frontal lobes. Hence, according to the theory of dissociated control, the process of hypnosis involves some degree of inhibition of frontal lobe activity. This idea is consistent with the clinical neuropsychological evidence: frontal lobe damage is associated with problems in the planning and regulation of behaviour and in the inhibition of automatic responses. Consequently, a hypnotized subject behaves a little like a patient with frontal lobe damage, responding in a genuinely automatic and involuntary manner to the suggestions and instructions of the hypnotist.

A small number of studies have provided evidence in support of this theory (for example, Bowers and Woody, 1996; Miller and Bowers, 1993), including some neurophysiological and neuropsychological findings (see Gruzelier, Chapter 23, this volume) suggesting, for example, that during hypnosis frontal lobe activity, especially on the left side, is attenuated in highly susceptible subjects. However, not all the available evidence is consistent with the theory (see, for example, Kirsch, Burgess and Braffman, 1999) and a number of conceptual problems have been identified (see Kirsch and Lynn, 1998).

Sociocognitive Processes in Hypnosis

Sociocognitive theories of hypnosis reject the idea that hypnotic responses are produced by a trance state or 'special processes' such as dissociation or dissociative control. Instead, these altered experiences are explained by the same factors that produce non-hypnotic experience and behaviour. The theories that have been developed differ in the emphasis that they give to different psychological process. The most commonly cited sociocognitive processes identified in the hypnosis literature are described below.

Absorption

Although sociocognitive theorists reject the classic notion of a special trance state as an explanatory concept, the idea of trance may still have some value in its weaker sense, namely an everyday experience when one is deeply absorbed in something – for example, a book, a film, some music or a daydream. In Chapter 12 Tellegen and Atkinson describe this state of absorption as one in which there is '. . . almost total immersion in the [imaginal] activity, with indifference to distracting stimuli in the environment' (p. 227).

In support of this, Crawford (Chapter 21, this volume) has provided neurophysiological evidence that hypnosis is characterized by a state of focused attention. The evidence for this has recently been critically reviewed by Jamieson and Sheehan (2002). Evidence has also accumulated that a tendency to engage in absorptive experiences in everyday life, as measured by self-report questionnaire (see Tellegen and Atkinson, Chapter 12), is correlated with hypnotic susceptibility, but the relationship is quite low and unstable (Kirsch, 1991; Milling, Kirsch and Burgess, 2000).

Role enactment

From the standpoint of role theory, Sarbin (Chapter 3, this volume; Sarbin and Coe, 1972) proposed that hypnotic responding results from taking on the social role of the hypnotized subject. As discussed below, this has often been misinterpreted as role playing and compliance. However, Sarbin and Coe have been careful to use the phrase 'role enactment' rather than 'role playing'. People enact the role of the hypnotized subject just as they enact other social roles (professor, student, parent, spouse and so on). Thus, the idea of role enactment does not imply that the person is faking or engaging in deception. Foreshadowing the idea that hypnotic responding might be related to absorption, Sarbin (Chapter 3) also put forward the idea of role *involvement* as a predictor of hypnotizability. According to Sarbin, the responsive subject is one who becomes sufficiently involved in the hypnotic role to be able to experience alterations that are suggested.

Imagination

Barber, who has been one of the major figures in the 'non-state' approach to hypnosis over the last half-century, considered imagination (or the ability to fantasize realistically) to be one of the central features of his understanding of hypnosis (see Barber, Spanos and Chaves, 1974). This thesis is supported by the consistent finding that individuals with a well-developed capacity for vivid fantasy ('fantasy-proneness') tend to score higher on scales of hypnotic suggestibility. Fantasy-proneness is closely related to absorption, but seems to be a more reliable predictor of hypnotic suggestibility.

Response expectancy

Another contender for a theory of hypnotic responding is response expectancy (Kirsch, Chapter 10, this volume, 1991), the anticipation of an automatic reaction, which is widely believed to be the basis of the placebo effect. Kirsch notes that hypnotic inductions are like placebos in that they do not contain any specific ingredients. For example, mesmeric inductions involved 'passes' over the body with magnets or just the hands; Charcot's inductions consisted of pressure on the forehead, oriental gongs and lights; whilst modern inductions usually emphasize relaxation. Thus, the only essential component seems to be the subject's belief in the procedure. The experiences and behaviour of hypnotized subjects also seem to be related to their expectations. For example, Mesmer's subjects convulsed, whereas those of later hypnotists relaxed. Finally, response expectancy has been found to be the strongest correlate of response to suggestion (Kirsch, Silva, Comey and Reed, 1995). Kirsch considers that response expectancy is part of the essence of hypnosis and not simply a byproduct. He and his colleagues (Wickless and Kirsch, 1989) have demonstrated experimentally how responsiveness to hypnotic suggestion can be modified by manipulating the subject's expectancy.

Expectancy theory has generated considerable research, primarily among non-state theorists. One weakness of the theory may be its ability to account for individual differences in suggestibility and the stability of suggestibility over time. This criticism may be more apposite now with growing research evidence of differences between high and low susceptibility at the neurophysiological and neuropsychological level. Also, most correlations between expectancy and hypnotizability are modest at best (see, for example, Shor, 1971). However, Kirsch (1991) has acknowledged that there may be an ability factor that is orthogonal to expectancy.

Strategic enactment

In contrast to state theorists, many sociocognitive theorists tend to regard the hypnotic subject as an active participant in the hypnotic interaction. He or she is not simply 'letting things happen' but is actively striving to deploy his or her cognitive skills to create the responses and experiences suggested by the hypnotist. Thus, Spanos (1991) conceived hypnotic responding as involving a process of 'strategic enactment'. So, for example, the subject who successfully responds to the suggestion of arm levitation does not wait for the arm to rise but actually lifts the arm, attempting to create, through imagination, the feeling that it is being pulled up. In responding to the suggestion of analgesia, a subject may adopt an appropriate strategy such as self-distraction rather than simply wait for the suggestion to take effect. A strategy such as attention switching, that inhibits recall, may be adopted when responding to a suggestion of post-hypnotic amnesia. Although responses are often experienced by susceptible subjects as 'automatic' or 'involuntary', this is interpreted as an attribution on the subject's part that arises from the expectations generated by the hypnotic context.

Spanos and his colleagues have taken this line of reasoning a logical step further. Unlike special trait theorists, who consider hypnotic susceptibility to be a fixed individual characteristic, they have argued that it is modifiable and that individuals low in susceptibility can be trained to increase their scores. Essentially, this involves educating subjects in the correct attitude and approach to hypnotic suggestion. Accordingly, Spanos and his colleagues have developed a training programme, the Carleton Skills Training Program (CSTP), which is available in published form (Gorassini and Spanos, 1999). Individuals undergoing this training are encouraged to adopt positive attitudes and expectations about hypnosis and are trained in the strategic enactment approach to a range of suggestions. It is claimed that this leads to a permanent increase in hypnotic suggestibility. However, critics such as Bowers and Davidson (1991) consider that 'naturally' highly susceptible subjects owe their high scores on susceptibility scales to cognitive processes that are different to those deployed by subjects who have been trained on the CSTP. In support of this criticism one may cite laboratory studies showing that 'natural' highs and lows differ on certain neuropsychological tests and neurophysiological activity both in and outside of the hypnotic context (see, for example, Gruzelier's review in Chapter 23).

Compliance

Another possibility is that the responsive hypnotic subject is simply being compliant – that is, knowingly pretending. For example, in response to a suggestion of arm levitation he or she may consciously raise the arm, while claiming that the response is involuntary. Or in response to suggested analgesia, he or she may be aware of the pain but deny this and suppress any pain behaviour. At least one theorist, Wagstaff (1981, 1991), considers that compliance is a major component of hypnotic responding. Others, however, point to evidence that hypnotized subjects are not merely pretending (see, for example, Perugini *et al.*, 1998).

The sociocognitive account of hypnotic induction

If the concept of a 'trance state' can be dispensed with, what is the role of the hypnotic induction? This is still considered to be important by sociocognitive hypnotists, as the presence of this procedure defines the context as one in which 'hypnotic suggestions', rather than 'suggestions without hypnosis', or what is sometimes referred to as 'waking suggestions' are being administered. However, the purpose of the induction is not to guide the subject into a trance state but to enhance his or her sense of expectation and motivation. If the induction procedure fulfils these aims (and defines the context as 'hypnosis') then the content of the induction is not so important.

Laboratory research has demonstrated that the gains in suggestibility that are achieved when the traditional induction routines are used are matched by 'motivating instructions' (Barber and Calverley, 1963a, 1963b), suggestions to become more alert while engaging in an energetic activity (Bányai and Hilgard, 1976), and 'dummy' or 'placebo' inductions (Kirsch, 1991). In fact, the gains in responsiveness due to an induction are, in the psychological laboratory at least, quite modest and not obtained in all individuals (Braffman and Kirsch, 1999). Nevertheless, traditional relaxation induction procedures may be preferable in clinical contexts, as, for many clients, they may enhance treatment outcome to some degree.

Convergence of Approaches

It is fair to say that the 'state versus non-state' (or 'special process versus sociocognitive') debate has been quite polarized and, certainly in the second half of the twentieth century, fiercely contested on both sides. However, like many controversies in the social sciences, with the accumulation of research has come the recognition that the distinction is not as clear-cut as much of the literature suggests (see Kirsch and Lynn, 1995). The various accounts are not mutually exclusive, and a comprehensive theory of hypnotic phenomena must draw on concepts from both sides (see, for example, Nadon, 1997; Brown and Oakley, 2004). Intriguingly, for example, Barber (1999), in contrast to his earlier strong anti-state stance, now argues that a small percentage of highly susceptible subjects, whom he describes as 'amnesia-prone', correspond to the highly susceptible–highly dissociative individuals conceived in state accounts of hypnosis. Whether this idea will gain general acceptance remains to be seen (see, for example, Lynn, Meyer and Shindler (2004) for a critical analysis). Nevertheless, the way forward lies not in compromise but in acknowledging the complex range of psychological processes that are involved in the activity designated as 'hypnosis'.

Hypnosis in Therapy

Hypnotherapeutic approaches typically involve induction and deepening methods that emphasize mental and physical relaxation, as well as suggestions and imagery aimed at encouraging desired changes in perception, feelings, thinking and behaviour. The patient may also be encouraged to practise self-hypnosis in order to rehearse relaxation and other self-control methods. Hypnosis may also be employed in an analytic or psychodynamic fashion, using suggestions and guided imagery techniques to explore possible difficulties and conflicts that underlie the presenting problems. This application of hypnosis is often based on the very simple idea that hypnosis somehow facilitates access to unconscious processes.

Although hypnosis originally evolved as a healing procedure, it is only in the last 30 years that serious attempts have been made to evaluate its therapeutic application in a systematic manner. Several reviews of this work are available (see below) including a recent meta-analysis review by Flammer and Bongartz (2003).

In their working party report for the British Psychological Society, Heap *et al.* were able to conclude the following:

> Enough studies have now accumulated to suggest that the inclusion of hypnotic procedures may be beneficial in the management and treatment of a wide range of conditions and problems encountered in the practice of medicine, psychiatry and psychotherapy. In many cases, however, the relative contribution of factors specific to hypnosis is as yet unclear, and often the influence on outcome of the measured hypnotic susceptibility of the patients is small or insignificant. (Heap *et al.*, 2001, p. 9)

The following is a brief summary of the findings to date.

1 Hypnosis and self-hypnosis may have a significant beneficial effect in reducing general anxiety, tension and stress (Schoenberger, 2000), and in treating insomnia (Anderson, Dalton and Basker, 1979; Stanton, 1989) but probably no more so than for other relaxation and self-regulation procedures.
2 There is good evidence that hypnotic procedures are effective in the management and relief of pain due to medical conditions and in assisting in the alleviation of pain, discomfort and distress due to medical, surgical and dental procedures, and in childbirth (Montgomery, DuHamel and Redd, 2000; Patterson and Jensen, Chapter 28, this volume).
3 There have been a number of clinical trials demonstrating that hypnotherapeutic procedures may be effective in alleviating the symptoms of a range of psychosomatic complaints such as tension headaches and migraine (Alladin, 1988; Holroyd and Penzien, 1990; ter Kuile *et al.*, 1994); asthma (see the review of clinical studies by Hackman, Stern and Gershwin, 2000); gastrointestinal complaints such as irritable bowel syndrome (Galovski and Blanchard, 1998; Gonsalkorale, Miller, Afzal and Whorwell, Chapter 27, this volume); warts (DuBreuil and Spanos, 1993); and possibly other skin complaints such as eczema, psoriasis and urticaria (Shertzer and Lookingbill, 1987; Stewart and Thomas, 1995; Zachariae, Øster, Bjerring and Kragballe, 1996).
4 Hypnosis may be at least as effective as other comparable methods for giving up smoking (see the review by Green and Lynn, 2000). Meta-analyses by Law and Tang (1995) and Viswesvaran and Schmidt (1992) give mean abstinence rates for hypnosis at 23 per cent and 36 per cent respectively.
5 Several studies have indicated that the inclusion of hypnotherapeutic procedures in a weight reduction programme may significantly enhance outcome, especially in the long term (see Bolocofsky, Spinler and Coulthard-Morris, 1985; Kirsch, Montgomery and Sapirstein, Chapter 26, this volume; Levitt, 1993).

The above general findings on adult patients may be extended to children (see the review by Milling and Costantino, 2000).

Accounts have been published (for example, Heap and Aravind, 2002; Rhue, Lynn and Kirsch, 1993) documenting the use of hypnosis as an adjunctive therapeutic procedure in the treatment of psychological disorders such as depression, sexual dysfunction and disorder, anorexia and bulimia nervosa, speech and language disorders, post-traumatic stress disorder and phobias; it is likewise useful in sports psychology. However, to date there have been too few systematic studies to enable us to state with confidence whether hypnosis makes a significant contribution in such treatment.

Legal and Forensic Issues

There are a number of reasons why hypnosis is sometimes considered by legislators and those working in the civil and criminal justice systems. For example, in certain countries (for example, Norway, Austria and Israel; see Hawkins and Heap, 1998) the practice of hypnosis is legally restricted to professions such as medicine, dentistry and psychology. In such countries the use of hypnosis for the purposes of entertainment is also legally proscribed whereas in other countries, such as the UK, there are rules and guidelines about its conduct.

Occasionally, legal cases arise in which the plaintiff (claimant or complainant) alleges that, during hypnosis, he or she has suffered physical or psychological harm due either to the negligence of the hypnotist (for example, during therapy or a performance of stage hypnosis) or a criminal action on the hypnotist's part – typically sexual assault. There are accounts of both types of case in the academic literature (for example, Heap, 1995a, 1995b, Chapter 31, this volume; Hoëncamp, 1989; Kleinhauz and Beran, 1984). In the historical literature there is also the occasional reference to an allegation by a defendant that he committed a crime 'while under hypnosis'. The implication in these criminal cases is that the hypnotic subject is 'at the mercy of the hypnotist's will'. There is a theoretical and experimental literature on this theme (see, for example, Laurence and Perry, 1988), the consensus appearing to be that hypnosis has no unique properties in this regard.

Finally, based on the assumption that hypnosis has the property to enhance memory, hypnotic procedures have been used to attempt to assist witnesses of crimes to recall, with greater detail and accuracy, what they observed. This application of hypnosis has been the subject of much controversy. First, it is unclear on theoretical grounds why hypnosis should improve recall; second, there is very little reliable experimental evidence to show that, beyond properties common to a range of methods (concentration, relaxation, contextual reinstatement by imagery and so on), hypnosis has any special facility to improve recall; and, third, it is considered that hypnosis may carry the risk of encouraging believed-in confabulation and fantasies on the part of the eye witness (see American Medical Association, Chapter 29, this volume). A similar controversy has arisen concerning the use of hypnosis to 'recover repressed memories' during therapy (Conway, 1997; Ofshe and Watters, 1994).

Conclusions

This overview reveals stages in the evolution of modern hypnosis that reflect the cultural and scientific attitudes and practices that prevailed at various times. First, we have its origins as a healing practice, namely mesmerism, rather than a normal psychological process or phenomenon. The setting for this is eighteenth-century France in the Age of Enlightenment and, although Mesmer explained his procedures by reference to an imaginary entity – namely an invisible fluid that he called 'animal magnetism' – he endeavoured to relate this to ideas and discoveries from the natural sciences of that time.

Next, we see the application of more critical thinking and the shedding of superfluous practices such as mesmeric passes and crises. Alongside this comes the development of psychological, rather than physical, explanations for the observed phenomena. Hypnosis then emerges not primarily as a treatment but as a psychological phenomenon for scientific study in the laboratory with normal individuals. Accordingly, theorizing becomes grounded in existing mainstream psychology and its related disciplines and, correspondingly, there is more systematic investigation of the therapeutic effectiveness of hypnosis in the form of controlled clinical trials than anecdotal evidence.

This process continues to evolve with, for example, the application of theories and research grounded in current neurocognitive approaches and neurophysiological models that are investigated by brain imaging techniques.

In this volume, we have selected a sample of essays that reveal how a scientific approach to understanding hypnosis as a psychological phenomenon has emerged over the last 70 years. We also include a selection of reports on clinical applications and on legal and forensic issues. We hope that this sample of essays will prove useful not only to those readers who are already familiar with the subject, but also to those new to the field and who are keen to be more informed.

References

Alladin, A. (1988), 'Hypnosis in the Treatment of Head Pain', in M. Heap (ed.), *Hypnosis: Current Clinical, Experimental and Forensic Practices*, London: Croom Helm, pp. 159–66.

Anderson, J.A.D., Dalton, E.R. and Basker, M.A. (1979), 'Insomnia and Hypnotherapy', *Journal of the Royal Society of Medicine*, **72**, pp. 734–39.

Bányai, E.I. and Hilgard, E.R. (1976), 'A Comparison of Active-Alert Hypnotic Induction with Traditional Relaxation Induction', *Journal of Abnormal Psychology*, **85**, pp. 218–24.

Barber, T.X. (1999), 'A Comprehensive Three-dimensional Theory of Hypnosis', in I. Kirsch, A. Capafons, E. Cardeña-Buelna and S. Amigó (eds), *Clinical Hypnosis and Self-Regulation: Cognitive-Behavioural Perspectives*, Washington, DC: American Psychological Association, pp. 21–48.

Barber, T.X. and Calverley, D.S. (1963a), 'The Relative Effectiveness of Task Motivating Instructions and Trance Induction Procedure in the Production of "Hypnotic Like" Behavior', *Journal of Nervous and Mental Disease*, **137**, pp. 107–16.

Barber, T.X. and Calverley, D.S. (1963b), 'Toward a Theory of Hypnotic Behavior: Effects on Suggestibility of Task Motivating Instructions and Attitudes Toward Hypnosis', *Journal of Abnormal and Social Psychology*, **67**, pp. 557–65.

Barber, T.X., Spanos, N.P. and Chaves, J.F. (1974), *Hypnosis: Imagination and Human Potentialities*, New York: Pergamon.

Bolocofsky, D.N., Spinler, D. and Coulthard-Morris, L. (1985), 'Effectiveness of Hypnosis as an Adjunct to Behavioral Weight Management', *Journal of Clinical Psychology*, **41**, pp. 35–41.

Bowers, K.S. and Davidson, T.M. (1991), 'A Neodissociative Critique of Spanos's Social-Psychological Model of Hypnosis, in S.J Lynn and J.W. Rhue (eds), *Theories of Hypnosis: Current Models and Perspectives*, New York: Guilford, pp. 105–43.

Bowers, K.S. and Woody, E.Z. (1996), 'Hypnotic Amnesia and the Paradox of Intentional Forgetting', *Journal of Abnormal Psychology*, **105**, pp. 381–90.

Braffman, W. and Kirsch, I. (1999), 'Imaginative Suggestibility and Hypnotizability: An Empirical Analysis', *Journal of Personality and Social Psychology*, **77**, pp. 578–87.

Brown, R.J and Oakley, D.A. (2004), 'An Integrative Cognitive Theory of Hypnosis and High Hypnotisability', in M. Heap, R.J. Brown and D.A. Oakley (eds), *The Highly Hypnotizable Person: Theoretical, Experimental and Clinical Issues*, London: Routledge, pp. 152–86.

Coe, W.C. and Sarbin, T.R. (1991), 'Role Theory: Hypnosis from a Dramaturgical and Narrational Perspective', in S.J. Lynn and J.W. Rhue (eds), *Theories of Hypnosis: Current Models and Perspectives*, New York: Guilford, pp. 303–23.

Conway, M.A. (1997), *Recovered Memories and False Memories*, Oxford: Oxford University Press.

Crawford, H.J., Macdonald H. and Hilgard, E.R. (1979), 'Hypnotic Deafness: A Psychophysical Study of Responses to Tone Intensity as Modified by Hypnosis', *American Journal of Psychology*, **92**, pp. 193–214.

DuBreuil, S. and Spanos, N.P. (1993), 'Psychological Treatment of Warts', in J.W. Rhue, S.J. Lynn and I. Kirsch (eds), *Handbook of Clinical Hypnosis*, Washington DC: American Psychological Association, pp. 623–43.

Flammer, E. and Bongartz, W. (2003), 'On the Efficacy of Hypnosis: A Meta-analytic Study', *Contemporary Hypnosis*, **20**, pp. 179–97.

Freud, S. (1959), 'Charcot', in E. Jones (ed.), *Sigmund Freud: Collected Papers*, New York: Basic Books, pp. 9–23. First published 1893.

Freud, S. (1961), 'The Ego and the Id, in J. Strachey (ed. and trans.), *The Standard Edition of the Complete Psychological Works of Sigmund Freud*, Vol. 19, London: Hogarth Press, pp. 12–59. First published 1923.

Fromm, E. (1979), 'The Nature of Hypnosis and Other Altered States of Consciousness: An Ego-Psychological Theory', in E. Fromm and R. Shor (eds), *Hypnosis: Developments in Research and New Perspectives*, New York: Aldine, pp. 81–103.

Fromm, E. (1992), 'An Ego-Psychological Theory of Hypnosis, in E. Fromm and M.R. Nash (eds), *Contemporary Hypnosis Research*, London: Guilford, pp. 131–48.

Galovski, T.E. and Blanchard, E.B. (1998), 'The Treatment of Irritable Bowel Syndrome with Hypnotherapy', *Applied Physiology and Biofeedback*, **23**, pp. 219–32.

Gill, M.M. and Brenman, M. (1959), *Hypnosis and Related States: Psychoanalytic Studies in Regression*, New York: International Universities Press.

Gorassini, D.R. and Spanos, N.P. (1999), 'The Carleton Skill Training Program for Modifying Hypnotic Suggestibility: Original Version and Variations', in I. Kirsch, A. Capafons, S. Amigó and E. Cardeña-Buelna (eds), *Clinical Hypnosis and Self-Regulation Therapy: A Cognitive-Behavioral Perspective*, Washington, DC: American Psychological Association Books, pp. 141–77.

Green, J.P. and Lynn, S.J. (2000), 'Hypnosis and Suggestion-based Approaches to Smoking Cessation: An Examination of the Evidence', *International Journal of Clinical and Experimental Hypnosis*, **48**, pp. 195–224.

Hackman, R.M., Stern, J.S. and Gershwin, M.E. (2000), 'Hypnosis and Asthma: A Critical Review', *Journal of Asthma*, **37**, pp. 1–15.

Hawkins, P. and Heap, M. (1998), *Hypnosis in Europe*, London: Whurr Publishers.

Heap, M. (1995a), 'Another Case of Indecent Assault by a Lay Hypnotherapist', *Contemporary Hypnosis*, **12**, pp. 92–98.

Heap, M. (1995b), 'A Case of Death Following Stage Hypnosis: Analysis and Implications', *Contemporary Hypnosis*, **12**, pp. 99–110.

Heap, M., Alden, P., Brown, R.J., Naish P.L.N, Oakley, D.A. Wagstaff, G.F. and Walker, L.J. (2001), 'The Nature of Hypnosis: Report Prepared by a Working Party at the Request of the Professional Affairs Board of the British Psychological Society', Leicester: British Psychological Society.

Heap, M. and Aravind, K.K. (2002), *Hartland's Medical and Dental Hypnosis* (4th edn), London: Churchill Livingston/ Harcourt Health Sciences.

Hilgard, E.R. (1979), 'Divided Consciousness in Hypnosis: The Implications of the Hidden Observer', in E. Fromm and R.E. Shor (eds), *Hypnosis: Developments in Research and New Perspectives* (2nd edn), New York: Aldine, pp. 45–79.

Hilgard, E.R. (1986), *Divided Consciousness: Multiple Controls in Human Thought and Action: Expanded Edition*, New York: Wiley.

Hoëncamp, E (1989), 'Sexual Coercion and the Role of Hypnosis in the Abused Therapeutic Relationship', in D. Waxman, D. Pedersen, I. Wilkie and P. Mellett (eds), *Hypnosis: The Fourth European Congress at Oxford*, London: Whurr Publishers, pp. 160–74.

Holroyd, K.A. and Penzien, D.B. (1990), 'Pharmacological versus Non-pharmacological Prophylaxis of Recurrent Migraine Headache: A Meta-analytic Review of Clinical Trials', *Pain*, **42**, pp. 1–13.

Hull, C. (1933), *Hypnosis and Suggestibility*, New York: Appleton Century Crofts.

Jamieson, G.A. and Sheehan, P.W. (2002), 'A Critical Evaluation of the Relationship Between Sustained Attentional Abilities and Hypnotic Susceptibility', *Contemporary Hypnosis*, **19**, pp. 62–74.

Kirsch, I. (1991), 'The Social Learning Theory of Hypnosis', in S.J. Lynn and J.W. Rhue (eds), *Theories of Hypnosis: Current Models and Perspectives*, New York: Guilford, pp. 439–65.

Kirsch, I., Burgess, C.A. and Braffman, W. (1999), 'Attentional Resources in Hypnotic Responding', *International Journal of Clinical and Experimental Hypnosis*, **47**, pp. 175–91.

Kirsch, I. and Lynn, S.J. (1995), 'The Altered State of Hypnosis', *American Psychologist*, **50**, pp. 846–58.

Kirsch, I. and Lynn, S.J. (1998), 'Dissociation Theories of Hypnosis, *Psychological Bulletin*, **123**, pp. 100–15.

Kirsch, I., Silva, C.E., Comey, G. and Reed, S. (1995), 'A Spectral Analysis of Cognitive and Personality Variables in Hypnosis: Empirical Disconfirmation of the Two-factor Model of Hypnotic Responding', *Journal of Personality and Social Psychology*, **69**, pp. 167–75.

Kleinhauz, M. and Beran, B. (1984), 'Misuse of Hypnosis: A Factor in Psychopathology', *American Journal of Clinical Hypnosis*, **26**, pp. 283–90.

Laurence, J-R. and Perry, C. (1988), *Hypnosis, Will & Memory: A Psycho-Legal History*, New York: Guilford.

Law, M. and Tang, J.L. (1995), 'An Analysis of the Effectiveness of Interventions Intended to Help People Stop Smoking', *Archives of Internal Medicine*, **155**, pp. 1933–41.

Levitt, E.E. (1993), 'Hypnosis in the Treatment of Obesity', in J.W. Rhue, S.J. Lynn and I. Kirsch (eds), *Handbook of Clinical Hypnosis*, Washington DC: American Psychological Association, pp. 533–53.

Lynn, S.J., Meyer E. and Shindler K. (2004), 'Clinical Correlates of High Hypnotisability', in M. Heap, R.J. Brown and D.A. Oakley (eds), *The Highly Hypnotizable Person: Theoretical, Experimental and Clinical Issues*, London: Routledge, pp. 187–212.

Miller, M.E. and Bowers, K.S. (1993), 'Hypnotic Analgesia: Dissociated Experience or Dissociated Control?', *Journal of Abnormal Psychology*, **102**, pp. 29–38.

Milling, L.S. and Costantino, C.A. (2000), 'Clinical Hypnosis with Children: First Steps Toward Empirical Support', *International Journal of Clinical and Experimental Hypnosis*, **48**, pp. 113–37.

Milling, L.S., Kirsch I. and Burgess, C. (2000), 'Hypnotic Suggestibility and Absorption: Revisiting the Context Effect', *Contemporary Hypnosis*, **17**, pp. 32–41.

Montgomery, G.H., DuHamel, K.N. and Redd, W.H. (2000), 'A Meta-analysis of Hypnotically Induced Analgesia: How Effective is Hypnosis?', *International Journal of Clinical and Experimental Hypnosis*, **48**, pp. 138–53.

Nadon, R. (1997), 'What this Field Needs is a Good Nomological Network', *International Journal of Clinical and Experimental Hypnosis*, **45**, pp. 314–23.

Nash, M.R. (1991), 'Hypnosis as a Special Case of Psychological Regression', in S.J. Lynn and J.W. Rhue (eds), *Theories of Hypnosis: Current Models and Perspectives*, New York: Guilford, pp. 171–94.

Norman, D.A. and Shallice, T. (1986), 'Attention to Action: Willed Control of Behavior', in R.J. Davidson, G.E. Schwartz and D. Shapiro (eds), *Consciousness and Self-regulation*, New York: Plenum, Vol. 4, pp. 1–18.

Ofshe, R. and Watters, E. (1994), *Making Monsters: False Memories, Psychotherapy and Sexual Hysteria*, Berkeley CA: University of California Press.

Orne, M.T. (1962), 'Hypnotically Induced Hallucinations, in L.J. West (ed.), *Hallucinations*, New York: Grune & Stratton, pp. 211–19.

Orne, M.T. (1972), 'On the Simulating Subject as a Quasi-control in Hypnosis Research: What, Why and How?', in E. Fromm and R.E. Shor (eds), *Hypnosis: Research Developments and Perspectives*, Chicago: Aldine-Atherton, pp. 399–443.

Perugini, E.M., Kirsch, I., Allen, S.T., Coldwell, E., Meredith, J., Montgomery, G.H. and Sheehan, J. (1998), 'Surreptitious Observation of Responses to Hypnotically Suggested Hallucinations: A Test of the Compliance Hypothesis', *International Journal of Clinical and Experimental Hypnosis*, **46**, pp. 191–203.

Rhue, J.W., Lynn S.J. and Kirsch I. (1993), *Handbook of Clinical Hypnosis*, Washington DC: American Psychological Association.

Sarbin, T.R. and Coe, W.C. (1972), *Hypnosis: A Social Psychological Analysis of Influence Communication*, New York: Holt, Rhinehart and Winston.

Schoenberger, N.E. (2000), 'Research on Hypnosis as an Adjunct to Cognitive-Behavioral Psychotherapy', *International Journal of Clinical and Experimental Hypnosis*, **48**, pp. 154–69.

Shertzer, C.L. and Lookingbill, D.P. (1987), 'Effects of Relaxation Therapy and Hypnotisability in Chronic Urticaria', *Archives of Dermatology*, **123**, pp. 913–16.

Shor, R.E. (1959), 'Hypnosis and the Concept of the Generalised Reality-orientation', *American Journal of Psychotherapy*, **13**, pp. 582–602.

Shor, R.E. (1962), 'Three Dimensions of Hypnotic Depth', *International Journal of Clinical and Experimental Hypnosis*, **10**, pp. 23–38.

Shor, R.E. (1971), 'Expectations of Being Influenced and Hypnotic Performance', *International Journal of Clinical and Experimental Hypnosis*, **19**, pp. 154–66.

Spanos, N.P. (1986), 'Hypnotic Behaviour: A Social Psychological Interpretation of Amnesia, Analgesia, and "Trance Logic"', *Behavioral and Brain Sciences*, **9**, pp. 449–67.

Spanos, N.P. (1991), 'A Sociocognitive Approach to Hypnosis', in S.J. Lynn and J.W. Rhue (eds), *Theories of Hypnosis: Current Models and Perspectives*, New York: Guilford, pp. 324–63.

Spanos, N.P. and Hewitt, E.C. (1980), 'The Hidden Observer in Hypnotic Analgesia: Discovery or Experimental Creation?', *Journal of Personality and Social Psychology*, **39**, pp. 1201–14.

Stanton, H.E. (1989), 'Hypnotic Relaxation and Insomnia: A Simple Solution?', *Hypnos: Swedish Journal for Hypnosis in Psychotherapy and Psychosomatic Disorders*, **16**, pp. 98–103.

Stewart, A. and Thomas, S.E. (1995), 'Hypnotherapy As a Treatment for Atopic Eczema in Adults and Children', *British Journal of Dermatology*, **132**, pp. 778–83.

ter Kuile, E.G., Spinhoven, P., Linssen, A.C.G., Zitman, F.G., Van Dyck, R. and Roojimans, H.G.M. (1994), 'Autogenic Training and Cognitive Self-hypnosis for the Treatment of Recurrent Headaches in Three Different Subject Groups', *Pain*, **58**, pp. 331–40.

Viswesvaran, C. and Schmidt, F. (1992), 'A Meta-analytic Comparison of the Effectiveness of Smoking Cessation Methods', *Journal of Applied Psychology*, **77**, pp. 554–61.

Wagstaff, G.F. (1981), *Hypnosis, Compliance and Belief*, Brighton: Harvester Press.

Wagstaff, G.F. (1991), 'Compliance, Belief and Semantics in Hypnosis: A Non-state, Sociocognitive Perspective', in S.J. Lynn and J.W. Rhue (eds), *Theories of Hypnosis: Current Models and Perspectives*, New York: Guilford, pp. 362–96.

Wickless, C. and Kirsch, I. (1989), 'Effects of Verbal and Experiential Expectancy Manipulations on Hypnotic Susceptibility', *Journal of Personality and Social Psychology*, **57**, pp. 762–68.

Zachariae, R., Øster, H., Bjerring, P. and Kragballe, K. (1996), 'Effects of Psychological Interventions on Psoriasis: A Preliminary Report', *Journal of the American Academy of Dermatology*, **34**, pp. 1008–15.

Part I
The Birth of Modern Hypnosis

[1]

QUANTITATIVE METHODS OF INVESTIGATING HYPNOTIC SUGGESTION [1] *

Part I

By CLARK L. HULL
YALE UNIVERSITY

IN the preface to the fourth edition of his well known work on hypnosis[2] Moll expresses the opinion that little or nothing remains to be discovered in the field of hypnotic phenomena (Symptomatology). He says: "Very little has been added to our knowledge of these questions during the last few years, and *it would appear that this branch of hypnotic research is fairly exhausted,* though of course, it may one day happen that it will have to go through a searching revision which will prove instructive." [3] The history of science shows that similar views have been put forward from time to time in the various fields of scientific research, always to be disproven by subsequent events. Moll's pessimistic prediction most certainly will be no exception. It is one of the purposes of the present article to show that the possibilities of research in hypnotism not only are not exhausted but that, comparatively speaking, they have as yet scarcely been touched.

Perhaps the most effective way of establishing such a thesis as that just put forward, is to demonstrate the possibilities of fruitful research by concretely pointing them out. This it is proposed to do to the extent of outlining over a hundred typical experimental projects from this rich field.[4] It is hoped that this concrete exhibition, at once of our ignorance regarding the major hypnotic

---

1 These outlines are not in all cases the result of the unaided efforts of the author. They have been evolved in connection with an extensive cooperative research program carried on at the University of Wisconsin under his leadership. The outlines thus represent in many cases, the result of the combined suggestions and criticisms from a number of different persons. In most cases the identity of the individual contribution has been lost in the complex give and take of cooperative thinking. The author hereby expresses his sincere appreciation to all those earnest young people who have so loyally associated themselves with him in the attempt to establish hypnotism on a genuinely scientific basis.

* Manuscript received February, 1929.

2 Moll, Albert. *Hypnotism.* Charles Scribner's Sons, New York, 1913.

3 Italics ours.

4 Outlines of forty somewhat analogous projects in waking suggestion have been given in a previous article: Quantitative Methods of Investigating Waking Suggestion, this Journal, July, 1929.

phenomena and of its remedy, will ultimately bring about an increasing number of exact and carefully controlled scientific investigations of hypnotism.

It is scarcely an exaggeration to say that the present state of hypnotic knowledge is a scientific scandal. It will be recalled that Mesmer was a contemporary of Benjamin Franklin. During the period of something over a century and a half since Franklin's kite experiment (1752), electricity has developed into one of the most exact and quantitative sciences in existence. After approximately the same period (Mesmer propounded to the scientific world his views on animal magnetism in 1775), we find hypnotism for the most part still languishing in the hands of charlatans and mystery mongers. Except for a little notable work performed during the last decade, scarcely anything of scientific significance has been done for a century. During this period almost nothing has been accomplished save the more or less imperfect correction of experimental blunders committed by earlier workers.

It is not as if this remarkable backwardness in the development of hypnotism as a science had been due to lack of attention. Actually throughout this long period there has been continuous and widespread experimental activity in this field. The meager scientific results from all this really immense expenditure of human energy has resulted to a considerable extent from the workers wasting their time in mere dabbling. For the most part they contented themselves with repeating the classical experiments: inducing the trance, producing catalepsies, analgesias, post-hypnotic amnesias, and acts by post-hypnotic suggestion, but without significant variation from the procedures employed thousands of times before by previous experimenters. To a large extent this is true even today. There are signs, however, that this long period of sterility is rapidly drawing to a close. It is the hope of the author that the following suggestions of experimental procedures will aid in hastening the renaissance in hypnotic research which seems to be on its way.

Outlines of Experimental Projects and Procedures [5]

1. It is obvious to all who have had any experience in putting people into the hypnotic trance, that some persons are far more

[5] The reader should bear in mind that these outlines are not intended to be complete or final but merely suggestive, both as regards problems and methods of experimental solution. Many problems permit several modes of solution and many of the experimental methods described may be used with appropriate modifications to solve a variety of problems. Moreover, the limitations of space make it impossible to indicate in any detail or completeness the experimental safeguards necessary to be observed.

susceptible than others. Indeed, occasional individuals appear to be quite uninfluenced by the hypnotic technique. This last is particularly paradoxical since most psychological processes, such as the ability to perform the various types of learning, are found to some, though varying, degree in all normal individuals. Moreover, it is known that the quantitative distribution of most human abilities is strictly continuous, approaching the normal or Gaussian form. In this connection it becomes a matter of some interest to know the form of the distribution of susceptibility to the trance, particularly at that point of the scale where the minimal positive response passes over—apparently—into complete failure to respond.

For this problem to be solved in a satisfactory manner, a large homogeneous group of psychologically naïve subjects is needed. To secure a measure of susceptibility to the trance each subject should be subjected to a standard trance procedure by a single experimenter, lasting say twenty minutes. The measure of individual susceptibility should be the time required to induce a given standard of response. Of the various hypnotic phenomena available as a criterion for this purpose, probably the final closure of the lids is the best, because (1) lid closure is one of the most generally obtainable responses and (2) it can be observed and recorded most readily. The subject should be instructed very definitely not to close his lids voluntarily but only as the result of the suggestion.

The time required to induce final closure could be taken with the aid of a good stop-watch. Since the lids frequently close for a few seconds at a time before final closure takes place, a watch with a double stop attachment should be used, the one hand being stopped at each apparent closure and released again every time the lids open. The reading at the stop marking the final closure would then be the time required. In case it were desired to secure a record of the various temporary closures, this could be secured readily by using a kymograph provided with a time marker and a magnetic signal marker, the latter connected with a battery and a key. An assistant could watch the subject's eyes and press on the key during the period of each closure. The smoked-paper record would then show the detailed history of the closures.

A dot distribution could be constructed from the time scores made by the subject, each subject being represented by a dot. These results could then be subjected to various forms of statistical treatment to determine whether the subjects giving positive responses taken alone constitute a "normal" group, or whether the individuals showing no response are required in order to complete the "slow" end of the presumably Gaussian distribution surface, and so on.

2. The differences in susceptibility to the trance noted under project No. 1 raise various questions: Are the differences in trance susceptibility due to an inherited organic positive or negative suggestibility? Or are they expressions of a more or less specialized set of socially conditioned habits? Are they due to differences in the personalities of the subjects? Are they significantly related to other aspects of the subjects' behavior, particularly such as may be sampled by psychological tests? The degree of correlation between trance susceptibility and various test scores should have considerable significance as to the essential nature of the particular process taken as the criterion of the trance.

Among the tests which it might be well to try for this purpose are one or two of the better verbal "intelligence" tests, the Kent-Rosanoff association test, an introversion-extroversion test and a considerable variety of tests presumably depending upon waking suggestibility and ideo-motor action, the stimulus of the latter being understood as originating outside the subject's organism. Some of these are: the tendency to move imitatively when watching some one making strong muscular effort; the tendency when the subject is standing with the eyes closed to sway forward when given quiet but continuous suggestions that he is doing so; the tendency, when holding a small bob suspended by a thread, to gradually make it swing in a direction indirectly suggested; the inability to unclasp the hands, to bend the arm, or to take the foot from the floor when told emphatically that it can not be done.

The classification of trance susceptibility in this case might be based on the number of subjects from a group like that of project No. 1, who report respectively (1) complete amnesia, (2) partial amnesia, and (3) no apparent amnesia, at the end of the standard 20-minute trance procedure. With this classification there might be computed either the bi-serial r, the tetrachoric correlation coefficient, or the coefficient by the four-fold-table method. If, on the other hand, the criterion of lid closure as described under project No. 1 should be employed, the ordinary Pearson correlation coefficient could be utilized.

3. If a criterion of trance susceptibility were used in project No. 2 which would permit of the computing of the Pearson correlation coefficient, the results from that investigation would make it possible to organize a test battery for estimating susceptibility to the trance, the several tests of which could be accurately

weighted by a multiple regression equation. The criterion as described under project No. 2 would also permit of the organization of a battery but its weighting would be very rough and crude. Such batteries as these, especially if the hypnotic score itself were included, might also be very useful in forecasting numerous vocational aptitudes involving suggestibility. It is possible that this trait or combination of traits is much more significant in various occupations, especially those primarily dealing with people, than is generally realized.

4. Pierre Janet has suggested that hypnotics are especially susceptible to fatigue. It would be an easy matter to test the truth of this assertion by testing on the ergograph a group of subjects like that suggested in projects No. 1 or No. 2 and then correlating the fatigability as shown by the ergograph with the degree of trance susceptibility. Appropriate corrections would, of course, need to be made to render comparable the rate of fatigue for people of different muscular equipment.

5. There is some reason to believe that individuals in an advanced state of general muscular fatigue have an increased susceptibility to the trance. Divide a large homogeneous group of naïve volunteers into two equally susceptible sections as nearly as this can be done by means of a battery of tests such as described under No. 3. Lacking the test battery, the subjects could be arranged according to chance. Let the individuals of one group take a long walk which will pretty thoroughly exhaust them. At once following this, subject them to the standard twenty-minute hypnotic technique. Subject the second or control group to the standard hypnotic technique with everything else constant except that they shall not be fatigued. The fatigued subjects should not know or suspect that fatigue is a part of the hypnotic experiment. Probably use trance susceptibility criteria of both projects No. 1 and No. 2. Compare the mean susceptibility to trance of the two groups and determine the statistical reliability of the difference found between the means.

6. Occasional observations suggest rather strongly that persons suffering from loss of sleep are especially susceptible to the trance. This problem could be solved by methods analogous to those described under No. 5. The loss of one night's sleep by the experimental group would be a convenient unit of privation to employ.

7. Certain drugs are said to increase suggestibility and to favor susceptibility to the trance. Among those worthy of investigation may be mentioned alcohol, chloral, ether, chloroform, and mor-

phine. Perhaps most promising of all is scopolamine. An experimental squad of subjects and a comparable control squad of subjects as described under No. 5 would be desirable. In addition it is imperative that a control dose, if possible indistinguishable by the subjects from the actual drug, should be administered to the control group.

It would be especially interesting to test the influence of various drugs upon subjects who had proven refractory to ordinary suggestion. Divide a group of such refractory subjects into two comparable squads and treat as described in the preceding paragraph.

8. It is quite evident to even casual observation that most persons, when about to submit to the hypnotic technique, are in a state of considerable emotional excitement. This may be easily seen, for example, in the beating of the arteries of the neck. This raises the question as to whether the presence of strong emotional excitement facilitates or retards the tendency to fall into the trance.

A large group of subjects such as described under No. 2 should have their emotional reactions recorded as described under No. 25 throughout the initial twenty-minute standard trance procedure. In this manner the mean and the range of intensity of the several emotional reactions should be determined respectively for the three divisions of subjects as regards susceptibility to the trance. A comparison of these means should at least show whether the excitement characteristic of persons about to go into the trance the first time is a favorable or an unfavorable symptom.

9. Subjects who fail to go into the trance often report later that they more or less deliberately resisted the suggestions. On the other hand, tales are sometimes told of traveling hypnotists who are able to hypnotize individuals who at the outset are aggressively defiant. Moreover, subjects responding positively in waking suggestion experiments often report having at first resisted. Some light might be thrown on this problem by securing systematic reports from the various subjects at the conclusion of experiments like Nos. 1, 2, and 8, as to whether they resisted. The percentage of subjects reporting resistance in the various susceptibility groups might indicate something as to the influence of resistance on susceptibility.

It would also be of great interest to see whether the resisting subjects showed more or less than average amounts of the emotional reactions investigated by No. 8.

Unfortunately verbal reports of the nature mentioned above are very easily influenced by various subsequent, and hence irrelevant, factors such as whether or not the subjects actually went into the trance. Probably a much more promising method than that just described would accordingly be for a second experimenter to instruct half of the subjects in a set-up like No. 1 or No. 2, definitely to resist the suggestion. It would be preferable if the hypnotist should himself know nothing about this until after the experimental work should be finished. The mean susceptibility scores of the instructed and the uninstructed groups might easily furnish a useful index of the rôle of voluntary resistance in producing refractoriness to the hypnotic technique.

10. Since the time of Braid, one of the very common methods of inducing the trance is to ask the subject to look fixedly at some bright object held rather close to the eyes and somewhat above, in such a position that the latter are under a certain amount of muscular strain. This is ordinarily accompanied by specific verbal suggestions. Now it is known that verbal suggestions alone will induce the trance. The question arises as to what extent, if any, the optical fixation in itself contributes to inducing the trance.

The solution of this problem calls for three comparable squads of naïve subjects. With one group have S look fixedly at the bright object. These subjects should not know that the experiment has anything to do with hypnosis. Accordingly some fictitious but plausible explanation of the purpose of the experiment should be given. With the second group the verbal sleeping suggestion should be given without the optical fixation of the bright object. With the third group both fixation and verbal suggestion should be given as in the usual technique. In all cases the period should be twenty minutes. The criterion of trance susceptibility used in No. 1 and No. 2 could be employed. Compare the mean susceptibility of the three groups, and the differences between the means with the probable errors of the differences. If the differences between the means appear fairly large but are less than two and a half or three times the size of their probable errors, add continuously to the number of subjects in the respective squads until the P.E.'s become as small as desired.

11. From experiments carried out in his laboratory in Petrograd, Pavlov has come to the conclusion that sleep is a highly universal internal inhibition. Here we are concerned mainly with the fact that he has noted certain intermediate states between the waking and sleeping states which he believes to be of the same nature as the hypnotic trance. These experiments should be repeated with human subjects.

Set up a conditioned reflex in which the kneejerk is conditioned to the tone of a tuning fork of 256 d.v. and conditioned not to

powers and the other that he is a crude amateur. Subjects from the respective squads will be tested for trance susceptibility in a random order. The hypnotist should not know of the plan of the experiment until it is completed.

15. Various procedures for facilitating the induction into the trance have been employed and advocated from time to time. The relative effectiveness of these various methods should be susceptible of experimental comparison by such methods as described under No. 10 above. Some of the alternative questions which thus present themselves are: (a) Is it advantageous to precede the formal giving of the trance suggestion by a description of the hypnotic behavior which the subject will show? (b) Is there any advantage in letting a new subject see some other person be put into the trance previous to attempting a first time? (c) Is it more effective in general to use an aggressive commanding manner or to employ a quiet, gentle, and insinuating manner? Do some personalities (possibly as revealed by suitable tests) respond better to one manner and some to the other? (d) Is it more effective to experiment on a subject by himself or to have a number of sympathetic persons present? (e) Is it better to have the subject stand or to sit reclining in a comfortable chair?

16. It has been observed repeatedly that subjects who show few or no signs of going into a trance, particularly after prolonged application of suggestion, often show marked effects and even fall into an amnesic trance spontaneously after the experimenter has discontinued his efforts and begun on a second subject in the presence of the first. The question arises as to how much of this apparent after-discharge is due to a genuine perseveration of suggestion and how much is due to the indirect action of the suggestion being administered to the second subject. It is well known, for example, that susceptible subjects frequently fall into a trance while observing hypnotic suggestions being given to another person.

The problem might be attacked in the following manner: A large group of naïve subjects who are known to be refractory should be divided into comparable groups. The individuals of one group, following the standard trance procedure in each case, would be left sitting quietly in a chair for twenty additional minutes while the experimenter talks uniformly about the weather, say, with a trained assistant in quiet monotonous tones. The individuals of the second squad would follow their standard trance suggestion by twenty additional minutes, during which they sit quietly the same as the first squad, only in this case the experi-

respond to ten neighboring tones up the scale and ten down, such as 426, 160, 640, and so on. All stimuli and responses will be recorded automatically on smoked paper. After the conditioning and differential inhibition have been set up, try the following: Sound the 256 d.v. fork and record the extent of the kneejerk; now sound in succession at five-minute intervals the various neighboring tones in random order. If the dog results hold with humans, the lids should begin to droop after a few stimulations of these negatively conditioned tones. The degree of drooping of the lids might also be recorded by means of the method described under No. 19.

When the lids are closed to varying degrees, the subject should be tested in various ways for suggestibility, amnesia, etc. If amnesia develops, determine whether recall can be effected in a subsequent trance of the usual kind. It would also be of interest to know whether there is any correlation between susceptibility to this phenomenon and to the ordinary trance.

12. Whether Pavlov's theory turns out to have any truth or not, there is excellent reason to believe that the hypnotic trance is characterized by a great diminution of the spontaneous thinking activity. It is possible that resistance to suggestion consists in the subject continuously telling himself subvocally that he is not going into the trance, and by this self-stimulation counteracting the stimuli furnished by the experimenter. If this is true, it might be possible to prevent this type of resistance by otherwise engaging the speech apparatus in monotonous but irrelevant activity such as counting in a low tone. This could be tried out on a squad of refractory subjects, a control squad of the same type also being run.

13. Some persons seem to be much more successful in giving trance suggestions than others. Exactly what the factors determining this personal suggestive potency are and the range of variability among various persons is of importance. This should be determined with respect to age, sex, size of body, quality of voice, aggressiveness of manner, and so on. A matter of some interest is whether certain subjects are more susceptible to one type of experimenter and other subjects to another type of experimenter. This problem could be solved by methods analogous to that described for No. 8, this JOURNAL, p. 160, vol. XXIV.

14. How potent is the fact that a hypnotist has a reputation for being an expert in facilitating the induction into the trance? This problem could be solved by having two squads of naïve subjects. Instruct one squad that the hypnotist is world-famous for his

menter will give strong suggestions to an assistant trained to resist for some minutes but finally to yield. The tendency of the eyes to close in each case can be recorded mechanically on a kymograph by a second assistant who observes the subjects from a concealed position, perhaps by means of a laboratory telescope.

17. Verbal reports from certain subjects indicate that the phenomenon mentioned under No. 16 may be especially characteristic of subjects who deliberately resist the direct suggestions of the trance technique. A squad of subjects who have recently gone into an amnesic trance for the first time (to make sure that they are really hypnotically susceptible) may be instructed by a third person to resist the suggestions. Those who succeed will be left quietly in their chairs the same as the second group of No. 16 and their lid behavior recorded. If, now, they rather uniformly show tendencies to lid closure, it will raise some presumption that the phenomenon of No. 16 is in part, at least, a matter of primary resistance. If, in addition, verbal reports secured from those subjects of No. 16 show a conspicuously larger proportion of admitted resistance where S's fell into a spontaneous trance following the trance technique than where they did not, the presumption would be considerably strengthened.

18. It is a well known fact that if susceptible subjects, either through self-instruction or instruction by another, deliberately resist the suggestion of a hypnotist to perform a given act, the act will be much slower in appearing; it will usually be weaker and perhaps modified in character, or it may not appear at all. It is a question of some interest whether the conflict between the two tendencies takes place centrally, as Sherrington found with spinal dogs, or whether it takes place in part at least as a struggle between antagonistic muscles.

Some light might be thrown on this problem by making exact tracings of the behavior of the two dominant muscles in an antagonistic group, one of which should contract to execute the suggested movement. Rough results could be secured by taking mechanical tracings from the bulging or hardening of the respective muscles or muscle groups involved. More satisfactory results could be secured by recording the action currents from the respective muscles in question by means of the capillary electrometer or the Einthoven string galvanometer. Coupled with this should be an exact tracing of the gross behavior of the bodily part, the movement of which is being suggested. In this way it could be determined in any given case whether the failure of the part to react explicitly is due (a) to failure of innervation of the appropriate muscles, (b) too feeble innervation, or (c) a vigorous innervation of the appropriate muscles due to hetero-suggestion, but which is counterbalanced by an equally vigorous innervation of the antagonistic muscles, presumably by auto-suggestion.

19. We have characteristic curves which represent the progress of various psychological processes such as learning and forgetting. In this connection we may raise the question of the typical curve of the onset of the trance. Does it take place more rapidly at the beginning, the middle, or the end? Is there an initial period of latency and at the end an after-discharge, as seems to be the case in waking suggestion? Does this vary characteristically for the different stages of hypnotic training?

These problems are probably not susceptible of solution for the trance in general, but instead must be solved separately for the several major trance phenomena. As has been suggested more than once previously, the closure of the lids offers special advantages, chiefly because the several stages of their closure are not only open to observation but especially because their behavior may be recorded with precision. This may be effected quite easily by attaching a small piece of aluminum foil to the lid by means of a drop of glue. To the aluminum is attached a light thread which is led through small guides to a very light glass lever which will trace on smoked paper a faithful record of the lid's activities, enlarging three or four times. After two or three minutes the person no longer feels the attachment to his eye and will often ask if it has not come detached. Such a device would record the exact progress of the closure from beginning to end, thus giving the desired curve automatically.

20. The curve of recovery from the trance may be considered for the present purpose to begin at the point when the trance suggestions cease and to extend to a point at which trance phenomena can no longer be detected. In this latter case specific exception must be made of the influence of post-hypnotic suggestions on the one hand and of the relatively permanent increase in susceptibility to the trance which results from repeated hypnotization, on the other.

So far as the phenomenon of lid behavior goes, this problem may be investigated by securing lid tracings very much as in No. 19. The subjects in this case should be brought into a deep trance and then allowed to wake spontaneously. Casual observations would indicate that in the case of the trance the period of after-discharge or persistence of the influence of the suggestion, even where no special suggestion of persistence is made, is much longer than is the case with waking suggestion.

21. A second aspect of this problem, but one in which the lid technique is not adequate, is seen in the familiar case where the subject is told to wake at a signal such as the snapping of the finger. In such cases the subject's eyes usually open instantly, yet there is reason to believe that the subject is for some time thereafter by no means free of the trance. Perhaps the most striking indication of this is the fact that the subject will go into a trance so much more quickly at once following a trance than he will after a longer interval, as well as a generally heightened susceptibility to heterosuggestion immediately after seemingly completely waking from a trance.

This observation gives us the clue of the method of measurement upon the basis of which we shall plot our curve of diminution. Use as subjects persons who have been hypnotized so many times that they no longer show any increase in susceptibility from repetitions of the trance. Put them into the trance by a standard technique, and after a given period following eye closure wake them by a standard waking technique. After varying periods, repeat the trance technique and record the length of time required to produce eye closure, for example. Suggested times would be: 1 sec., 20 sec., 5 min., and 30 min. Only one test should be made following a given trance. It would be well to separate the trances by as much as a week.

A second technique for determining the curve of the diminution of suggestibility following the superficial "waking" from the trance would be to base it on the increasing time required to induce by means of suggestion a given amount of swaying forward while standing and apparently awake. The movements in this case could be recorded automatically by means of the special recorder for postural movements described in an earlier paper.[6] In this second case the subject should probably be put into the trance in a standing posture.

22. Subjects often themselves report, upon being questioned, that they are not fully awake even when they appear superficially to be so. It would be of some interest to secure reports of such internal observations and compare them with the objectively determined curves secured as described. At what point in the recovery to normal suggestibility does the subject regard himself as *fully* awake?

23. It is a well known fact already referred to (No. 20) that successive repetitions of the trance usually facilitate the induction

6 *Op. cit.*

of the trance on a later occasion. The extent to which this is true and the shape of the practice or learning curve of the acquisition of this particular form of habit may readily be determined. Let the experimenter use a standard hypnotic technique. An assistant provided with a suitable stop watch (see No. 1) could note and record the time required to induce the trance on each occasion. Probably the best criterion here also would be the required time to induce lid closure. Separate curves should be plotted from distinct groups of subjects (a) in which the trances are given every day and (b) when given once per week, to reveal influence of spacing repetitions.

A second problem related to that just mentioned concerns the speed with which acts not necessarily associated with the trance, such as the falling forward of the head until the chin practically rests upon the chest, can be acquired after the ordinary trance is well established, as compared with setting it up at the very beginning. Curves based upon time required to induce a given amount of reaction could be plotted. Graphic tracings of the head movements themselves could be secured easily by the postural movement recording device.

24. No. 23 is concerned with what appears superficially to be a phase of habit formation. It is a matter of some interest to know whether the increased susceptibility to the trance acquired through repetition is, like ordinary habits, lost through disuse, and if so, the curve of its diminution. This should probably be investigated by means of several squads of subjects of tested comparability as to susceptibility to the trance, amount of trance training, and so on. The criterion in this case might be the rate of lid closure as in those projects previously sketched.

25. As pointed out in No. 8, there is usually considerable emotion present the first time a subject is exposed to the trance technique. There is reason to believe that the intensity of this emotional reaction diminishes with the successive repetitions of the trance. This latter process, if existent, would then be a process of adaptation or a kind of negative learning. It should be possible to measure the rate of the diminution of emotional reactions for successive trances and from these data to plot the curve with precision.

Among the emotional reactions which are promising for this purpose are:

I. Breathing, as recorded on smoked paper by means of a pneumograph. A number of different indices of emotional reaction which may be used are the following:

A. Change in the inspiration-expiration ratio.

B. Increase in the variability of the inspiration-expiration ratio.

C. Increase in the variability of the time consumed by individual inspiration-expiration cycles.

D. Increase in the variability of the depth of breathing.

E. Increase in the total up-and-down movement of the pneumograph per unit time.[7]

II. The galvanic conductivity of the skin, the so-called galvanic skin reflex. With the aid of an assistant and suitable apparatus, this may be recorded on smoked paper parallel with the pneumograph tracings.

A. The extent of rise in conductivity.

B. The time required to return to normal.

III. The pulse beat, as recorded on smoked paper by the Erlanger-Meek sphygmograph. The following reactions are worth investigation:

A. The fall in the amplitude of the pulse tracing.

B. The increase in variability in the height of the individual pulse beats.

C. The increase in the variability of the time consumed by the individual pulse beat. These latter, if necessary, may be measured by means of a microscope with a graduated scale in the eyepiece.

D. The general increase in the heart rate over the prehypnotic rate.

All of these reactions may be recorded simultaneously on a single piece of smoked paper. The subjects should first be thoroughly accustomed to the recording apparatus before anything is said about the trance. Then, each time a normal record should be taken preceding the trance. Trances should be repeated regularly, say once per week, until the emotional reactions have ceased to decline. Separate curves might be plotted from each of the eleven quantitative indices listed above.

26. As an important by-product from the investigation sketched under projects 8 and 25 may be mentioned the possibility of plotting a curve which would show the characteristic degree of the several emotional responses for the different stages of the trance: the period of anticipation, the period of latency after overt suggestion begins, periods when the subject reports being startled at feeling himself going in and as a result partially recovers spon-

[7] This is measured with precision by the linear oscillometer. This instrument is described in *J. Exp. Psych.*, 1929, Vol. XII, pp. 359–361.

taneously, the period when the deep trance is reached while resting quietly, the period of warning that he is about to be wakened, and finally the period of actual waking.

27. In current practice, post-hypnotic amnesia is probably the most characteristic symptom of hypnosis. As such it deserves especially full investigation.

Bramwell has quite rightly raised the question as to whether the post-hypnotic amnesia for trance events, which is such a common phenomenon of hypnotism, tends to be inherent in the trance state or whether it is, like most other trance phenomena, itself the result of suggestion either directly or in some obscurely indirect manner. If thoroughly naïve subjects, who had never heard of this aspect of suggestion, could be secured, this extremely important but difficult problem might yield to experimental attack. It should at least be possible to determine experimentally the proportion, if any, of subjects professing no knowledge of hypnotic phenomena who show the amnesia where no direct suggestion of any kind has been given. The subjects should be put into the trance, probably by the method in which the eyes are kept open. Use catalepsy, analgesia, and post-hypnotic suggestion as tests of the attainment of the trance. Ten minutes after the termination of the trance, have all subjects fill out in writing a skillfully prepared form containing adroit questions calculated to reveal any waking knowledge of the trance events without actually suggesting the events. Probably one of the most critical of the tests is whether S recalls the act carried out post-hypnotically, and if so, whether he recalls why he did it, *i.e.*, the giving of the post-hypnotic suggestion. The writer ventures the prediction that the percentage of spontaneous amnesia appearing under such circumstances will prove comparatively small.

28. It is a matter of common observation that many subjects who do not show spontaneous post-hypnotic amnesia develop it quite readily after it has been suggested. The question arises as to whether this suggested amnesia is the same phenomenon as the spontaneous form. One method of attacking this problem would be to compare the time required by the two types of amnesic subjects to relearn standard nonsense paired-associates memory material in the waking state which had just been learned in the trance state to two perfect reproductions, say. A further procedure would be to compare the time required to relearn the paired associates a *second* time twenty-four hours later. Perhaps the most promising method of detecting a qualitative difference between the two types of amnesia would be to compare the agreement between

the original-learning and the relearning difficulty of the individual paired associates by the method described under No. 36. In this connection it might be illuminating further to compare the types of amnesia with the performance, under comparable conditions, of subjects instructed to simulate an amnesia of about the same degree. Presumably the behavior of the group showing directly suggested amnesia would more closely resemble the simulation group.

29. It has been shown by Strickler that paired associates learned in the trance require approximately 50 per cent of the original learning time to relearn fifteen minutes later in the waking state. The question rises as to whether this amount of amnesia as measured by the relearning method is peculiar to the verbal type of memory material. An excellent comparison could be made by having subjects learn numerous stylus mazes to a given degree of perfection—say three successive perfect runs—and then relearn fifteen minutes later. Relearn a second time twenty-four hours later. Half of the original learning should be done in the waking state and half in the trance. Special precautions must be taken to protect the results from constant errors due to practice effects, differences in difficulty of the mazes, and so on.

30. Two very different things are popularly taken as evidence of memory. One is the reinstatement of a pattern of reaction previously performed or rehearsed by the subject, such as the execution of a tennis stroke learned last season. The second is exemplified by the verbal description of the stroke. In this latter case the action is in no remote sense like that of a reinstatement—one is mainly executed by the arm, the other by the tongue. Now the test for amnesia ordinarily made is of the second type—we ask the subject to report to us symbolically what he did (or experienced) during the trance. There is a little reason to suspect that this second phase of memory is more susceptible to the amnesia of the trance than the first.

A method of securing some light on the problem thus suggested would be to have two comparable squads of subjects learn a series of stylus mazes in the trance, one squad being directed to do the learning by systematically counting the alleys and otherwise aiding themselves in the learning by their symbolic processes, whereas the other squad would be instructed not to count or to aid themselves in any similar manner. Compare the time required by the respective squads to relearn in the waking state immediately after the trance learning.

A variant of the above method would be to have the same individual learn one set of mazes one way and another set the other way, but otherwise as above. By this method special precautions should need to be taken to eliminate constant errors due to practice effects, differences in maze difficulty, and so on.

31. A characteristic form of memory which it seems possible may not be subject to the usual amnesia is the generalized skill which subjects develop through practice. Thus a subject who learns a large number of series of nonsense paired associates will usually learn the later series in less than half the time required to learn the earlier ones. Now most good hypnotic subjects will show by the test of recall a nearly complete post-hypnotic amnesia for the material thus learned. Will there also be a similar confinement of the increased skill or facility in learning to the trance where it was acquired, or will this function equally or in part in subsequent learning done in the waking state? The basic method of solution would be to give an initial test of the activity in question in the waking state, then give a fairly extended period of memorizing training in the trance, which would be followed by a second testing period in the waking state. If there is no transfer from trance to waking, then the practice curve of the final waking test period will be a simple continuation or extension of the practice curve begun by the preliminary practice period. If, on the other hand, there is complete transfer of acquired skill from the trance to the waking state, the curve of the final testing period will be continuous with the trance practice curve. Almost any other activity showing marked practice effects, such as continuous addition, speed in tapping, cancelling A's, and so on, could be used for this purpose quite as well as the rote learning.

32. That hypnosis should produce a genuine post-hypnotic amnesia not due to suggestion in any ordinary sense is rendered fairly probable by the fact that genuine amnesias appear to result from emotional shocks, blows on the head, and other traumas of a similar type. But just why a trance *per se* should produce an amnesia is something of a mystery. One is tempted to invoke the principle of redintegration as an explanatory principle. Some experiments seem to show, for example, that material learned in one experimental sitting is relearned with greater difficulty in a new sitting than it is in the original one. The only difference in the two cases of learning just cited would appear to be in the incidental parts of the stimulus patterns furnished by the surroundings. In the case of the waking and trance states, one is tempted to wonder whether the *internal* component of the stimulus pattern is sufficiently different in the two conditions to interfere with

recall. Unfortunately for this conjecture, if such a factor were operative, it should present as much resistance to going from the normal state to the trance as from the trance to the normal. While casual observation does not furnish much support for such an expectation, the theoretical considerations are of sufficient weight to make it desirable that the possibility of a real, though moderate, amount of amnesia from the normal state to the trance, should be investigated. This could be done by reversing Strickler's procedure, learning material in the waking state and after an hour testing half the series for recall in the trance state and a comparable half in the waking state. The principle of redintegration would lead us to expect a less perfect recall in the trance state.

33. One of the most remarkable things about amnesias in general and post-hypnotic amnesias in particular is the ease with which they may be made to disappear without any relearning. Subjects who show complete post-hypnotic amnesia as tested by recall *seem* to remember trance events perfectly in the following waking state if the hypnotist will merely tell them before waking that they will remember everything. Certain *a priori* consideration, however, leads one to suspect that careful measurement might reveal a substantial residue of amnesia after it has supposedly been removed by suggestion. For example, it is often impossible, even in the waking state, at once to remove a suggestion that a subject's fingers can not be unclasped, by giving a counter suggestion. Heterosuggestion is often unable to remove psychotic symptoms which are presumably due to some form of autosuggestion; and when immediately effective, the influence of the curative suggestion is too often transitory. This problem might easily be investigated by learning standard paired associates in the trance, then test for recall immediately in the waking state after having suggested perfect post-hypnotic memory. Control series would be run where the subject is tested in the trance state after a similar interval. If the amnesia is not entirely banished, there should be a larger score of failures to recall in the waking state than in the trance.

A second form of this experiment, which might easily yield quite different results, would be to compare the two after twenty-four hours.

34. It is a matter of considerable importance in the understanding of post-hypnotic amnesia to know whether its degree is to any extent dependent upon the strength of the associative tendencies themselves. This problem may be approached by having subjects learn in the trance series of comparable nonsense paired associates

to one perfect recitation. Have other series overlearned to the extent of twice the repetitions necessary for one perfect recitation and still other series three times overlearned. In all cases test for recall in the waking state immediately after the conclusion of the original learning and then relearn. If post-hypnotic amnesia is a function of the strength of the associative tendencies, there should be less amnesia with each increase in the thoroughness of the original learning. If not, then the indication would be that post-hypnotic amnesia is almost purely an inhibitory phenomenon.

35. A further question bearing on the essential nature of post-hypnotic amnesia is whether it combines in a summative manner with ordinary forgetting. Suppose a subject shows 50 per cent post-hypnotic amnesia at once after waking, for barely learned nonsense series. Suppose further that time enough elapses so that he would show 25 per cent loss if tested in a subsequent trance. Will the subject at this point show a waking loss of 75 per cent (the sum of the 25 per cent and the 50 per cent) or will he still show only the 50 per cent due to the amnesia? What will be the waking score when the true forgetting loss alone reaches 50 per cent? This problem may be solved by methods analogous to those already described. If post-hypnotic amnesia is purely an inhibitory phenomenon, we should not expect it to combine in a summative manner with the results of ordinary forgetting.

36. The various items of nonsense material as they appear in the experimental series present markedly different degrees of difficulty for the learning process. The same is true of the several *culs de sac* of a stylus maze. And on relearning after a period of forgetting, those points which caused most difficulty in the original learning series are very apt again to cause most difficulty. In other words, there is quite a high correlation between the original learning and the relearning series as regards the difficulty presented by the several elements composing the series. This is as should be expected because in the original learning the difficult parts are only just barely learned, whereas the easier parts are considerably overlearned. During the period of forgetting the barely learned parts naturally sink below the threshold of recall more readily and so require more reinforcement. But in the case of post-hypnotic amnesia as tested directly after thorough trance learning, all of the associative tendencies are present in sufficient strength to evoke recall if the test should be made in the trance state. The question arises as to whether the evident inhibition of these tendencies in the waking state acts as a kind of flat load placed on the associative connections (as is evidently the case with the true for-

getting process) pressing each individual associative process backward toward its threshold approximately an equal distance from its true trance level; or whether it is merely a capricious interference, singling out certain segments for inhibition without much or any regard for its true associative strength; or lastly, whether it is simply a leveling tendency, reducing all the associative connections to an approximate equality of impotence.

This problem might be investigated by using numerous series, each of twenty paired nonsense associates. Learn in the trance to four perfect recitations. Then relearn half the series at once in the waking state, and the other half in the trance state, the latter after the lapse of enough time to require approximately the same amount of relearning as that produced by post-hypnotic amnesia. Have a similar squad of hypnotically susceptible subjects learn the same material in the waking states and at once *pretend* to relearn half of it in the same state and relearn the other half after the lapse of enough time to require about the same amount of true relearning. For each series learned by each subject compute the correlation between the number of promptings on the corresponding paired associates for the original learning and for the relearning. N of the correlation formula would be twenty or the number of paired associates in the series. There will thus be one coefficient for each series learned. If either the second or third possibility suggested above should hold true, we would expect that the central tendency of the correlation coefficients for the amnesic relearning should hover around zero. If, on the other hand, the first possibility proves true, the correlations should be positive and comparatively high, comparable with those from true forgetting. Lastly, if the amnesic relearnings should show consistently high correlations, and the simulated amnesic relearnings should run consistently low, we should have a precise and objective method for detecting simulation.

37. A further means of examining the nature of post-hypnotic amnesia would be to take detailed records of the emotional reactions (see No. 25) during the learning process. There is reason to believe that if the stimuli were not presented in too rapid succession, fairly characteristic emotional reactions would be called out by certain parts of each series, and that these would tend to reappear on relearning. It would be illuminating to know whether these emotional reactions escape the usual post-hypnotic amnesia as tested by immediate relearning in the waking state, and if so, to what extent as compared with a suitable control series. This would be shown for any given type of emotional reaction by corre-

lating the magnitude of its manifestation at the several parts of each learning series with that at the corresponding points in the relearning of the same series.

38. Another question bearing on the essential nature of post-hypnotic amnesia relates to whether it is an inhibition which is fixed in some sense at the time of learning (as would be the case if it were a simple redintegrative phenomenon) or whether it is a more shallow process operating according to the suggestion which chances to be operating at the time of relearning. If the latter be the case, amnesia might be shifted to material really learned in the waking state, provided time enough could elapse so that the subject would forget which particular series, out of a large number, were learned in the respective states. Control series should be run where the confusion mentioned above would not enter. In case the true amnesia should prove consistently to be more deeply seated, as suggested by the first hypothesis, the experiment might lead to a useful method of detecting simulation. Presumably simulation would follow the second rule, though this would need to be determined experimentally by running a squad of simulators.

39. It has long been known that subjects usually show an amnesia for acts carried out as a result of post-hypnotic suggestion if tested shortly after. The question arises as to the profundity of this amnesia as compared with the post-hypnotic amnesia of the same individual. This problem might be investigated by having subjects directed in the trance to open an experimental book specially provided for the purpose and to memorize some paired associates of a series shown on a certain page during a four-minute period. Half the series should be learned in trances and half by post-hypnotic suggestions, the latter five minutes after the termination of the trance. In order to avoid the complications of retroactive inhibition, only one type of learning should be attempted at any given séance. The beginning and end of the learning should be indicated to the subject by appropriate signals. In the case of the trance learning, subject should be wakened at once after the learning. The amount of retention in both series should be tested after fifteen minutes, one hour, and one day, using separate series for each time interval.

40. Pavlov states that he encountered quite constantly in his experiments on dogs a state intermediate between sleep and waking. In its extreme form the state is said to be characterizes by the suppression of conditioned reflexes, the dog even failing to eat the offered meat. In less extreme cases the food may be neglected

(a failure of a "natural" conditioned reflex to respond) though the saliva may flow, but in diminished quantity, at the presentation of an artificially conditioned stimulus such as a buzzer. If the state which Pavlov considers hypnotic in his dogs is really the same in essence as that called hypnosis in man (as Pavlov evidently believes),[8] then we should expect a corresponding disappearance and diminution of human conditioned reflexes when tested in a true trance state. To test Pavlov's theory it will accordingly be necessary only to set up in a number of hypnotically susceptible subjects, in the *waking* state, a considerable variety of conditioned reflexes, the strength of which should be measured both in the waking and the trance states. If no disappearances and no particular diminutions take place in the trance, a formidable presumption will be created in favor of the view that Pavlov's phenomena are not particularly related to the hypnotic trance.

41. There is reason to believe that in the trance the spontaneous thinking (symbolic-verbal) processes are largely in abeyance. Evidence of value might be secured, throwing at least indirect light on the matter, by comparing the ease of setting up the various conditioned reflexes in the trance and normal state when (a) S is counting subvocally, (b) adding mentally continuously, (c) gripping a dynamometer, (d) while in a voluntary tension of all the muscles of the body, and (e) while relaxed as profoundly as possible.

42. Still further evidence concerning the nature of post-hypnotic amnesia may be furnished by determining whether conditioned reflexes set up in the trance will function in the following waking state. In this, separate comparisons should be made for reactions (a) which are voluntary (like the flexion finger reflex), (b) which are semi-voluntary (like breathing and winking), and (c) which are non-voluntary (such as the galvanic skin reflex, heart action, etc.).

43. If it should prove possible to set up genuine delayed and trace conditioned reflexes in man, their use might offer an interesting additional means of exploring the mechanism of post-hypnotic amnesia. Set up a trace conditioned reflex in the trance in which the response takes place five minutes after the stimulus. Administer the stimulus, then wake the subject and observe whether the response follows in the waking state, and if so, any modifications which are characteristic as to time of appearance, intensity of reaction, and so on. Run suitable control series.

---

8 Pavlov, I. P. *Conditioned Reflexes.* Pp. 265, 267, 404ff.

44. It is a well known fact that with men as well as dogs, if a conditioned reflex is used without reinforcement a number of times, experimental extinction will take place so that the stimulus will no longer evoke the response. This fact offers still another means of exploring the mysteries of post-hypnotic amnesia. Set up in the waking state a strong conditioned reflex to the kneejerk or some emotional reaction, say, and then bring it to an advanced state of experimental extinction in the trance, well below zero. At once wake the subject and when fully awake apply the stimulus and see whether this inhibitory habit obeys the ordinary law of post-hypnotic amnesia or whether it escapes the amnesic influence and inhibits the reflex. Several other forms of negative habits have been elaborated by the reflexologists, such as differential inhibition and conditioned inhibition, which should prove useful in this connection.

45. Set up a strong conditioned reflex in the waking state of a bell to the kneejerk. In the trance set up a strong homogeneous conditioned reflex in which a red flash evokes the kneejerk. Then present both stimuli together (a) in the trance state and (b) in the waking state. If there is no interference by post-hypnotic amnesia, responses in each case should be stronger than that evoked by either stimulus alone. But if post-hypnotic amnesia is operating the response to the combined stimulus in the waking state should be perceptibly weaker than that in the trance.

A negative variant of this experiment would be to bring the trance component of the above homogeneous conditioned reflex considerably below zero by means of experimental extinction. Then present both stimuli together as indicated above both in the trance and the waking states. If post-hypnotic amnesia is not operating in this field, the response in both cases should be zero or very small, but if it is operating, then the response in the waking state should be larger than in the trance state.

46. It has long been known that if a given learning activity is followed by another, particularly if the second is of the same type of material, the subsequent recall of the first is diminished. This is known as retroactive inhibition. The question arises as to whether material learned in the waking state, followed by learning similar material in the trance state, will be recalled any worse than if it were followed merely by a quiet sleeping trance of the same duration. Run a second (control) series in which the original learning is followed by learning done in the waking state. If post-hypnotic amnesia operates on the mechanism of retroactive inhibition, there should be no difference between recall where waking

learning is followed by the learning trance from that when followed by the quiet trance; but both should show a markedly better recall than where followed by waking learning. If, on the other hand, post-hypnotic amnesia does not operate in this case, recall where waking learning is followed by quiet trance should be best and where followed by trance learning should be equal to where followed by waking learning. If, however, post-hypnotic amnesia is partially operating, as seems most likely, the recall where normal learning is followed by trance learning will be intermediate between where followed by quiet trance and by waking learning.

[2]

A PREFACE TO THE THEORY OF HYPNOTISM

BY ROBERT W. WHITE
Harvard University

Hypnotism has been the object of wonder and speculation ever since its promotion by Mesmer more than a century and a half ago. Oddly enough, the interest shown by ordinary people and by literary men has only rarely been matched among scientists. Science is the outgrowth of human curiosity, but the trained scientist often appears to be the least curious of mortals because he has imposed upon himself such rigorous conditions for satisfying his need. Thus in 1784, when Mesmer's cures were the talk of Paris, a commission of scientists dismissed his findings on the ground that the phenomena, though real, were the result of imagination, hence not of the physical stuff with which science could safely deal. Branded with this scarlet letter, ejected from the better consulting rooms, hypnotism was destined to wander for a hundred years in the slums of medical practice, from which disgrace she was not rescued until the eminent neurologist Charcot picked her out of the gutter, examined her reflexes, and pronounced her worthy of a place in medical research. More recently, through similar good offices by Hull, she has been allowed to enter the portals of experimental psychology, where in the last fifteen years she has begun to live down her reputation, learn the manners of the laboratory, and speak the language of polite science. Yet so recent is her social ascent that even in contemporary studies of hypnotism there occasionally seems to linger the atmosphere of magic and darkened rooms rather than the clear light of reason.

It is psychology's misfortune that hypnotism has only just now been admitted to a place among its methods and problems. For hypnotism is one of the few experimental techniques applicable to human beings whereby it is possible to produce major changes in the organization of behavior. Without discomfort or danger to the subject, provided certain precautions have been taken, it is possible to effect an extensive alteration in those patterns of experience which constitute the self and in those controls of behavior which we know as volition. Had it used a technique which really affected volition instead of the method of fleeting observation pursued with such slender profit by Ach and Michotte, the experimental psychology of will might have survived and prospered. With the aid of hypnotism it is possible to reproduce, artificially and temporarily, the diverse symptoms of hysteria, or with equal ease to make a manageable laboratory model of compulsion neurosis. By the same means, one can create an artificial "complex," make it effectively "unconscious," and, for the first time under controlled conditions with known antecedents, study the irruption of unconscious strivings into the normal stream of behavior and the methods of defense set up against them. Since no two people respond to hypnotic technique exactly alike, an avenue is opened up for the study of individual differences in the control and organization of behavior. Furthermore, hypnosis as a social situation offers an excellent opportunity to understand more clearly the influence one person can have upon another; it provides an experimental method for building out from Le Bon's intuitions concerning group behavior and carrying forward a study which does not grow less important in our time. With the aid of hypnotism, in short, it is possible to investigate a variety of difficult but extremely significant psychological problems. To complain that the more complex processes of human behavior are inaccessible to experimental technique is certainly premature.

In view of this promise of things to come, it is important to keep a sharp and critical eye roving over the theory of hypnotism. The foundations hastily laid in the days of animal magnetism may give way unexpectedly under the superstructure which is now beginning to arise. The writer believes that certain basic misconceptions have secretly lodged themselves in the theory of hypnotism like termites boring in the sills. The central difficulty, as he will try to show, is the stubborn persistence of mechanical ideas and mechanical figures of speech to describe what is essentially a human situation involving a delicate interplay of human strivings. Modern students of hypnotism, he believes, have rarely taken the trouble to shake out of their minds such notions as animal magnetism, trance states, and ideo-motor action. Despite the sad object-lesson of Charcot, most cautious of scientists who nevertheless came to a series of wrong conclusions because he overlooked the subtleties of indirect suggestion, they have failed to consider exactly what the hypnotist communicates to his subject, exactly how the subject understands it, and exactly what he tries to do about it. Before it can make its proper contribution to the understanding of behavior, hypnotism must become a sophisticated chapter in social psychology. Only then will it be possible to study the nature of the hypnotic state without confusing the issues from the very start.

Facts Which Require Explanation

To begin with, we shall review briefly the facts that any theory of hypnosis is called upon to explain. What are the characteristics which make hypnosis a perennial object of wonder and amazement? Three things appear to create surprise. One of these is that the hypnotized person can effectuate suggestions lying outside the realm of ordinary volitional control; he can do things that he could not possibly do in the normal state. No less surprising, however, is the way a hypnotized person carries out those suggestions lying within the realm of volition. Stiffening the arm or clasping the hands are actions that anyone could perform volitionally, but in hypnosis they occur without benefit of volition, unaccompanied by the experience of intention, yet at times so strongly that the subject seems unable to arrest them when he tries. Furthermore, hypnotic actions are carried out with a curious lack of humor and self-consciousness, often with an air of abstraction and drowsiness, and they do not seem to have the claim over subsequent memory to which their recency and importance entitle them. Finally, it is a constant source of amazement that these rather drastic effects can be brought about simply by talking. If a person suffered a head injury, took a drug, or was worked into a state of violent emotion, radical changes in the control of behavior would be expected as a matter of course, but no one can believe that mere words entering the ears of a relaxed and drowsy subject can be sufficient cause for the changes which actually take place. It will repay us to consider each of these items in a little more detail.

1. *Hypnotic transcendence of voluntary capacity* is strikingly illustrated by insensitivity to pain. One of the most dramatic chapters in the history of hypnotism is its use by James Esdaile about 1845 as an anaesthetic in major surgical operations. There is still no more convincing way to persuade a sceptic that hypnosis is "real" than by showing that ordinarily painful stimuli can be endured without signs of pain. Carefully controlled experiments

designed to exclude every possibility of error have reaffirmed the reality of this phenomenon and have shown that the inhibition extends to such non-voluntary processes as pulse rate and the galvanic skin reaction (5; 25). Along somewhat different lines, recent experiments show that muscular strength and resistance to fatigue are at least somewhat increased (33) and that recall is substantially improved in consequence of hypnotic suggestions (26; 30). There is still some reason to believe that older claims concerning the production of blisters, cold sores, and digestive reactions are not without foundation, although the investigation of these topics has suffered from a lack of control experiments (10; 11; 21). Whatever the ultimate decision upon one or another of the latter claims, there is no danger in concluding that hypnotic suggestion can produce a number of effects beyond the realm of volition, and that among these effects is an increased control over autonomic functions. The implication of these facts for a theory of hypnotism will be considered in a later section.

2. It is not necessary, however, to depend upon these facts of transcendence in order to demonstrate that hypnotic behavior differs from voluntary. If we confine ourselves to actions which could perfectly well be performed intentionally, there is still a *distinct difference in the way they are performed* in response to hypnotic suggestion. When retrospection is possible, as often happens after relatively light hypnosis, a crucial difference in the accompanying experience can be recognized. Janet reports that a patient, ordinarily suggestible, one day declared that the suggestion "did not take." "I am quite ready to obey you," she said, "and I will do it if you choose: only I tell you beforehand that the thing did not take" (12). This patient clearly recognized the difference between obedience, when one intentionally carries out another person's command, and suggestion, when the action executes itself without the experience of intention, even in defiance of it.

Bleuler, describing his experiences when hypnotized, said, "I felt my biceps contracting against my will as soon as I attempted to move my arm by means of the extensor muscles; once, on making a stronger effort to carry out my intention, the contraction of the flexors became so energetic that the arm, instead of moving outward as I had intended, moved backward on the upper arm." "At other times," he said again, "I felt that the movement was made without any active taking part by my ego, this being especially marked with unimportant commands" (8).

One of the writer's subjects reported himself as "quite marvelling at the way my arm stayed up, apparently without volition on my part. I was still aware of myself off in a corner looking on." Observations such as these could be multiplied indefinitely, but further emphasis is scarcely necessary. It is sufficient to remember that subjects after light trances can almost always give evidence concerning their susceptibility, and that their own spontaneous criterion is whether or not they had the feeling of collaborating in the production of the suggested actions. Though there is a hazy borderland between intentional and automatic acts, in the majority of cases subjects can readily discriminate between the two. Hypnotic suggestion not only transcends the limits of volitional control but also dispenses with volition when bringing about actions which normally lie within those limits.

Subsequent report is frequently impossible because of post-hypnotic amnesia. Even so there is an appreciable difference between hypnotic behavior and the everyday intentional performance of like actions. For one thing, the subject's manner differs from the ordinary: he seems literal and humorless, he shows no surprise and makes no apology for bizarre behavior, he appears entirely un-self-conscious, and very often he acts abstracted, inattentive, almost as if he were insulated against his surroundings. Braid's notion of monoideism serves very well to describe the impression a hypnotized person makes on an outside observer. For another thing, hypnotic behavior does not seem to occupy a proper place in the subject's memory. He disclaims recollection of recent and often very complicated actions which in the ordinary way he seems to have every reason to remember. Thus, whether we choose an introspective criterion or whether we prefer external observation, we are entitled to be surprised at the difference between hypnotically suggested actions and similar actions intentionally performed.

3. *The procedure by which hypnosis is made to occur does not seem adequate to produce such an effect.* So great is this discrepancy that for many years it was customary to assume a magnetic force, an invisible fluid, or some similar powerful agent, passing from the operator into the subject. With the decline of such theories there has been a tendency to argue that the phenomena of

hypnosis are after all not unique, that under suitable conditions they can all be duplicated without resort to a hypnotic procedure. It is known, for example, that under stress of excitement and violent emotion people surpass by a wide margin their usual levels of muscular strength and endurance. In like circumstances there is often a considerable degree of anaesthesia for the pain of fairly serious injuries. Hypermnesia occurs during free association, in drowsy states, and in dreams. Many actions which cannot be initiated by themselves without the experience of intention take place quite involuntarily when embedded in a context of other actions, as in playing a game. Perhaps these claims are justified; perhaps there is no phenomenon in the repertory of hypnotic suggestion which cannot be produced in some other way. But, even if this be true, we are not exempt from explaining why the hypnotic procedure, which does not create excitement and violent emotion, which does not put one to sleep, which makes no use of free association, which virtually excludes a context of other actions, and which especially with practice requires very little time, brings about so momentous an effect. It is legitimate to be surprised at the power of hypnotic suggestion.

The task which confronts a theory of hypnosis is roughly defined by the three foregoing peculiarities. Any such theory must explain how (1) the hypnotic procedure brings about (2) the non-volitional performance of acts that ordinarily require volitional assistance and (3) the performance of acts outside the normal range of volition.

Hypnotic Behavior as Goal-Directed Striving

When Charcot discovered that it was possible to reproduce the symptoms of hysteria by means of hypnosis he surmised that the two phenomena were closely related, indeed that they were aspects of the same underlying condition. This dubious bond, however, was not sufficient to keep hypnosis and hysteria long on an equal footing of medical interest. Thus it happened that the theory of hypnotism lingered at the Salpêtrière stage, while the theory of hysteria advanced steadily from Charcot's time to the present, becoming at last the basis for a new understanding of all neurotic conditions and the starting-point for modern dynamic psychology. The central insight which transformed the theory of hysteria was the idea that symptoms spring from strivings, that neurosis is an outcome of conflict among fundamental impulses rather than a damaged state of the nervous system. Such a view would have been impossible without the still more basic insight that large parts of a person's striving may take place unconsciously, forming no part of his organized picture of himself and his intentions. In psychopathology these once radical notions have gradually worked their way to acceptance.

The benefits of this progress have been largely withheld from the theory of hypnotism. Two concepts, *automatism* and *dissociation,* once useful in understanding hysteria but long since modified, reshaped, and animated with dynamic ideas, have persisted in a peculiarly literal and lifeless form in hypnotic theory. Automatism, invoked to explain the non-volitional character of hypnotic behavior, implies that hypnotized persons are helpless executants of the operator's will as this is expressed in verbal suggestion. Dissociation, called upon to account for amnesia, post-hypnotic phenomena, and those instances when impressions seem to be excluded from awareness or when intentions fail to govern motor processes, implies the subject to be in a state of temporary fragmentation such that different parts of his behavior take place independently without their usual communication. These ideas deserve the respect which is due to first approximations, but their prolonged survival keeps the theory of hypnotism in swaddling clothes when it should be grown to adult stature.

The concept of striving, so useful in other parts of psychology, needs to be applied in thoroughgoing fashion to the behavior of the hypnotized person. This application may be embodied in the following statement: *hypnotic behavior is meaningful, goal-directed striving, its most general goal being to behave like a hypnotized person as this is continuously defined by the operator and understood by the subject.* This point of view is not original with the present writer, having been previously maintained by Rosenow (23), Lundholm (15), Pattie (19; 20), and Dorcus (4), who have found it more satisfactory in explaining the facts subsumed under both automatism and dissociation. The hypnotized person is seen not as an almost inanimate object, upon which strange effects can be wrought by touching the right levers or tapping the right lines of cleavage, but as a human being who hears and understands and who tries to behave in the different ways which are proposed to him. The adoption of such an hypothesis should not, of course, depend upon one's general preferences in psychological theory. It is the argument of the present paper that hypnotic behavior, on the face of it, can be adequately described and adequately understood in no other way than as goal-directed striving.

1. Automatism. We shall examine first the reasons for preferring the concept of striving to that of automatism. Hypnotists, who write the theories of hypnosis, have preferred to allocate all the striving to themselves. Certain facts, to be sure, have always stood up to combat this attitude of omnipotence. Many people cannot be hypnotized at all, and no careful operator embarks on his enterprise without assuaging the subject's natural fears and building up a feeling of confidence—without trying, in other words, to set at rest antagonistic strivings. It has long been known, furthermore, that hypnotized subjects can successfully resist, often if not always, suggestions which are repugnant to their own deeper tendencies. But in spite of these hints, hypnotists have rested comfortably with the idea that subjects, unless activated to some kind of resistance, functioned as passive instruments through which words were transformed into actions. Such a view is maintained by Hull in the following words:

> A true suggestion response is one in which the subject's own symbolic processes, instead of becoming active either in facilitating or resisting the tendency to action naturally arising from the experimenter's words, remain passive so far as the particular act suggested is concerned. . . . This withdrawal of the subject's symbolic activities would naturally leave his muscles relatively susceptible to the symbolic stimulation emanating continuously from the experimenter (11, *397*).

This theory, which is admittedly a moderized version of ideomotor action, requires considerable bolstering before it can explain how the hypnotist's symbolic stimulation, even when in full possession of the subject's muscles, can bring about effects which the subject's own symbolic activities are powerless to achieve. But it becomes still more inadequate when one recollects that hypnotized persons carry on long trains of activity, improvise details, exert themselves to calculate and remember, and in general produce a complex pattern of behavior for which the initial suggestion is certainly not a sufficient cause or a sufficient explanation. Hypnotized subjects make substantial spontaneous additions to what is stated in the suggestion, a fact which marks the difference between automatism and a goal-directed striving to act as if hypnotized.

The shortcomings of automatism may be illustrated by a few examples which could be multiplied indefinitely. Prince (22), Burnett (2), and others have reported experiments in which it was suggested to subjects that they perform difficult mental feats such as adding three-place numbers in their heads or making unusual calculations like the number of seconds intervening between 10:43 and 5:13 o'clock. These and similar calculations were successfully made without awareness when other matters occupied the focus of attention. Even if they had been done without this complicating feature, they would strain to the breaking-point any acceptable meaning of automatism. School teachers will surely not agree that, when they ask children to solve a problem of addition, a "natural tendency" arises from their words which, in the absence of outright resistance, gets the problem solved. To take another example, Erickson (6) has reported a number of experiments in which post-hypnotic suggestions were framed in very general language, the details of their execution being left to the subjects. For instance, a subject was told that he would be bored by a conversation and that while trying to appear interested he would look around for distractions which might be used to end the tedium. The subject executed the suggestion in spite of hindrances interposed by the assistants, choosing an appropriate distraction and calling to his aid unconscious irony and a telling slip of the tongue. Once more the concept of automatism seems totally out of place; the hypnotized person plays altogether too active and too discriminating a part to be regarded in this light.

It is unnecessary to linger over this question except to point out again the backwardness of hypnotic theory and its subjection to outworn concepts. The automatism theory arose at a time when there were supposed to be two distinct levels of behavior, the level of purposive volitional striving and the level of reflex machinery. Since hypnotic behavior clearly did not belong to the volitional level, it had to be classified as some kind of automatism. This arrangement was no more than a recognition of the fact that such behavior took place without the experience of intention, that it seemed to the subject himself to occur of its own accord. In recent years, however, the dichotomy of levels has completely broken down: goal-directed striving no longer necessarily implies either awareness or intention, and nothing, therefore, can be gained by trying to force hypnotic phenomena into the automaton category. Hypnotic theorists may well follow the lead of psychopathologists in putting aside such concepts as ideomotor action.

2. *Dissociation.* In spite of its honorable place in history, the concept of dissociation has a distinctly harmful effect on present thinking about hypnotism. In another place the present writer and Shevach (32) have reviewed in detail the several ways in which dissociation has been invoked to account for the phenomena of hypnosis. They were led to conclude that it aptly describes only certain limited aspects of hypnosis and that it no longer deserves to be considered a key concept for understanding this state. A crucial advance in the theory of hysteria came when Freud added the notion of striving to Janet's dissociation.

> We do not derive the psychic fission from a congenital lack of capacity on the part of the mental apparatus to synthesize its experience, but we explain it dynamically by the conflict of opposing mental forces, we recognize in it the result of an active striving of each mental complex against the other (9).

The theory of hypnotism is entitled to a similar advance: when the hypnotized person acts in a dissociated fashion it is because the suggestion is so framed that separated strivings are required to carry it out.

Once again we must justify this view by an appeal to hypnotic phenomena, by showing that the behavior which exemplifies dissociation can be better understood as goal-directed striving. At first glance it might seem that if a subject is made blind by suggestion, this fact is well described as a dissociation of his visual system. Similarly, if one leg is rendered insensitive to pain or if the events of the trance are wiped out of memory, it seems not inappropriate to refer to dissociated systems. Again, the posthypnotic performance of two simultaneous tasks surprises us mainly because of the apparent isolation of functions which we expect will interfere with each other. But a closer scrutiny of just what can be produced by hypnotic suggestion puts the problem in a new light. It is quite easy, for instance, to dissociate not visual function as a whole but simply the perception of one person in a crowded room, or the perception of face cards in a spread-out pack, or any other quite arbitrary fragment of the visual field. Memory for the hypnotic trance is similarly divisible; the subject may be made to forget all but one incident, or to forget only one. For such phenomena the concept of dissociation yields rapidly diminishing returns. When the system which is dissociated ceases to be a plausible biological unit and becomes an arbitrary grouping of items plastic to whatever suggestion the hypnotist happens to make, and freely changeable at his whim, then the hypothesis of striving fits the facts much more closely. "When you suggest an insensitivity," as Lundholm (16) puts it, "your suggestion sets up an impulse to behave as if the insensitivity obtained."

There is still further reason for doubting the value of dissociation and preferring the concept of striving. Dissociation implies a real insulation of one system from another, a boundary marked by amnesia and lack of interaction. It is very easy to show, however, that the dissociated system is not insulated at all but instead exerts a constant influence on the total behavior. To take one example, let five of a dozen white cards on the table be marked with a small cross; then suggest to the subject that he cannot see the marked ones, and ask him to count the cards. His total of seven can be arrived at only if he apprehends the cross-marks and skips those cards in his count. Such experiments work so well that onlookers become distrustful, but the very same subjects can be exonerated from complicity by suggestions that cause them clearly to transcend their voluntary capacity.

It has been argued thus far that the concept of a goal-directed striving to act like a hypnotized person accounts for the facts of hypnosis better than the notions of automatism and dissociation. Automatism was held to be invalidated by the presence of substantial spontaneous additions to what is stated in the suggestions. Dissociation was discredited by two findings: (1) the biologically implausible, arbitrary, changeable nature of the systems alleged to be dissociated, and (2) the active participation of the supposedly insulated items in the total pattern of behavior. It remains to point out certain ways in which the rejected concepts have corrupted the theory of hypnotism and to show that the striving hypothesis makes a favorable difference.

3. Application of goal-directed striving. A typical instance of hypnotic suggestion, often used for purposes of demonstration, is catalepsy or suggested immobility of one of the limbs. The operator declares that the extended arm has become rigid, that it is impossible to move it, that if the subject now makes the attempt he will find he cannot move it. What happens is described as follows by McDougall:

And now the patient will fail to achieve a forbidden movement not merely because he cannot or will not make the necessary effort, but because, when he tries to make the movement and succeeds in innervating the proper muscles, the antagonistic muscles come into play and prevent the movement. At this stage, then, there is manifested a certain splitting of the personality, a conflict of one part against another: the muscles of one set obey the one part, the conscious willing subject; the antagonistic muscles obey some other part of the personality, which understands and is subservient to the commands and suggestions of the operator (7).

We are entitled to wonder, in reading this account, whether a dissociation exists anywhere except in the thoughts of the operator. One set of muscles, we can agree, "understands and is subservient to" his suggestions, but we do not need to assume that the other set is differently disposed, for it, too, has precisely obeyed his command to try and his suggestion to fail. Realizing this, we can abolish altogether the fiction that the patient is divided and that the operator has spoken separately to the two parts. It appears instead that the hypnotized person has fully understood the operator's intention and has subserviently enacted a pattern of behavior which consists of stiffening the arm, then trying and failing to bend it. The subject is not dissociated, nor is one part of him functioning as an automatism; he is striving to behave like a hypnotized person, as this has just been defined by the operator.

It is important to notice that in substituting this hypothesis for the older ones we are not explaining away the mystery of hypnosis nor accusing the subject of deception. Often the hypnotized person exhibits surprise, sometimes even alarm, when he discovers that the suggestion has taken effect and that what he conceives to be his will cannot break up the pattern set by the operator. What he does not realize, however, is that it was not "truly" his will to overcome the suggestion. Had it been "truly" his will, he would have succeeded, and been pronounced an insusceptible subject, as happens in many cases. But if the motive of behaving like a hypnotized person is regnant, the operator's command to try to overcome a suggestion calls for a token display of will which the subject secretly hopes will not prevail. There can be no justification for assuming that he does not understand the operator's hopes and intentions, or for supposing that one command can be isolated from the total pattern and attached to a separate part of his personality. The vain struggle of the hypnotized person is an instance of willing when you do not want your will to succeed, a situation in which we need not be surprised to find volition singularly ineffective.

On the other hand, even in this simple example we do not propose to minimize the difference between hypnotic behavior and voluntary compliance in a wide-awake, alert state. The subject's surprise, the changes in his experience of intention, the unwitting character of his collaboration, all serve to remind us that hypnotic behavior, the striving to behave as if hypnotized, takes place in an *altered state of the person.* This assumption becomes still more necessary when we consider those phenomena which transcend the usual limit of volitional control. Our hypothesis declares that anaesthesia, for instance, is a striving to behave as if part of the body were devoid of feeling. We know that in the normal state, let us say in the normal hour at the dentist's, such a striving is doomed to failure. As we shall see in a later section, it is impossible to dispense with the idea of a hypnotic state which permits certain types of striving to achieve unusual success. Our present argument claims no more than that hypnotic behavior, if looked squarely in the face without preconceptions about the state, inevitably appears to be a goal-directed striving.

We shall now pass directly to the end of the hypnotic trance and to the post-hypnotic phenomena which have played so great a part in experimental studies. It is here that the notions of automatism and dissociation have worked their most disastrous effect. Let us consider as an example the experiments of Messerschmidt (18) designed to test the alleged independent operation of conscious and subconscious activities. It was suggested to a subject in hypnosis that upon being awakened he would perform subconsciously a stated mental task. After the awakening he was assigned a second task which in the nature of the case had to be performed simultaneously with the subconscious task, permitting the investigator to measure interference between the two. Erickson and Erickson (7) have recently exposed the serious misconception which underlay this work. Messerschmidt supposed that she could initiate one task by suggestion given in hypnosis, then wake the subject with amnesia and set in motion a second task dissociated from the first. So firm was her belief in the reality of this dissociation that she did not feel it necessary to conceal from the hypnotized subject that a second task would be added after waking. In reality, therefore, she gave a single post-hypnotic suggestion to perform two simultaneous tasks, one of which was described forthwith and the other defined a little later. The net result of this experiment was to disprove dissociation between two tasks wrongfully assumed in the first place to be dissociated. As the Ericksons point out, "to suggest to the hypnotized subject that he will do one task 'subconsciously' and another task 'consciously' will serve only to elicit post-hypnotic performances of both tasks and not a waking performance of one, despite the greater degree of conscious awareness of it, which itself constitutes an additional post-hypnotic response."

This example brings us to the verge of a far-reaching new insight into the nature of post-hypnotic behavior. The argument of the Ericksons' paper, as it happens, rests with the statement that when a subject executes a post-hypnotic suggestion he falls into "a spontaneous self-limited post-hypnotic trance" having various demonstrable properties. Let us take the one remaining logical step and declare that the state which follows upon the operator's command to awaken is itself a suggested state. Hypnotists glibly and none too modestly assume that their subjects wake up merely because they tell them to do so. The command to awaken, however, is a perfect example of post-hypnotic suggestion. The subject is told, in effect, that to behave like a hypnotized person now means to act as if he were wide awake, except that any suggestions already given are to be considered as more nearly embodying the operator's intentions than remarks which he may forthwith introduce. There will be no more suggestions, and the subject must open his eyes, move about, and join in normal conversation. Just how and when he really emerges from the hypnotic state we can say only after we have looked more closely at the nature of that state. At this point we maintain merely that a subject just awakened from hypnosis is still striving to behave like a hypnotized person, that his attempt to act awake, an attempt which is not always entirely successful, must be considered a specimen of post-hypnotic suggested behavior.

Similar considerations apply to post-hypnotic amnesia. Although the degree of forgetting can be much greater than we would expect in the absence of an altered state of the person, the starting point of post-hypnotic amnesia is a striving to behave as if the events of the trance were forgotten. Often when the hypnosis has been light this fact is apparent to the subjects themselves. Following is a sheaf of spontaneous remarks made when subjects with suggested post-hypnotic amnesia were afterwards asked what they could remember of the trance:

(a) I feel that if I thought hard enough I could remember, but I just can't get down to business.

(b) I haven't any inclination to go back over it.

(c) Something is holding back my memory.

(d) My mind doesn't want to think.

(e) I notice I have a lot more trouble trying to recall. I get as far as the eye suggestion and then my thoughts go off into something else.

(f) I do remember but I can't say, I can't think of the word. . . . (Later) I could remember it without being able to say it. Something inside me said, "You know what it is all the time." I partly knew and partly didn't.

These subjects all say essentially the same thing—not that they could not remember, but that they could not make the effort or sustain the activity of remembering. The striving to remember is inhibited by the antagonistic striving to act as if the trance were forgotten, and the subject secretly sides with the latter tendency which he rightly understands as corresponding to the hypnotist's real desire.

It will be seen from the foregoing remarks that the argument of this section runs as follows: the subject is ruled by a wish to behave like a hypnotized person; his regnant motive is submission to the operator's demands; he fully understands at all times, in a well-conducted experiment, what the operator intends; and his behavior is a striving to put these intentions into execution. Let us briefly examine one more experiment the implications of which are radically changed by this hypothesis.

Wells (28) argues that a hypnotized subject of good moral character can be forced by suggestion to commit a real crime. Not wishing to lie to his subject, Wells after putting him into hypnosis described explicitly each step of the experiment. He was told that upon waking he would take a dollar from the experimenter's coat which he would wrongly perceive as his own; he would then forget this episode, but on finding the dollar in his pocket would wrongly recall that it belonged to him and would spend it; finally, he would forget that he had ever been hypnotized. This experiment was completely successful; for several days the subject argued vehemently with accusing friends that he had never been hypnotized and never stolen a dollar. What conclusions can be drawn?

At the beginning the subject understood the whole procedure exactly as the reader understands it; he must have been perfectly aware that taking the dollar was part of the operator's intention. Wells assumes that somewhere along the way the subject's understanding becomes divided, that he loses the initial connection among his ideas, that the taking of the dollar becomes separated from the larger purpose of the experiment and therefore can be viewed in the light of a criminal action. The thing which makes this assumption possible is the concept of dissociation, the idea that by suggesting an amnesia it is possible literally to divide the mind into insulated parts and to hold communication with them separately. If instead we apply the concept of the present paper, it appears that the subject strove to behave like a hypnotized person as Wells defined it to him, that he acted as if he were dissociated because this was part of the definition, and that no proof has here been furnished that a subject could be forced to commit a crime if he had reason to suppose that it really was a crime.

Whatever the merits of this question, it cannot be decided until hypnotism becomes, as was remarked before, a sophisticated chapter in social psychology, with attentive consideration for the interplay of motives and intentions between subject and hypnotist. The subject knows what is going on, infers the intentions and hopes of the operator, and he does his best to oblige. Even when we urge him beforehand to resist us, or afterwards coax him to remember what we have ordered him to forget, he decides as best he can what we really want and he strives to give it to us.

The hypothesis of goal-directed striving, however, does not and cannot alone explain the phenomena of hypnotism as these were outlined in a previous section. It cannot tell us how the hypnotized person transcends the normal realm of volition, how his experience of intention is altered, or how the procedure for inducing hypnosis leads to such important changes. So far we have argued only that hypnotic behavior looks like a goal-directed striving; we must now consider how this striving achieves its unexpected degree of success.

HYPNOSIS AS AN ALTERED STATE OF THE PERSON

In a recent review of experimental hypnotism P. C. Young (35) calls attention to sharp differences of opinion as to the nature of the hypnotic state. In one camp he places those who adhere to a conational hypothesis similar to the one advanced in the previous section. On the other side he puts those who contend that the profound organic changes which result from hypnotic suggestion argue for an important alteration in the behavior mechanism. The factors involved, Young believes, can be diagnosed better "from experiments on simple sensory experience than from those on the more spectacular, but more complicated, autonomic processes." Reviewing a number of contradictory reports, he finds that "the weight of testimony seems to point to an actual change in the content of sensed stimulations as the result of hypnotic suggestion, rather than merely to a changed attitude towards the stimulations sensed." Much evidence has been accumulated showing that the hypnotized person can execute suggestions which in a normal waking state would lie well outside the realm of his volitional control. These findings offer a formidable obstacle to theories which depend wholly on conation. "After all," Young continues, "these explanations amount to saying that the subject is playing a game with the experimenter and with himself. They would put the inhibition or dissociation (if dissociation is admitted) at a very high integrative level." In view of the kind of changes which can be produced, it seems to him unlikely that the explanation belongs at this level.

All theories which involve an interaction of factors are destined to pass through a long adolescence of storm and stress. The human mind seems to abhor complexity, preferring to nail its colors to the mast and go down fighting for some simple and sovereign explanation. Arguments over body and mind, heredity and environment, biology and culture, appeal to something in human nature which is not the shrewd and dispassionate search for truth. The theory of hypnotism will never prosper until, outgrowing the dialectic dichotomy of "striving" and "state," it considers the possibility of interaction. There is no law of nature which declares that hypnosis may not be at one and the same time a goal-directed striving and an altered state of the organism. On the contrary, it is upon this view of the matter that we should insist, because only in this way is it possible to reconcile the otherwise conflicting data. The hypothesis of goal-directed striving, moreover, gives us a new and valuable perspective in which to study the hypnotic state. It is to be regarded as a state in which certain kinds of striving, normally associated with volition, take place without the usual volitional experiences and achieve effects outside the usual realm of volition. Its chief peculiarity is its effect on goal-directed striving.

Ever since the concept of magnetic force fell into disrepute, it has been assumed that hypnotic technique created an altered state of the person. At one time or another a long list of distinguishing characteristics has been assigned this state, but here modern research has taken a heavy toll. Reviewing the literature in 1926, Young (34) dismissed catalepsy, post-hypnotic amnesia, and exclusive rapport of subject with operator, showing that all of these are the result of suggestion and do not necessarily appear if appropriate suggestions are not made. To the discard pile Hull (11) in 1933 added the lowering of sensory thresholds, pointing out that, while subjects believe themselves to possess whatever heightened sensitivities have been suggested to them, actual measurement fails to reveal a significant departure from normal levels. Even more important than these findings is the demonstration, through a convincing series of experiments, that hypnosis is not a form of sleep. Older writers, bent upon reassuring timid clients, made much of the outward likeness between sleep and hypnosis, and suggestions of drowsiness appear in the great majority of techniques for inducing the latter state. In reality, however, there is little resemblance between the two. In a very neat experiment Bass (1) has shown that the knee jerk and the voluntary pressing of a key in response to a bell, actions which disappear quite early in true sleep, remain unchanged throughout a deep hypnotic trance. Other investigators have measured pulse and respiration rates, brain potentials, and electrical resistance of the skin in hypnotized persons, finding that none of these measurements shows the changes characteristic of sleep (3; 13; 14). Physiologically the hypnotized subject is awake, not asleep, a fact which appears less remarkable when one recalls the feats of problem-solving and calculation which have been known to take place in hypnosis.

The trend of research has thus been to denude the hypnotic state of its once extensive vesture of distinguishing characteristics. What remains of its former majesty? "The answer is simple," writes Hull (11): "the only thing which seems to characterize hypnosis as such and which gives any justification for the practice of calling it a 'state' is its generalized hypersuggestibility. The difference between the hypnotic state and the normal is, therefore, a quantitative rather than a qualitative one." Responsiveness to suggestions emanating from other people, to "prestige suggestion," is a very common phenomenon, but this is not the distinguishing mark; "the essence of hypnosis lies in the fact of *change* in suggestibility . . . in the experimental fact of a *shift* in the upward direction which may result from the hypnotic procedure." "Hypnotic hypersuggestibility has a relative and not an absolute significance."

In these statements hypnosis is reduced to its barest possible meaning: a state of relative hypersuggestibility brought about by certain artificial techniques. Simple as it sounds, this definition easily covers the essental phenomena: insensitivity to pain, increased muscular capacity, amnesia and hypermnesia, non-intentional performance of actions usually requiring volition, all these are instances of hypersuggestibility. But it would be unduly hopeful to suppose that the elevation of this particular unifying concept would much simplify the task before a theory of hypnotism. The concept of suggestion may be admired for its versatility but not for its defining power. If by calling hypnosis suggestion we brought to our aid a number of well-formulated facts concerning non-hypnotic phenomena, our thinking would be considerably straightened and broadened. Unfortunately such is not the case, and the theory of hypnotism is left to face its task much as before.

There are two ways in which the nature of the hypnotic state may be profitably investigated. The first way is to study its characteristics directly, asking ourselves how it differs from the normal, comparing the range and quality of hypnotic behavior with that of a person trying to execute voluntarily the same acts. The other way is to consider how hypnosis is brought about and how it is terminated, to examine the significance of the procedure and to deduce therefrom the nature of the state produced. Inasmuch as both speculation and experimentation have been more active along the first than along the second line, it is appropriate to emphasize the benefits which might accrue from a more searching scrutiny of the hypnotic procedure. We shall first, however, look briefly at the better-tilled field, undertaking not to review it but merely to point out, in the spirit of a preface, the problems involved and the apparent trend of the findings.

The most impressive phenomena of hypnosis are those in which there is a transcendence of voluntary capacity. The high attracting power of these phenomena has drawn attention away from the true nature of the problems and led to fantastic speculations about the release of hidden powers. Little has been said about the limitations of hypnotic behavior, the things which are done less well in hypnosis than in the normal state. The hypnotized person lacks alertness and humor; he is literal and serious in his execution of the operator's wishes, seems to have lost all sense of the ludicrous, pursues one goal with disproportionate intensity, and pays little attention to matters and impressions which lie outside this purpose. He seems to have a contracted frame of reference, and above all he lacks initiative, lying perfectly quiet and even dropping off to sleep if the operator stops proposing lines of action. It may well be that suitable tests of performance demanding alertness, decisions, and quick complex judgments would outline a sphere of achievement in which hypnotized persons made reliably poorer scores. The hypnotic state is not a super-state; it is simply an altered state.

Perhaps the best way to conceive of this problem is to use a topographical analogy. Suppose we draw two regions, one including the behavior which can be produced, the functions which can be controlled, in the hypnotic state, the other enclosing the capacities of the normal state. These two regions, of course, will overlap, but not completely coincide; at either edge of the diagram will be a zone which belongs to only one region. To this statement we may add the conception that in light hypnosis the overlap with the normal region is at its greatest, growing progressively less as the subject passes toward profound somnambulism. It may now be stated that the task of research is to establish the detailed geography of these regions, to find out on the one hand exactly what capacities can be transcended, on the other what powers are distinctly reduced, and in both cases the measurable extent of these changes.

Research into these matters has not been idle; at least one important general statement can be drawn from the accumulated results. It appears to be approximately true that the boundary of functions which can be more effectively controlled under hypnosis lies parallel to the boundary for normal volition. Certain functions which lie wholly outside the realm of volitional influences are also inaccessible to hypnotic suggestion, but others which may be regarded as semi-voluntary can be surprisingly transcended in the hypnotic state. Let us take as an example Sears' (25) investigation of hypnotic anaesthesia. Here the attempt was made to abolish various normal reactions to a painful jab on the calf of the leg by suggesting that the leg was anaesthetic. Verbal report, facial flinch, and changes in respiration, all of which are at least partly voluntary, were almost completely eliminated, but the characteristic rise in pulse rate was reduced only 77 per cent, variability of pulse 50 per cent, and the galvanic skin reaction no more than 22 per cent. These achievements of hypnotic suggestion, of course, greatly exceed the capacities of the normal state; in a control experiment Sears was able to show that "voluntary inhibition of reaction to pain does not present a picture even remotely resembling the reaction under true hypnotic anaesthesia." But it will be noticed that the further one gets from a volitional function the smaller is the effect of hypnotic suggestion. A similar trend can be observed in experiments on the extent of post-hypnotic amnesia. Hull, under whose direction the experiments were performed, summarizes the results as follows:

> [The subjects] uniformly deny any recollection of trance events, *i.e.*, as tested by general symbolic recall, amnesia is 100 per cent. By detailed specific recall this amount of amnesia is reduced for nonsense material probably to about 97 per cent. By the relearning method amnesia falls to approximately 50 per cent. Manual habits learned in the stylus maze show by the relearning method an amnesia also of about 50 per cent. With specific training in arithmetical addition and general training in memorizing nonsense material the amount of post-hypnotic amnesia is reduced to zero (11, *155*).

Thus as one passes from specific learned content to the more remote results of practice, the effectiveness of hypnotic suggestion declines. To this conclusion we may add one more observation, that of Lundholm (15), who showed that with suggested blindness a flashing light elicited the usual pupillary reflex but no eye-movements, whereas with suggested hallucination of a flashing light there were eye-movements but no pupillary reflex. The trend of all these observations is clear. Hypnotic behavior can in many respects transcend the limits of volitional control, but it remains somehow related to those limits; its own limits seem always to lie at a not-too-great distance beyond those of volition.

We have seen in this section that hypnosis must be conceived as an altered state of the person the chief peculiarity of which is a change in the success achieved by certain kinds of striving. If in some respects the hypnotized person is inferior to his best normal self, in others he distinctly transcends the usual boundaries of volitional control. But this transcendence appears less remarkable, and perhaps ultimately less bewildering, when we notice that it consists of a roughly measurable pushing out of those boundaries in certain directions rather than a capricious disregard for their existence. The hypnotic alteration of the person is neither unintelligible nor immeasurable.

SIGNIFICANCE OF THE PROCEDURE FOR INDUCING HYPNOSIS

It is difficult to think about hypnosis without thinking about the procedure by which it is induced and terminated. A close inspection of these procedures might well be expected to reveal the nature of the hypnotic state. That it has not already done so is doubtless due to the extraordinary variety of methods for which success is claimed, the wide range of techniques to which one or another operator pins his faith. The first task is to factor out the features which are common to all these methods. There appear to be at least two features which are almost if not quite universal, which certainly assist the process of inducing hypnosis even if they are not completely indispensable: these are (1) relaxation and the reduction of sensory input, and (2) the presence of an operator who administers the suggestions. So obvious are these conditions that they often escape the searching examination they deserve.

We may pause for a moment to defend the assertion that these factors are well-nigh universal in hypnotic techniques. As regards the first, it is true that people can be hypnotized in a standing position and without closing the eyes. Hull, in fact, considers such a method under certain circumstances "perhaps the most effective of any," but this effectiveness depends on the following instructions:

> I direct him to look steadily into my eyes and to think of nothing but sleep, to relax his muscles all over, even so much that his knees bend a little and his legs scarcely hold him up (11, *32*).

Relaxation is thus included, even with the upright posture, and reduction of sensory input is achieved by steady optical fixation. Wells (27) uses a technique designated "waking hypnosis," the success of which must be apparent to all who have witnessed it, but even here, although suggestions of drowsiness and sleep are scrupulously avoided, the subjects are instructed to close their eyes and to attend carefully to the operator. It can be safely stated that nine out of ten hypnotic techniques call for reclining posture, muscular relaxation, and optical fixation followed by eye closure. The presence of an operator who administers the suggestions is similarly well-nigh universal. The possibility of auto-hypnosis cannot be denied, but there are very few procedures for self-hypnosis which do not start with training by an operator. It is apparently much easier to talk yourself into getting better and better if someone else has first suggested it to you.

Let us now briefly rehearse a standard hypnotic technique to see exactly what takes place. In the first place, the operator must make the subject willing to participate in the event; he must make sure of the favorable motives without which hypnosis cannot take place, for he is certain to fail "if a pattern of needs is aroused which dispose the subject unfavorably toward hypnosis" (31). Having elicited a willingness to be hypnotized, he asks the subject to lie down and relax his muscles, perhaps darkens the room, fatigues and then excludes vision, and lowers his voice to a quiet monotone. Vision thus becomes inoperative, kinaesthesis is much reduced by immobility, and audition is more or less focussed on a single stream of impressions. The operator meanwhile talks about drowsiness and sleep; but it is doubtful whether these remarks function as true suggestions, since the steps already taken are exactly those which anyone might use to permit drowsiness and sleep to overtake him in their own natural way. The onset of a little real drowsiness would appear to be an indispensable condition for producing hypnosis for the first time, although trained subjects can pass into the state without these leisurely preliminaries.

At this point the operator introduces his first unmistakable suggestion, such as that the eyelids are stuck down and cannot be opened. If on trial this proves to be the case, the subject is regarded as being in the hypnotic state. It should be observed, however, that there are not two but rather four possible outcomes of this first real suggestion. The first is that the subject will open his eyes when challenged to try, in which case it will be admitted that hypnotism has failed. Another outcome is that the subject will make the attempt, perhaps in a rather vigorous manner with visible movements of the surrounding musculature, but fail to open his eyes. A third possibility is that the subject will make no apparent effort to open the eyes; he will have to be urged repeatedly to try, and in the end make perhaps some slight flicker in the surrounding muscles as a token to satisfy the operator. These two outcomes correspond to what the author has called elsewhere (29) the active or alert and the passive type of hypnotic trance. The subject in the passive state may be regarded as essentially too drowsy to move; drowsiness has progressed far enough so that he is distinctly disinclined to be disturbed. The fourth outcome is a total failure to respond; the subject acts as if he had heard nothing, and awakens with a start when gently shaken. He has been really asleep, hence not in any kind of hypnotic state, and his amnesia will be complete.

It is implied in this description that there is a continuum from the wide-awake state through drowsiness to sound sleep. The hypnotist, in order to succeed, must bring his subject a short distance along this continuum to a light drowsiness, but must stop him there and prevent him from getting more sleepy; otherwise he will go into the passive trance or drop off to sleep altogether. We know from many studies that the hypnotized person is not asleep, that his bodily state is not that of real sleep. Nevertheless, it appears that a dash of drowsiness, so to speak, is essential in producing the hypnotic state, and in no other way can we explain the reported good effects of sedative drugs when other methods of hypnotizing have failed (24).

We are now in a position to understand the importance of the hypnotist and to explain why he is all but indispensable in bringing on the hypnotic state. Apart from the instruction he gives and the motivational state he brings about—both of which might be essentially present without him—he serves the very vital purpose of keeping the subject awake, allowing him to relax and give himself up to drowsiness but at the same time "pegging" this drowsiness in a light stage and preventing a lapse into real sleep. A person may learn through practice to catch himself at this state and thus become adept at self-hypnosis, but a beginner almost invariably needs assistance if he is to arrive and remain at that curious point halfway between sleepiness and alertness. The first function of the hypnotist, then, is to keep the subject from sliding around on the sleep continuum.

This he does in the course of executing his second function, which is to keep up a moderate degree of auditory input while the other senses remain relatively closed. Subjects rightly complain that they do their best to go to sleep but are prevented from doing so by the operator's stream of talk. We must remember at this point that it is not a matter of indifference what the operator says: the urgent character of his words, their power to keep the subject attentive in spite of his drowsiness, lies not in their volume, not even in their relative volume, but in the fact that they consist of requests, commands, and suggestions which in turn convey the wishes and intentions of the hypnotist. By the measures which he takes to exclude distraction, and especially by his words, the operator tries to maintain a state of mono-motivation, a focal press of dominance, and the subject is given little alternative except to continue the deference which made him susceptible in the first place or else to display a resistive autonomy which under the circumstances could hardly be distinguished from aggression. In short, the operator's words, far from being lifeless syllables, are loaded with his hopes and wishes; they act on the subject with the force of another's hopes and wishes which through him may be either gratified or frustrated. We cannot understand hypnosis without bearing in mind the motivational field in which it takes place. The dual function of the operator is to prevent the deepening of drowsiness and to keep regnant the wish to behave like a hypnotized person.

The importance of relaxation and the restriction of sensory input probably lies in their relation to drowsiness. When we know more about drowsiness and can state more precisely the changes which go with it we shall be able to advance considerably our knowledge of the hypnotic state. Here we shall offer only one very general hypothesis: the peculiarities of hypnotic behavior discussed earlier, the involuntary feeling, the literal, humorless manner, the un-self-consciousness, inattentiveness, and poor subsequent memory, can all be plausibly related to the changes which take place in drowsiness. When a person is drowsy, his images and experiences tend to become more vivid, more concrete, and more absolute. Abstract processes and complex frames of reference seem to be highly vulnerable to fatigue. The operator avails himself of this vulnerability, reduces as far as possible the perceptual supports which might serve to sustain a wider frame of reference, bids the subject relax his mind as well as his body, and thus encourages drowsiness to take a small toll from the higher integrative processes.

It is significant that one of the commonest complaints of unsusceptible subjects is that they could not forget the situation as a whole, could not stop thinking how absurd it was to be lying there on the couch, what their friends would say afterwards, how unreasonable the suggestions sounded, how humiliated they would be to have their wills overcome. Such comments, in so far as they are not simply signs of unfavorable motivation, imply that the frame of reference has refused to contract, that in spite of external circumstances there remains an internal alertness to "other considerations" which is the opposite of drowsiness and the enemy of successful hypnosis.

It would be profitable to follow up the idea that hypnosis involves some slight degree of functional decortication, of a kind, however, which is produced by relaxation and quieting rather than by drugs, operation, or strong emotion. All thinking along this line must be limited, of course, by two facts, that the hypnotized person is in no true sense asleep and that he remains capable of fairly active mental operations. There would appear to be enduring value, nevertheless, in the hypothesis of lowered functioning, of activity a little removed from the alert, wide-awake, self-conscious level which we ordinarily consider the best of all possible mental states. Physiology has accustomed us to the idea that the highest centers are mainly inhibitory in function, so that their withdrawal tends to release the energy of more primitive processes. Psychopathology has accustomed us to the notion that unconscious strivings may possess a peculiarly direct communication with the autonomic system, as in the psychosomatic disorders, and even with certain functions of the cerebro-spinal system, as in conversion hysteria. It may well be that hypnotic behavior lies somewhere between the level of volition and the level of unconscious strivings, enjoying some of the privileges of the latter in the way of extended control. The two hypotheses here discussed, the creation of an unusually weighted motivational field and the production of a moderate degree of disinhibition, while they by no means exhaust the problems of hypnotism, point the direction in which the scientific caravan should move.

In an earlier section it was proposed that the manner of terminating hypnosis required rather drastic reconsideration. The command to awaken must be regarded as itself a post-hypnotic suggestion which constrains the subject, still docile to the operator's wishes, to start acting as if he were awake. We need not assume that he issues from the hypnotic state in the fraction of a second required for the operator's signal. But the new suggestion which the hypnotist has unwittingly given involves certain conditions which of themselves gradually wipe out the hypnotic state, the more rapidly, no doubt, when there are no further post-hypnotic suggestions waiting to be performed. Upright posture must be assumed, the eyes must be opened, conversation must be made, and the hypnotist relinquishes his position as sole speaker and focal press of dominance. This withdrawal of all the conditions deemed essential for producing hypnosis in the first place makes it impossible for the subject to keep his frame of reference contracted and to remain in the hypnotic state, even though, as is often the case, he would prefer to do so. Just as it is the hypnotic situation as a whole, rather than specific suggestion, which puts the subject gradually into the hypnotic state, so it is the post-hypnotic situation as a whole, rather than the command to awaken, which gradually brings him out of it.

Summary

In the forward march of psychological theory hypnotism has fallen to the rear, unable to shed the conceptual baggage of a past age. The present paper has attempted to lighten this load so that hypnotism will be encouraged to take its place as a chapter in social psychology and as a means of investigating the structure of personality.

A theory of hypnotism is called upon to explain the following facts: (1) that the hypnotized person can transcend the normal limits of volitional control, (2) that he behaves without the experience of will or intention, without the self-consciousness, and without the subsequent memory which under the circumstances one would expect, and (3) that these changes in his behavior occur merely because the hypnotist says so.

As a first step it is proposed that hypnotic behavior be regarded as a meaningful, goal-directed striving, its most general goal being to behave like a hypnotized person as this is continuously defined by the operator and understood by the subject. Such a view replaces the older notions of automatism and dissociation which have persisted in a peculiarly rigid and unenlightened form to the great detriment of hypnotic theory. Reasons for preferring the hypothesis of goal-directed striving are found by a direct inspection of typical hypnotic phenomena. The application of the hypothesis puts several of these phenomena in a quite new light, particularly the post-hypnotic behavior which has played such a prominent part in experimental studies. The subject, it is held, is ruled by a wish to behave like a hypnotized person, his regnant motive is submission to the operator's demands, he understands at all times what the operator intends, and his behavior is a striving to put these intentions into execution. In order to explain the peculiar character and surprising success of the hypnotic striving, however, it is necessary to conceive of hypnosis as an altered state of the person.

The hypnotic state can be profitably investigated in two ways: (1) directly, by comparing the range and quality of hypnotic behavior with that of a person trying to perform voluntarily the same acts, and (2) indirectly, by considering how it is brought about and terminated. The first problem has been the topic of considerable investigation in which it is possible to discern a definite and important trend: hypnotic transcendence of the usual boundaries of volitional control consists of a roughly measurable pushing out of those boundaries in certain directions rather than a capricious disregard for their existence. As one passes from semi-voluntary functions such as respiration and eye-movements to completely involuntary acts like pulse, pupillary reflex, and galvanic skin response, the effects of hypnotic suggestion grow smaller.

The procedure for inducing hypnosis has received little attention as a means of studying the nature of the hypnotic state. The two factors which appear to be common to all techniques are (1) relaxation and a reduction of sensory input, and (2) the presence of an operator who administers the suggestions. The operator is indispensable because he prevents the subject from passing from light drowsiness into real sleep and because he maintains a continuous motivational pressure, a focal press of dominance. Relaxation and the restriction of sensory input are conducive to drowsiness, and this in turn may be conceived as a slight lowering of functional level the effect of which is disinhibitory, so that in certain ways the range of actions accessible to the hypnotic striving is increased. It is at all events along such lines, keeping step with advances in psychopathology, physiology, and motivation, that the theory of hypnotism should press forward.

REFERENCES

1. BASS, M. J. Differentiation of the hypnotic trance from normal sleep. *J. exp. Psychol.*, 1931, 14, 382–399.
2. BURNETT, C. Splitting the mind. *Psychol. Monogr.*, 1925, 34, No. 2.
3. DAVIS, R. C., AND KANTOR, J. R. Skin resistance during hypnotic state. *J. gen. Psychol.*, 1935, 13, 62–81.
4. DORCUS, R. M. Modification by suggestion of some vestibular and visual responses. *Amer. J. Psychol.*, 1937, **49**, 82–87.
5. DYNES, J. B. An experimental study in hypnotic anesthesia. This JOURNAL, 1932, **27**, 79–88.
6. ERICKSON, M. H. Experimental demonstrations of the psychopathology of everyday life. *Psychoanal. Quart.*, 1939, 8, 338–353.
7. ERICKSON, M. H., AND ERICKSON, E. M. Concerning the nature and character of post-hypnotic behavior. *J. gen. Psychol.*, 1941, **24**, 95–133.
8. FOREL, A. *Hypnotism and psychotherapy.* New York: Rebman, 1907.

9. Freud, S. The origin and development of psychoanalysis. *An outline of psychoanalysis,* ed. by J. Van Teslaar. New York: Modern Library, 1925.

10. Frick, H. L., Scantlebury, R. E., and Patterson, T. L. The control of gastric hunger contractions in man by hypnotic suggestion. *Amer. J. Physiol.,* 1935, **113,** 471.

11. Hull, C. L. *Hypnosis and suggestibility: an experimental approach.* New York: Appleton-Century, 1933.

12. Janet, P. *Psychological healing.* (Trans. by E. & C. Paul.) (2 vols.) London: Allen & Unwin, 1925.

13. Jenness, A., and Wible, C. L. Respiration and heart action in sleep and hypnosis. *J. gen. Psychol.,* 1937, **16,** 197–222.

14. Loomis, A. L., Harvey, E. N., and Hobart, G. Brain potentials during hypnosis. *Science,* 1936, **83,** 239–241.

15. Lundholm, H. An experimental study of functional anesthesias as induced by suggestion in hypnosis. This Journal, 1928, **23,** 337–355.

16. Lundholm, H. Laboratory neuroses. *Character & Pers.,* 1933, **2,** 127–133.

17. McDougall, W. *Outline of abnormal psychology.* New York: Scribners, 1926.

18. Messerschmidt, R. A quantitative investigation of the alleged independent operation of conscious and subconscious processes. This Journal, 1927–1928, **22,** 325–340.

19. Pattie, F. A. A report of attempts to produce uni-ocular blindness by hypnotic suggestion. *Brit. J. med. Psychol.,* 1935, **15,** 230–241.

20. Pattie, F. A. The genuineness of hypnotically produced anesthesia on the skin. *Amer. J. Psychol.,* 1937, **49,** 435–443.

21. Pattie, F. A. The production of blisters by hypnotic suggestion: a review. This Journal, 1941, **36,** 62–72.

22. Prince, M. *Clinical and experimental studies in personality.* Rev. ed. Cambridge, Mass.: Sci-Art, 1939.

23. Rosenow, C. Meaningful behavior in hypnosis. *Amer. J. Psychol.,* 1928, **40,** 205–235.

24. Schilder, P., and Kauders, O. *Hypnosis.* (Tr. by S. Rothenburg.) New York and Washington: Nervous and Mental Disease Pub. Co., 1927.

25. Sears, R. R. An experimental study of hypnotic anesthesia. *J. exp. Psychol.,* 1932, **15,** 1–22.

26. Stalnaker, J. M., and Riddle, E. L. The effect of hypnosis on long-delayed recall. *J. gen. Psychol.,* 1932, **6,** 429–440.

27. Wells, W. R. Hypnotizability versus suggestibility. This Journal, 1931, **25,** 436–449.

28. Wells, W. R. Experiments in the hypnotic production of crime. *J. Psychol.,* 1941, **11,** 63–102.

29. White, R. W. Two types of hypnotic trance and their personality correlates. *J. Psychol.,* 1937, **3,** 279–289.

30. White, R. W., Fox, G. F., and Harris, W. W. Hypnotic hypermnesia for recently learned material. This Journal, 1940, **35,** 88–103.

31. White, R. W. An analysis of motivation in hypnosis. *J. gen. Psychol.,* 1941, **24,** 145–162.

32. White, R. W., and Shevach, B. J. Hypnosis and the concept of dissociation. (In preparation.)

33. Williams, G. W. The effect of hypnosis on muscular fatigue. This Journal, 1929, **24,** 318–329.

34. Young, P. C. Hypnotism. *Psychol. Bull.,* 1926, **23,** 504–523.

35. Young, P. C. Experimental hypnotism: a review. *Psychol. Bull.,* 1941, 38, 92–104.

Part II
Theories of Hypnosis: The Altered State Debate

[3]

CONTRIBUTIONS TO ROLE-TAKING THEORY: I. HYPNOTIC BEHAVIOR [1]

BY THEODORE R. SARBIN

University of California

This paper attempts to construct from a social psychological standpoint a workable theory of hypnosis. Briefly stated, it essays to demonstrate that hypnosis is one form of a more general kind of social psychological behavior, namely, role-taking.

That a theory based on social psychological considerations is necessary arises from the obvious social psychological nature of the hypnotic situation. The patent dependency of hypnosis on interpersonal relations calls for a theory which is more continuous with social psychological formulations than with outworn physiological speculations (25) or revived mentalistic entities (46). Moreover, the search for shorter and more efficient psychotherapeutic measures (together with the former widespread use of hypnosis in the treatment of the hysterias) suggests a reconsideration of hypnosis in the treatment of certain behavior disorders. Such treatment will be less abused if it rests on a more substantial theoretical framework than formerly. In addition, the potential value of hypnosis as a tool for social science and medical research demands a careful evaluation of the nature of hypnosis. Thus appropriate allowances will be made for the perturbations in the experimental field introduced by the use of hypnosis as a research instrument.

Observations Which Must Be Accounted For

A theory of hypnosis must account for many phenomena subsumed under a single label. These phenomena and the conditions which elicit them may be grouped for our purposes into these four classes: (1) the apparent discontinuity or dissociation of behavior; (2) the apparent automaticity of response; (3) the disjunction between the magnitude of the response and the procedure which instigates the response; and (4) individual differences in responsiveness to hypnotic induction procedures. These four types of observations are briefly elaborated below.

Apparent discontinuity. In hypnosis the subject appears to be in a state which is discontinuous from events prior to the initiation of the hypnotic induc-

[1] A preliminary form of this paper was read at the 1946 meetings of the Western Psychological Association. Most of the experimental and clinical work reported in this paper was begun during the author's tenure as a postdoctoral fellow of the Social Science Research Council, 1941–43. The author expresses his gratitude to his colleague, Dr. Harrison G. Gough, and to Dr. R. W. White of Harvard University for critically reading the manuscript.

tion procedure. From introspective accounts and from observers' protocols it seems that stimuli are perceived by a markedly altered organism and that the responses are quantitatively and qualitatively different from those in the pre- and post-hypnotic periods. Some of the more dramatic items of conduct which lead to the acceptance of the inference that the subject's behavior is discontinuous (dissociated) are: anesthesia, amnesia, post-hypnotic compulsive behavior, hypermnesia and various somatic effects such as the inhibition of gastric contractions. To those who are content only with a superficial examination of hypnotic phenomena it appears that hypnotic subjects can perform acts which violate the limits of everyday behavior. When the data are inspected more closely, however, we find that the changes in behavior which do occur involve chiefly the skeletal musculature—*i.e.,* voluntary responses. Responses which are involuntary, such as PGR, blood pressure shifts, and pupillary reflexes are less amenable to verbal instructions, and the limits are extended not too far from the limits of waking behavior (43). Later we shall show that those responses involving the skeletal musculature require no further explanation than that the subject is taking the role of the hypnotic subject as understood by him as a result of his previous interactions with similar social psychological situations. The extension of the limits of behavior involving the autonomic functions is understood in terms of the conception of the organism as-a-whole—a conception which is now generally accepted in sophisticated psychological theory.

Apparent automaticity. Most of the early theorists were thrown off the trail of a really workable theory of hypnosis by the manner in which acts are carried out under hypnotic stimulation. The word "trance" has been used to express this meaning. In most instances the subject appears to act like an automaton. There is an apparent absence of volitional activity. The experimenter throws out commands which seem to be accepted by the subject without critical consideration. He is often slow, stuporous, and seems to be exerting a great deal of effort to perform simple acts. Retrospective accounts reveal a distinction between obedience as found in everyday behavior and the automatic acceptance of commands without the subjective experience of intent. In addition to accounting for this apparent automaticity, a workable hypnotic theory must account for many acts which are added spontaneously by the subject without the benefit of instruction from the experimenter. Unlike physiologically-oriented theories, the role-taking theory considers these observations under the concepts of role-enactment and role perception.

The disjunction between the magnitude of the response and the procedure which instigates the response. This aspect of hypnosis is probably responsible for the popular association of hypnosis with magic. The experimenter (or therapist) merely talks to the subject. How, then, can such marked changes in behavior occur merely as a result of verbal instructions? The need for explaining this observation would be less urgent if the stimuli were of the same order of magnitude as are found in extreme stress, fatigue, toxicosis, narcosis, or febrile conditions. In a later section we shall point out how verbal instructions may help the subject focus on and enact a role which may have markedly altered somatic components.

Individual differences in response to hypnotic induction procedures. The observation which has received the least attention from the theorists and experimenters is (at least to this writer) the most obvious one, *viz.,* individual subjects respond differently to the same hypnotic procedures. As is well known, many subjects cannot be hypnotized at all, some will exhibit mild cataleptic reactions, and still others will exhibit all the classical responses of hypnosis. Furthermore there is a great deal of variation in the manner in which directions are accepted (or rejected) by subjects who are apparently hypnotized to the same degree. As anyone who has taken the role of a hypnotist knows, and as Brenman (7) has concluded from her analysis of various induction procedures, little or no relationship exists between the subject's performance and the specific innovations which are introduced into the hypnotic instructions. Since the induction procedure *per se* cannot account for the differential responsiveness of subjects, this leaves the subject *as a person* as the more fruitful focus of study.

These four types of observations may be combined into a question, the answer to which will provide us with a more definitive theory of hypnosis: What are the characteristics of those individuals who, in response to hypnotic induction procedures, exhibit conduct which is apparently discontinuous and apparently automatic?

SOME CONCURRENT THEORIES

It is unnecessary to take time out to flog the dead horse of dissociation theory. Numerous experiments and sophisticated observations have led to the unmistakable conclusion that the hypnotized subject is not composed of various psychophysiological systems that can be dissociated one from the other. White and Shevach (45) have written a thoroughgoing analysis of the concept of dissociation and have concluded that the natural cleavages in the nervous system postulated by Janet are nonexistent.

A number of writers cling to the conditioned response theory to explain hypnosis. Historically the conditioned response theory stems from this simple explanation: The word is the conditioned stimulus and acts as an efficient stimulus. This is no more than a streamlining of the old ideomotor hypothesis. In 1933 Hull stated it this way: ". . . the withdrawal of the subject's symbolic activities would naturally leave his muscles relatively susceptible to the symbolic stimulation emanating continuously from the experimenter . . ." (21, p. 397). From such a conclusion (which seems naïvely to regard the subject as a spinal animal) Welch has recently presented an hypothesis and an experiment which purport to give credence to the conditioning theory (9, 42). Taking as his point of departure the most commonly used induction procedure, Welch says:

"If the subject analyzed himself in some naïve fashion, he might say, 'When the hypnotist said I felt A, I felt A; when he said I felt B, I felt B; and now he says I feel X, I feel X.' At this point the generalization has extended to the point that whatever the hypnotist says the subject feels, he, within limits, actually feels" (42, p. 361).

On the basis of his hypothesis that hypnosis is a kind of generalized conditioning, Welch and his co-workers performed a learning experiment (in which, incidentally, none of the subjects was hypnotized) based on this experimental analogue. ". . . a word flashed on a screen was used as analogous to the spoken word of the hypnotist, and followed by the phenomenon for which the word was a symbol. Thus the word 'music' was followed by the playing of music. After a certain number of trials the word 'electric shock' was flashed on the screen and was not re-inforced." His findings were summarized thus: ". . . in a group of 15 subjects, 11, or

73 per cent gave a (PGR) response greater than to any other stimuli."

That Welch has demonstrated a type of abstract conditioning is not to be denied. But he has not shown that this type of conditioning is the important feature of hypnosis. In the first place, many subjects can be hypnotized without using the analogous procedure. If a subject comes into a hypnotic experiment with certain self-perceptions and role-taking skills, it is possible for him to become hypnotized without the usual monotonous delivery and so-called reinforcement. In an unpublished study (36) the present author has shown that some subjects can be hypnotized with these instructions: "Make yourself comfortable in this easy chair. I'll step out of the room for a few minutes so you can relax. When I come back I will count to ten, you will close your eyes and go into a hypnotic sleep." Even if we could accept the analogy between the Welch experiment and hypnosis, there is no answer to the question: Why did the other 27 per cent not condition? If Welch could show that a correlation existed between "abstract conditionability" and hypnotizability, we should still have to fit this correlation into a more comprehensive framework based on an understanding of the antecedents of these individual differences.

Eysenck and Furneaux (12, 13, 17) have also reported some studies which are related to the ideomotor principle. Using a factorial approach, they isolated three factors from a series of psychomotor and other tests. The first, primary suggestibility, is highly correlated with hypnotizability and is best measured by the postural sway test. The second factor, secondary suggestibility, is unrelated to hypnotizability. The third factor, unrelated to the previous two, also predicts susceptibility to hypnosis, and is measured by a test of heat illusion. They conclude that susceptibility to hypnosis is an innate characteristic (presumably on the grounds that psychomotor traits are inborn). This writer would declare this conclusion a *non sequitur*. That hypnotizability and certain traits are shown to be related is an acceptable conclusion, but to posit that this relationship is based on inherited factors is not continuous with the data. Below we try to fit these data into our conceptual framework.

Perhaps the most widely accepted hypothesis at the present time is a conative one which places the phenomena of hypnosis at a high integrative level. A number of writers have contributed evidence to support such a theory, notably Dorcus (10), Lundholm (28), Rosenow (32), Pattie (31), White (43), and Sarbin (37). The most systematic presentation of this hypothesis has been offered by White. He defines hypnosis as "meaningful, goal-directed striving, its most general goal being to behave like a hypnotized person as this is continuously defined by the operator and understood by the subject." This approach purports to look upon the hypnotic subject as a functionally intact human organism who is very much in contact with stimulus objects and events, trying to conduct himself in certain meaningful ways rather than in the manner of a spinal animal.

White's theory deals with three of the previously identified four sets of observations. It looks first upon the apparent automaticity as a form of striving: the subject tries to behave in an organized manner, following instructions as he understands them. The apparent discontinuity is treated in terms of measurable extensions of the boundaries of volitional control. How the goal-directed striving makes possible this extension of the limits is subject to speculation in terms of "disinhibition of the higher centers." The importance of the procedure for inducing hypnosis is analyzed in terms of relaxation, reduction of sensory input, drowsiness, and a contracted frame of reference. This procedure produces an altered state of the organism which makes possible the success achieved by the striving. The theory fails to provide an explanation for differential susceptibility beyond that due to motivational factors, such as need for submissiveness and deference.

This analysis places the striving in a context beginning with the experiment itself. It fails to recognize explicitly that the subject comes into the hypnotic situation with certain pre-conceptions about the experiment, the experimenter, and even about such items as the place in which the experiment is being conducted. It does not make clear that the subject also comes into the hypnotic setting with certain self-perceptions, and that these self-perceptions will operate toward the subject's being successful or not in his striving to behave "in ways defined by the operator." White's analysis would be more tenable if there were no individual differences in responding to the operator's instructions. Relaxation, drowsiness, and reduction of sensory input—time-consuming processes—obviously would not be involved with those subjects who responded immediately to the command: "Go into a hypnotic sleep."[2] The observable differences in individuals, not only in the depth of hypnosis, but also in the kind and quality of spontaneous additions to the operator's directions, suggest that we look into the reactional biography of the subject and into the evolution of the stimulus setting for clues as to the nature of hypnosis.

THE ROLE-TAKING HYPOTHESIS

To fill the gap in White's goal-striving theory, another hypothesis is herewith introduced. Hypnosis is a form of a more general kind of social psychological behavior known as role-taking. In the hypnotic experiment the subject strives to take the role of the hypnotized person; the success of his striving is a function of favorable motivation, role-perception, and role-taking aptitude. This orientation breaks completely with the tradition of looking on hypnosis as some strange phenomenon for which it is necessary to invent psychophysiological constructions. Rather it is placed in continuity with other social psychological conceptions.[3]

[2] In a personal communication, R. W. White has extended his theory as follows: "It would have been better, I think, to develop at more length the idea of a contracted frame of reference, or, as I would now prefer to put it, a contracted frame of activation. What has to be explained is how the hypnotic suggestions achieve their peculiar success, and I think the explanation should include two things: first, the presence of a single ruling motivation, and second, the exclusion (by quieting) of all promptings and even of the sensory avenues to such promptings that might set up competing processes. In this contracted field of activation there may be conceived to take place a deep vertical activation, reaching to the affective and autonomic levels, of those processes which are suggested. In contrast to this would be the relatively horizontal activation of everyday life where different processes tend to act together or check each other.

"This (monoideism) appears to me to be the pre-dynamic form of what now looks like the best hypothesis for the nature of the hypnotic state. For present purposes some such term as monomotivation would be more suitable. This view of the matter makes possible a fruitful comparison between hypnosis and other states, such as great fear or excitement, in which volition is transcended. All such states are monomotivational but in the sense that one extremely powerful motive or one strong preoccupation momentarily towers over all other processes. Hypnosis achieves the same relative effect at low dynamic intensities, quieting the competitors rather than heightening the chief process."

[3] The concept of role-taking has been described in a previous paper (34). In brief, role-taking may be summarized as follows: (1) Role-enactment depends upon prior ex-

To adopt a frame of reference that departs from dependence on traditional formulations, and to provide a logical link between the observations and theory, we point to another area of conduct which is apparently automatic, apparently discontinuous, elicited by relatively simple verbal instructions, and characterized by individual differences in performance: to wit, the drama. Introspective accounts and observers' reports of stage actors taking roles reveal a kind of behavior which may be characterized in much the same way as hypnosis. The apparent discontinuity, for example, has been established as an important factor in dramatic role-taking. The actor's stage behavior appears to be dissociated or discontinuous from his "normal personality." In Archer's classical study of acting (2) some actors report losing themselves completely in certain roles so that they are relatively unaware of the audience or of other physical or social objects. The role may even carry over to off-stage statuses. The introspective accounts of actors taking roles are often undifferentiated from the accounts of hypnotic subjects (36).

Allen cites Oesterreich who collected a number of observations on this point. One such observation is reproduced here: "Martersteig compares the personality of the theatrical character to a self suggested to the actor by hypnotism, and states that the waking remainder of the actor's consciousness (*Bewusstseinsrest*) can observe the actions of the hypnotic self, as though it were another person, at one time feeling anxiety with regard to them, at another time allowing them to have full play" (1, p. 123).

It appears that the stage director stands in the same relationship to the actor as the hypnotist does to the subject. The statuses or positions are defined beforehand, the specific role-behaviors are dictated by the attempts of each participant to validate his status (27). In short, the participants interbehave with each other in ways that are appropriate to each position—provided, of course, that such interbehavior can be incorporated by each participant in his self-concept. Because acting has not been burdened with the incubus of dissociation or ideomotor theory, we are not amazed at the frequent marked changes in skeletal and visceral behavior which occur merely because the director tells the actor what to do. The analyst of dramatic acting does not seem to be concerned with such pseudoproblems as the search for a one-to-one constancy relationship between the magnitude of the stimulus (the director's verbal instructions) and the magnitude of the response (the complicated verbal, motor, and visceral reactions of the actor).

From this preliminary description we submit that the role-taking of the stage actor and the role-taking of the hyp-

perience, either symbolic or overt, in order to build up a perception of a given role. (2) Role-taking is organismic, that is to say, it embraces the entire organism, not merely the voluntary reaction-systems. (3) Role-taking occurs with various degrees of participation of the self in the role (this may also be described as levels of consciousness). (4) The perception and enactment of roles is variable inter-individually, intra-individually, and culturally—both qualitatively in terms of the role-behaviors that go to make up any given role, and quantitatively in terms of the number of roles available to an individual or group. (5) Role-taking is a complex form of conduct and can be condensed into significant symbols. (6) Role-taking can be understood as coordinate with the self; a self-concept, phenomenal self, self-dynamism, or ego must be postulated in order to understand role-behavior, in fact, any social psychological behavior. To these may be added another item, (7) statuses or positions, which are established in various ways and which define what roles are appropriate and expected. (See also Cameron [8], especially Chapter IV, and a forthcoming book by the writer, *The Psychology of Role-Taking*.)

notic subject embody the same characteristics: (a) Favorable motivation—the actor's self-concept and his perception of the part to which he is assigned must be congruent; if it is not, then his performance is unconvincing or he pays a terrific psychological price. (b) Role-perception—the actor must first perceive the role he is to play—this is achieved partly by the actor's own experiences with similar stage or real-life roles, partly by the director's definition of the role. (c) Role-taking aptitude—needless to say, some actors can take a role more completely than others. Compare, for example, the performance of Barrymore as Hamlet with the efforts of a high school senior.

notic subjects become so involved in the role that perception becomes over-focalized and many self-other observations are by-passed. From those studies of acting which have come to this writer's attention, it would seem that there is a great deal of overlap with hypnotic role-taking in this dimension, but there would be, on the average, less participation of the self in the role of actors as compared with hypnotic subjects. Below is a schematization of this dimension of role-taking, in which acting is placed at a relatively high level of differentiation of self from role. The overlapping in the drawing is intentional. Not only is the relationship of acting to hypnosis shown but these forms of role-taking are placed in a larger setting the better to illustrate what is meant by this dimension.[3a]

states of ecstasy; mystical experiences;
role and self undifferentiated

hysterias

hypnosis

"heated" acting

technical acting;
role and self are differentiated

Young (46) has criticized such conceptions of hypnosis by saying that the subject is playing a game with himself and with the experimenter. This criticism is invalid because it does not consider an important dimension. In the two types of role-playing there is a quantitative difference along a continuum which we may characterize as the "conscious-unconscious" dimension. We may ask, how conscious is the actor of his surroundings, of stimulus-objects, and of himself as compared with the hypnotized subject? Or, to put it in terms more continuous with the present study, what is the relative degree of participation of the self in the role (or in Mead's terms, of the "I" in the "me")? Some actors and some hypnotic subjects become so involved in the role that perception becomes over-focalized and many self-other observations are by-passed.

In the last few paragraphs we have tried to orient the reader away from the necessity of physiologizing about hypnosis by showing the similarity of hypnosis and acting. Thus we can conceive of hypnosis as being continuous with other social psychological events. At this time we submit certain observations to lend support to the central hypothesis, *viz.*, hypnotic role-taking is dependent on at least three factors—

[3a] This discussion of the role-taking process is given more detailed treatment in a forthcoming article: Sarbin, Theodore R. and Farberow, Norman L. "Contributions to Role-Taking Theory: II. A Clinical Study of Self and Role."

favorable motivation, role-perception, and role-taking aptitude.

Favorable motivation. The most complete paper on this topic has been contributed by White (44). He reviews the studies which have attempted to demonstrate the relationship between hypnotizability and motivational variables. The obtained correlations have for the most part not been significantly different from zero. In his own study White finds a small but positive correlation between hypnotizability and the need for deference (.42), and also a small but negative correlation with the need for autonomy (−.42). ". . . there is a great deal of individual variation in the tendencies which are awakened, so that manifest needs like *passivity, exhibitionism, sex,* or *aggression* may sometimes occupy the foreground. . . . There is [also] reason to believe that three latent infantile needs sometimes function as motivating forces favorable to hypnosis: the need for *love,* . . . the tendency for *passive compliance,* . . . and the wish to participate in *omnipotence*. . . ." He concludes with this significant statement. "It is doubtful whether the analysis of motivational factors can be pushed further except by the intensive study of the subjects as individuals"[4] (44, p. 161).

In terms which are more continuous with those of contemporary social psychology, White's conclusion may be restated as follows: If the subject's perception of the self (self-concept) and his perception of the role (here, the role of the hypnotized subject) are not disjunctive or incongruent, then he may be said to be favorably motivated.

One example is herewith presented to facilitate understanding of this formulation. The author gave a lecture and demonstration of hypnosis to a group of undergraduates. The class instructor had previously pointed out (to the author) several students whom he thought would make good subjects. One of these was a young woman of 21 whom he characterized as being dominated by the need for exhibitionism. She had volunteered, along with several others, to be a subject. She responded to the usual induction procedures and served as the main subject to demonstrate the usual signs of hypnosis, catalepsy, rigidity, hallucinations, post-hypnotic compulsive behavior, amnesia, age-regression (to a period when she could only understand and speak another language), etc. At the end of the meeting those subjects who had passed the usual hypnotic tests were asked if they would participate in an experiment in the author's laboratory. She volunteered along with the others. An appointment was made for a week later. She came with some friends at the appointed hour. But instead of being the easily-hypnotized subject of the week before, she was extremely resistant and showed external signs of anxiety and conflict. After about 30 minutes the experiment was terminated. In an interview which followed, the subject said, "I could not understand why, but every time you said my eyes were getting heavier, I would try harder to keep them open. When you said I would cooperate, I seemed to say to myself, 'I mustn't do this.' " Further questioning revealed that when she had discussed the demonstration with her parents, her father had expressed vehement disapproval of her submitting herself to such indignities, and had instructed her not to participate again. At the time, she thought she gave his instructions little attention, but as the time drew near for keeping the appointment, she became

[4] The psychoanalytic theories of hypnosis have contributed little to a systematic understanding of hypnosis *except* in the area of motivation. The transference phenomena (14, 38) can be readily translated into the language of social psychology.

more and more anxious. "You know, I always try to please my father."

In this instance we can say that for the first experiment the subject was favorably motivated. Her self-concept (dominated by the need for exhibitionism, if the instructor's appraisal was correct) and the perception of the role of the hypnotized subject were not disjunctive. In the second experiment the self-concept carried another characteristic—of greater valence than the need for exhibition—the maintenance of her father's approval. The role of the hypnotized subject was incongruent with her self-perception, which perception had been modified by interaction with her father. Although she had demonstrated before that she could perceive the role of the hypnotic subject, and could enact it with great fidelity, she could not focus on the role because of her changed self-perception.

In clinical experience this writer has found that as a patient achieves a set of self-perceptions which makes dependency ego-alien, resistance to hypnosis as a therapeutic aid increases. One patient, near the termination of therapy, was faced with blocking involving her school work. This same symptom had cleared up earlier after a few hypnotic sessions. When it was suggested that hypnosis be used as an auxiliary therapeutic technique, she was resistant to the idea. She said: "I know it worked before, but I would rather work this through on a more mature basis." Janet (24) long ago made the same observation, but related it to different concepts.

Role-perception. This concept was first introduced by G. H. Mead (29) and later by Moreno (30) in his studies of the psychodrama. In order to enact a dramatic or psychodramatic role, it is necessary for the subject to have a perception of the role. (The words "image" and "preconception" are used by other writers to express the same idea [22].) Through various media of communication, such as parental instruction, motion pictures, novels, comic strips, radio stories, rumors and folktales, role perceptions are built up.[5] The role of the father, the role of the teacher, the role of the policeman, etc., are built up from interaction with others in the social environment. When the subject enters the hypnotic situation, then, he comes not only with various self-perceptions, but also with various role-perceptions, among them the role of the hypnotic subject. The announcement of the experiment and the directions of the operator serve as stimuli which elicit the perception of the role. The validity of this conception is suggested by at least three kinds of observations: (1) trance states of certain primitive and religious groups, (2) the role-playing of young children, and (3) clinical and experimental studies.

Trance states. In many cultures trance states mark a *rite de passage.* As an illustration we cite one of Benedict's studies. She has described how, among the Plains Indians, an individual will experience many of the phenomena, including hallucinations, which are usually subsumed under the term hypnosis. The content of the hallucinations is relatively constant within groups but highly variable between groups. The role of the tranced subject is perceived from interaction with his own group. "The tranced individual may come back with communications from the dead describing the minutiae of life in the hereafter, or he may visit the world of the unborn, . . . or get information about coming events. Even in trance the individual holds strictly to the rules and expectations of his culture, and his experience is as locally patterned as a

[5] In a paper now in preparation the author analyzes in greater detail how the established principles of perception may be applied to role-perception.

marriage rite or an economic exchange" (6, p. 77). In brief, the perception of the trance role is built up in social interaction.

Role-playing of young children. Space prevents the identification of the numerous studies which have been reported dealing with the fantasy-roles observed in young children. One can condense the findings for the purposes of this paper into this general statement: The roles which emerge in the fantasy and play activities of young children are dependent upon their being able to perceive other-roles (4, 5, 8, 15). Some of the studies of imaginary companions are especially illuminating (18).

Hartley *et al.* have recently reported a pioneering study in an attempt to understand how children perceive ethnic group roles and parental roles. As might be expected, children begin to have role-perceptions at an early age and there are levels of complexity in their formulations of role-perception (20).

Clinical and experimental studies. Dorcus *et al.* (10) have reported a study which shows clearly that college students—who make up most of the experimental population—are not naïve subjects as far as hypnosis is concerned. For example, of 669 students questioned, 79 per cent answered yes to the question: Is hypnosis possible? To the question, Could you be hypnotized?, 36 per cent said yes, and 15 per cent answered in the affirmative in regard to the possibility of hypnotic amnesia. These data may be interpreted to signify that most college students (the usual experimental population) have a perception of the role of the hypnotic subject. Not all who have such a role-perception, however, can enact the role. The proportion of college students who are successfully hypnotized is much less than would be expected from the Dorcus *et al.* data.

In an unpublished study (36) the author asked a sophomore class to write descriptions of what takes place in hypnosis. This assignment was made a week before the lecture and demonstration of hypnosis. Volunteers from this class were subject to the induction procedure described by Friedlander and Sarbin (16). The spontaneous acts, introduced by the subjects without instructions from the experimenter, were noted. Of the 12 subjects who volunteered, six subjects were classified as "good" subjects. The spontaneous additions of four of these subjects could have been predicted from their descriptions of the week before. For example, one subject spontaneously awakened from the trance each time she was given a task which called for opening her eyes. Upon a later perusal of her paper, we read "A person's eyes must be closed in order to be in a hypnotic trance." Another subject was non-hypnotizable on the first attempt. On the second trial he performed all the classical tests. His role-description contained the statement: "It takes time to learn to be hypnotized. Most people can't be hypnotized the first time." A third subject performed all the tests satisfactorily, except where she was asked to rise from her chair and write on the blackboard. She was resistant to all suggestions when on her feet. Her paper contained this statement: "The subject has to be reclining or sitting." The fourth subject was extremely stuporous, slow-moving, and unable to perform any of the tests. He required a vigorous shaking in order to wake him from the trance. His paper contained the sentence: "Hypnosis is like a deep sleep, the hypnotizer talks in a low voice and you go into a deep sleep." Of the remaining six subjects, all had a correct perception of the role. Their failure to enact it could be attributed either to unfavorable motivation or to a lack of role-taking aptitude (*v. infra*). These observations lend support to the notion that variations in role-perception influence role-enactment.

In a clinical study of 10 adult patients in a hospital ward, a standard hypnotic procedure was used except that the operator avoided any mention of the word hypnosis or trance. The words relaxation and restful state were substituted. By any of the usual criteria none of these patients was hypnotized. Five of them fell asleep, however. Later the same subjects were told that hypnosis was to be attempted. They were told about the phenomena of hypnosis, the manner in which it is induced, and the possible therapeutic outcomes. The same induction procedure was used as before but the words hypnosis and hypnotic trance were reinstated. Three of the ten subjects responded to the usual hypnotic tests. Thus certain conditions leading to the perception of the role were prerequisite for enacting the role of the hypnotized subject.

Role-taking aptitude. Since motivational factors are necessary but not sufficient to account for the phenomena of hypnosis, and since role-perception does not automatically lead to role-enactment, a role-taking aptitude is postulated. However, since it is impossible to separate the motivational from the aptitudinal factors in studying hypnosis, White has suggested an experimental design (44). To a certain extent this design controls the factor of motivation and allows for an approximate isolation of the hypnotic aptitude. White recommends that all completely unhypnotizable subjects be eliminated for the reason that subjects with unfavorable motivations will thereby be discarded. The remaining subjects may be placed in two groups—somnambulists, showing marked amnesia, hallucinations and anesthesia, and light trance subjects who show eyelid and limb catalepsy. "It can be postulated that the first group possesses the hypnotic aptitude to a marked degree, the second to a moderate degree. There should accordingly be significant differences between their average scores on tests which measure the hypnotic aptitude." This design was adopted in a study conducted at the University of Chicago by the author on an original sample of 70 undergraduate volunteers. All were given the Minnesota Multiphasic Personality Inventory. All were subject to the same induction procedures. Of the 70, 36 were discarded as non-hypnotizable subjects. All verbalized a role-perception (variations in role-perception were not considered). Of the remainder, 16 fell into the category of somnambulistic subjects, and 18 in the category of light trance subjects. Of the various scales on the test, the Hy (hysteria) scale differentiated the two groups. Using a T-score of 55 as a cutting point, the following four-fold table depicts the results.

	Somnambulists	Light trance
55 and above	12	4
Below 55	4	14

The chi-square value is significant to .01. (The mean T-score of the somnambulists was 60, of the light trance subjects, 51.) Thus a scale which differentiates hysterical patients also differentiates hypnotic subjects. This finding recalls that part of Charcot's theory which regards hypnosis as an artificially induced hysteria. However, none of the subjects was known to be a hysterical patient. We are led to the same conclusions made by clinicians for many years—the good hypnotic subject and the hysterical patient have something in common. We would suggest the role-taking aptitude.

Auxiliary support is given to this conclusion in a study reported by Lewis and Sarbin (25). Here hypnotic subjects were told to imagine eating a meal at a time when they were having gastric hunger contractions. We found a high correlation between the depth of hypnosis (Friedlander-Sarbin scale) and the ability to inhibit hunger contractions. Those who could take the role of the eater—to use an expression of Moreno's—who could imagine themselves ingesting food, initiated a set of internal responses which resulted in the cessation of the gastric contractions. Subjects who could not be hypnotized, who could not take the role either of the hypnotic subject, or of the eater in imagination, showed no cessation of gastric contractions. That role-taking is organismic is demonstrated here.

When we say that the role-taking aptitude is organismic we refer back to our "observations which must be accounted for." We repeated the question raised by the laity and by other theorists: How can such marked changes in behavior result from such apparently innocuous stimuli? [7] It is probably not far from the truth to say with Goldstein (19) that any act involves the entire organism. When an individual places himself in the hypnotic situation—when he takes the role of the hypnotic subject—he does so organismically. When the subject acts *as if* he is ingesting food, his actions are total. The variation in his bodily responses, of course, will vary with the completeness and intensity of the role-taking.

A further comment is required about the organismic basis of the role-taking aptitude, especially as seen in acts which transcend normal limits. In the case of actors taking a stage role there are some who will enact the role without a preliminary warming-up process, while others require "preparation." In this warming-up or preparatory process the director helps the actor perceive some of the necessary attributes of the role. This might be considered a kind of covert practice in role-taking. In hypnosis the frequent lengthy induction may serve the same purpose, especially where the subject requires time to shift to the type of attentional behavior which is a component of the hypnotic role. Relaxation, diffuseness, and uncritical passivity as components of the role may be perceived by the subject as a result of the experimenter's instructions. When the subject aptly takes the hypnotic role (whether immediately, or after warming up *via* the induction procedures) a shift occurs from a sharp, alert, objective and critical attitude to a relatively relaxed, diffuse, and uncritical one. Because the alert orientation is highly valued and supported in our society some coaching or "preparation" is required for certain subjects. They must shift their focus to a relaxed, diffuse orientation which (as in the case of mystical states, for example) allows for more active motor-involvement and more intense affectivity. The variations in intensity or completeness with which one takes a role, and the concurrent motor and autonomic effects, are probably related to the subject's ability to

[7] A philosophical digression is in order here. Scientists, no less than laymen, are influenced and limited by their historical and cultural horizons. Growing up in an intellectual environment in which a dichotomy is made between mind and body, between mental events and physical events, scientists are "amazed" when they observe events which are not congruent with the dichotomy. When a scientist's *eidos* is freed from the necessity of fractionating behavior into the dichotomy dictated by 17th century dualism, then he can regard human behavior as organismic. Why should social psychological events not serve as conditions for altering predominantly biological activities? No one is amazed when respiratory changes are observed in attention experiments, or BMR's of westerners become more like those of orientals when living under specified oriental conditions, etc.

utilize *as-if* formulations. It is to this notion that we now turn.

THE *AS–IF* FORMULATION

Upon what does the role-taking aptitude depend? In a prior paragraph we noted the apparent relationship between the role-taking of the drama and role-taking in hypnosis. Mr. Arbuthnot, the actor, in taking the part of Hamlet, acts *as if* he is Hamlet and not Mr. Arbuthnot. The hypnotic subject acts *as if* he is an automaton (if automaticity is included in his role-perception). As a preliminary postulate we can say that the role-taking aptitude depends upon the subject's participation in *as-if* behavior. That this has a more general application is seen from a logical analysis of Rosenzweig's "triadic hypothesis" (33). In this statement, hypnotizability as a personality trait, repression as an ego-defense, and impunitiveness as a response to frustration are shown to be related. These may be considered *as-if* structures. We have already noted the *as-if* character of hypnosis. In repression the subject acts *as if* an event threatening to the self had not occurred. In the impunitive response to frustration, similarly, the subject acts *as if* the frustrating event were no longer frustrating. The *as-if* formulation may be seen not only in the drama, in hypnosis, but in fantasy, play, and, in fact, all imaginative behavior. Imaginative behavior is *as-if* behavior (40). Some data have been put forward by Jacobson (23), Schultz (39), Arnold (3), and others which may be put to use in formulating our theory. From the proposition that all imaginative behavior is *as-if* behavior, we may state that role-taking aptitude depends upon imagination. The following statements give at least initial validity to this proposition.

In a series of carefully controlled studies Jacobson (23) was able to demonstrate the influence of the subject's imagining certain events upon bodily functions. For example, in a condition of relaxation, a subject was told to imagine elevating his arm. The electrical recording showed activity in the muscles which were involved. Schultz (39) reports many instances of the influence of imagination on various muscular and vascular characteristics. Varondenck (41) tells how imaginary processes (implicit) can spill over into overt muscular movements during the act of imagining. Common experience verifies the same notion. In imagining a former embarrassing situation we can feel our ears reddening and our faces flushing; in imagining a former painful experience we may involuntarily withdraw from the direction of the imagined stimulus, or in imagining something extremely unpleasant or disgusting we may experience nausea.

Arnold has written the most complete analysis of the relationship between hypnosis and imagination (3). According to her hypothesis, ". . . in hypnosis the individual is actively striving to imagine what the hypnotist describes, and in so doing gradually narrows down his focus and relinquishes control of his imaginative processes. . . . The individual focuses on a situation and actively selects the sensations which he will perceive; he actively focuses on possible situations in imagining, on symbols in logical thinking; and he refocuses on past experiences in remembering. Such focussing . . . is merely directed more efficiently, more intensely, during hypnosis than in waking life, and determined by the hypnotist instead of by the subject himself" (3, p. 127). This writer would amend the last statement to read: The focussing is determined by the hypnotist only insofar as the subject's self-perceptions and role-perception permit such direction. This amendment would follow from a careful consideration of the data Arnold presents from her own experiment which reveals the individual character of the subject's own imagining over and above the directions of the experimenter.

Although Arnold's views are more sophisticated than most previous theories, we are left without any anchorage point for understanding differential responsiveness. The numerous experiments cited by Arnold show the influence of imagination on behavior and the kinds of experimental and clinical situations appear to be of the same kind as the hypnotic situation. But what of the answer to the all important social-psychological question: What are the characteristics of those individuals who are *not* able to focus and thus cannot produce changes in overt or covert behavior?

In Arnold's data is concealed a partial answer to this question. She reports an experiment in which the postural sway technique is used. She tested the hypothesis that a suggestion is acted upon only if the subject actively imagines it. The subjects were told to imagine falling forward. The amount of postural sway was recorded. Comparisons were made between the amount of sway and the reported vividness of imagery. Her conclusion was: The more vivid the imaginative process, the more pronounced the overt movements. From this conclusion and from the long-accepted conclusion about the relationship between the postural sway test and hypnotizability a correlation between vividness of imagery and hypnotic depth could be posited. We could then deduce that hypnotic role-taking depended upon imaginative (*as-if*) processes.[8] One might fit the previously mentioned findings of Eysenck and Furneaux into this formulation. Subjects who score high on postural sway tests and test of heat illusion are able to imagine vividly in these sense modalities. *A fortiori,* the experiment of Sarbin and Madow (37) may be cited in which the depth of hypnosis and the Rorschach W/D ratio were shown to be correlated. The W or Whole response purportedly indicates a more active imagination.

How, then, does the role-taking theory apply to the four sets of observations previously identified as requiring explanation?

The apparent automaticity is apparent only. The subject varies his responses to the hypnotic situation in terms of his perception of the role of the hypnotized subject. If his perception includes automaticity, then he will act like an automaton.

The apparent discontinuity of behavior is also apparent but not real. The subject's behavior is continuous with his pre-experimental behavior—modified only by his enactment of the role of the hypnotic subject. Such "discontinuous" behavior as amnesia, post-hypnotic compulsions, etc., can be understood in terms of the subject's perception of the role, of his facility in *as-if* behavior and of the degree of participation of the self in the role.

The apparent disjunction between the magnitude of the response and the procedure for eliciting the response is a pseudo-problem. The magnitude of the response is not dependent upon the procedure except insofar as it coincides with the role-expectations of the subject. What appears to be a disjunction is a vestigial remnant of an outmoded psychology which sought to find constancy between phenomenal experience and stimulus events. If the subject has an adequate perception of the role, if this perception is not incongruent with

[8] Clinically, the writer has never found an adult with eidetic or vivid imagery who was not a good hypnotic subject. In a personal communication D. W. MacKinnon reports the same observation.

his self-perceptions, and if he has an appropriate amount of the role-taking aptitude, then he will produce all the dramatic phenomena of hypnosis merely because "the operator talks to him." If he does not or cannot perceive the role, if the role is not congruent with his self-perceptions, and/or he does not have a sufficient amount of the role-taking aptitude or skill, then he will not respond to the operator's commands. Thus differential responsiveness is declared to be a function of these three variables.

SUMMARY

The known facts about hypnosis were grouped in four classes of observations: (1) apparent automaticity, (2) apparent discontinuity, (3) disjunction between the magnitude of the stimulus and the magnitude of the response, and (4) differential responsiveness. Because of the obvious dependence of the first three factors upon the fourth (differential responsiveness) this question was formulated: What are the characteristics of those individuals who, in response to hypnotic induction procedures, exhibit conduct which is apparently discontinuous and apparently automatic?

We sought to demonstrate that concurrent theories of hypnosis were tradition-bound: trying to explain hypnotic behavior in terms of conditioning, heredity, or vague neurological formulae. In order to establish a logical link between hypnosis and another form of social psychological conduct which is accepted without resorting to traditional formulations, we first indicated the similarity between role-taking in the drama and role-taking in hypnosis. We postulated that success in taking a dramatic role or hypnotic role depended upon favorable motivation, a perception of the role, and role-taking aptitude. The chief difference in the two forms of role-taking was the degree of participation of the self in the role (levels of consciousness).

The main portion of our presentation attempted to establish the validity of these conceptions. Favorable motivation was re-defined as congruence between the subject's self-concept and the role of the hypnotic subject. Role-perception is derived from the individual's interaction with various media of communication: the manner in which role-perception influences role-enactment is indicated. Finally, a role-taking aptitude is postulated. From our present state of knowledge this aptitude is probably dependent upon or continuous with the ability of the subject to use *as-if* formulations. Various research and clinical findings were introduced to supply a groundwork for the initial validity of the argument.

REFERENCES

1. ALLEN, A. H. B. *The self in psychology.* London: Kegan Paul, Trench, Trubner & Co., 1935.
2. ARCHER, W. *Masks or faces?* New York: Longmans, Green & Co., 1889.
3. ARNOLD, M. B. On the mechanism of suggestion and hypnosis. *J. abn. soc. Psychol.,* 1946, **41**, 107–128.
4. AXLINE, V. *Play therapy.* Boston: Houghton-Mifflin Co., 1947.
5. BACH, G. Young children's play fantasies. *Psychol. Monogr.,* 1945, **59**, No. 2.
6. BENEDICT, R. Anthropology and the abnormal. *J. gen. Psychol.,* 1934, **10**, 59–82.
7. BRENMAN, M., & GILL, M. M. *Hypnotherapy.* New York: International Universities Press, 1947.
8. CAMERON, N. *The psychology of behavior disorders.* Boston: Houghton-Mifflin Co., 1947.
9. CORN-BECKER, F., WELCH, L., & FISICHELLI, V. Conditioning factors underlying hypnosis. *J. abn. soc. Psychol.,* 1949, **44**, 212–222.
10. DORCUS, R., BRETNALL, A. K., & CASE, H. W. Control experiments and their relation to theories of hypnosis. *J. gen. Psychol.,* 1941, **24**, 217–221.
11. DYMOND, R. A scale for the measurement of empathic ability. *J. consult. Psychol.,* 1948, **13**, 127–133.

12. EYSENCK, H. J. Suggestibility and hysteria. *J. Neurol. Psychiat.*, 1943, **6**, 22–31.
13. ——, & FURNEAUX, W. D. Primary and secondary suggestibility. *J. exp. Psychol.*, 1945, **35**, 485.
14. FERENCZI, S. *Sex in psychoanalysis.* Boston: Richard G. Badger, 1916.
15. FLUGEL, J. C. *Man, morals, and society.* New York: International Universities Press, 1944.
16. FRIEDLANDER, J. W., & SARBIN, T. R. The depth of hypnosis. *J. abn. soc. Psychol.*, 1938, **33**, 453–475.
17. FURNEAUX, W. D. Prediction of susceptibility to hypnosis. *J. Personal.*, 1946, **14**, 281–294.
18. GREEN, G. *The day dream.* London: Univ. of London Press, 1923.
19. GOLDSTEIN, K. *The organism.* New York: American Book Co., 1939.
20. HARTLEY, E. L., ROSENBAUM, M., & SCHWARTZ, S. Children's perceptions of ethnic group membership. *J. Psychol.*, 1948, **26**, 387–398.
21. HULL, C. L. *Hypnosis and suggestibility.* New York: D. Appleton-Century, 1933.
22. ICHHEISER, G. Misunderstandings in human relations—a study in false social perception. *Amer. J. Sociol.*, 1949, **55**, Part 2.
23. JACOBSON, E. *Progressive relaxation.* Chicago: Univ. of Chicago Press (rev. ed.), 1938.
24. JANET, P. *Major symptoms of hysteria.* New York: Macmillan Co., 1907.
25. KUBIE, L. S., & MARGOLIN, S. The process of hypnotism and the nature of the hypnotic state. *Amer. J. Psychiat.*, 1944, **100**, 611–622.
26. LEWIS, J. H., & SARBIN, T. R. Studies in psychosomatics: the influence of hypnotic stimulation on gastric hunger contractions. *Psychosom. Med.*, 1943, **5**, 125–131.
27. LINTON, R. *The cultural background of personality.* London: Routledge & Kegan Paul, Ltd., 1947.
28. LUNDHOLM, H. An experimental study of functional anesthesias as induced by suggestion in hypnosis. *J. abn. soc. Psychol.*, 1928, **23**, 337–355.
29. MEAD, G. H. *Mind, self, and society.* Chicago: Univ. of Chicago Press, 1934.
30. MORENO, J. L. Role tests and role diagrams of children. In *Psychodrama,* New York: Beacon House, 1946, Vol. 1.
31. PATTIE, F. A. The production of blisters by hypnotic suggestions: a review. *J. abn. soc. Psychol.*, 1941, **36**, 62–72.
32. ROSENOW, C. Meaningful behavior in hypnosis. *Amer. J. Psychol.*, 1928, **40**, 205–235.
33. ROSENZWEIG, S., & SARASON, S. An experimental study of the triadic hypothesis: reaction to frustration, ego-defence, and hypnotizability. *Character & Pers.*, 1942, **11**, 1–19.
34. SARBIN, T. R. The concept of role-taking. *Sociometry,* 1943, **6**, 273–285.
35. ——. Rorschach patterns under hypnosis. *Amer. J. Orthopsychiat.*, 1939, **11**, 315–318.
36. ——. Studies in role-taking (unpublished).
37. ——, & MADOW, L. Predicting the depth of hypnosis by means of the Rorschach test. *Amer. J. Orthopsychiat.*, 1942, **12**, 268–270.
38. SCHILDER, P., & KAUDERS, O. Hypnosis. *Nerv. ment. Dis. Monogr. Ser.*, 1927, No. 46.
39. SCHULTZ, J. *Das Autogene Training* (Konzentrierte Selbstentspannung), Leipsig, 1932.
40. VAIHINGER, H. *The philosophy of 'as-if.'* London: K. Paul, Trench, Trubner & Co., Ltd., 1924.
41. VARENDONCK, J. *The psychology of day dreams.* London: George Allen & Unwin, Ltd., 1921. Pp. 367.
42. WELCH, L. A behavioristic explanation of the mechanism of suggestion and hypnosis. *J. abn. soc. Psychol.*, 1947, **42**, 359–364.
43. WHITE, R. M. A preface to the theory of hypnotism. *J. abn. soc. Psychol.*, 1941, **36**, 477–505.
44. ——. An analysis of motivation in hypnosis. *J. gen. Psychol.*, 1941, **24**, 145–162.
45. ——, & SHEVACH, S. Hypnosis and the concept of dissociation. *J. abn. soc. Psychol.*, 1937, **42**, 309–328.
46. YOUNG, P. C. Hypnotic regression—fact or artifact? *J. abn. soc. Psychol.*, 1940, **35**, 273–278.

[MS. received January 11, 1950]

[4]

THE NATURE OF HYPNOSIS: ARTIFACT AND ESSENCE[1]

MARTIN T. ORNE

Harvard University and Massachusetts Mental Health Center

THE most meaningful present-day theories of hypnosis interpret hypnotic phenomena along three major lines: (*a*) desire on the part of the subject to play the role of a hypnotized subject (Sarbin, 1950; White, 1941), (*b*) increase in suggestibility (Hull, 1933), and (*c*) a further less well-defined category that is called by White "an altered state of consciousness" and by others, "cortical inhibition" (Pavlov, 1923), dissociation (Weitzenhoffer, 1953), etc. depending on their theoretical orientations.

The heuristic model of hypnosis that underlies this paper incorporates these three aspects. One of the hypotheses of the paper holds that much hypnotic behavior results from the subject's conception of the role of the hypnotic subject as determined by past experience and learning, and by explicit and implicit cues provided by the hypnotist and the situation. These varied role conceptions appear to be the source of most if not all of the inconstant patterns of behavior seen in the hypnotic state.

An increase in suggestibility may be viewed as an increase in motivation to conform to the wishes of the hypnotist. A second basic hypothesis to be tested thus proposes that, although increased motivation may be a constant accompaniment of the trance state, such increased motivation is by no means a phenomenon unique to hypnosis but can be seen to operate in other experimental and life situations with equal force.

By experimentally controlling these two elements, role-playing and increased motivation, it is possible to investigate their sufficiency for explaining all aspects of the trance state and the extent to which still other concepts, such as an altered state of consciousness, are required.

The third aspect of hypnosis, the altered state of consciousness, presents the greatest problem for investigation, yet it has been felt necessary to include the concept in all attempts to explain the phenomenon. This residual aspect, which remains after increased motivation and role-playing are accounted for, may be regarded as the "essence" of hypnosis, with reference to which increased motivation and role-playing appear as artifacts.

Three related experiments are presented. The first is devoted to the effects of "role-play artifact" on the manifestations of hypnosis commonly seen clinically. It demonstrates that much of the complex phenomenon which we call hypnosis may result from (*a*) the subject's preconceptions of what hypnosis is, (*b*) implicit cues by the hypnotist as to what he thinks it should be, and (*c*) the particular techniques of trance induction. The second experiment demonstrates an aspect of role-play artifact that is introduced by a concrete experimental situation. It investigates cues that an experimental design may give about the role the subject is expected to play and demonstrates that in some instances an experimental result may more reasonably be accounted for on this basis than by invoking "trance effects." The third experiment is concerned with the effect of "motivation artifact" upon performance. It examines the claims of increased physical capacity in hypnosis and tests the hypothesis that this may be accounted for by increased motivation.

Table 1 gives a schematic representation of the author's working model of the hypnotic state.

[1] This investigation was supported in part by a postdoctoral research fellowship from the Public Health Service.

I would like to thank Robert W. White for his encouragement and guidance and Milton Greenblatt for his support and his cooperation in the use of the facilities of the Massachusetts Mental Health Center. I am greatly indebted to Donald O'Connell, for his help in the pilot studies, and Ronald Shor and Theodore X. Barber for their invaluable assistance in running the first two experiments reported here. In addition, thanks are due Peter D. Watson for his aid in preparing and editing the manuscript. Finally, I would like to express my appreciation to Abraham H. Maslow of Brandeis University, Philip Nogee of Boston University, William McGill of the Massachusetts Institute of Technology, E. G. Boring and Ray Hyman of Harvard University, and the respective departments of psychology for making their classes available to me.

TABLE 1
SCHEMATIC REPRESENTATION OF A WORKING MODEL OF HYPNOSIS

Situation of trance induction	"Role-Play Artifact" (cognitive component) +	"Increased Motivation Artifact" (conative component) +	Essence of Trance
Creation of situation to maximize: 1. Desirability of entering trance 2. Expectation that trance can be achieved 3. Respect and trust for operator 4. Restriction of extraneous stimuli 5. Focusing of attention	1. Expectations of *S*s a. preconceptions b. cues from trance induction 2. Cues from Experimenter a. explicit b. implicit 3. Cues from experimental situation	The sources of increased motivation are not defined They represent a major area of future inquiry Probably some aspects will prove to be a component of "essence"	Uncertain
All techniques have the further qualities of: 1. Concrete suggestions in vivid simple language 2. "Suggestions" utilizing the perception of subjective events as their basis 3. Suggestions of gradually increasing difficulty to insure successful responses 4. Praising (rewarding) explicitly or implicitly the subject's positive responses			

PRECONCEPTIONS OF HYPNOSIS AND THEIR EFFECT ON TRANCE MANIFESTATIONS

The states induced by Mesmer (Binet & Féré, 1888; Boring, 1950), Coué (1922, p. 83), Wells (1923), Schilder (1956), and others are all hypnosis, yet their descriptions of how hypnosis characteristically manifests itself are very different. The common characteristics of these varied states that bring them all under the heading of "hypnosis" would appear to include: posthypnotic amnesia, apparent inability to use a given motor system when a functional paralysis is suggested, various sensory illusions including positive and negative hallucinations of all sensory modalities, apparent memory disturbances or improvements as well as reported increased control over autonomic nervous system functions. Whether all of these phenomena are necessarily part of hypnotic behavior will be discussed below. In any event, hypnosis is evidently characterized by the ability of the subject (*S*) in this special state to experience changes that are not normally found in response to similar cues in everyday life.

What, then, determines the particular trance manifestations that an *S* shows on entering hypnosis? In terms of the model presented here, the answer may lie in role-play artifact. From this viewpoint, *S*s who enter trance are motivated to play the role of the hypnotized *S*, and the precise manifestations of this role depend upon their perception of what it entails. Behavior of the *S* in trance is then determined by the *S*'s preconceptions about how a hypnotic *S* acts, and the cues, both explicit and implicit, as to the desired behavior which the hypnotist communicates in the process of trance induction.

To test this hypothesis that conceptions about hypnosis held prior to entering the hypnotic state affect an *S*'s trance behavior, a pilot study and a main experiment were conducted in which volunteer *S*s were given the erroneous prior impression that catalepsy of the dominant hand (with the other hand flaccid) is a typical feature of hypnosis. This behavioral item was chosen because it satisfied a number of criteria. It is sufficiently unusual to have been reported had it ever been observed as a spontaneous characteristic of hypnosis; it is easily recognizable so that judgments of its presence or absence are unequivocal; and it is sufficiently plausible as a characteristic associated with hypnosis that it would be accepted as such by the *S* population.

Especial care was exercised to eliminate possible effects of the bias of the experimenter by making it impossible for him to influence the results. It is easy to suggest to an *S* by implicit cues that he manifest catalepsy as part of the hypnotic state. Perhaps catalepsy of one hand might also be suggested during induction of the trance. Selection of catalepsy of the *dominant* hand avoids this possibility, as the experimenter had no way of knowing whether the subject was right- or left-handed until he asked for this information after the data on catalepsy had been gathered.

Pilot Study

An introductory psychology class at the Massachusetts Institute of Technology was given a lecture on hypnosis. Prior to the lecture, and without the knowledge of the class, two students had been hypnotized and given the posthypnotic suggestion that upon entering the trance subsequently, they would manifest catalepsy of one hand, the dominant hand. One student was right-handed and one student was left-handed. The class was then given a 25-minute lecture on the nature of the hypnotic state, at which point volunteers were called for in order to demonstrate the phenomenon. Of the 11 students who volunteered, the two who had been previously hypnotized were selected in a fashion that appeared random. They were again placed in trance, in a manner that appeared to be the initial trance induction, and simple trance phenomena were demonstrated, including one-handed catalepsy. Attention was called to the fact that the right-handed student had catalepsy of the right hand, and the left-handed student had catalepsy of the left hand. Immediately following this procedure, three more students from the same group of volunteers, who had not been hypnotized previously, were placed in trance.

A class of psychology students at Harvard were subsequently given the same kind of a lecture and demonstration, following which four *S*s were hypnotized and tested for one-handed catalepsy.

All three of the M.I.T. experimental *S*s gave good trance results, and all showed catalepsy of the dominant hand. One *S* was left-handed. Of the four Harvard students who were hypnotized immediately after observing three demonstration *S*s with catalepsy of the dominant hand, three manifested catalepsy of the dominant hand and one, catalepsy of both hands. All *S*s were right-handed.

Main Study

In order to make it impossible for the experimenter to communicate his desire that the *S* demonstrate unilateral catalepsy, the main study was performed in a rigorous "blind" fashion. In this instance matched classes were used, each of which had received a lecture and demonstration of hypnosis. In one class the hypnotic demonstration included catalepsy of the dominant hand, while in the other this was omitted. The *S*s were then tested in small groups, with members of both groups mixed randomly. The experimenter thus had no way of knowing which subjects should manifest one-handed catalepsy.

Procedure

The procedure of the pilot experiment was repeated with members of the introductory psychology course at Boston University with the inclusion of the control group. Instead of asking for volunteers, three *S*s were employed who were introduced to the class as having taken part in prior research. The same three *S*s were used for both sections of the course, to which essentially identical lectures were given. The demonstrations differed only in that in one section the three *S*s manifested unilateral catalepsy, while in the other section this was not demonstrated. No students from either class were hypnotized at that time. Volunteers were solicited and subsequently tested in such a way that the experimenter had no way of telling which lecture they had attended until after the completion of the experiment.[2] All but two *S*s were tested by an experimenter who was not at the lectures.

Trance depth was rated by the experimenter and an observer. The degree of consensus was high and in no case was there more than a one point difference. In case of disagreement both ratings are recorded. The ratings are rough clinical estimates based on the phenomena

[2] One of these *S*s was tested the evening of the lecture. The remaining *S*s were tested approximately one month after the lecture.

TABLE 2
TRANCE BEHAVIOR IN THE EXPERIMENTAL AND CONTROL GROUPS

Subject	Catalepsy		Trance Depth	Dominant Hand
	R.	L.		
Experimental group				
1. M.S.	+	0	4	R.
2. M.K.	+	+	4	R.
3. R.L.	+	0	4	R.
4. C.L.	0	0	2	R.
5. S.T.	0	0	3	R.
6. A.L.	0	+	3	L.
7. O.B.	+	0	3	R.
8. S.R.	+	+	5	R.
9. B.T.	+	0	4	R.[a,b]
Control group				
1. D.L.	0	0	4	R.
2. W.O.	0	0	4	R.
3. M.R.	+	+	3	R.
4. L.P.	+	+	3	L.
5. B.Z.	0	0	3	R.
6. L.V.	0	0	4–5	R.
7. M.O.	+	+	3	R.
8. A.T.	0	0	3	L.[b]
9. W.M.	0	0	1–2	R.

[a] This *S* was tested the evening of the lecture when he appeared unannounced along with a group of *S*s who had previously volunteered. The experimenter did not know which class the *S* had attended until after the experiment was over.

[b] *S*s tested by author. I was not aware of which class these *S*s had attended, in fact, I did not know until subsequently that they had been at the lectures.

which could be elicited from the *S*s. A rating of 1 indicated no response; 2 implied eye-closure and only partial hand levitation without a positive response to "challenge" suggestions, i.e., you cannot open your eyes, or you cannot bend your elbow; 3 referred to positive responses to all challenge suggestions but inability to achieve hallucinations or posthypnotic phenomena; 4 was used to denote those *S*s who responded to suggested hallucinations, gave simple posthypnotic phenomena, but did not achieve a good posthypnotic amnesia; 5 referred to "somnambulists" who could achieve all hypnotic phenomena easily, including complete amnesia.

Results

Of the nine *S*s in the experimental group, five showed catalepsy of the dominant hand. Two showed catalepsy of both hands, and two showed no catalepsy. None of the control group showed catalepsy of the dominant hand, but three out of the nine *S*s showed catalepsy of both hands. Table 2 gives a summary of the findings.

Discussion

The item of behavior that was used is known not to occur spontaneously; its occurrence is significant if it is found at all. The results of the pilot and main experiments may be regarded as confirming the hypothesis that trance behavior is affected by the individual's conceptions about hypnosis held prior to entering the hypnotic state.

It would not be expected that all *S*s would show this behavior. No truly naive *S* population is available, and many of the *S*s had observed hypnosis prior to the demonstration. Some *S*s should therefore have sufficient prior information to have formed very strong conceptions unlikely to be altered by the relatively mild attempt to manipulate these ideas experimentally.

That three of the nine *S*s in the control group spontaneously manifested catalepsy of both hands is readily understood in view of the repeated testing for catalepsy, which they apparently interpreted as a cue to manifest the behavior. None of the control *S*s, it should be emphasized, manifested unilateral catalepsy, indicating that no such desire was communicated by the hypnotist to the *S*.

This study has demonstrated for a single behavior item that trance behavior is affected by individual preconceptions about hypnosis. The results can be extrapolated to account for the apparently fixed qualities, not stemming from cues given by the hypnotist, that are reported in practically all present-day descriptions of hypnosis.

Thanks to the media of mass communication, it is relatively easy for a particular view of hypnosis to have gained wide currency and thus be found as a part of the general knowledge in which the *S*s share. Such novels as *Mario and the Magician* (Mann, 1931) and *Trilby* (DuMaurier, 1895) have had very wide audiences and are known indirectly to almost all members of our culture. Uncounted articles and features about hypnosis have been disseminated to all levels of society. The picture of hypnosis that emerges in all of these is that of a passive *S* in a sleeplike state who has amnesia for the events occurring in hypnosis, and responds only to the hypnotist's suggestions. According to Dorcus, Brintmall, and Case (1941), 79% of the student sample that they studied accepted hypnosis as possible, 71% had discussed hypnosis with someone, 54% had read about it, and 29% had actually seen a hypnotic trance at one time during their lives.

In the context of group tests for "suggestibility," in order to screen *S*s, the investigators asked 57 students in elementary psychology courses: "Have you observed any other demonstrations of hypnosis; if so, where and when?" and "What have you read about hypnosis?" Only 12 *S*s denied both having read about hypnosis and having had any chance to see the phenomenon previously; 18 *S*s had seen hypnosis demonstrated in some form, and 23 had somehow read about it.

In the context of the questionnaires used in the above studies, "having read about hypnosis" meant specific reading in the scientific sense. In questioning well over 200 student *S*s about their knowledge of hypnosis, the author failed to find one who did not have a very clear-cut notion about the nature of hypnosis, and who could not define the trance in a fashion similar to that found in dictionaries. Furthermore, they had all read something about hypnosis and could recall having done so, once it was made clear that this included nonscientific sources. The normal *S* population thus knows the meaning of the word hypnosis prior to taking part in any study.

Cues Implicit in an Experimental Design

An *S* participating in an experiment is aware that his responses are being recorded for specific purposes—that there is a *raison d'être* for the experiment—and he frequently has some idea of what these purposes are. How this knowledge affects the *S*'s behavior depends upon the motivational structure that he brings to the experimental situation. The participation of the college student volunteer in psychological studies is usually due, not to the relatively low monetary remuneration but, rather, to his interest in taking part in scientific research, which in turn is likely to be based, at least in part, on a desire to further "progress in science" by his participation. Since the experimenter is perceived as knowing what he is doing, furthering "progress in science" may well be equated with "making the experiment work" or, in more sophisticated terms, having his individual performance support the hypothesis of the experiment. Thus, when the *S* is motivated to comply with the wishes of the experimenter, his responses are readily influenced by what he perceives to be the basic hypothesis of the experiment.

Typically, the experimenter's hypotheses are not stated explicitly to the *S* because of the very considerations just mentioned. But unstated hypotheses may be conveyed implicitly by the experimental procedure itself, through what will be called here the "demand characteristics of the experimental situation." It should be understood that a person may fail to perceive fairly clear demand characteristics either because of lack of past experience or because of an inability to generalize from it.

Demand characteristics thus conceived appear central to much psychological work. Experimental situations vary widely in the extent to which they convey the purpose and the hypothesis of the experimenter. If an *S* can describe a hypothesis being tested, of which he is supposedly unaware, the experimental arrangements have significant demand characteristics. The obvious way to test for their presence is to ask the *S* about his perception of the experiment and its purpose. Usually, however, *S*s are reticent about revealing their notions about the purpose of the experiment.

It is reasonable to assume that the student *S* population has some sophistication in regard to the philosophy of experimentation. They are aware that if an *S* is not told the purpose of an experiment he ought to remain naive in regard to it, lest his knowledge influence his performance. At the same time they understand the necessity for an experimental *S* to be "honest" in his response to the experimental situation and to questions about it. For these reasons, *S*s are motivated to avoid recognizing explicitly the purpose of an experiment even though it may be clearly communicated by its design. Thus, the response to the direct question "What do you think this is about?" tends to be "I don't know." The *S*'s behavior may nevertheless clearly betray an implicit awareness of the relevant factors, and he may even verbalize them after the experiment in a "bull session" with his friends. We deal, therefore, with "knowledge" not readily available to consciousness which must be elicited in a clinical fashion. As in the case of other such material, the boundaries of consciousness may be expected to vary with the situation. When, however, a clinical approach is used in an inquiry and the *S* is pressed, one may be amazed—or horrified—by the *S*'s ability to formulate one's hypotheses in a lucid and at times highly sophisticated fashion. Unfortunately, the so-called inquiry is usually a most casual procedure.

While the demand characteristics of experimental situations probably have wider significance than is generally recognized, they are particularly significant for hypnotic experiments. Hypnotic *S*s tend to be particularly cooperative, almost eager participants. Furthermore, one of the assumptions of the present research for which there is extensive observational support is that the hypnotic state as such increases the motivation of the *S* to comply with the wishes ("suggestions")—both explicit and implicit—of the experimenter. The extent to which compliance can take place depends upon the demand characteristics in the experimental situation. The usual problem of demand characteristics (difficult enough to control in other fields of psychology because of the unconscious cooperation between *S* and experimenter) is thus compounded in hypnotic research.

In order to investigate the influence of the demand characteristics of an experimental procedure, a recent study (Ashley, Harper, & Runyon, 1951) was repeated with minor variations to be described. This experiment attempts to demonstrate a further dimension of the Bruner-Goodman (1947) effect, which has been the center of major controversy in recent years. Bruner and Goodman's basic tenet was that the perceiver's values alter his perception. There is no question that the perceiver's *previous experiences* may affect perception. A dispute, however, centers about whether *values* as such are significant variables affecting perception.

In order to show "clearly and unequivocally that the perceiver can contribute to the organization of his perception in a structured stimulus-situation," Ashley, Harper, and Runyon (1951) argue it would be necessary to have a special situation. They state: "The Bruner and Goodman type of experiment would do this *if* the rich group and the poor group were identical in every other respect—in terms of their experience with money, their life histories, their physiological conditions, in short, if the sole difference between the two groups was that only one group had the psychological organization . . . of rich people and the other group the psychological organization of poor people." They go on to say: "Actually for our problem, it is irrelevant whether the *S*s are economically as well as psychologically rich or poor, or whether they are only psychologically rich or poor. In either case, a difference in performance of the two groups would reflect a difference in the perception due to the psychological organization of the perceivers" (p. 565).

In order to obtain two groups identical in every respect but for their perception of their economic status, they used hypnosis. While the *S* was in trance, artificial life histories were induced—one rich and one poor—each followed by induced amnesia. In essence, then, they view the situation as if two identically matched groups were available—one rich, and one poor. It is assumed that because amnesia was induced for the preceding state, the *S* is again naive and that the only difference is in respect to his perceived economic status.

The final sentences of their rationale are particularly interesting. "Even though we do not know fully what happens when we hypnotize a person, if we do hypnotize him and tell him he is rich and he behaves in one way in the coin-matching situation, and then, a few moments later, we tell him he is now poor and he behaves in another way, *we can conclude that the observed difference is due to a change in his psychological organization*" (Ashley et al., 1951, p. 565).[3] The authors in fact conclude from their data that the psychological organization (including the wants, needs, interests, attitudes, and values) of the person contributes to the figural organizations of his perceptions.

It is unquestionably true that observed differences in coin-size judgments are due to

[3] Italics mine.

changes in psychological organization. The question with which we are concerned, however, is whether these changes in psychological organization relate to the actual experiencing of the feelings of being rich or poor, or whether they reflect the demand characteristics of the experimental procedure. The hypothesis to be tested is that the demand characteristics of the experiment are largely responsible for the results obtained by Ashley et al. (1951).

Disregarding the theoretical framework of the study, this is what actually took place: An individual was told—in hypnosis—that he was very poor, then—again with amnesia in hypnosis—that he was very rich and, subsequently, with another hypnotically induced amnesia, that he was himself. In each of these states he was required to make a series of coin-size judgments. The authors' interpretation rests largely on the assumption that hypnotic amnesia is truly the same as not knowing. Granted this, one would be justified in ignoring the fact that the procedure of coin-size estimation is repeated and that economic status is hypnotically induced. However, data are available that lead one to question this assumption.

One of the few specific experiments dealing with posthypnotic amnesia directly is a study by Strickler (1929), who compared the relearning of nonsense material in the posthypnotic state with induced amnesia with the learning time required for the material not previously learned. He concludes that "the posthypnotic amnesia ordinarily met with, which appears superficially to be a complete wiping-out of memory, is by no means complete."

Even more relevant are the data obtainable in hypnotic age-regression. Here we are dealing with an induced amnesia in hypnosis for what purports to be all material learned after a given age. All studies of hypnotic age-regression have shown that some material persists no matter how "real" the regression appears.

In the investigator's prior work (Orne, 1951), it was possible to show that an individual regressed to age six was able to comprehend English, though he himself pointed out in German that he could not understand it. Historically, the *S* was unable to understand English at age six. Another *S* could spell without error "I am conducting an experiment which will assess my psychological capacities." Another was able to give the square root of four, and so on. Furthermore, if we test for amnesia in a more subtle fashion, it is easy to demonstrate in the wake state or in trance that no true ablation of the material for which the *S* has amnesia exists, despite his subjective feeling of being unable to remember.

The fallacy of the assumption that knowledge for which the *S* has amnesia does not influence his behavior can be seen in any posthypnotic suggestion. The *S* firmly denies recall yet assiduously persists in the suggested behavior. The phenomenon is well known in response to an explicit cue; it would seem rather absurd to deny it in response to an implicit one.

A pilot study was therefore conducted that replicated all essential characteristics of the Ashley, Harper, and Runyon experiment, with the addition, however, of a careful inquiry after the completion of the experiment. The procedure was patterned after the inquiries commonly performed as part of the Rorschach test, which seek answers to a series of questions without providing the *S* with a cue as to the answers expected. 1. The subject's perception of the experimental task was elicited by a general question, "What do you think this experiment was about?" 2. The *S*'s perception of the purpose of the investigation was elicited by questions such as "What do you think this experiment is trying to prove or demonstrate?" 3. *S*'s perception of the experimenter's hypothesis was elicited by direct questioning, with such questions as "What do you think I hope to find?" 4. The *S* was also asked about his own hypothesis concerning the study—what he, on the basis of what he knew about the experiment, would predict the results to be. 5. The final question related to his beliefs about his own performance with the question, "What do you think your experimental behavior demonstrates?"

The following hypotheses were formulated:

1. The subject in an experiment is usually able to express some demand characteristics of the procedure, if careful inquiry is conducted and his initial resistance is penetrated in a clinical fashion.

2. The majority of subjects may perceive the same demand characteristics in the experi-

ment and these may be the same as the hypothesis being tested.

3. These demand characteristics rather than the experimental variables may be the major determinant of the subject's behavior.

a. If the majority of subjects perceive the same demand characteristics, then subjects who fail to perceive them should not show the behavior characteristic of the group.

b. If the demand characteristics are the determinant of subjects' behavior, it is possible for an experimental design that omits a crucial aspect of the original independent variable to elicit similar responses to the extent that the same demand characteristics are present.

Pilot Study

The pilot study was designed to test the first two hypotheses.

Procedure

The Ashley, Harper, and Runyon study was repeated in all essential details with four undergraduate *S*s, with the addition of appropriate inquiry. Equipment employed in the original Bruner-Goodman study (1947) was used for making the coin-size estimations. Unlike the procedure of Ashley, Harper, and Runyon, however, the coins were presented on the *S*'s left palm which he was permitted to hold beside the box. He was not permitted to remove the coin from his palm.

All *S*s used in this study had demonstrated their ability to manifest all of the usual deep trance phenomena including responsiveness to posthypnotic suggestions and the ability to experience what appeared to be total amnesia when this was suggested.

The procedure, briefly stated, was as follows: After the *S* was placed in trance, amnesia for his own life history was induced. He was then given a pseudo-life history which was essentially the same as that described by Ashley, Harper, and Runyon. The poor state was induced first, then the rich state, and finally the normal state. The *S* judged coin sizes in all three states. The same *S* was run with both imagined coins and with real coins presented in all three states. Also in all three states, he was given brass slugs which were called "lead," "silver," "gold," and "platinum." The brass was of a very whitish color so that it could conceivably have been the appropriate metal.

Results

The results are summarized in Figure 1b, which presents the subjects' average coin-size estimates. The data are essentially identical to those obtained by Ashley, Harper, and Runyon (see Fig. 1a). The data on the size estimates of "slugs" successively called silver, gold, and platinum were also similar to those presented by Ashley, Harper, and Runyon in their series using a lead slug. All of the four subjects were able to describe correctly the purpose of the experiment and the hypotheses of the investigator who originally designed the experiment.

Discussion

The data from the pilot study imply that the present procedure effectively reproduces that of Ashley, Harper, and Runyon. Both in terms of the quantitative results and the observed behavior of our *S*, no significant differences emerge.

The only essential difference between these data and those obtained by Ashley, Harper, and Runyon relates to the inquiry procedure. The results confirm the first two hypotheses. 1. The *S* in an experiment is able to express some demand characteristics of the procedure, if careful inquiry is done and his initial resistance is penetrated in a clinical fashion. 2. The majority of *S*s may perceive the same demand characteristics of the experiment and these may be the same as the hypothesis being tested. However, the third hypothesis has yet to be dealt with.

It is interesting to note that two of the four *S*s who were specifically questioned about this point denied vehemently that they were influenced during the experiment by an awareness of the experimenter's hypothesis. But the *S*'s verbalization during inquiry cannot be accepted at face value. As long as the *S* recognizes and is able to verbalize the demand characteristics of the experiment, they may play a significant role in his experimental behavior, although to demonstrate that they do so requires supporting evidence. It is with this further evidence that the main study is concerned.

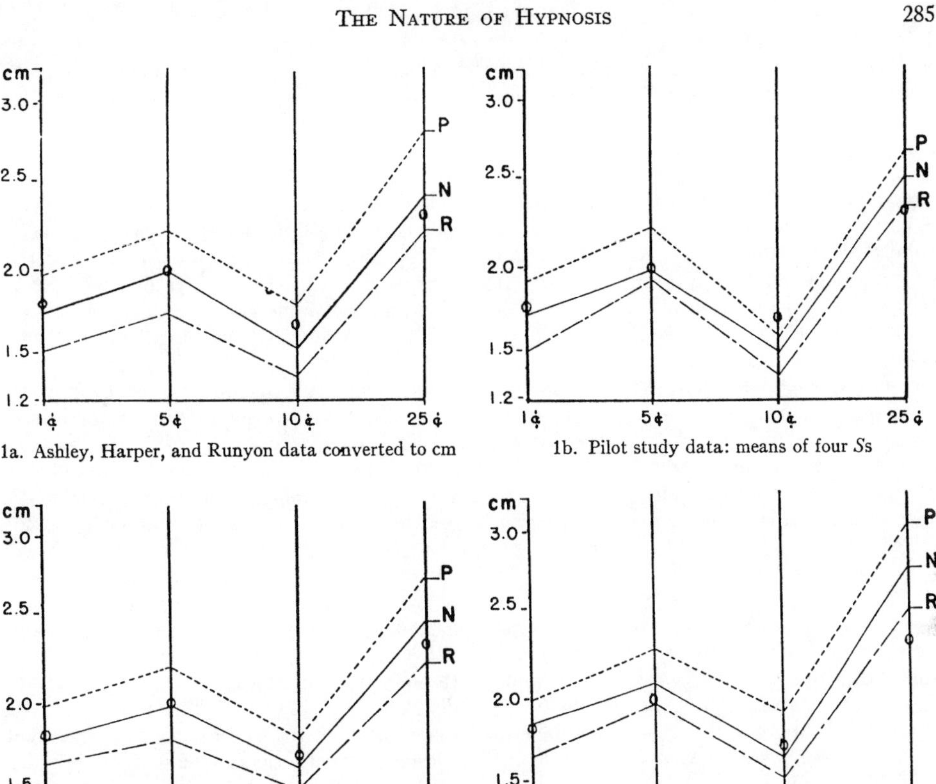

1a. Ashley, Harper, and Runyon data converted to cm

1b. Pilot study data: means of four *S*s

1c. Mean performance of "real" *S*s ($N = 7$)

1d. Mean performance of "fake" *S*s* ($N = 10$)

FIG. 1. COMPARISON OF ASHLEY, HARPER, AND RUNYON DATA WITH DATA FROM PRESENT REPLICATIONS (Legend: [R] = Rich; [P] = Poor; [N] = Normal; [O] = Actual coin size)

* One *S* (B. S.) was highly atypical and therefore excluded. See Fig. 2(b) for his performance.

Main Experiment

While the data found in the pilot study are consistent with the hypothesis that the demand characteristics of the experimental procedure may determine behavior, they are open to several serious objections.

The greatest single problem relates to the technique of inquiry and the interpretation of the data obtained in this fashion. It is important to have an objective method of rating how well the *S* perceives the demand characteristics of the experimental situation. The study was therefore designed so that the *S*'s inquiry would be rated by independent judges who did not have available to them the *S*'s data, but who would only have the opportunity of reading transcripts of the inquiry.

Another problem is a bias inherent in the inquiry procedure. Some *S*s who do not perceive the demand characteristics while engaged in the formal experimental procedure may perceive them during the inquiry. In such a case, and if the demand characteristics rather than the experimental variables determine the response, then the inquiry may indicate that the *S* should have responded a certain way when in fact he did not. However, the reverse should not occur.

The question still remains as to whether the *S*'s perception of the demand characteristics is responsible for his behavior, or whether it is due to the operation of the "intended" experimental variables. This question was dealt with by including a control group that could not conceivably be construed as experiencing a "psychologically rich and poor state." If it could be demonstrated that a group of *S*s who do not experience the "rich and poor state" but are exposed to the demand characteristics of the procedure also show the data reported, it would be justifiable to attribute the results to the demand characteristics rather than to a presumed change in the psychological organization of the individual because of being "psychologically rich and poor." The control group thus permits inferences without reliance on the inquiry.

A group of *S*s who were not in hypnotic trance and did not manifest amnesia should provide such a control group. They would, of course, have to go through the same procedure as the "real trance" group. Such a group of *S*s would be asked to "play act" being in hypnosis and go through the whole procedure as if they were real *S*s. This group of *S*s would not truly consider themselves as psychologically rich or poor. In these *S*s no amnesia could be induced, and their behavior would clearly be that of a group of persons acting under three different sets of instructions—act as though you were poor, rich, and yourself.

This type of procedure is open to an important objection. Experimenter bias could play a major role. While the procedure and the wording of instructions would be the same, it would be possible unwittingly to include a variety of cues which could differentially shape the behavior of the two classes of *S*s. A blind technique is thus necessitated, in which the experimenter would not know which *S*s were "real" and which were "fake."

Such a stratagem presupposes that a "fake" *S* can simulate hypnosis sufficiently well to deceive the experimenter. However, there is a widely held opinion in the literature that it is impossible to simulate hypnosis successfully (Jenness, 1944; Stokvis, 1955). Cursory attempts by the author to have *S*s fake trance showed that the *S*'s efforts were half-hearted and obviously transparent.

In the usual faking situation, the experimenter knows that the *S* is faking, and the *S* is aware that the experimenter knows it; the usual purpose of this situation is to demonstrate the difficulties of fooling an experienced hypnotist. Clearly, the experimenter is not really expecting the *S* to be able to carry out his task effectively, and the *S* is aware of this. Thus, the *S*, who is anxious to please the experimenter, is in actuality motivated to give an unsuccessful performance. Furthermore, since the *S* is aware that the experimenter knows that he is acting, the *S* feels, with good cause, that it is impossible to deceive the hypnotist. There is a marked tendency to smile during induction procedure and in response to suggestions that might be construed as foolish, as well as to ask "How am I doing?" at intervals. Any suggestions that evoke even mild discomfort are followed only briefly and half-heartedly.

Most classical texts and modern authorities agree that hypnosis cannot be faked easily and "if a subject attempts to fake, tests for anaesthesia will permit ready recognition" (Estabrooks, 1948; LeCron & Bordeaux, 1947, p. 103; Mayer, 1951). However, the author has, upon two occasions, been taken in by *S*s who had apparently faked their way through the procedure and who subsequently disclosed the fact. In discussions with other hypnotists, he found that all who had had considerable experience could recall similar instances.[4] These experiences are usually explained by stating that such *S*s must really have been in the trance state or they would not have been able to act as well as they had, a view that is supported by the literature on hypnosis. The report of the *S* that he has not really been in hypnosis is thus lightly passed over, since "subjective reports are really not reliable." It is the author's opinion that it is dangerous to ignore the conviction of the *S*, expressed in good faith, that he did not experience the amnesia or anaesthesia or any other trance phenomena that he appeared to have experienced; and that it is indeed possible to construct a situation that would facilitate the successful "faking" of a hypnotic trance.

To do so it is necessary to motivate the *S* to

[4] In this respect, it is interesting to note that Pattie (1937) was sufficiently concerned with being deceived by a faking *S* that he asked each *S* to sign a statement "I, realizing that the experiment performed on me will probably be published in a scientific journal, solemnly declare that I was not faking or imitating the hypnotic trance but that I was genuinely hypnotized and do not remember the events of the experimental periods."

act the part of a hypnotic *S*—not to go into a trance—and for him to believe that it is possible to convince the hypnotist that he really is in trance. Accordingly, a situation was set up in which the *S* knew that the hypnotist would not know in advance whether or not he was really in trance. Further, it was so structured that the *S* would perceive the desire of the experimenters for him to do a successful job of faking. Finally, the situation was presented as a challenge that provided ample motivation for the *S* to tolerate unpleasant suggestions or tests.[5]

Training of Subjects

College students from Harvard and Brandeis were used as *S*s. All *S*s had been present during a lecture about hypnosis and a demonstration of the phenomenon given by the author in the context of an introductory psychology course. All *S*s were volunteers who agreed to take part in the study at the time of the lectures. No *S*s were paid. All had also been tested and rated by investigators other than the author for "suggestibility," in at least one screening session. All *S*s in the real trance group had further training with the author's associates. In order to satisfy criteria for depth of trance, they had to manifest the ability to respond to all the usual hypnotic suggestions with special emphasis on analgesia, visual hallucinations, negative auditory hallucinations, amnesia induced by suggestion, and simple posthypnotic suggestions.

The fake group of *S*s was drawn from the same population as the others but did not have special training in entering trance beyond the first screening session. They were all informed of their task in the manner described below.

The experimental procedure was administered to all the *S*s by the author, and he was given no information or cues by his associates as to which group any *S* might belong. Nor was he informed of the number of real and of fake *S*s. There were seven real *S*s and 11 fake *S*s.

Special Procedure for Faking Subjects

Prior to the experiment, the faking *S*s were told by an investigator other than the hypnotist:

> We're doing a study in which we would like you to take part. You recall some time ago you volunteered as a subject for some hypnotic experiments. We would like you not to go into a hypnotic trance; however, Dr. Orne, who will be working with you, will not know whether you are a real or a fake subject. He will go through trance induction with you, and then several tests and an experiment. We would like you to act as if you were entering a trance, but I don't want you to go into a trance. Your job is to fake the whole thing and to try to fool Dr. Orne. He knows that I may have some people trying to fake their way through the experiment but he has no idea who they are. I would like you, as a special favor, to try to do the best possible job of fooling him; to really convince him that you are in trance. This is quite difficult but a very important part of the experiment. I am trying to find out whether people are capable of doing this successfully. One of the tests which he will do with you will involve a harmless but somewhat painful electric shock. After the trance part, which you will have been faking, he will ask you some questions about it. Again, I don't want you to let on that you have been faking, and I want you to try to answer these questions as though you had been in hypnosis. Please keep on playing this part until I give you a signal. After the signal you can tell him what really happened. The signal will be that I will turn off the light on a box which will be on the table in front of you. I am sure that you will be able to do a good job of it.

The *S*s usually objected by saying that they did not know how a hypnotized *S* would act. They were told that although this feeling was understandable, others had been able to carry it off and that besides, they themselves had seen other *S*s go into a hypnotic trance during a previous demonstration.

The motivation for the *S* to act the role of the hypnotized individual is fairly clear. The author had been presented to the *S*s as an authority in the field of hypnosis and they had been taken into confidence by one of his associates in an attempt to fool him. Thus, on the one hand they were contributing to the advance of knowledge, on the other, they would have the pleasurable experience of "putting one over" on one of their teachers.

[5] After the completion of this study a previous reference to the use of a faking subject as a form of control was encountered. In an experiment on hypnotic pain suppression, Dynes (1932) asked a member of the psychology department to talk to *S*s privately and have them fake a trance the next time. The *S*s thought that he knew nothing of the plan and carried out the request to fake. However, Dynes himself did know and reports no difficulty in distinguishing this state from the real trance. It would have been interesting to know whether Dynes would have found it quite so easy to distinguish the behavior had he not known in advance.

Experimental Procedure

At the experimental session the *S* was exposed to trance induction. The Erickson hand levitation technique as described by Wolberg (1948) was used. After the *S* appeared to be in trance, a series of tests were done such as: hand clasp, analgesia, negative auditory hallucination, and positive visual hallucination.

When these tests had been completed, the *S* was told that his name would appear on his forehead and that he would feel it as though it were there in Braille. After this suggestion had been accepted, he was informed that if he would wipe this off he would forget everything about himself. Once he had accepted the suggestion of total amnesia, the rich state and the poor state was induced in a fashion identical to that used by Ashley et al. (1951). The *S* was then asked to make coin-size judgments of a penny, nickel, dime, and quarter, again using the original Bruner-Goodman box. He was required to make six coin-size judgments of each coin in each state. The final set of judgments was made in his normal state, but with the suggestion that he had no recollection of anything that had happened since he entered trance. The rich and poor states were randomized as well as the order of the coins. A balanced design could not be achieved in respect to coin order because of the number of *S*s used, but it was approximated as far as feasible. The hypnotist-experimenter did not know the key to the order and was merely told in each instance which state he was to run first and with which coin to start.

The procedure, used by Ashley, Harper, and Runyon and in the pilot study, of estimating the size of the lead slug which was called lead, silver, gold, and platinum, was omitted.

At the completion of the coin-size judgments, an inquiry was performed as previously described. This inquiry was the same for all *S*s. At the completion of the inquiry, both in the hypnotic and wake states, the light of the Bruner-Goodman apparatus was turned off, which was the signal for the fake group to tell what really happened. If the *S*s were real, this had no meaning to them, and the experiment was completed. Those of the fake group were asked a series of questions as to whether or not they had been in trance. They were also asked about their performance, why they had acted as they did on some points, and if and when they felt anxious. Finally, they were asked whether they thought that they had given themselves away; if so, when and why. All of these inquiries were completely tape recorded and transcribed so that, subsequently, judges could rate what each subject perceived as the hypothesis being tested.

Results

1. *Objective Findings–Group Results.* Figure 1 displays a comparison between the present data and those of Ashley, Harper, and Runyon (Fig. 1a); in Fig. 1c, the results of the hypnotic *S*s are averaged in the manner described by Ashley, Harper, and Runyon; in Fig. 1d, the results of the "fake" *S*s are averaged in the same manner. All three graphs present essentially the same configuration. In all cases the judgments in the poor state are the largest, judgments in the rich state smallest, while judgments in the "normal" state fall between.

2. *Results for Individual Subjects.* Figures 2a and 2b give the results for each "real" or "fake" *S*. *S*s varied widely in their response to the experimental task, not all of them yielding a configuration that corresponds to the group average. While Ashley, Harper, and Runyon unfortunately do not give their individual results, they report considerable variation.

3. *Comparison of Judges' Ratings with Objective Categorization.* Using analysis of variance for each individual *S*, it is possible to test statistically whether there are significant differences between *S*'s coin-size estimates in any combination of the three states and the direction of significant differences. Ignoring the "normal" judgments, the possibilities reduce to three categories: no significant differences between rich and poor, poor significantly larger than rich, and rich significantly larger than poor. Each *S*'s coin-size judgments were classified into one of the three categories on the basis of statistical analysis considering differences not significant at the .05 level as no difference.

The transcribed postexperimental inquiries were given to two independent judges to rate the *S*'s perception of the hypothesis being tested at the time of the experiment in terms of the same three categories. The judges had no contact with the *S*s or each other. Table 3 shows a comparison in terms of the

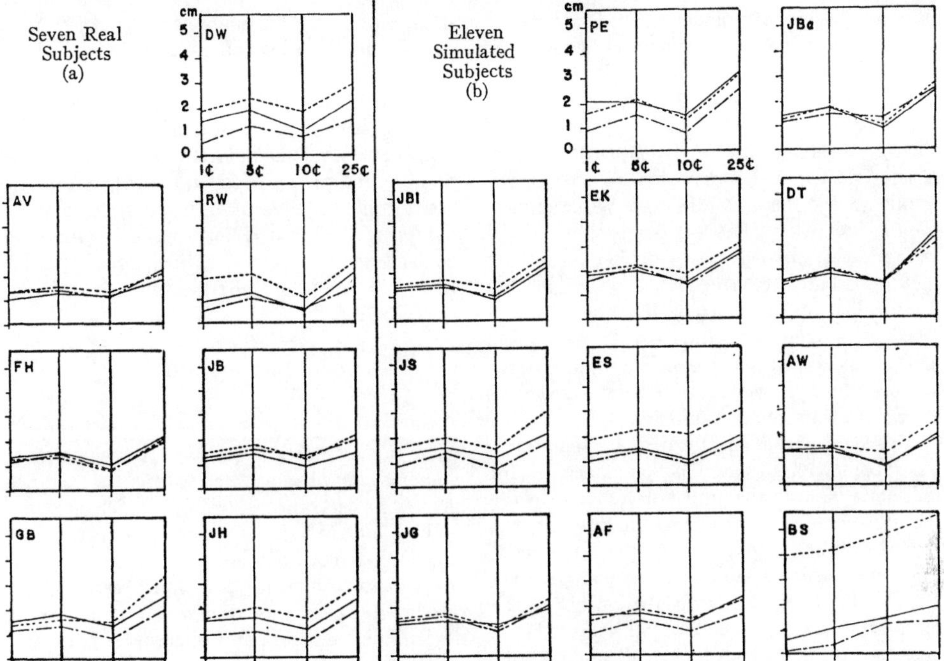

FIG. 2. GRAPHS OF INDIVIDUAL SUBJECTS
(Legend: [-----] = Poor; [——] = Normal; [—·—] = Rich)

TABLE 3

A COMPARISON OF JUDGED AND ACTUAL CATEGORIES OF RESPONSE

Subject	Major Categories		
	J1	J2	Actual
G. B.	II	II	II
F. H.	II	II	I
J. H.	II	II	II
A. U.	II[a]	I	I
R. W.	II	II	II
D. W.	II	II	II
J. Ba.	I	I	I
P. E.	II	II	II
J. Bl.	II	II	II
J. G.	I	I	I
A. W.	II	II	II
E. S.	II	II	II
J. S.	II	II	II
D. T.	I	II	I
A. F.	II	II	II
E. K.	II	II	II
B. S.	II	II	II

NOTE.—Key to symbols: I. No significant difference; II. Poor significantly larger than rich; III. Rich significantly larger than poor.

Two judges were used (J1 and J2). Note that no *S* actually belongs in Category III and that neither judge placed any *S* within it.

[a] Judge undecided about I or II here but chose II as better estimate.

three categories between the ratings of the two judges and the individual's responses. There is a high degree of correspondence between the judges' ratings and *S*'s performance.

Testing the null hypothesis of no systematic correspondence between judges' rating and *S*'s coin-size judgments leads to its rejection for each judge (.015, Fisher Exact Test); combining the significance levels of the two judges leads to an over-all significance of less than .01.

Discussion

The data obtained from the seven hypnotized *S*s are essentially identical to the findings of Ashley, Harper, and Runyon, and virtually indistinguishable from the performance of the 11 stimulating *S*s. These results confirm the hypothesis that it is possible for an experimental design that omits a crucial aspect (hypnotic amnesia) of the original dependent variable to elicit similar responses as long as the same demand characteristics are present.

The subjective experience of members of the simulating group was radically different from that of the *S*s in deep trance. The *S*s readily described their conscious efforts to "second guess" what the experimenter would expect of them if they were actually in hypnosis. The data obtained from the simulating group are the result of a concerted effort on the part of the *S*s to respond in a way identical to hypnotized *S*s. The subjective experience of the hypnotized group was different. While clinical inquiry revealed the *S*s' perception of the author's expectations, they denied that these factors had any effect upon their performance. This denial on the part of the hypnotized *S* does not, of course, mean that their perception of the experimental purpose was unimportant. It does mean, however, that they themselves were not aware of its significance.

An investigation of the demand characteristics perceived by each *S* may account for individual results that did not conform to the group average, as an examination of the judges' ratings confirms. It was discovered that the inquiry procedure had not been refined sufficiently to permit prediction of the *S*s' performance in the "normal" state. However, performance in the "rich" and "poor" states could be predicted with a high degree of accuracy from the judges' ratings of the *S*'s perception of the experimental purpose. No *S* reversed the expected trend by making his coin-size judgments larger in the rich state than in the poor state. No *S* was rated by either judge as having perceived this to be the hypothesis of the experiment. Twelve subjects made the coin-size estimates significantly larger in the poor state than in the rich state. All 12 *S*s were rated by both judges as having perceived this to be the author's hypothesis. Five *S*s failed to significantly differentiate their coin-size judgments between the rich and poor state. Of these five subjects, four were rated by either one or both judges as having failed to perceive the demand characteristics of the experiment.

The inquiry data thus support Hypothesis *3a*, that if the majority of *S*s perceive the same demand characteristics, then *S*s who fail to perceive these demand characteristics should not show the behavior characteristic of the group.

The present experiments do not bear on the validity of the Bruner-Goodman effect. The Ashley, Harper, and Runyon experiment was used, rather, as an example of a study that appears methodologically sound, but in which demand characteristics seem to be the major determinant of the *S*'s performance. The implications seem clear: demand characteristics may determine behavior in hypnotic experiments. Before an effect can legitimately be attributed to hypnosis, it is necessary to demonstrate that it is not primarily a function of demand characteristics. Such proof appears to require the use of blind techniques and adequate inquiry.

THE INFLUENCE OF MOTIVATION ON HYPNOTIC BEHAVIOR[6]

In studying the nature of the hypnotic trance, the question arises as to which phenomena are primary and consistent components of the trance state and which are secondary derivatives. Let us postulate that increased motivation is a constant accompaniment of the hypnotic state. The present phase of the research was designed to show that certain phenomena long viewed as part and parcel of the hypnotic state may more parsimoniously be viewed as derivatives of increased motivation, and can be reproduced *pari passu* by other motivational techniques that have no direct relationship to hypnosis.

For years it has been claimed that there is an increase in physical capacity during the trance state. In part this claim has been based on casual observation, the favorite example being that of the stage hypnotist who places a subject in deep trance across two chairs and permits one or more individuals to stand or sit upon him. This "experiment," with variations, is often cited as irrefutable evidence for increased physical capacity. Another group of frequently cited observations are those concerning the ability of the subject to maintain his hand in an outstretched position for extended periods of time without evidence of fatigue. On the basis of this type of data, estimates of greatly increased physical capacity have been made (McDougall, 1926; Moll, 1904).

An early study by Nicholson (1920, p. 89) maintained that "during the hypnotic sleep the capacity for work seemed practically end-

[6] This experiment was originally reported in German (Orne, 1954).

less." Unfortunately, no quantitative data were given, and the study was poorly controlled. In a meticulous investigation, Williams (1930) showed no difference between hypnotic and wake states in the ability to maintain the arm in an outstretched position. However, this study failed to employ suggestions to the effect that the arm would not get tired and could not drop. In another similar investigation, using an ergograph and employing appropriate hypnotic suggestions, Williams (1929) found a 12 to 16% increment in the trance. More recently, Roush (1951) showed an increment in performance in hypnosis significant at better than the .05% level using the arm dynomometer, the hand dynomometer, and hanging by the hands, as measures of fatigue.

All the experiments performed by psychologists in the laboratory have followed orthodox scientific methods insofar as a standard set of instructions was given to the *S* to hold a weight, pull an ergograph, or perform a similar task in both the nonhypnotic and hypnotic states. The better experiments used the usual ABBA arrangement to control fatigue or practice effects. Any increment in performance was defined as an increase in capacity due to trance. It is necessary here to question the logic on which the interpretation of these results is based. While these experiments undoubtedly show that instructions given in trance state result in increased performance over that achieved by the same instructions in the wake state, they do not necessarily show an increase in capacity. Alternatively, the *S* may be more willing to exert himself while in hypnosis. The governing factor could be the increase in the *S*'s motivation to comply with the experimenter's request rather than an increased capacity to comply. The instructions, while identical in wording, may be experienced as quite different by the *S* in hypnosis and the waking state. The request to hold a weight at arm's length, given in trance, may be a highly motivating cue or "suggestion," especially if the *S* is told that he is to feel very powerful and not fatigued. The identically worded request in the wake state is perceived as a request by the experimenter and may be followed if good rapport exists between experimenter and *S*. However, as the discomfort of the task increases, the *S* becomes increasingly disinclined to comply. Viewed in this context, the reported experimental results do not necessarily imply that physical capacity is in fact increased in trance but, rather, that the trance state increases performance.

Procedure

Nine *S*s in deep trance were asked to hold a kilogram weight at arm's length. This was done in such a way as to derive maximal benefit from the peculiar nature of the trance state. Thus the *S* was told to hallucinate a table, and only after the table was both seen and felt by the *S* was the suggestion given that the right arm would feel no fatigue and no pain.

All the standard tests of deep trance were met in each *S*. A kilogram weight was placed in the *S*'s right hand, and the *S* was instructed to place it on the imagined table, to continue holding it with his fingers, and under no circumstances to drop it or his arm. Continuous suggestions were given to the effect that he would be able to hold onto the weight, that his arm would not get tired, etc., and that he would continue to see the table. The end point was when the *S* was no longer able to hold up his arm and began to come out of trance. At that point he was reassured, told to drop the weight, and deep trance suggestions were again given. After some minutes, and having made certain deep trance was again established, the *S* was awakened with a carefully induced posthypnotic amnesia. The *S* was not told the length of his performance.[7] For the second part of the experiment, which was done within half an hour of the first, the *S*, not now under hypnosis, was instructed as follows:

> This is a most important part of our experiment. It is very important for us to know your endurance and

[7] In the preceding section it was pointed out that the posthypnotic amnesia induced in hypnosis is not tantamount to an ablation of memory. One may be justified in assuming that the *S*s do not know their hypnotic performance, not because of the amnesia but, rather, because they were never informed of the length of time they held the weight in hypnosis. A common belief that the *S* in hypnosis has a perfect sense of time would lead to the conclusion that this is not an adequate safeguard. Fortunately, a very thorough study of the time sense under hypnosis was conducted by Guenther Klaus in a doctoral dissertation (University of Freiburg, Germany, 1948) which demonstrates unequivocally that the time sense is not improved by hypnosis.

TABLE 4
COMPARISON OF SUBJECTS' PERFORMANCE IN HYPNOTIC AND WAKE STATE

Subject	Hypnosis		Waking	
	Minutes	Seconds	Minutes	Seconds
1	4	05	5	33
2[a]	4	40	6	25
3	4	38	8	06
4 (*a*)[b]	6	05	3	29
(*b*)	5	50	10	02
5	7	07	7	57
6	10	05	16	00
7	4	52	5	49
8	5	20	5	32
9[c]	4	57	2 (*a*)	10
			5 (*b*)	09

[a] This experiment was performed in 1950. In 1957, it came to my attention that this *S* feels that he simulated completely throughout this experiment. At the time, I was totally unaware of this possibility and the *S* was in trance by all the usual criteria.

[b] *S* dropped the weight after 3′ 29″ in the wake state. The next day, care was taken to motivate him adequately. While the hypnotic performance was only 15″ below the previous day, his wake performance now exceeded 10′.

[c] This *S* suddenly dropped the weight without warning in the wake state after 2′ 10″. She was encouraged and after a 20′ time lag again held the weight. This time her performance was 5′ 09″. This performance in itself is better than her hypnotic performance of 4′ 57″; however, it might seem that the waking performance was better than this, as the 2′ 10″ period was not given credit.

physical capacity. What I want you to do is a very difficult task. It does not look difficult but it is. I want you to hold this kilogram weight at arm's length. Your hand will get tired and it will take great effort to do this. There is a natural tendency to drop the weight if your hand gets tired. However, it is vital that we get your true capacity. Surprisingly enough, our female subjects have been able to hold the weight for T minutes. [The time T given would be his previous performance during hypnosis rounded off to the nearest half minute.] Our male subjests have been able to hold the weight at least T + ½ minutes. I realize that this is a difficult and painful task. Just to make it interesting we will try a game. At T minus 2 minutes we will start you off at 5 cents. At T minus one and a half, we will double that and make it 10 cents. At T minus one, 20 cents. At T minus one half, 40 cents. At T, 80 cents and at T plus one half, $1.60.

Then the *S* was told that while we could not afford to pay over $1.60, we were, of course, interested in how long he could actually hold the weight. One final point was explained to him:

While we often feel that we are so tired that we cannot go on, this is not really true. One can rarely be so tired as not to be able to continue for 30 seconds. Accordingly, I would like you to give me one-half minute's notice before you actually drop the weight.

Results

Table 4 gives the results for the nine *S*s tested. All but one *S* in the wake state immediately exceeded hypnotic performance. This *S* held the weight for 6 min. 5 sec. in trance, a very remarkable performance, but in a subsequent wake state dropped the weight after only 3½ min. The exception demonstrates very clearly that it is necessary to ego-involve the person in the task and to convince him of his ability to do it. He reported that the seven minutes that had been given as an illustration of "average performance" had seemed so long, and his hand became so tired after three minutes that he felt convinced that he would be unable to come even close to the average, so therefore "why bother to try?" The next day the *S* was more carefully motivated and encouraged. He was then able to hold the weight for over 10 minutes.

Discussion

This experiment does not purport to prove that there is no increase in physical capacity in the trance state. Because of the motivating nature of the trance state, and the operational difficulty in obtaining equal motivational states, it becomes a technical impossibility to prove conclusively whether increased physical capacity is produced or not. The data, however, do show that the usually observed increase in performance of trance *S*s may be accounted for by motivational difference.

From a theoretical viewpoint the reinterpretations to which this study had led seem most significant. As long as we believe physical capacity to be in fact increased by the simple expedient of the induced trance, it becomes necessary to look for the focus of the trance in something neurophysiological. If, on the other hand, we can understand the apparent increase in physical capacity observed during the trance state in terms of differences of motivation, we are then led to view hypnosis in psychological terms. It is clear that this study says nothing about why the trance tends to increase motivation nor does it even prove that this is so. It merely shows that adequate motivation in the wake state leads to levels of performance equal or better than those found in the trance.

An objection that might be raised takes the form of the question as to what would happen if similar motivational techniques were used in the trance state to those in the wake state. But this question has little bearing on the essential point. If application of these techniques should produce a trance performance greater than the wake performance, it could be interpreted as the result of combined effects of ego-motivation and the postulated increased motivation associated with hypnosis. If, on the other hand, performance in trance were not greater it could be argued that the type of ego-motivation used is not germane to the trance state.

It may, finally, be argued that the *S* in the wake state is, in fact, still in hypnosis, since the same experimenter who induced hypnosis conducts the second phase. Perhaps *S*s performed better in the wake state because of the demand characteristics of the experiment, i.e., my expectation that they should do so! It is not easy wholly to refute this argument. That all previous studies are open to the same criticism does not answer the question. The clinical observation that the *S* does not look, act, or feel in any way the same in the hypnotic part and the waking part appears much more relevant. Nevertheless, I hope sometime to repeat the study with the aid of another hypnotist who believes in "the power of hypnosis" and who, therefore, expects *S* to do better in hypnosis than in the wake state. If it were possible for me to enable *S*s subsequently to exceed their hypnotic performance, it would go far toward removing this objection, of which I was aware during the collection of data. A different way to check the results would compare the performances of "fake" and "real" *S*s, using the strategy developed in the section entitled Cues Implicit in an Experimental Design.

Real vs. "Fake" Hypnotic Subjects

The "real-fake" technique, a method of enabling *S*s to simulate hypnosis, was developed to demonstrate the effect of role-play artifact on trance behavior. Differences between the real and faking *S* that cannot be accounted for by the faking situation may be viewed as characteristic of hypnosis. Some behavior shown by both groups may, of course, also be a true characteristic of hypnosis since the fact that someone is able to simulate a given type of behavior does not indicate that it is not genuine in the nonsimulating group. For example, that it is fairly easy to simulate the compulsive quality of the trance does not imply that this quality is not germane to hypnosis. However, assertions that volitional capacities can be transcended in hypnosis would seem to require showing that faking *S*s cannot produce similar performances.

The present use of real and faking *S*s in a blind design appears to offer several advantages. It permits a rigorous control, in terms of behavior, of inquiry procedures designed to elicit demand characteristics of experiments. In the faking situation, the variable assumed to be the cause of the behavior can be omitted. If such behavior still occurs, it can then be accounted for adequately by the implicit demands of the situation. In this respect the technique may have useful application in other areas of psychology. With respect to hypnosis itself, the technique permits a rigorous control of experiments that claim to demonstrate transcendence of volitional capacities. It also helps to eliminate many biases almost universally present in hypnosis research and throws into relief certain differences between the "real" and "faking" groups which can then be attributed to the hypnotic state. These differences may be highly germane to the essence of hypnosis and seem to have been obscured by the overwhelmingly impressive nature of the phenomenon.

The Faking Subject

The situation of the simulating *S* may be viewed as one where he can (*a*) contribute to research by pleasing one experimenter and (*b*) satisfy different other needs by fooling another experimenter. The possibility of simultaneously satisfying usually incompatible needs leads to a state of peculiarly high motivation. Thus, he is highly motivated to play the role of a hypnotized *S* and continues to do so even in the face of great discomfort, without, however, the alteration of consciousness and the subjective experience found in hypnosis.

It had been anticipated that there would be differences in the clinical appearance of the two groups of *S*s, both when going into trance and while in trance. Since the hand levitation technique (Wolberg, 1948) was used to induce trance, it was expected that the "faking" *S*s would lift their hands in a manner clearly indicating active volition rather than permitting the hand to rise slowly and gradually in response to a subjective feeling of lightness. Similar differences were anticipated in respect to eye-closure. When the inability to bend the extended right arm was suggested, differences were expected in the *S*'s attempts to do so. The *S*'s responses to negative auditory hallucinations and positive visual hallucinations, analgesia and anesthesia, pseudo identities in the trance, and amnesia for the trance were all expected to be means of differentiating the two groups. The discovery that most of the simulating *S*s did not differ behaviorally from those in deep trance came therefore with considerable surprise. True, it was possible to distinguish most of the "faking" group from the "real" group, but this discrimination was based on a clinical diagnosis with an inordinate amount of subjective uncertainty and about 20% error. With prior knowledge that an *S* is simulating hypnosis it is very easy for the observer to discern cues that reveal the "faking" nature of the "trance" behavior. Without such prior knowledge, these cues are obscure and judgments can be made only with a great deal of subjective uncertainty.[8] If it seems obvious to the experimenter that the *S* is faking, systematic error would again be introduced, and could affect the results. In such cases it seems desirable to discard the subject from the experiment, as was done in two instances in the present study.

Response to Pain in "Fake" and "Real" Subjects

Traditionally, hypnotists have viewed the induction of analgesia for highly painful stimuli as the best test for clearly distinguishing simulating *S*s from the *S*s in deep trance. The author expected, therefore, to find that reactions to pain would distinguish between the "real" and "fake" groups.

The technique for producing pain for testing hypnotic analgesia which the author had been using routinely involves forcible flexion of the two terminal phalanges of the little finger and pressure of the experimenter's thumbnail on the dorsal aspect of the middle of the second phalanx of the *S*'s little finger. These techniques failed to discriminate between the two groups. The "faking" group reported pain but indicated that they had had little or no difficulty in suppressing their reaction.

In order to provide a more painful, though still safe, stimulus a Harvard inductorium was employed. Standard Grass silver electrodes were applied to the sides of the index fingers and fixed with adhesive tape. It was found that the "faking" group flinched less and tolerated more pain than the "real" group. Actually, almost all of the *S*s tolerated the maximal stimulation that could be applied by the inductorium.

Another procedure, not particularly painful in itself, was designed to maximize anxiety about pain. Negative auditory hallucinations were induced and at the same time an analgesia of one hand. A match was then lighted close to the *S*'s ear and held under the third finger of this extended "pain insensitive" hand long enough to produce painful heat without causing a second degree burn. The experimenter tested the time interval on himself each time in order to determine what constituted a safe but painful stimulus. In no instance was an *S* ever subjected to a blistering burn. Again it was found that there were no noticeable differences between the simulating group and the deeply hypnotized *S*s. However, postexperimental inquiry revealed that the simulating group experienced a high level of anxiety and some pain during the procedure, while those in trance felt little or no discomfort.

To summarize the results of these informal experiments with pain, no clear-cut behavioral differences between "real" and "fake" *S*s have as yet been found, no matter what type of stimulus was employed. However, on post-experimental inquiries a very real difference was found in the *S*'s attitude toward this part

[8] The experimenter is currently attempting to study systematically the cues perceived as indicative of faking by an observer who knows that the *S* is simulating to see if consistent patterns appear. However, results thus far indicate that observers who had experience with observing faking *S*s, knowing that they were simulating, did not thereby become more able to discriminate in the absence of such knowledge.

of the experiment and in his report of subjective pain.

Differences Between "Real" and "Fake" Subjects

The faking *S*'s condition is characterized by the presence of faking behavior and the absence of hypnosis. If we wish to regard true hypnotic behavior as the difference between what can be observed in faking and real *S*s, it is necessary to take into account the characteristics of the faking *S*s introduced by the act of simulating.

One of the observed differences is related to an attempt by the simulating group to avoid commitments whenever possible. In some aspects, the situation of the simulating group is analogous to that of the malingerer, although the motivation to malinger is different and usually stronger. The person who is simulating a disease attempts to give the appropriate behavioral and symptomological manifestations without subjectively experiencing the symptoms that would be present with the actual disease. The real hypnotic group is more akin to the hysteric who reacts to subjectively real symptoms without organic pathology. Rorschach studies on malingerers in the military service (Rosenberg & Feldberg, 1944; Ross, 1944) reveal a typical syndrome. The most significant aspect is a marked constriction of the record, with occasional bizarre responses, a feature that is understandable as an attempt to avoid giving oneself away in the face of an unknown situation while attempting to appear cooperative. Applied to the present situation, these features suggest a tendency for the simulating group to avoid responding whenever possible and when forced to respond in an unstructured situation to give the safest possible answer. Just this occurred. In the replication of the Ashley, Harper, and Runyon study, it was observed that the "faking" *S*s would tend to be more hesitant in giving a false life history after being told that they were rich or poor. This reluctance cannot be considered a particularly meaningful finding for the theory of hypnosis, since it should rather be attributed to the psychological situation analogous to malingering, and not to the presence or absence of hypnosis.

Differences observed which may be attributed to the presence or absence of trance were with respect to: (*a*) congruence, the appropriateness of a response to the apparent level of trance, and (*b*) trance logic, the apparently simultaneous perception and response to both hallucinations and reality without any apparent attempts to satisfy a need for logical consistency.

The "fake" *S*s tended to exhibit behavior that was incongruous with what clinically appeared to be the depth of trance. For example, an *S* who responded very slowly to hand levitation was given the suggestion that he could hear only my voice. This negative auditory hallucination was tested by rubbing the thumb against the first two fingers of the hand close to the *S*'s ear and asking him "do you hear anything but my voice?" A response congruent with the *S*'s behavior of slow hand levitation and in a medium trance would be either no response or a *slight* nod or shaking of the head. Frequently, a repetition of the question would be required to elicit even a nod of the head. An *immediate* and emphatic *verbal* denial of any auditory perception other than my voice was considered a typical incongruent response—incongruent both in respect to speed and modality of response.

The most reliable criterion, as it turned out, may be termed trance logic.[9] It refers to the ability of the *S* to mix freely his perceptions derived from reality with those that stem from his imagination and are perceived as hallucinations. These perceptions are fused in a manner that ignores everyday logic. A good example of this process is the reaction of many *S*s in hypnosis who see a hallucination of a person sitting in a chair and describe it as "This is very peculiar, I can see Joe sitting in the chair and I can see the chair through him." This type of reaction, when made spontaneously, was absolutely diagnostic of the "real" *S*. Unfortunately, it did not occur spontaneously in every *S*; it was found, however, that "fake" *S*s *never* gave such a response.

In order to obtain the same type of data

[9] This seems intimately related to primary process thinking or autistic thinking. To avoid the developmental, pathological, and theoretical implications of these concepts a new phrase seems preferable to describe the clinically observable phenomenon.

that had proved to be so characteristic of hypnosis, a special situation was devised. Throughout the experiments, one of the co-experimenters was in the room with the *S* and the author, taking notes. At the beginning of the experiment he sat to the side of the *S*, well within his visual field. Once the *S*'s eyes were closed, the co-experimenter rose very silently and walked behind the *S* out of the *S*'s visual field. Subsequently, the *S* was instructed to open his eyes while still in deep trance and a hallucination of the associate sitting in the chair was induced. This hallucination was facilitated by the fact that during the initial part of the experiment, just prior to the *S*'s closing his eyes, the associate was actually sitting in the chair. After the hallucination appeared to be fully accepted by the *S*, and he appeared to be responding to the hallucination as though it were actually the associate, he was instructed to turn around and look at the associate now behind him with the question, "Who is that behind you?" Almost invariably the "real" *S* would look at the associate, then quickly turn back to look at the empty chair, and back at the associate. After looking back and forth between the hallucinated and the "real" associate, the *S*s indicated verbally that they were perceiving two images of the same person.[10] When asked about this, they tended to give bland responses such as "mirrors" or a "trick." Though they seemed somewhat confused, they did not become seriously disturbed.

The "fake" group, in most cases, either refused to see anyone behind them, or claimed that they could not recognize the person. Occasionally, they admitted recognizing the associate behind them and then claimed that the hallucination had vanished. (This reaction, while unusual among the real group, is occasionally found, especially if the *S* did not fully accept the initial hallucination.) Of approximately 30 "faking" *S*s, only two acted as if they saw two images of the same individual. The others, when asked during post-experimental inquiry about the reason for their response, gave a very significant answer. They stated that I had instructed them to hallucinate, the associate in the chair and therefore, when I asked who the individual behind them was, they had to deny seeing him, or if they saw him, recognizing him. After all, there was only one such individual and I had already told them that they were supposed to see him sitting in the chair. This logical conclusion determined the response given by simulating *S*s; it did not occur to the overwhelming majority of the "real" *S*s who saw two images without any difficulty. This finding appears to represent a valid and significant difference. The "real" *S* responds to a subjectively real image of the associate in the chair. When asked about an objectively real image of the same individual, he is able to perceive this as well. He can respond to perceptions that are subjectively real and determined by the suggested environment, as well as to his actual perceptions of the real world, without attempting to satisfy a possible need to make them logically compatible. The absence of expression of a need for logical consistency seems, at this point, to be one of the major characteristics of hypnosis.

Because it is my belief that the "essence" of hypnosis will be found in the subjective experiences of the *S*, I have become increasingly interested in a series of techniques attempting to obtain data about the actual feelings and experiences of the *S*. In the future, I intend to develop inquiry procedures that will include "casual conversation" with another *S* who, in reality, is an investigator. It is hoped to elicit cooperation from the *S*'s friends. Casual preliminary attempts using such procedures indicate that material obtained in this way may be quite illuminating and not accessible to direct inquiry by the experimenter.

A POINT OF VIEW TOWARD HYPNOSIS

While much of the research described here appears to be explaining away the hypnotic phenomenon, the intention is rather to differentiate its valid and significant aspects from what might be termed artifact. One of the problems inherent in any study of hypnosis is that of its definition. There is high consensus of opinion about what constitutes hypnosis in terms of a variety of scales. However, the

[10] This situation was originally discussed by Milton H. Erickson in a personal communication.

essential characteristics have remained obscure. A great many investigators have become impressed and fascinated by the apparent transcendence of normal physiological capacities in hypnosis. The present research program has made me increasingly skeptical of the experimental data that purport to support this view. However, clinical data obtained both by others and myself seem to show in a dramatic way that responses can be evoked in some *S*s which they themselves could not perform voluntarily. Such phenomena seem to be limited to *S*s who have a peculiar disposition in this direction. For example, authenticated cases of hypnotically induced blistering have been achieved only in individuals with previous dermatological histories.

One might hypothesize that the capacity to produce marked physiological alterations in hypnosis is confined to persons who have a readiness to somatize in the organ system being investigated, which will usually have been demonstrated by a history of similar pathology occurring spontaneously. Such findings do not preclude the possibility, of course, that a transcendence of normal volitional capacities in some areas may eventually be established in the laboratory as unequivocally due to hypnosis.

Aside from the controversial issue of such changes in physiological capacities, it appears that a universal effect of hypnosis on any *S* in deep trance can be delineated in terms of his subjective experience. Experience, after all, is not to be taken as an ephemeral or unimportant aspect of hypnosis but, rather, as extremely significant and, to the *S*, dramatic and striking.

Any *S* who has experienced deep trance will unhesitatingly describe this state as basically different from his normal one. He may be unable to explicate this difference, but he will invariably be quite definite and certain about its presence. Thus, one of the characteristics of hypnosis is that in deep trance the *S* experiences the state as discontinuous from his normal waking experience (though not always in the intermediate stages of trance). Hypnotic trance differs from pathological states, which may also be discontinuous, in that the *S* enters and leaves the state in accordance with previously established "rules of the game."

Another aspect of this altered subjective state is one which the *S* describes as an inability to resist a cue given by the hypnotist. (Interestingly enough, if the *S before entering the trance* decides not to follow a specific suggestion he is able to resist it.)[11] The uniformity with which this compulsive quality is reported tends to make us accept it as a characteristic of hypnosis. However, it will not emerge as a difference in behavior between real and faking *S*s.

Finally, an important attribute of hypnosis is a potentiality for the *S* to experience as subjectively real suggested alterations in his environment that do not conform with reality. In trance, the waking distinction between an imagined idea and what is perceived externally to the organism fades, and images may be perceived as originating from external reality. Thus, the waking individual, no matter how hard he tries to imagine that he saw someone sitting opposite to him, might at best be able to evoke some kind of imagery but would always be aware of the distinction between this and reality. The *S* in deep hypnosis may well be unaware of the distinction, though at some level he will always be able to discriminate.

In sum, the principal features of the hypnotic state are seen as changes in the subjective experience which are characterized by (*a*) discontinuity from normal waking experience, (*b*) a compulsion to follow the cues given by the hypnotist, (*c*) a potentiality for experiencing, as subjectively real, distortions of perception, memory, or feeling based on "suggestions" by the hypnotist rather than on objective reality, (*d*) the ability to tolerate logical inconsistencies that would be disturbing to the individual in the wake state.

SUMMARY

This paper has attempted to delineate some aspects of hypnotic phenomena which can be

[11] However, suggestions that are inconsistent with the basic "rules of the game" governing the implicit contract between hypnotist and *S*, as seen by the *S*, are, as a rule, not followed: e.g., antisocial and self-destructive acts, or any other suggestions running counter to basic ego needs or superego inhibitions.

rigorously tested and established. The hypothesis that the subject's "knowledge" regarding behavior in hypnosis influences his own hypnotic behavior was supported by an experiment. Students were exposed to a demonstration and lecture on hypnosis in which catalepsy of the dominant hand was mentioned as a common feature of trance behavior. Five out of nine volunteers exhibited this phenomenon under hypnosis. No students in a control group, who were given a similar lecture and demonstration but with no mention of catalepsy, showed the phenomenon.

An experiment performed by Ashley, Harper, and Runyon, which depends on hypnotic amnesia to explain the results, was repeated with the inclusion of a control group of subjects. These were subjects who simulated hypnosis but who were otherwise exposed to the same experimental situation as the hypnotic subjects. The behavior of the simulating group was indistinguishable from that of the "real" group, and both were indistinguishable from the results of the original study. Some doubt is thus cast on an explanation of the results in terms of hypnotic amnesia, and support is lent to the hypothesis that the demand characteristics of the experimental procedure may be a significant determinant of subject behavior.

In another experiment it was found that motivated subjects in the wake state held a weight at arm's length for a longer period of time than they did while in the hypnotic state. This result casts doubt on the notion that enhanced physical capacity is a primary characteristic of the trance state.

Differences between "real" and "fake" subjects were investigated. The major difference appears to be a tolerance by the "real" subject of logical inconsistencies.

It was concluded that in the absence of objective indices of hypnosis the existence of trance may be considered a clinical diagnosis. Until an invariant index of hypnosis can be established, such a diagnosis must be confirmed by the subject's report of alterations in his experience, since the real focus of hypnosis appears to lie in the subjective experience of trance.

REFERENCES

ASHLEY, W. R., HARPER, R. S., & RUNYON, D. K. The perceived size of coins in normal and hypnotically induced economic states. *Amer. J. Psychol.*, 1951, **64**, 564–592.

BINET, A., & FÉRÉ, C. *Animal magnetism*. New York: Appleton, 1888. (Trans.)

BORING, E. J. *A history of experimental psychology*. (2nd ed.) New York & London: Appleton-Century-Crofts, 1950.

BRUNER, J. S., & GOODMAN, C. C. Value and need as organizing factor in perception. *J. abnorm. soc. Psychol.*, 1947, **42**, 33–44.

COUÉ, E. Self mastery through conscious autosuggestion. *N. Y. Amer. Library Serv.*, 1922. P. 83.

DUMAURIER, G. *Trilby*. New York: Harper, 1895.

DYNES, J. B. An experimental study in hypnotic anesthesia. *J. abnorm. soc. Psychol.*, 1932, **27**, 79–88.

ESTABROOKS, G. E. *Hypnotism*. New York: Dutton, 1948.

HULL, C. L. *Hypnosis and suggestibility*. New York & London: Appleton-Century, 1933.

JENNESS, A. Hypnotism. In J. McV. Hunt (Ed.), *Personality and behavior disorders*. New York: Ronald, 1944. P. 470.

LECRON, L. M., & BORDEAUX, J. *Hypnotism today*. New York: Grune & Stratton, 1947. P. 103.

MCDOUGALL, W. *Outline of abnormal psychology*. New York: Scribner's, 1926.

MANN, T. *Mario and the magician*. Lowe-Porter (Trans.) New York: Knopf, 1931.

MAYER, L. *Die Technik der Hypnose*. Munich: J. F. Lelumanns Verlag, 1951. Pp. 142–143.

MOLL, A. *Hypnotism*. (5th rev. ed.) New York: Scribner's, 1904.

NICHOLSON, N. C. Notes on muscular work during hypnosis. *Johns Hopkins Hosp. Bull.*, 1920, **31**, 89.

ORNE, M. T. The mechanism of hypnotic age regression: An experimental study. *J. abnorm. soc. Psychol.*, 1951, **46**, 213–225.

ORNE, M. T. Die Leistungsfähigkeit in Hypnose und im Wachzustand. *Psychol. Rdsch.*, 1954, **5**, 291–297.

PATTIE, F. A., JR. The genuineness of hypnotically produced anesthesia of the skin. *Amer. J. Psychol.*, 1937, **49**, 435–443.

PAVLOV, I. P. The identity of inhibition with sleep and hypnosis. *Sci. Monthly*, 1923, **17**, 603–608.

ROSENBERG, S. G., & FELDBERG, T. M. Rorschach characteristics of a group of malingerers. *Rorsch. Res. Exch.*, 1944, **8**, 141–158.

ROSS, Y. D. The use of the Rorschach method in the Canadian Army. *Rorsch. Res. Exch.*, 1944, **8**, 159–161.

ROUSH, E. S. Strength and endurance in the waking and hypnotic state. *J. appl. Physiol.*, 1951, **3**, 404–410.

SARBIN, T. R. Contributions to role taking theory: I. Hypnotic behavior. *Psychol. Rev.*, 1950, **57**, 255–270.

SCHILDER, P. *The nature of hypnosis*. Gerda Corvin (Trans.) New York: International Universities Press, 1956.

STOKVIS, B. *Hypnose in der Aerztlichen Praxis*. New York: S. Karger Basel, 1955.

STRICKLER, C. B. A quantitative study of post-hypnotic amnesia. *J. abnorm. soc. Psychol.*, 1929, **24**, 108–119.

WEITZENHOFFER, A. *Hypnotism.* New York: Wiley Press, 1953.

WELLS, W. R. Experiments in "waking hypnosis" for instructional purposes. *J. abnorm. soc. Psychol.*, 1923, **18**, 389–404.

WHITE, R. W. A preface to a theory of hypnotism. *J. abnorm. soc. Psychol.*, 1941, **36**, 477–506.

WILLIAMS G. W. The effect of hypnosis on muscular fatigue. *J. abnorm. soc. Psychol.*, 1929, **24**, 318–329.

WILLIAMS, G. W. A comparative study of voluntary and hypnotic catalepsy. *Amer. J. Psychol.*, 1930, **42**, 83–95.

WOLBERG, L. R. *Medical hypnosis.* Vol. I. New York: Grune & Stratton, 1948.

Received January 22, 1958.

[5]

Toward a Scientific Explanation of "Hypnotic" Behavior

Theodore X. Barber

During recent years, Weitzenhoffer (361, 362, 363), Gill and Brenman (165), Orne (277), Shor (327, 329), and Hilgard (186) have presented theories on the topic *hypnosis.* Although these recent theories and those proffered during the past century by such investigators as Braid (89), Bernheim (79), Moll (267), and Bramwell (92) differ in many respects, *they seem to be in agreement with respect to basic theoretical concepts and fundamental assumptions.* Both the recent and the nineteenth century formulations pivot around the construct *hypnosis* (or *hypnotic state* or *trance*) and appear to explicitly or implicitly accept the following interrelated "hypnotic state" assumptions: (a) there exists a state of consciousness—the hypnotic state or trance—which differs from both the waking and the sleeping state; (b) the hypnotic state can be elicited by many procedures, especially by those commonly termed *hypnotic inductions;* (c) the hypnotic state is a causal factor in producing suggested analgesia, hallucination, age regression, amnesia, and other hypnotic phenomena; (d) the greater the degree or depth of the hypnotic state, the more readily are hypnotic phenomena elicited.

The formulation developed in the present text differs radically from those mentioned above in that *it does not posit a "hypnotic state" and does not accept the "hypnotic state" assumptions* (115, 299).[1] The present formulation lays aside the construct *hypnotic state* for several reasons, including the following:

1. The construct *hypnotic state* and the "hypnotic state assumptions" are entangled in circular reasoning (25). As pointed out in Chapter 1, the presumed hypnotic state is directly or

[1] Although the present formulation and that previously presented by Sarbin (311, 315, 317) differ in several important respects, they are in agreement that constructs such as *hypnosis* or *hypnotic trance* are unnecessary and misleading in this area of inquiry.

indirectly inferred from responses to suggestions and is then used circularly to account for responses to suggestions.

2. Theoretical formulations which pivot around the constructs *hypnosis* or *hypnotic trance* fail to meet essential criteria for useful scientific theories—they cannot be tested empirically and thus can be neither confirmed nor disconfirmed (293). Such theories cannot be tested because their central construct—*hypnosis* or *hypnotic state* or *trance*—has no clearly defined referents or clearly defined limits and can be used in an *ad hoc* manner to "explain" every conceivable empirical finding. For instance, how would "hypnotic state" theories account for experimental data indicating that a higher level of response to test-suggestions for body immobility, thirst hallucination, and selective amnesia is elicited when the subjects are told that it is easy rather than difficult to perform well on assigned tasks (52)? "Hypnotic state" theorists would presumably explain these findings by arguing that hypnotic trance is satisfactorily produced when the subjects are told that it is easy to perform well on the tasks and is not produced when the subjects are told that it is difficult. However, suppose that the experimental data had indicated the opposite conclusion, namely, that a higher level of response is elicited when the subjects are told that it is difficult rather than easy to respond. "Hypnotic state" theorists could also explain these findings, arguing in an *ad hoc* manner that hypnotic trance is more satisfactorily produced when subjects are told that it is difficult rather than easy to respond. How would "hypnotic state" theories account for data demonstrating that a substantial proportion of subjects, who have *not* received a "hypnotic induction procedure" or "task motivational instructions" and who appear to be awake, manifest high "base-level" response to suggestions of analgesia, hallucination, amnesia, etc. (38, 39)? It appears that "hypnotic state" formulations, such as those of Wells (368), Weitzenhoffer (361, 362, 363), Hilgard (186) and Tart and Hilgard (345), can account for such anomalous data by positing that subjects who appear to be awake while manifesting a high level of response to suggestions have spontaneously slipped into a hypnotic state or a state of waking hypnosis.[2]

[2] Tart and Hilgard (345) recently presented experimental data to buttress the contention that control subjects, who have not been

Since the construct *hypnosis* can be used in an *ad hoc* manner to "explain" every conceivable empirical finding, it is questionable whether it actually explains anything at all. Furthermore, since theories which pivot around the construct *hypnotic state*

exposed to a hypnotic induction procedure, may "spontaneously slip into hypnosis." These authors worked with subjects who had previously shown high response to suggestions under a waking-imagination condition. The subjects were retested for suggestibility under a treatment that included the following: (a) the subjects were urged not to "drift off" into a borderline state (between sleep and wakefulness) or into a state of light hypnosis; and (b) they "were immediately brought back to full wakefulness by rousing them" whenever they said that they were "drifting off." Typically, the subjects failed to show a high level of suggestibility under this treatment in which they were maintained in a fully aroused condition. Tart and Hilgard concluded from these data that "in order for *S* to respond well to suggestibility tests under waking-imagination conditions, he had to slip into a borderline or hypnotic state." Tart and Hilgard noted that their conclusion was based on the assumption that "*S*'s report that he feels hyponotized to some degree is primary data about the presence or absence of hypnosis, if not a criterion of hypnosis." However, as pointed out in Chapter 6 of the present text, subjects' report that they "feel hypnotized" has been shown to be functionally related to a series of denotable antecedent variables including (a) their pre-experimental conceptions of what hypnosis is supposed to involve, (b) the degree to which they responded to suggestions, (c) the phrasing and tone of the questions that are submitted to them to elicit their testimony, and (d) whether or not the experimenter states or implies that he thinks they were hypnotized. Although subjects' testimony that they did or did not experience hypnosis has been shown to be functionally related to a series of antecedent variables, it now remains to be demonstrated, *it should not be assumed,* that subjects' testimony is also functionally related to the presence or absence of a "special state of consciousness"—a hypnotic state of trance.

Chaves (104a) has recently outlined an even more basic difficulty with the notion that control subjects "spontaneously slip into hypnosis":

"If the subjects do, indeed, slip in and out of hypnosis as readily as is implied by Tart and Hilgard and if the hypnotic state is relevant to behavior, it would seem that much research in psychology has been negated since very few if any investigators control for this variable. Carried to its logical conclusion, it would be necessary for all experimenters in psychology—irrespective of whether they are studying learning, reaction time, psychophysics, psychophysiology, or whatever—to periodically insure that their subjects had not

can use *ad hoc* reasoning to account for all possible experimental outcomes, they can be neither proved nor disproved.

It is incumbent upon theorists who speak in terms of *hypnosis* (or equivalent terms such as *hypnotic state, trance*, and *hypnotized*) to delineate criteria for inferring the presence of "hypnosis" which are independent of the behaviors that this presumed "state" is supposed to explain. After they have delineated non-circular criteria, it is incumbent upon them to demonstrate that "hypnosis" or the "hypnotic state" is an instrumental factor in eliciting the phenomena discussed in this text. Although it is conceivable that "hypnotic state" theorists may some day delineate non-circular criteria for their major construct, it does not necessarily follow that they will also be able to demonstrate that the "hypnotic state" is a relevant factor in eliciting (a) suggested analgesia, hallucination, amnesia, and other responses to test-suggestions; (b) "hypnotic" or "trance-like" appearance; (c) reports of unusual experiences; and (d) testimony of having been hypnotized. The data presented in this text indicate that these behaviors, which have been traditionally labeled as *hypnotic*, will be shown to be a function of a set of denotable antecedent variables *that are very similar to those that play an important role in a wide variety of test-situations*. This set of instrumental antecedent variables includes, for example, the subjects' attitudes and expectancies with respect to the specific test-situation, their motivation to cooperate and to try to perform maximally on assigned tasks, and the tone and wording of the suggestions and of the questions used to elicit subjective reports.

It needs to be emphasized that, although theories which pivot around the construct *hypnotic state* have been extant for more than 100 years, criteria for "hypnotic state" have *not* been delineated which are independent of the phenomena that this presumed state is said to produce. Consequently, it has not been

---

slipped into hypnosis. Until further evidence has been provided, Tart and Hilgard's contention, that 'The fact that E has not administered an induction procedure should not be taken as insuring that *S* is wide awake and in a normal state,' must remain open to question. More specifically, constructs such as 'normal state' and 'hypnosis,' as used by hypnotic state theorists, must be unambiguously and nontautologically denoted before questions pertaining to 'spontaneous hypnosis' can be seriously entertained."

demonstrated that a unique state of consciousness that differs from waking and also differs from sleep ("the hypnotic state") can account for even a small proportion of the variance in so-called "hypnotic" behaviors.

The failure of "hypnotic state" theories to account satisfactorily for observed events suggests the possibility that such theories may suffer the same fate historically as the theories of the "ether" in physics and the theory of "phlogiston" in chemistry (217). During the nineteenth century a hypothetical substance (the ether) was postulated by all competent authorities to explain the transmission of those forces (electric, magnetic, gravitational) which one material object exerts on another located at a distance (135). Although there was diversity of opinion as to the properties of the ether, it was generally conceived as filling all space and as possessing such unusual properties as extreme tenuity, absolute continuity, and high rigidity and elasticity. Various attempts to observe the presumed effects of the ether (e.g., the Michelson-Morley experiment) were unsuccessful and the concept *ether* was gradually abandoned when it became clear that it was unnecessary for the explanation of any observed phenomenon. Similarly, to explain the phenomena of combustion, eighteenth century chemists postulated a unique substance—phlogiston—which was supposed to be given off when a substance burned. The notion of phlogiston was maintained for many years by resorting to *ad hoc* reasoning to "explain" incongruous findings. For instance, to explain data indicating that, during combustion, some substances lost weight and other substances gained weight, theorists argued that phlogiston possessed both a positive weight and a negative weight (109). After Lavoisier provided an alternative, empirically-based formulation that explained the phenomena of combustion without resorting to *ad hoc* arguments, the construct *phlogiston* was gradually abandoned. Similarly, it appears to the author that (a) the construct *hypnosis* and the "hypnotic state assumptions" that were mentioned at the beginning of this chapter are not only unnecessary but also misleading; and (b) the phenomena which have been supposedly "explained" by postulating an unusual state of consciousness ("hypnotic state") can be explained more satisfactorily by an alternative approach that does not postulate a unique "state." Let us now briefly summarize the main features of the alternative approach that has been presented in this text.

AN ALTERNATIVE TO "HYPNOTIC STATE" THEORY

The essential features of the alternative approach are as follows:

1. First, the phenomena that are to be explained (dependent or consequent variables) are specified and methods for measuring each phenomenon are delineated.
2. Next, antecedent (independent) variables that might be functionally related to the phenomena to be explained are specified and methods for measuring each antecedent variable are delineated.
3. Functional relations holding between the antecedent and consequent variables are determined experimentally.
4. Investigations are conducted to show that the lower-order empirical generalizations (which formulate the functional relations between antecedent and consequent variables) can be subsumed under a smaller number of higher-order theoretical principles. Deductions are made from the higher-order principles and are tested empirically.

Each of these features of the alternative approach will now be discussed in turn.

Dependent (Consequent) Variables— The Phenomena to be Explained

We began by delineating four sets of dependent variables—behaviors subsumed under the topic *hypnosis* that require explanation.

One set of dependent variables was labeled as *response to test-suggestions.* This set includes overt acts and verbal testimony that are elicited by specific suggestions intended to produce specific effects—e.g., suggestions for limb rigidity, hallucination, and amnesia. We constructed a scale (the BSS) which included a representative sampling of responses to test-suggestions and which assessed two dimensions of response—overt motoric responses and verbal reports that the suggested effects were experienced. In Chapter 3 we presented psychometric data—reliabilities, norms, and a factor analysis—indicating the usefulness of the scale in measuring response to test-suggestions. We also delineated methods for measuring responses to other types of test-suggestions (which are not included in the BSS) such as suggestions for analgesia, age regression, time distortion, and deafness (46, 51, 57, 67).

Three additional sets of behaviors that are subsumed under the topic *hypnosis* were labeled as *"hypnotic" appearance, reports of unusual experiences,* and *testimony of having been hypnotized.* In Chapter 6 we specified methods for quantifying these three sets of dependent variables.

Independent (Antecedent) Variables

Having specified the "hypnotic" behaviors that require explanation and having delineated methods for measuring them, we asked: What are the effective antecedent variables in eliciting these behaviors? Since experimental data indicated that the behaviors that are to be explained are more effectively elicited in situations described as *hypnosis,* we asked, more specifically: Which of the many antecedent variables present in "hypnotic" situations are relevant and which extraneous in eliciting a high level of response to test-suggestions, "hypnotic"-like appearance, reports of unusual experiences, and testimony of having been hypnotized? To answer this question it was necessary first to specify each important class of independent variables that is present in situations traditionally termed *hypnotic.* Several sets of antecedent variables were delineated including the following:

1. A set of subject variables such as subjects' attitudes and expectancies with respect to the test-situation.

2. A set of procedural variables such as the specific wording of the test-suggestions, the tone of voice, pitch, and inflections used in presenting the test-suggestions, and the specific wording and tone of the questions used to elicit subjective reports.

3. A second set of procedural variables that are commonly

subsumed under the label *hypnotic induction procedure* such as statements which define the situation as "hypnosis," motivational instructions, and repetitive suggestions of relaxation, drowsiness, and sleep.

4. A set of experimenter variables such as the experimenter's attitudes, expectancies, and "biases."

Functional Relations Between Antecedent and Consequent Variables

A series of experiments were conducted to delineate lawful relations between the independent and dependent variables listed above. Somewhat different combinations of antecedent variables appeared to be instrumental in eliciting each of the four sets of dependent variables ("hypnotic" behaviors). To summarize these complex antecedent-consequent relations in the space available, it is necessary to speak in very general terms. In general, then, the following eight antecedent variables appeared to be functionally related to the four sets of "hypnotic" behaviors.

1) Subjects' Attitudes toward the Test-Situation. 2) Subjects' Expectancies Concerning their own Performance. A series of experiments demonstrated that subjects' behavior during a "hypnosis" experiment and their postexperimental testimony of having had unusual experiences and having felt hypnotized is dependent, in part, on their *pre*-experimental attitudes toward the test-situation and their *pre*-experimental expectations (self-predictions) concerning their own performance (58, 60, 123, 258). Furthermore, experimental manipulations of subjects' attitudes and expectations produce dramatic changes in response. For instance, if an attempt is made by a prestigeful person to produce negative attitudes and expectations in subjects who have previously manifested high response, these subjects now show very little if any response to test-suggestions of the type traditionally associated with the word *hypnosis* (45).

3) Wording and Tone of Specific Suggestions. Direct suggestions that specified events are occurring or will occur—e.g., "Your arm is heavy," "You cannot stand up," "You will forget" —play a very important role in eliciting "hypnotic" behaviors.

When the eight test-suggestions included in the BSS are administered directly, without special preliminaries ("base-level" condition), two important findings are obtained: (a) most subjects manifest some "hypnotic" behaviors (responding positively to at least two of the eight test-suggestions); and (b) some subjects (about 16% to 27%) manifest *many* "hypnotic" behaviors, passing at least five of the eight test-suggestions and thus exhibiting, for example, limb heaviness, thirst hallucination, body immobility, selective amnesia, and postexperimental or "posthypnotic" response, (31). Also, suggestions that one will hear or see objects that are not present, and that one is going back to an earlier chronological age, are sufficient *by themselves* to elicit testimony of having experienced "auditory hallucination," "visual hallucination," and "age regression" in a substantial proportion of unselected subjects (42, 57). Specifically, when volunteer subjects were tested under "base-level" conditions (without a "hypnotic induction procedure" or "task motivational instruction"), (a) one of every two who received direct suggestions for auditory hallucination testified that they clearly heard the suggested sounds; (b) one of every three who received direct suggestions for visual hallucinations testified that they saw the suggested object clearly; and (c) three of four who received suggestions for age regression testified that they were in another place and at an earlier time. Also, the majority of experimental subjects who received direct suggestions for time distortion testified that time had slowed down (51); when subjects perceive the experimental situation as having an apparent purpose, most of them respond positively to direct suggestions to carry out ostensibly harmful or dangerous acts (98, 263, 281); and a substantial proportion of subjects who receive direct suggestions for amnesia testify that they have forgotten the experimental events (59). Similarly, a variety of physiological effects can be produced by "direct suggestions *per se*": direct suggestions given without special preliminaries to allergic individuals have been shown to produce and also to inhibit an allergic response (196); direct suggestions designed to produce effortless fixation have resulted in improved visual acuity in myopic subjects (202, 203); and direct suggestions to try to accelerate or to decelerate the heart have produced augmented and reduced cardiac rate in normal individuals (206). In brief, although many variables enter into the elicitation of "hypnotic" behaviors, the importance of *direct suggestions per se* needs to be heavily underscored.

It is not sufficient, however, to speak simply of "direct suggestions *per se*." The exact wording of the suggestions or instructions and the tone of voice in which they are presented also play important roles. For instance, quite different results are obtained when suggestions for amnesia are worded in different ways—say, permissively ("Try to forget") versus peremptorily ("You will not remember!"), (59). Also, if a suggestion is presented in a firm tone of voice (with the implication that the experimenter wants and expects the subject to respond) a greater degree of responsiveness is obtained than if the same suggestion is presented in a lackadaisical tone (with the implication that the experimenter does not especially care if the subject accepts the suggestion) (44).

4) Task Motivational Instructions. As noted above, "base-level suggestibility is often underestimated. Under "base-level" conditions (without special preliminaries) most subjects are responsive to some test-suggestions and some subjects manifest a high level of response. This "base-level" responsiveness can be enhanced by administering instructions of the type we have labeled as *task motivational* which typically include exhortative statements to try to experience the suggested effects together with statements that others have performed well and that the subject too can perform satisfactorily. Task motivational instructions augment responsiveness to a wide variety of test-suggestions including, for example, the eight test-suggestions of the BSS and suggestions intended to produce a reduction in pain reactivity, heightened learning-cognitive proficiency, hallucination, dreaming on a specified topic and amnesia (34, 38, 40, 41, 42, 59, 69, 70).

5) Definition of the Situation. The extent to which subjects exhibit behaviors traditionally labeled as *hypnotic* depends in part on how the situation is defined to them. For instance, a higher level of response to test-suggestions is obtained when the situation is defined as "a test of imagination" rather than as "a test of gullibility" (50). Also, with other variables held constant or counterbalanced, a higher level of response to test-suggestions is obtained when the subjects are told that they are participating in a "hypnosis" experiment rather than in a "control experiment involving a test of imagination" (52).

6) *Relaxation-Sleep Suggestions.* With other variables held constant or counterbalanced, subjects are more prone to exhibit "hypnotic" behaviors when they have received repeated suggestions of relaxation, drowsiness, and sleep (54, 55). This finding is open to more than one interpretation.

A traditional interpretation is that repetitive suggestions of relaxation, drowsiness, and sleep tend to produce a hypnotic state and the hypnotic state in turn gives rise to a high level of response to suggestions to manifest "hypnotic" behaviors such as body immobility, analgesia, hallucination, and amnesia. This interpretation is open to all of the criticisms mentioned in Chapter 1 and at the beginning of the present chapter. Furthermore, the "hypnotic state" interpretation would be compelled to resort to *ad hoc* reasoning to explain data such as the following: (a) suggestions of relaxation, drowsiness, and sleep tend to facilitate responsiveness to test-suggestions even when they fail to give rise to relaxation or drowsiness and even when they result in heightened arousal and activation rather than in relaxation (63); (b) when the situation is explicitly or implicitly defined to subjects as "hypnosis," repeated suggestions to become more and more alert and activated appear to be as effective in facilitating response to test-suggestions as repeated suggestions of relaxation, drowsiness, and sleep (238).

An alternative interpretation is that repeated suggestions of relaxation, drowsiness, and sleep facilitate response in that they emphasize to the subject that he is in a "hypnosis" situation, that the experimenter is making a serious attempt to "hypnotize" him, and, since he is being "hypnotized," high response to suggestions is possible, is desired, and is expected. This alternative interpretation can be tested empirically with a group of children of whom some are and some are not acquainted with the culturally-defined implications of the word *hypnosis.* If the interpretation is correct, repetitive suggestions of relaxation, drowsiness, and sleep (a) should facilitate base-level response to test-suggestions in children who are familiar with the traditional connotations of the word *hypnosis,* that is, who have learned that suggestions of relaxation, drowsiness, and sleep give rise to hypnosis and that hypnosis gives rise to high suggestibility; and (b) should not augment base-level response to test-suggestions in children who have not as yet learned that suggestions of relaxation, drowsiness, and sleep are supposed to give rise to hypnosis and to high suggestibility.

7) *Wording and Tone of the Inquiry.* The subjects' testimony—for example, testimony that they had unusual experiences, felt hypnotized, and were unable to resist the suggestions—varies with ostensibly "slight" changes in the wording of the inquiry. For instance, subjects give incongruent testimony when asked, "Did you experience the hypnotic state as basically similar to the waking state?" and "Did you experience the hypnotic state as basically different from the waking state?" Similarly, whether or not subjects testify that they could resist the suggestions depends in part on whether they are asked, "Did you feel you could resist?" or "Did you feel you could not resist?" The inconsistencies in testimony that are produced by seemingly "slight" changes in the wording of the inquiry appear to be due to at least two factors: (a) in some instances the subject is simply acquiescing with the implications of the experimenter's questions; and (b) in some instances the subject finds his experiences complex or ambiguous, is uncertain how to classify them, and is consequently willing to accept the categories for classifying his experiences which are implicitly offered to him by the specific wording of the experimenter's questions (64).

The experimenter's tone of voice and vocal inflections also appear to influence the subject's testimony. For instance, whether or not subjects who have received suggestions of amnesia state that they have forgotten is dependent in part on the tone and inflection used by the experimenter in asking them questions such as "Do you remember?" The question "Do you remember?" can be asked in a tone of voice and with inflections implying that the subject cannot and should not remember or it can be asked in a different way with the implication that the subject is permitted to and can remember (22).

8) *Experimenter Role.* Most of the independent variables discussed above, which play a role in eliciting "hypnotic" behaviors, are under the control of the experimenter. It is the experimenter

who defines the situation, who administers the instructions and suggestions, and who conducts the inquiry. Speaking metaphorically, the experimenter can be viewed as a funnel through which most of the important antecedent variables must filter before they affect the subject.

As mentioned above the degree to which the subject exhibits "hypnotic" behaviors is dependent in part on the experimenter's tone of voice and inflections and the way in which he phrases the test-suggestions and the inquiry questions. When the experimenter's role is permitted to vary, "hypnotic" behavior can be viewed from a transactional frame of reference, that is, the degree to which the subject exhibits "hypnotic" behaviors influences the role of the experimenter and the role the experimenter adopts in turn influences the subjects' behavior (14). For instance, when suggestions for age regression have been administered and the experimenter's role is allowed to vary, subjects will behave more or less in an age regressed manner depending on whether the experiment treats them as children or as adults (348).

Although subtle qualities of the experimenter's role appear to influence performance, we do not know to what extent the personal characteristics of the experimenter—his age, sex, ethnic background, and personality characteristics—interact with the characteristic of subjects to affect their behavior. Also, we lack empirical data pertaining to the effects exerted by the experimenter's attitudes, expectancies, or "biases." However, it is clear that with few exceptions investigators working in this area have had very strong "expectancy biases" (304). For instance, with few exceptions, investigators have expected more dramatic or "better" results with "hypnotized" subjects than "awake" subjects. In some studies these expectancies were apparently so strong that a waking comparison group was not used; apparently it was assumed that non-hypnotized subjects could not or would not perform "hypnotic" behaviors. In other instances, it seems that in expecting better results under the hypnotic treatment, investigators may have inadvertently (a) given suggestions in an emphatic and expectant manner to hypnotic subjects and in a hesitating, less forthright, and less effective manner to the controls; (b) conducted the inquiry differently for hypnotic and nonhypnotic groups; and (c) varied their procedures in other subtle ways.

Further studies are clearly needed to assess the effects of biased experimenter expectancies. For instance, experimenters should be led to expect that some of their subjects, selected at random, will obtain high scores on a standarized scale of suggestibility (say, the BSS) and that other subjects will obtain low scores. The data available at present (35, 72) suggest two hypotheses:

1. Experimenters tend to obtain results in line with their expectancies *if they are permitted to vary their procedure*, for example, if they can vary their tone of voice when they are administering the instructions, suggestions, or inquiry questions.

2. Biased expectancies on the part of the experimenter exert a non-significant effect on the results *when the experimental procedures are rigorously standardized across subjects,* for example, when the test-suggestions are administered to all subjects by a tape-recording of the experimenter's voice and when the inquiry is conducted by written questionnaires.

Convergence and Interaction of Variables. "Hypnotic" behaviors are multidetermined; each of the behaviors traditionally labeled as *hypnotic* is functionally related to more than one of the antecedent variables listed above. For instance, the extent to which subjects manifest a *"hypnotic"-like appearance*—e.g., limpness-relaxation, lack of spontaneity, and general passivity—depends in part on their pre-experimental attitudes and expectations with respect to "hypnosis" and also depends in part on the suggestions for relaxation, drowsiness, and sleep included explicitly in the hypnotic induction procedure and implicitly in the definition of the situation as hypnosis. Along similar lines, at least five classes of variables affect subjects' postexperimental *testimony of having been hypnotized* (58, 64); (a) their pre-experimental conceptions of what hypnosis involves; (b) their pre-experimental expectations as to how deeply they will be hypnotized; (c) the extent to which they respond to test-suggestions during the experiment (subjects who respond to test-suggestions often use this fact as evidence that they were hypnotized); (d) the specific wording of the questions used to elicit their testimony; (e) whether the experimenter states or implies that he believes they were hypnotized.

The antecedent variables listed above not only converge but also *interact* to produce "hypnotic" behaviors. For instance, complex interactions have been demonstrated experimentally among the following three antecedent variables: (a) *the definition of the situation* (as "hypnosis" or as "a control experiment involving a test of imagination"); (b) *motivational instructions;* and (c) *statements that it is easy to respond* (54). It also appears likely that each of these three antecedent variables interacts with other antecedent variables such as subjects' pre-experimental attitudes and expectations. In brief, the data available at present indicate that (a) the effect of a given antecedent variable upon "hypnotic" behaviors depends upon the qualitative and quantitative properties of other antecedent variables that are simultaneously present; and (b) to attain a thoroughgoing explanation of "hypnotic" behaviors we need to delineate the many complex interactions that occur among all important antecedent variables.

Toward a Theoretical Integration

The search for broad principles that can explain a wide variety of empirical facts is an important goal of science. Scientific theories aim to account for the greatest number of empirically-established relations between antecedent and consequent variables with the smallest number of broad principles.

Although, with respect to the topic *hypnosis,* the specification of lawful antecedent-consequent relations is still at a relatively early stage, a sufficient number of functional relations have been established to justify serious endeavors toward an overall theoretical integration. We need to continue an active search for new variables and new relationships among variables while, at the same time, endeavoring to conceptualize the domain of empirical facts parsimoniously.

An important task, then, is to subsume the empirical generalizations that are at hand under a smaller number of broader principles. There are clearly many paths toward this goal (91, 150, 151, 212, 213, 248, 249). For instance, in one grand sweep we could formulate a series of propositions that might serve to unify the empirical data. Hilgard's recent text on hypnotism (186) follows along this path. The final chapter of Hilgard's text presents 17 propositions (e.g., "The hypnotic state is characterized by various partial dissociations") which aim to account for the data he had presented in the preceding chapters. Similarly, Shor (327, 329) has presented 22 propositions to explain the topic *hypnosis* (e.g., "Hypnotic depth may be defined as some complex of depth along three conceptually separate dimensions: (a) the dimension of hypnotic role-taking involvement, (b) the dimension of trance, and (c) the dimension of archaic involvement"). Such attempts at broad-scale theory construction may serve some useful purposes. However, we are in agreement with Koch (212, 213), Marx (248, 249), and others that, at the present stage of the development of psychology, it is more fruitful to proceed toward broad theoretical principles *by a series of gradual inductive-deductive steps which allow concepts to be closely tied to empirical data* rather than by attempting, in one stroke, to formulate a broad-scope theory. The issues involved here, which are far too many and too complex to discuss in the brief space available, have been succinctly stated by Marx (247):

> The potential usefulness of theoretical structures of so high a degree of abstraction need not be denied. Nevertheless the most immediate need of psychology would rather plainly seem to be the careful development of a large number of low-level empirical laws and low-order theories based upon the use of intervening constructs of the more operational type. Higher-order theoretical generalizations may then be built upon a sound empirical framework . . . rather than developed from above, as has too often been attempted in the past and is encouraged by the premature emulation of theoretical models based upon highly abstract physical pattern.

There is a method available by which we could proceed by gradual inductive-deductive steps, *always adhering closely to empirical data,* to unify many of the empirical generalizations presented in the text under a smaller number of broader principles. This method is based on the following considerations.

Taken *in toto,* the 70 empirical generalizations proffered in the text state that "hypnotic" behaviors are functionally related to at least eight classes of antecedent variables, namely, to Subject's Attitude toward the Test-Situation, Subject's Expectations of His Own Performance, The Wording and Tone of Specific Suggestions, Task Motivational Instructions, Definition of the Situation, Relaxation-Sleep Suggestions, Wording and Tone of Inquiry, and the Role of the Experimenter. *We could subsume many of the empirical generalizations under a smaller number of broader principles if we could show experimentally that the eight major independently-defined antecedent variables that enter into the empirical generalizations can be subsumed under a smaller number of more broadly-defined variables.* The reader may have noted in previous chapters and earlier in this chapter that we have proposed several types of investigations that could help to demonstrate that the number of independently-defined antecedent variables can be reduced to a smaller number of broader variables. Let us summarize three types of empirical investigations that might be helpful.

1. We may be able to demonstrate empirically that (a) variations in the Definition of the Situation—e.g., definition of the situation as "hypnosis," as a "test of imagination," or as "a test of gullibility"—produce different attitudes, expectancies, and motivations toward the test-situation and toward the experimental tasks; and (b) differences on the latter three variables (different "task-attitudes," "task-expectancies," and "task-motivations") give rise to different levels of response. These relationships could be demonstrated empirically in investigations which include three steps: First, the situation is defined to the subjects—e.g., as "hypnosis" or as a "test of imagination." Next, utilizing recently-developed methods that ingeniously assess how the subjects construe the test-situation (338), an assessment is made of subjects' task-attitudes, task-expectancies, and task-motivations. Finally, the subjects are tested for response to test-suggestions. Experiments along these lines may be able to confirm propositions such as the following:

(a) Subjects who are more responsive to test-suggestions when the situation is defined as "hypnosis" rather than as a "test of imagination" view the former situation rather than the latter as one in which it is more appropriate or more acceptable to perform unusual behaviors and to experience unusual effects (task-attitude).

(b) Subjects who are more responsive to test-suggestions when the situation is defined as "hypnosis" rather than as a "test of imagination" view the former situation more than the latter as one in which they will find it not only possible but also rather easy to respond to suggestions and to experience unusual effects (task-expectancy).

(c) Subjects who are more responsive to test-suggestions when the situation is defined as "hypnosis" rather than as a "test of imagination" view the former situation more than the latter as one in which they should not resist but instead should cooperate and try to perform the suggested behaviors and try to experience the suggested effects (task-motivation).

If propositions of this type are supported by empirical studies, we may be able to subsume the variables that we have labeled as *Definition of the Situation* under the more broadly-defined variables that we have labeled as *Task-Attitude, Task-Expectancy,* and *Task-Motivation.*

2. We may be able to demonstrate empirically that the variable we have labeled as *Relaxation-Sleep Suggestions* can also be subsumed under the three broader variables discussed in the preceding paragraph. More specifically, we may be able to show experimentally that Relaxation-Sleep Suggestions exert their effects in that they emphasize to subjects that they are now in an unusual or unique situation (a "hypnosis" situation) in which it is appropriate to perform unusual behaviors (positive task-attitude), in which they will find it not only possible but also rather easy to perform the requested behaviors and to experience the suggested effects (positive task-expectancy), and in which they should not resist but on the contrary should cooperate and try to experience that which is suggested (positive task-motivation).

3. We may be able to show empirically that the experimenter significantly affects the subjects' behavior only when he is free to vary the manner in which he administers the instructions and suggestions and the way in which he conducts the inquiry. If this can be demonstrated, we may be able to subsume the class of variables that we have labeled as *Role of the Experimenter* under those labeled as *Tone and Wording of Suggestions* and *Tone and Wording of the Inquiry.*

In brief, it appears that by conducting a series of carefully-designed experiments we may be able to show that the effective antecedent variables can be reduced to a smaller number of more broadly-defined variables and, consequently, that the 70 empirical generalizations proffered in this text can be reduced to a smaller number of broader principles. Specifically, it appears possible that at least three of the eight important antecedent variables—Definition of the Situation, Relaxation-Sleep Suggestions, and Role of the Experimenter—can be subsumed under the remaining five variables, namely, under Task-Attitude, Task-Expectancy, Task-Motivation, Tone and Wording of Suggestions, and Tone and Wording of Inquiry. If this were accomplished, most of the empirical generalizations proffered in the text could be subsumed under five broad-scope principles which will state that *a substantial proportion of the variance in "hypnotic" behaviors is determined by (a) subjects' attitudes toward the specific test-situation, (b) subjects' expectations concerning their own performance on assigned tasks, (c) subjects' motivation to cooperate, not to resist, and to try to perform the suggested behaviors and to experience the suggested effects, (d) the tone and wording of the specific suggestions that are administered, and (e) the tone and wording of the questions that are designed to elicit reports of subjective experiences.*

Two additional considerations are relevant here:

1. The five sets of variables specified above are conceived as similar to those that operate *in many and possibly all situations in which specific tasks are to be performed.* It appears likely that when individuals are assessed on tasks of various types, for example, tasks involving learning ability or physical abilities, performance is determined in part by Task-Attitude, Task-Expectancy, Task-Motivation, Tone and Wording of Instructions or Suggestions, and Tone and Wording of the Inquiry. In brief, the proposed conceptualization views the performance of "hypnotic" behaviors as closely related to variables which play an important role in a wide variety of test-situations.

2. If the experimental program outlined above succeeds in showing that the independently-defined antecedent variables can be reduced to a smaller number, further research will be required to determine how much of the variance in "hypnotic" behavior can be accounted for by the reduced number of antecedent variables and to delineate additional variables that may account for the unexplained portion of the variance. Furthermore, if the experimental program demonstrates that, by reducing the number

of independently-defined antecedent variables, the empirical generalizations can be subsumed under a smaller number of broader principles, empirical and theoretical endeavors will still be at a very early stage. Further investigations will then be needed to test predictions that are deduced from the higher-order principles, to discard those principles which give rise to predictions that are not confirmed by empirical test, and to continue to formulate and test new principles until such time as the theoretical conceptualization closely covers the domain of empirical facts.

Future Prospects

The present text is an *approach* to an area of inquiry, not a closed treatise. The aim it hopes to fulfill is that of being a sufficiently systematic approach to move others to undertake continually more focused investigations which ask continually more penetrating questions. Implementation of the approach has barely begun. Intensive investigations are now required which focus on the following:

Consequent Variables. Further work is needed to objectify and to measure more precisely each of the major consequent variables that have been historically associated with the word *hypnosis,* for example, (a) overt responses to test-suggestions of analgesia, hallucination, age-regression, and amnesia, and (b) subjective testimony of having experienced the suggested effects, of having been hypnotized, and of having had unusual experiences. Further work is also needed to determine the degree of relationship between naturally occurring phenomena and "hypnotic" phenomena which bear the same name, asking questions such as: What criteria can we accept as indicating similarities and differences between non-suggested and suggested hallucination, analgesia, color blindness, blindness, deafness, and amnesia?

Antecedent Variables. Although we have delineated a series of antecedent variables that play a role in eliciting "hypnotic" behaviors, there is every reason to believe that other independent variables, as yet unspecified, also exert an effect. We need to continue an active search for further antecedent variables. We also need to delineate the effects of variables that appear to play a role but have not as yet been studied intensively such as the interpersonal relationship between subject and experimenter and the moment-to-moment subject-experimenter social interaction.

Relations between Antecedent-Consequent Variables (Empirical Generalizations). Research is needed to cross-validate each of the 70 empirical generalizations (which relate antecedent and consequent variables) that have been presented in the text and to determine the limits of each generalization, that is, to determine under what conditions the generalizations fail to account for empirical data. Further research is also needed to specify the complex interactions that occur among the independent variables that affect "hypnotic" behavior.

Parsimonious Conceptualization (Theory Construction). Endeavors are needed which aim toward a parsimonious codification of research findings. These endeavors will be successful to the degree that the empirically-established generalizations which relate antecedent and consequent variables are unified under a smaller number of broader principles and deductions are made from the general principles that are confirmed by empirical tests.

When the approach outlined in this text has been implemented —when we have attained a parsimonious conceptualization of all important antecedent-consequent relations—we may expect the following to occur:

1. A series of useful effects that have been traditionally associated with the word *hypnosis*—e.g., heightened learning-cognitive proficiency, enhanced physical endurance, heightened recall of earlier events, reduction of pain and anxiety in dental situations or in other situations involving noxious stimulation—may be produced much more simply and directly than at present, utilizing only the effective variables and excluding variables that are extraneous.

2. If the methodology outlined in the text helps to clarify the complex topic *hypnosis*, it may also help to clarify various other topics in psychology that are also complex and that appear rather mysterious or "unique"—e.g., such topics as *creativity, multiple personality, schizophrenia,* and *hysteria.* Investigators may find it fruitful to approach other complex or "unique" topics in the same way we have approached the topic *hypnosis,* that is, to hold in abeyance extant constructs and theories while proceeding

along the following lines. First, the overt and verbal behaviors that have been traditionally subsumed under the topic are denoted and measured. Also, antecedent variables (for example, factors in the subject's life history and in the hospital setting) which may be instrumental in eliciting the behaviors that are to be explained are denoted and measured. Next, functional relations are sought between antecedent and consequent variables. Finally, proceeding gradually and always adhering closely to empirical data, studies are conducted to show that the empirical generalizations which summarize the important antecedent-consequent relations can be subsumed under a smaller number of broader principles and that deductions can be made from the broad-scope principles that are confirmed by empirical test.

3. Principles developed in the study of "hypnosis" may be relevant to a deeper understanding of various topics in general psychology and in social psychology. Research in "hypnosis" is more than the study of one concrete "compartment" of human behavior. This area of inquiry offers rewarding possibilities for the study of the effects of language (verbal stimulation) on behavior and on physiological processes. It could also provide a deeper understanding of such broad psychological topics as *cognition, perception, emotion,* and *interpersonal relations.*

Although research in "hypnosis" promises to provide a broader understanding of human behavior, the reverse is also true—as psychologists working on other topics develop general principles, their principles should help us attain a deeper understanding of the topic *hypnosis*. Finally, the topic *hypnosis* may lose all of its aura, mystery, and separate status and become integrated into general psychology.

References

14. Barber, T. X. The concept of "hypnosis." *J. Psychol.*, 1958, *45*, 115–131.
22. Barber, T. X. Toward a theory of hypnosis: Posthypnotic behavior. *Arch. gen. Psychiat.*, 1962, *7*, 321–342.
25. Barber, T. X. "Hypnosis" as a causal variable in present-day psychology: A critical analysis. *Psychol. Reports*, 1964, *14*, 839–842.
31. Barber, T. X. Measuring "hypnotic-like" suggestibility with and without "hypnotic induction"; psychometric properties, norms, and variables influencing response to the Barber Suggestibility Scale (BSS). *Psychol. Reports*, 1965, *16*, 809–844.
34. Barber, T. X. The effects of "hypnosis" on learning and recall: A methodological critique. *J. clin. Psychol.*, 1965, *21*, 19–25.
35. Barber, T. X. Five attempts to replicate the experimenter expectancy bias effect. Harding, Mass.: Medfield Foundation, 1966. (Mimeo)
38. Barber, T. X., and Calverley, D. S. "Hypnotic" behavior as a function of task motivation. *J. Psychol.*, 1962, *54*, 363–389.
39. Barber, T. X., and Calverley, D. S. "Hypnotic-like" suggestibility in children and adults. *J. abnorm. soc. Psychol.*, 1963, *66*, 589–597.
40. Barber, T. X., and Calverley, D. S. The relative effectiveness of task motivating instructions and trance induction procedure in the production of "hypnotic-like" behaviors. *J. nerv. ment. Dis.* 1963, *137*, 107–116.
42. Barber, T. X., and Calverley, D. S. An experimental study of "hypnotic" (auditory and visual) hallucinations. *J. abnorm. soc Psychol.*, 1964, *63*, 13–20.
44. Barber, T. X., and Calverley, D. S. Effect of *E*'s tone of voice on "hypnotic-like" suggestibility. *Psychol. Reports*, 1964, *15* 139–144.
45. Barber, T. X., and Calverley, D. S. Empirical evidence for a theory of "hypnotic" behavior: Effects of pretest instructions on response to primary suggestions. *Psychol. Record*, 1964, *14* 457–467.
46. Barber, T. X., and Calverley, D. S. Experimental studies in "hypnotic" behavior: Suggested deafness evaluated by delayed auditory feedback. *Brit. J. Psychol.*, 1964, *55*, 439–446.
50. Barber, T. X., and Calverley, D. S. The definition of the situation as a variable affecting "hypnotic-like" suggestibility. *J. clin. Psychol.*, 1964, *20*, 438–440.
51. Barber, T. X., and Calverley, D. S. Toward a theory of "hypnotic" behavior: An experimental study of "hypnotic time distortion." *Arch. gen. Psychiat.*, 1964, *10*, 209–216.
52. Barber, T. X., and Calverley, D. S. Toward a theory of hypnotic behavior: Effects on suggestibility of defining the situation as hypnosis and defining response to suggestions as easy. *J. abnorm. soc. Psychol.*, 1964, *68*, 585–592.

54. Barber, T. X., and Calverley, D. S. Empirical evidence for a theory of "hypnotic" behavior: Effects on suggestibility of five variables typically included in hypnotic induction procedures. *J. consult. Psychol.*, 1965, *29*, 98–107.
55. Barber, T. X., and Calverley, D. S. Empirical evidence for a theory of "hypnotic" behavior: The suggestibility-enhancing effects of motivational suggestions, relaxation-sleep suggestions, and suggestions that the subject will be effectively "hypnotized." *J. Pers.*, 1965, *33*, 256–270.
57. Barber, T. X., and Calverley, D. S. Effects on recall of hypnotic induction, motivational suggestions, and suggested regression: A methodological and experimental analysis. *J. abnorm. Psychol.*, 1966, *71*, 169–180.
58. Barber, T. X., and Calverley, D. S. Fact, fiction, and the topic *hypnosis:* Multidimensional analysis of hypnotic behavior. Harding, Mass.: Medfield Foundation, 1966. (Mimeo)
59. Barber, T. X., and Calverley, D. S. Toward a theory of "hypnotic" behavior: Experimental analyses of suggested amnesia. *J. abnorm. Psychol.*, 1966, *71*, 95–107.
60. Barber, T. X., and Calverley, D. S. Toward a theory of hypnotic behavior: Experimental evaluation of Hull's postulate that hypnotic susceptibility is a habit phenomenon. *J. Pers.*, 1966, *34*, 416–433.
61. Barber, T. X., and Calverley, D. S. Toward a theory of hypnotic behavior: Replication and extension of the Hilgard-Tart study. Harding, Mass.: Medfield Foundation, 1966. (Mimeo)
62. Barber, T. X., Chauncey, H. H., and Winer, R. A. Effect of hypnotic and nonhypnotic suggestions on parotid gland response to gustatory stimuli. *Psychosom. Med.*, 1964, *26*, 374–380.
63. Barber, T. X., and Coules, J. Electrical skin conductance and galvanic skin response during "hypnosis." *Int. J. clin. exp. Hypn.*, 1959, *7*, 79–92.
64. Barber, T. X., Dalal, A. S., and Calverley, D. S. The subjective reports of hypnotic subjects. Harding, Mass.: Medfield Foundation, 1966. (Mimeo)
67. Barber, T. X., and Hahn, K. W., Jr. Physiological and subjective responses to pain producing stimulation under hypnotically-suggested and waking-imagined "analgesia." *J. abnorm. soc. Psychol.*, 1962, *65*, 411–418.
69. Barber, T. X., and Hahn, K. W., Jr. Experimental studies in "hypnotic" behavior: Physiological and subjective effects of imagined pain. *J. nerv. ment. Dis.*, 1964, *139*, 416–425.
70. Barber, T. X., and Hahn, K. W., Jr. Suggested dreaming with and without hypnotic induction. Harding, Mass.: Medfield Foundation, 1966. (Mimeo)
72. Barber, T. X., and Silver, M. J. Fact, fiction, and the experimenter expectancy bias effect. Harding, Mass.: Medfield Foundation, 1966. (Mimeo)

79. Bernheim, H. *Suggestive Therapeutics*. Westport, Conn.: Associated Booksellers, 1957. (Original date of publication: 1886.)

89. Braid, J. *Neurypnology: Or the Rationale of Nervous Sleep Considered in Relation to Animal Magnetism*. London: Churchill, 1843.

91. Braithwaite, R. B. *Scientific Explanation*. London: Cambridge Univ. Press, 1953.

92. Bramwell, J. M. *Hypnotism*. London: Grant Richards, 1903.

98. Calverley, D. S., and Barber, T. X. "Hypnosis" and antisocial behavior: An experimental evaluation. Harding, Mass.: Medfield Foundation, 1965. (Mimeo)

104a. Chaves, J. F. Hypnosis reconceptualized: An overview of Barber's theoretical and empirical work. Boston: Dept. of Psychology, Northeastern Univ., 1966. (Mimeo)

109. Conant, J. B. *On Understanding Science*. New York: Mentor Books, 1951.

115. Dalal, A. S. An empirical approach to hypnosis: An overview of Barber's work. *Arch. gen. Psychiat.*, 1966, *15*, 151–157.

123. Dermen, D., and London, P. Correlates of hypnotic susceptibility. *J. consult. Psychol.*, 1965, *29*, 537–545.

135. Eckart, C. Ether (in physics). In *Encyclopedia Britannica*. Chicago: Encyclopedia Britannica Inc., 1965.

150. Feigl, H. Existential hypotheses: Realistic versus phenomenalistic interpretations. *Philo. Sci.*, 1950, *17*, 35–62.

151. Feigl, H., and Brodbeck, M. *Readings in the Philosophy of Science*. New York: Appleton-Century-Crofts, 1953.

165. Gill, M. M., and Brenman, M. *Hypnosis and Related States*. New York: International Univ. Press, 1959.

186. Hilgard, E. R. *Hypnotic Susceptibility*. New York: Harcourt, Brace, & World, 1965.

196. Ikemi, Y., and Nakagawa, S. A psychosomatic study of contagious dermatitis. *Kyushu J. Med. Sci.*, 1962, *13*, 335–350.

202. Kelly, C. R. Psychological factors in myopia. Unpublished Ph. D. dissertation, New School for Social Research, 1958.

203. Kelly, C. R. Psychological factors in myopia. Paper read at *Amer. Psychol. Ass.*, New York, August 31, 1961.

206. Klemme, H. L. Heart rate response to suggestion in hypnosis. Topeka, Kans.: Veterans Administration Hospital, 1963. (Mimeo)

212. Koch, S. Clark S. Hull. In *Modern Learning Theory*. New York: Appleton-Century-Crofts, 1954. Pp. 1–176.

213. Koch, S. Epilogue. In S. Koch (Ed.) *Psychology: A Study of a Science*. (Vol. 3) New York: McGraw-Hill, 1959. Pp. 729–788.

217. Kuhn, T. S. *The Structure of Scientific Revolutions*. Chicago: Univ. of Chicago Press, 1962.

238. Ludwig, A. M., and Lyle, W. H., Jr. Tension induction and the hyperalert trance. *J. abnorm. soc. Psychol.*, 1964, *69*, 70–76.

247. Marx, M. H. Intervening variable or hypothetical construct? *Psychol. Rev.*, 1951, *58*, 235–247.

248. Marx, M. H. *Psychological Theory*. New York: Macmillan, 1951.

249. Marx, M. H. *Theories in Contemporary Psychology*. New York: Macmillan, 1963.

258. Melie, J. P., and Hilgard, E. R. Attitudes toward hypnosis, self-predictions, and hypnotic susceptibility. *Int. J. clin. exp. Hypn.*, 1964. *12*; 99–108.

262. Michael, A. M. Hypnosis in childbirth. *Brit. Med. J.*, 1952, *1*, 734–737.

263. Milgram, S. Behavioral study of obedience. *J. abnorm. soc. Psychol.*, 1963, *67*, 371–378.

267. Moll, A. *The Study of Hypnotism.* New York: Julian Press, 1958. (Original date of publication: 1889.)

277. Orne, M. T. The nature of hypnosis: Artifact and essence. *J. abnorm. soc. Psychol.*, 1959, *58*, 277–299.

293. Popper, K. R. *The Logic of Scientific Discovery.* New York: Basic Books, 1959.

304. Rosenthal, R. The effect of the experimenter on the results of psychological research. In B. A. Maher (Ed.) *Progress in Experimental Personality Research.* (Vol. 1) New York: Academic Press, 1964. Pp. 79–114.

311. Sarbin, T. R. Contributions to role-taking theory: I. Hypnotic behavior. *Psychol. Rev.*, 1950, *57*, 255–270.

314. Sarbin, T. R. Attempts to understand hypnotic phenomena. In L. Postman (Ed.) *Psychology in the Making.* New York: Knopf, 1962. Pp. 745–785.

315. Sarbin, T. R. Role theoretical interpretation of psychological change. In P. Worchel and D. Byrne (Eds.) *Personality Change.* New York: Wiley, 1964. Pp. 176–219.

317. Sarbin, T. R., and Andersen, M. L. Role-theoretical analysis of hypnotic behavior. In J. Gordon (Ed.) *Clinical and Experimental Handbook of Hypnosis.* New York: Macmillan, in press.

327. Shor, R. E. Hypnosis and the concept of the generalized reality-orientation. *Amer. J. Psychother.*, 1959, *13*, 582–602.

329. Shor, R. E. Three dimensions of hypnotic depth. *Int. J. clin. exp. Hypn.*, 1962, *10*, 23–38.

338. Spielberger, C. D., and DeNike, L. D. Descriptive behaviorism versus cognitive theory in verbal operant conditioning. *Psychol. Rev.*, 1966, *73*, 306–326.

345. Tart, C. T., and Hilgard, E. R. Responsiveness to suggestions under "hypnosis" and "waking-imagination" conditions: A methodological observation. *Int. J. clin. exp. Hypn.*, 1966, *14*, 247–256.

348. Troffer, S. A. H. Hypnotic age regression and cognitive functioning. Unpublished Ph.D. Dissertation, Stanford Univ., 1966.

361. Weitzenhoffer, A. M. *Hypnotism: An Objective Study in Suggestibility.* New York: Wiley, 1953.

362. Weitzenhoffer, A. M. *General Techniques of Hypnotism.* New York: Grune & Stratton, 1957.

363. Weitzenhoffer, A. M. The nature of hypnosis: Part II. *Amer. J. clin. Hypn.*, 1963, *6*, 40–72.

368. Wells, W. R. Experiments in waking hypnosis for instructional purposes. *J. abnorm. soc. Psychol.*, 1924, *18*, 389–404.

[6]

ALTERED STATES OF AWARENESS

ERNEST R. HILGARD, Ph.D.[1]

A man knows that he belongs to the human race because of his conscious experiences; the existentialists tell us that what he most dreads is death, which means the end to experience. He values his experiences, but he is frightened by some of them, too; in any case they provide for him the meaning of his life, his joys, his sorrows, his hopes, and his defeats. Why, then, are psychologists so timid in talking about conscious states, about awareness, when they are the initial subject matter?

The answer is, in one sense, simple: psychologists are trying to be scientists like other scientists, and they will do anything to be proper about it, even to the point of denying some of their subject matter. The early scientific psychologists, who did accept consciousness as their subject matter, so sterilized it through their formal methods of introspection that those who wanted an enriched psychology broke with that tradition. It was the behaviorist Watson who put a chapter on personality in his textbook, not the mentalist Titchener. But behaviorism proceeded then to deny consciousness and carried the revolt against sterility too far, so that new strictures arose against some of the topics of psychology. At the risk of some oversimplification, we may recognize three contemporary trends that represent efforts to be scientific about psychology and still to be open to its range of potential topics. One is a continuing battle for purism of the kind that Watson's behaviorism started. This now takes the form of an attack on intervening variables of all kinds, but particularly on what is called "reification," or making "things" out of traits or states or conscious experiences. This position we may call *contemporary behaviorism,* to note that it has changed some since Watson through the efforts of Skinner, Bandura, and others. A second tendency, at the other extreme, is to throw off preoccupation with scientific objectivity in order to celebrate human values and to revel in experience, hence to look for the outreaches of human potentiality, consciousness expansion, and rich encounters. There are many variants of this, but to use the name of a society dedicated to this standpoint, we may call this *humanistic psychology.* The third tendency is the more moderate one of throwing off the "you mustn't say" strictures of behaviorism without departing from objectivity, and without rejecting an enlightened operationism. Miller, Galanter, and Pribram (32) somewhat whimsically called such a position "subjective behaviorism," but I prefer to use an older term and call it *contemporary functionalism.* The older functionalist, typified by James Rowland Angell, was always willing to use consciousness, behavior, physiology, and mathematics, and I see no reason why the moderates of today should not recognize this ancestry. It does not mean that there have been no advances since Angell for this group, just as there have been advances since Watson for the avowed behaviorists.

THE PROBLEM OF STATES AND AWARENESS OF THEM

Skinner has been the spokesman for the empty organism, thus representing those who object to dealing with nonobservables in the form of either introspections or inferences. Some behaviorists permit verbal

[1] Department of Psychology, Stanford University, Stanford, California 94305. The research was conducted under Contract AF 49(638)-1436 with the Air Force Office of Scientific Research, and under a grant from the National Institute of Mental Health, U. S. Public Health Service (Grant MH-03859).

reports to serve as objective evidence for inner states, but Skinner is careful to have them refer to *stimuli*, not to states. For instance, in his book on verbal behavior: "Consider, for example, the complex tact, *I am hungry*. This is emitted under the control of relevant (usually private) stimuli" (44, p. 151).

Those who carry on the behaviorist tradition in the study of personality and social psychology attack *traits* and *states* as misleading ways in which to describe the continuities in personality (33), preferring always to point to specific learned behavior (2).

> From the viewpoint of social behavior theory the results viewed in this and previous chapters reflect the empirically unjustified assumptions of trait and state theory and not merely the limitations of measurements (33, p. 148).

Others carry the same general line of attack against descriptions of present awareness according to states of consciousness. In an avalanche of papers, Barber has taken a position against hypnosis as a state and prefers to write the word "hypnosis" in quotation marks as though it represented something mythical (3, 5). Sarbin, too, has taken up cudgels against named states of awareness; he finds myths not only in the concept of "hypnosis," but in "hallucination" and "schizophrenia" (38), and also "anxiety" (39).

The arguments of Skinner, Bandura, Mischel, Barber, and Sarbin deserve to be taken quite seriously, for they have all been able to go a long way toward advancing our understanding of important phenomena while embracing their position. I am prepared to recognize this, even though the general position is one that I cannot endorse.

So much for contemporary behaviorism. The other extreme, of variants on existentialism and humanistic psychology, not only is found in the popular movements of the time toward consciousness expansion, psychedelic experiences, and experimentation with drugs or Eastern religions, but is found also in the serious psychological literature. The forms are quite varied (8, 11, 30, 34, 37, 42). While there is something refreshing about this protest against "scientism," just where it will lead in producing a new paradigm for psychology is uncertain. The prior history of various returns to a "naive" or "phenomenalistic" psychology in the past does not augur well for its survival, even though it will doubtless have a leavening influence.

The middle ground—what I am calling contemporary functionalism—has had an interesting upsurge over the last 10 years. A careful historical analysis would probably find a growing distaste for stimulus-response concepts, already criticized by Dewey many years ago (13), but joined in by others from time to time (19, 32, 48). Information theory for a time appeared to provide a new model, at the time that other influences were converging to produce an emphasis upon a cognitive psychology. Mathematical models were precise but "neutral" on many of the classical issues. Computer simulation came in and made respectable new studies of thinking that appeared more promising than the earlier introspective ones. In any case, many voices began to be heard (14, 24, 31). Investigators began to turn to neglected fields of study, to attention, imagery, hallucinations, and other "subjective" phenomena which had earlier made behaviorists uncomfortable. Those who began to look into these neglected topics had themselves been brought up on behaviorism and operationism, and they did not find that they had to strain their scientific integrity or objectivity in redirecting the focus of their investigations. They merely had to have confidence that psychology's tools were now sharp enough, its position as a science firmly enough established, that they could venture into the study of "subjective" phenomena without loss of scientific status.

Thus psychologists do not march forward with a common front, but they veer toward a contemporary behaviorism, at one extreme, toward humanistic psychology at the other extreme, or to the middle ground of contemporary functionalism. I wish now, from the vantage point of the mid-position, to examine waking consciousness and its alterations in sleep and dreams and in hypnosis.

WAKING AS A COMPLEX STATE

By a normal waking state we mean one in which we can report accurately what is happening in the environment about us and can use this information to control our behavior. We do not do these things well when we are asleep, or drugged, or delirious. Under those other conditions most of us are willing to say that someone is in an altered state, even though the borderlines are hard to define.

A little reflection will show us that the waking state itself is far from simple. When we carry on a conversation, we are simultaneously listening and formulating a reply, and even while replying we are thinking of our next maneuver. Thus we are not doing just one thing at a time, and how many things we can do at once, and how well we do them, pose problems for experimental study. This is the kind of thing that sets the functionalist to work; subjective observation has set him some problems that he hopes he can solve by objective methods. His preference for operationism does not make him deny the problems. He performs experiments on listening to more than one conversation at a time, on one message to one ear and another to the other, on reciting aloud what is coming in over earphones, with informative results (10). It takes a little effort to remain alert, even when we are not very tired, and to avoid vacant staring we do a good deal of squirming about, chewing of pencils, lighting a pipe, adjusting clothing, or talking merely to eliminate silence. My point here, as against those who deny "states," is that I see no reason to deny that being awake is a state, even though it is hard to give it a fully satisfactory definition.

SLEEPING AND DREAMING AS ALTERED STATES

With the discovery of the rapid eye movement state of sleep (the REM state) and another state of sleep, defined negatively as non-rapid eye movement (the NREM state), we now understand quite well that there are at least three states where before we thought there were only two. That is, the sleep state is divided (in addition to several levels of depth) into two quite distinct states with different properties. But I should like to point out something here: it did not take electroencephalographic (EEG) studies to tell us that there were two states, such as waking and sleeping, even though it was sometimes hard to tell when a person was asleep (or merely playing possum). If he was trustworthy, he would tell you when he was simulating sleep, although sometimes, when really asleep, he might deny having been asleep. It is important to remember this when we come to the discussion of hypnosis, for the dismissal of hypnosis as a state because we don't know its physiology would be like dismissing sleep as a state *before* we knew its physiology. Lack of perfect correlation and ill defined border conditions do not prevent useful experiments from reaching satisfactory inferences through convergent operations (15).

Fortunately, the study of sleep and dreaming has advanced greatly since the discovery of REM sleep by Aserinsky and Kleitman (1), and the questions of "state" are essentially now empirical ones. Stoyva and Kamiya (47) have made a very useful contribution to the discussion of a strategy for the study of consciousness by citing in some detail the recent history of research on sleeping and dreaming. Extending the notion of convergent operations, they have shown how useful the interchange has been between the physiological indicators (chiefly, but not exclusively, EEG and REM) and dream recall. There would be no way of knowing whether the eye movements were related to dreaming except by asking the subject. At the same time there is no certainty with respect to the subject's reported dream content. Only by exercising ingenuity in relating the two kinds of data (physiological response and verbal report) can the true state of affairs be inferred. Some of the work of Kamiya (cited in 29) on the operant control of the EEG alpha rhythms is referred to as a further illustration of the usefulness of combining objective measures with verbal reports. Under the conditions in which the alpha is "on," the subject commonly reports that he is relaxed and not experiencing visual imagery: he usually finds long periods of time in continuous alpha to be quite pleasant (35). There are always some uncertainties and options in any single set of correspondences from two orders of data, but in this case there are three kinds of data—operant procedures, physiological indicators, and verbal reports—so that more complex convergences are possible, leading to greater confidence about the inferences to a "mental state." Here we have a very good illustration of contemporary functionalism in that the curiosity about the mental state is fully as great as that of any phenomenologist, yet the rules of scientific evidence are followed as faithfully as by the more classical behaviorist who does not wish to make inferences respecting states of consciousness.

Our "inventory" of states now adds up to the three-fold cycle of waking, REM, and NREM, through which everyone goes every day, and now another set (alpha and non-alpha) through which people also go, but which they can learn to control in the laboratory, or in certain kinds of exercises, as under a Zen master.

HYPNOSIS AS AN ALTERED STATE

Hypnosis is commonly considered to be a "state," perhaps resembling the state in which the sleepwalker finds himself, hence the term "somnambulist" as applied to the deeply hypnotized person. William James, in discussing the significance of suggestibility in hypnosis, endorsed the notion of a special state: "The suggestion-theory may therefore be approved as correct, provided we grant the trance-state as its prerequisite" (25, p. 601).

In a very lucid analysis of what happens during hypnotic induction and within the established hypnotic state, Kubie and Margolin (27) agreed with those who, like James, found it congenial to recognize the hypnotic state as an altered state of awareness. They pointed out that the usual hypnotic procedures (including immobilization and monotony) tend to cut off communications with the outside world, except for the voice of the hypnotist. The subject then confuses the hypnotist's words with his own thoughts. Following the steps of induction, in which the ego boundaries have been blurred, the established hypnotic state emerges, including a partial reexpansion of ego boundaries. Gill and Brenman (16), quoting this earlier analysis favorably, also distinguished between the fractionation of the ego in the induction phase and a reintegration within the established hypnotic state, although still at a partially regressed level.

As in the case of other "states" the conception of an established hypnotic state has not gone unchallenged. The two most vocal challengers are Barber and Sarbin. Barber stated, for example:

> Further research aiming to delineate the factors making for high response to suggestions should be careful not to confound the variable labeled as "trance" with such variables as instructions designed to produce positive motivation to perform well on assigned tasks and instructions or suggestions to perform the criterion behaviors. We can predict that when the varia-

bles discussed in this chapter are kept distinct and unconfounded, the variable labeled "hypnotic trance" will prove to be extraneous to producing "analgesia," "hallucinations," "amnesia," and so on (4, p. 472).

Sarbin, extending his earlier role-theoretical analysis in hypnosis in collaboration with Andersen, clearly rejected the concept of trance (or other "state" concepts):

> One feature that differentiates role-theoretical and other social psychological formulations of hypnosis from the more credulous theories is the nonemployment of the trance either as a descriptive device or as a mediational process (40, p. 342).

To get at the problem of the nature of hypnosis, we have conducted a number of experiments in our laboratory on hypnotically suggested analgesia. I wish to use them to illustrate the puzzling nature of these phenomena, and the futility of jumping to conclusions about task motivation, demand characteristics, or role enactment in accounting for the detailed events that occur.

Some of the preliminary accounts appeared in this journal (20), but a number of experiments since then have added quantitative sophistication to the suggestions there offered (17, 18).

My collaborators and I have used two methods to induce pain, and this fact in itself turns out to be important in order to avoid finality in interpreting and generalizing from experiments. The first method is that of the *cold pressor test,* in which a hand and forearm are placed in circulating ice water. When the water is actually at 0°C, an immersion period of 30 to 40 seconds is sufficient to produce intense pain (23, 49). The second method is that of *ischemic pain,* in which a tourniquet is applied above the elbow, the subject exercises for a time by squeezing a dynamometer, and then waits while the pain in the forearm rises (28, 45). The pain often does not begin right away, and there may be little or no pain for a matter of minutes, but then it begins to rise and eventually the forearm becomes excruciatingly painful, so that the tourniquet has to be removed.

Both of these pains lend themselves to lawful verbal reports. The courses of verbal reports on a scale from 0 up, with 10 the point at which they would very much wish to have the hand taken out of the water or the tourniquet removed; both fit a power function with time, in accordance with the psychophysical expectations found by Stevens (46) for so many sensory functions. Both kinds of pain can be reduced under the suggestion of hypnotic analgesia, the amount of reduction in pain correlating with the degree of susceptibility to hypnosis as measured by the standard hypnotic susceptibility scales. The correlations are of the order of $r = .50$ or .60, large enough to be adequately significant with the sizes of the samples that we use. These results suffice to indicate the reality of pain reduction under hypnosis; the correlation with measured hypnotic susceptibility indicates that the individual differences in susceptibility not only are enduring over time, but are predictive of measures not used in the original measuring scales, which had no strictly analgesia items, the most closely related being an item on anosmia to ammonia. There is nothing in what I have reported that would cause disagreement by Barber or Sarbin, except that Barber would wish to know whether induction of hypnosis was really necessary; both he and Sarbin accept the main point that there *are* persistent individual differences which are highly relevant to hypnotic-type responses.[2] Thus the question of "state" is not necessarily involved.

Accepting the logic of converging operations, we were desirous of having a meas-

[2] Barber commonly implies that the individual differences are motivational, but this is an inference on his part (4, p. 451), and others disagree (36).

ure of physiological response that correlated with the verbally reported pain. We used several measures of cardiac response and breathing, but, without going into the details, we found a repeatedly monitored measure of systolic blood pressure in the middle finger of the nonstimulated hand to be the most satisfactory.[3] For example, in experiments on cold pressor pain not involving hypnosis, but with water at four temperatures (15°C, 10°C, 5°C, and 0°C) we were able to demonstrate a correspondence between the rise in blood pressure both with time in the water and with temperature, the blood pressure curves paralleling very closely the verbally reported pain. We found the same relationship of rising blood pressure with reported pain in the ischemia experiment. So far there is a parallelism between the results with cold water and ischemia, but here the parallelism stops.

In replicated experiments in the ice water, using both waking controls and a control for hypnosis *without* analgesia as well as hypnosis *with* suggested analgesia, we found that blood pressure *rose more for the hypnotic analgesia condition* than for the waking condition, in the same subjects. Without further evidence, one might conjecture that the reports of hypnotic analgesia were not genuine, and that perhaps we had a kind of "lie detection" experiment here, with the higher blood pressure associated with the reports of "no pain" under hypnosis. However, the same effect was found for the low hypnotizables who were reporting as much pain as ever, so that this explanation is not satisfactory. Apparently there was some kind of excitement associated with the expectations engendered by the instructions, and this was communicated to those who were to become analgesic as well as to those who did not become analgesic. Also the shock of cold water may have had reflex effects uncontrolled by the hypnotic suggestions. The results show how generalizations from single experiments can be misleading, such as the interpretation that the analgesic effect owes to the relaxation and nonanxiety of the hypnotic subject (43). Our hypnotic subjects without instructions for analgesia were relaxed, too, but suffered pain, and if we use rise in blood pressure as indicating the opposite of relaxation, our most analgesic were the least relaxed and most anxious of all.

We also ran a carefully designed experiment using simulators to see the effect on their blood pressure as they deliberately attempted to "fool" the experimenter into believing that they were analgesic. This is possible in a short exposure to the ice water; a willing subject can be trained to act as though he feels no pain. The experiment (recently completed and as yet unpublished) was extremely carefully controlled to be sure that the experimenter had no knowledge as to whether or not his subject was a "true" hypnotic subject or a subject "simulating" hypnosis, but the subject, after the experiment was over, reported back to the staff member who had given the instructions for simulation in the first place. The ones posing as hypnotic subjects in no case found the pain relieved (though occasionally it was slightly reduced) while the subjects selected on the basis of prior evidence of analgesia felt no pain throughout the experiment. What about the blood pressure? There was a clear difference between the blood pressure under the analgesia conditions for the "true" and "simulating" subjects. Both increased their blood pressure over the waking condition, but the simulators increased theirs by an amount that was significantly greater than the amount by which the "trues" increased theirs. In terms of formal design,

[3] Credit for the blood pressure-measuring device, and for the ischemic pain experiments, goes primarily to John Lenox, who has kindly permitted me to refer to his work before he has had the opportunity to publish it. A number of the ideas in this paper have come from him and other collaborators in these experiments.

therefore, the experiment worked out all right, showing that "simulators" and "trues" differ, but the details remain to be explained. Let me now state some propositions regarding the relationship between blood pressure and pain and hypnosis: *1) When pain is felt in the cold pressor experiment in the normal waking state, there is a tendency for blood pressure to rise in an amount correlated with the amount of experienced pain. 2) In the cold pressor experiment combined with hypnotic instructions blood pressure may rise independent of the amount of felt pain.*

What this amounts to—and I wish to state this rather firmly—is that the cold pressor experiment is not a good place to look for physiological correlates of pain and of pain reduction under hypnosis. We have used far more subjects than earlier investigators and, I believe, more stringent controls. Our results make the findings of an experiment such as that of Barber and Hahn (7) not wrong but indecisive on the issues being studied.

Had we stopped with the cold pressor experiment, we would have made generalizations that were misleading, for the ischemic pain experiments turned out differently. In them, the highly susceptible subjects not only felt no pain under suggested hypnotic analgesia, for durations of ischemia half again as long as the time at which they were writhing in pain in the waking state, but *the blood pressure did not rise.* This is not a result of subject selection, for these subjects came from the subjects who had participated in the cold pressor experiment, where they responded as the others did. An effort to use the simulator design in this experiment failed: we were not able to coax or cajole or train simulators to deny pain long enough under the more severe stress of ischemia to serve the design of a simulation experiment. The end result is, of course, the same: showing the genuineness of the hypnotic analgesia for those subjects who can experience it. It shows also that the "demand characteristics" of the experiment, the motivation to please the experimenter, are not sufficient, *unless* the subject can really rid himself of the pain as a consequence of the hypnotic procedures. This leads to the third assertion about blood pressure and pain: *3) In the ischemic experiment, the failure of the blood pressure to rise, which is correlated with absence of a verbal report of pain, supports the reality of the hypnotic analgesia.*

These are the unexpected results that take the scientist off of the debating platform and send him back to the laboratory. Why should there be this difference between the effects of hypnosis on blood pressure in the cold pressor experiment and in the ischemia experiment? There are many variables, and these have to be explored: the time factors, the effects of temperature confused with the effects of pain in the cold pressor test, the amount of prior experience of the subjects. These are not matters for debate but for study. At the same time, even though these questions are open they do not deny the ultimate finding: highly susceptible hypnotic subjects, following hypnotic induction and with the suggestion of analgesia, felt no pain under circumstances in which they would normally feel excruciating pain, and their physiological responses also attested to the absence of pain.[4]

With these data before us we are ready to turn to the question of whether our subjects were in a "state" of hypnosis. It is very easy to lose the focus of theoretical argument. Very often the argument against "state" becomes an argument against the reality of the phenomena, and our experiments settle (unless they are subsequently challenged) the empirical reality of hypnotic pain reduction. I doubt that this is any longer at issue, because of the abun-

[4] The heart rate in ischemia also confirmed the absence of pain, although it served no better than blood pressure in the cold pressor experiment.

dant clinical evidence in addition to the laboratory evidence. But this is not the basic argument over "state." Our data would have to be supplemented by a demonstration that these same subjects, when not in a "state" of hypnosis, could not yield the phenomena. They do not yield them when they are awake; that is, these are not cases of people insensitive to pain. But would they yield them if exhorted, cajoled, their imaginations stirred up, their attention directed elsewhere? Here we are in difficult territory, because these are all methods of inducing the "state" (if such there be) in highly susceptible subjects. Actually the question is not a very decisive one, for surely people capable of producing hypnotic phenomena can produce them in various ways, through self-hypnosis, at a signal set up through posthypnotic suggestion, and so on. It would not matter very much whether, after demonstration of the ability to achieve hypnotic analgesia in the ischemic pain situation, a subject could do it without special induction procedures. I would expect him to—but he might do it by entering the state of hypnosis, and this is the nub of the question. Just as we know that he experiences pain by asking him, so we ask him about hypnosis. He might be lying in either case, but he usually tells the truth; in any case the experimenter exercises such ingenuity as he can to find out what is so. If he pushes the subject for the truth, as Bowers (9) did, the simulators will confess to falsifications, while the truly susceptible subjects will not. This led Bowers to conclude that many of the experiments designed to prove that task-motivated behavior was the equivalent of hypnotically suggested behavior prejudged the issue by accepting behavioral compliance as the criterion of similarity of response. His own experiments led him to believe that over and above this compliance hypnosis represents "an altered state within which suggestions have a peculiarly potent effect."

Careful interviews with subjects prior to and following hypnosis have begun to throw considerable light on the cognitive and affective features of the hypnotic involvement, and its relationship to experiences outside hypnosis (22). To deny the relevance of such observations because of preconceptions as to the appropriate methods of science is to throw away highly pertinent and illuminating data.

ALTERED STATES AS CATEGORIES *VS.* STATES AS CAUSES

The world is too complex and confusing to study all at once, so that scientists "stake their claims" through some sort of classification of phenomena. This persists in the names of fields of science such as physical sciences, life sciences, social sciences. Such classificatory schemes are in the interests of simplification and order and need not be divisive. Thus the separation of life sciences from physical sciences does not prevent the emergence of the fields of biochemistry or of biophysics, which resist classification in the old rubrics. But classification serves other purposes of more scientific relevance, as in distinguishing phases (ice, water, steam), with rules relating them and their transitions. The same is true in the classification of states of awareness. It is convenient to talk about waking and sleep, about sobriety and drunkenness, about reality orientation and reality distortion, without thereby disturbing objective reporting of what is known about the phenomena under study.

The main reason that these classificatory labels are objected to is that they occasionally run the danger of becoming explanations. The controversy over instincts that has gone on intermittently for a half-century illustrates this. Instinct was (and still is!) a convenient term for species-specific behavior, when used in a classificatory sense, to describe, for example, characteristic nest building of birds according to species. But if a pigeon returns home *be-*

cause of a homing instinct, we get into a little trouble, and there is some circularity, for the way we know it has a homing instinct is that it returns home. There still is no harm in pointing out that some pigeons have this instinctive tendency and others do not. The objection is not to instinct as a classificatory word but to instinct as an explanatory one.

This same argument holds for words like sleep and hypnosis. In drawing some parallels between their treatment, I am not endorsing the interpretation of hypnosis as a partial sleep, although that theory of Pavlov's continues to have supporters in many parts of the world. I am simply using sleep as a familiar illustration to justify ways of talking about hypnosis, which is less familiar.

If one wishes to argue that sleep is not a state, I have no quarrel with that, because then the argument is not over fact but over words. If sleep is not a state, then hypnosis is not a state either. But if sleep *is* a state, which I suppose most of us would accept, then maybe hypnosis is a state, too. Let us see where we are on empirical grounds.

Suppose we apply to sleep the same critical attacks that have been made on hypnosis. First, it is very difficult to define sleep; as Kleitman (26) pointed out, it is usually defined negatively as the opposite of wakefulness. It is hard to distinguish it from coma, for example, except by some sort of operational definition: you can be aroused from sleep, but not from coma. (This departs from a "state" definition and hence can be used to argue against sleep as a state.) Or suppose you build some sort of behavioral test for sleep, such as what the person tells you when you wake him up ("I must have been asleep, because I didn't hear you come in"), whether or not he reports a dream, or some more "objective" measures such as whether or not he snores or how loud a bell it takes to rouse him. These would not work out too badly, but they would be subject to the same criticisms as those leveled against hypnotic scales. For one thing, any of these measures can be "faked." A person can imitate snoring, even though he is not asleep; he can report a dream when he had none. Therefore, we do better to abandon the notion of "sleep," write the word in quotation marks, and stick to the input-output measures that we use in experiments concerned with the phenomena associated with a person who is lying in bed at night with his eyes closed.

Those who might wish to save sleep as a state, but still reject hypnosis, have another line of argument. Because of the EEG we now have a physiological definition of sleep and hence are on much more secure ground when we study, for example, the question of whether or not sleep-learning is possible. This is a good argument, but it does not completely escape the circularity that the EEG measures of depth of sleep can only be validated by behavioral measures. It turns out, in fact, that it is more difficult to be aroused from stage 1 than from "deeper" stages, if REMs are occurring in stage 1. This evidence comes not from physiology but from behavior, although, to the extent that there are lawful correlates, everything remains in order. It would be a great help to the researcher on hypnosis if there were physiological indicators, such as the EEG in sleep, to help define more precisely what condition the subject is in. The search for such indicators, as illustrated by our use of the blood pressure measures in relation to pain, is valid and should be pressed. But the question I am raising is this: would we have denied sleep as a "state" before the EEG measures were available? I think not. Perhaps hypnosis research lags behind sleep research by a decade or two. Hence I do not believe that the absence of clear physiological correlates of hypnosis is crucial in the answer to the question of whether or not it represents a state.

The temptation to use state as a cause

or an explanation is another matter. Even though snoring and dreams typically occur during sleep, it does not help very much to say that sleep causes them, for of course it is possible to sleep without snoring or dreaming. Still it does no harm to point out that their presence is *more likely* during sleep. This is an empirical question, and similar empirical questions arise in relation to hypnosis: is typical hypnotic behavior more likely when the conditions have been favorable for entering a hypothesized hypnotic state? The empirical answer is not as easy as might be supposed. In one of our investigations concerned with this problem we found that it was necessary to use careful designs to demonstrate rather small increments as a result of hypnotic induction (21). As Tart and I pointed out, the experimental design must take into account the following considerations: 1) many nonhypnotizable people are not going to change following attempted induction; 2) some highly susceptible subjects do not require induction to enter hypnosis and yield all the phenomena, and hence they do not change between waking suggestion and hypnosis; 3) the argument for change with induction therefore rests on a minority of subjects who respond only slightly to waking suggestion but are very responsive to suggestion after induction procedures. Under these circumstances, small groups of unselected subjects are quite likely to lead to no statistical difference attributable to induction, especially if extraneous demands toward increasing voluntary compliance are added in the nonhypnotic condition. While our conditions, favorable to detecting small changes, led to the conclusion that the effects of induction could be demonstrated, the matter is still subject to some empirical controversy (6). Although the question of the effects of induction continues to be of interest, it is not crucial to the question whether or not some subjects can enter a state of hypnosis. That has to be determined on more subtle grounds, using converging operations which will doubtless include subjective report, overt behavior, and physiological indicators.

Suppose the results turn out that there are phenomena associated with the hypnotic state that are not as likely when the subject is not in that state. It is possible to accept all of this without making the state of hypnosis the cause of the behavior, any more than sleep causes snoring or dreams.

Note also that the use of a classificatory rubric does not require that there be no differentiation within that rubric. Thus sleep turns out not to be one state but at least two (REM and NREM). This does not negate a differentiation between sleep and waking: both the REM subject and NREM subject are still asleep. I doubt if there will turn out to be just one state of hypnosis; subjects capable of deep relaxation under hypnosis are also capable of alert hyperactivity, and only careful study will reveal what it is that they have in common physiologically. But there is no harm in still defining the area of experimental study as that of hypnosis, just as the student of REM and NREM sleep still studies sleep.

It would be possible to go on to the definition of other kinds of altered states of awareness, such as those engendered by fever or by drugs. These cover a wide range from stupor to ecstasy. All the arguments over states as descriptive and as explanatory apply here as well. The work of Schachter and Singer (41) shows how careful we have to be before we assign emotional states on the basis of the kind of drug ingested. This does not require us to argue that emotion is a myth.

CONCLUSION

The arguments against altered states of awareness follow the pattern of scientific logic historically associated with American behaviorism, continuing today in some forms of contemporary behaviorism and social behavior theory. Those who take these positions tend to dislike traits and states and intervening variables generally, particularly if the names have survived from the subjective vocabulary of an earlier era. Revolt against this earlier behaviorism has taken two forms: a more extreme rejection in the form of humanistic psychology, and a milder corrective in the form of a modern functionalism, emphasizing convergent operations. The last method has worked well in the study of sleeping and dreaming, in the relating of subjective experiences to the control of the alpha rhythm, and there is no reason why it should not work well in the study of hypnosis. The method permits the identification and classification of states of awareness, without assigning to these states any unusual causal properties. The inference of a state is coherent with the kind of ordering of disparate data that advanced sciences ultimately achieve.

REFERENCES

1. Aserinsky, E., and Kleitman, N. Regularly occurring periods of eye motility, and concomitant phenomena, during sleep. Science, *118:* 273–274, 1953.
2. Bandura, A., and Walters, R. *Social Learning and Personality Development.* Holt, Rinehart, and Winston, New York, 1963.
3. Barber, T. X. "Hypnosis" as a causal variable in present-day psychology: A critical analysis. Psychol. Rep., *14:* 839–842, 1964.
4. Barber, T. X. Hypnotic phenomena: A critique of experimental methods. In Gordon, J. E., ed. *Handbook of Clinical and Experimental Hypnosis,* pp. 444–480. Macmillan, New York, 1967.
5. Barber, T. X. Reply to Conn and Conn's "Discussion of Barber's 'Hypnosis as a causal variable...'" Int. J. Clin. Exp. Hypn., *15:* 111–117, 1967.
6. Barber, T. X., and Calverley, D. C. Toward a theory of "hypnotic" behavior: Replication and extension of experiments by Barber and co-workers (1962–65) and Hilgard and Tart (1966). Int. J. Clin. Exp. Hypn., *16:* 179–195, 1968.
7. Barber, T. X., and Hahn, K. W., Jr. Physiological and subjective responses to pain-producing stimulation under hypnotically suggested and waking-imagined "analgesia." J. Abnorm. Soc. Psychol., *65:* 411–418, 1962.
8. Barron, F. *Creativity and Personal Freedom.* Van Nostrand, New York, 1968.
9. Bowers, K. Hypnotic behavior: The differentiation of trance and demand characteristic variables. J. Abnorm. Psychol., *71:* 42–51, 1966.
10. Broadbent, D. E. *Perception and Communication.* Pergamon, New York, 1958.
11. Bugental, J. F. The challenge that is man. J. Humanistic Psychol., *7:* 1–9, 1967.
12. Chaves, J. F. Hypnosis reconceptualized: An overview of Barber's theoretical and empirical work. Psychol. Rep., *22:* 587–608, 1968.
13. Dewey, J. The reflex arc concept in psychology. Psychol. Rev., *3:* 357–370, 1896.
14. Galanter, E., and Gerstenhaber, M. On thought: The extrinsic theory. Psychol. Rev., *63:* 218-227, 1956.
15. Garner, W. R., Hake, H. W., and Eriksen, C. W. Operationism and the concept of perception. Psychol. Rev., *63:* 145–159, 1956.
16. Gill, M. M., and Brenman, M. *Hypnosis and Related States.* International Universities Press, New York, 1959.
17. Hilgard, E. R. Pain as a puzzle for psychology and physiology. Amer. Psychol., *24:* 103–113, 1969.
18. Hilgard, E. R. A quantitative study of pain and its reduction through hypnotic suggestion. Proc. Nat. Acad. Sci. U. S. A., *57:* 1581–1586, 1967.
19. Hilgard, E. R. *Theories of Learning,* 1st ed. Appleton-Century-Crofts, New York, 1948.
20. Hilgard, E. R., Cooper, L. M., Lenox, J., Morgan, A. H., and Voevodsky, J. The use of pain-state reports in the study of hypnotic analgesia to the pain of ice water. J. Nerv. Ment. Dis., *144:* 506–513, 1967.
21. Hilgard, E. R., and Tart, C. T. Responsiveness to suggestion following waking and imagination instructions and following induction of hypnosis. J. Abnorm. Psychol., *71:* 196–208, 1966.
22. Hilgard, J. R. *Personality and Hypnosis: A Study of Imaginative Involvements.* University of Chicago Press, in press.
23. Hines, E. A., and Brown, G. E. A standard stimulus for measuring vasomotor reactions: Its application in the study of hypertension. Proc. Staff Meetings Mayo Clin., *7:* 332, 1932.
24. Holt, R. R. Imagery: The return of the ostracized. Amer. Psychol., *19:* 254–264, 1964.
25. James, W. *Principles of Psychology,* vols. 1 and 2. Holt, New York, 1890.
26. Kleitman, N. *Sleep and Wakefulness,* rev. ed. University of Chicago Press, Chicago, 1963.
27. Kubie, L. S., and Margolin, S. The process of hypnotism and the nature of the hypnotic state. Amer. J. Psychiat., *100:* 611–622, 1944.
28. Lewis, T., Pickering, G. W., and Rothschild, P. Observations upon muscular pain in intermittent claudication. Heart, *15:* 359-383, 1931.
29. Luce, G. G., and Segal, J. *Sleep.* Coward-McCann, New York, 1966.
30. Maslow, A. H. *Toward a Psychology of Being.* Van Nostrand, Princeton, N. J., 1962.

31. McClelland, D. C. The psychology of mental content reconsidered. Psychol. Rev., *62:* 297–302, 1955.
32. Miller, G. A., Galanter, E., and Pribram, K. H. *Plans and the Structure of Behavior.* Holt-Dryden, New York, 1960.
33. Mischel, W. *Personality and Assessment.* Wiley, New York, 1968.
34. Murphy, G. *Human Potentialities.* Basic Books, New York, 1958.
35. Nowlis, D. The control of EEG alpha through auditory feedback and the associated mental activity. Unpublished manuscript, 1968.
36. Orne, M. T. Hypnosis, motivation, and compliance. Amer. J. Psychiat., *122:* 721–726, 1966.
37. Otto, H. A., ed. *Human Potentialities: The Challenge and the Promise.* Warren H. Green, St. Louis, 1967.
38. Sarbin, T. R. The concept of hallucination. J. Personality, *35:* 359–380, 1967.
39. Sarbin, T. R. Ontology recapitulates philology: The mythic nature of anxiety. Amer. Psychol., *23:* 411–418, 1968.
40. Sarbin, T. R., and Andersen, M. L. Role-theoretical analysis of hypnotic behavior. In Gordon, J. E., ed. *Handbook of Clinical and Experimental Hypnosis,* pp. 319–324. Macmillan, New York, 1967.
41. Schachter, S., and Singer, J. E. Cognitive, social, and physiological determinants of emotional state. Psychol. Rev., *69:* 379–399, 1962.
42. Severin, F. T., ed. *Humanistic Viewpoints in Psychology.* McGraw-Hill, New York, 1965.
43. Shor, R. E. Physiological effects of painful stimulation during hypnotic analgesia under conditions designed to minimize anxiety. Int. J. Clin. Exp. Hypn., *10:* 183–202, 1962.
44. Skinner, B. F. *Verbal Behavior.* Appleton-Century-Crofts, New York, 1957.
45. Smith, G. M., Lawrence, D. E., Markowitz, R. A., Mosteller, F., and Beecher, H. K. An experimental pain method sensitive to morphine in man: The submaximum effort tourniquet technique. J. Pharmacol. Exp. Ther., *154:* 324–332, 1966.
46. Stevens, S. S. Matching functions between loudness and ten other continua. Percept. Psychophysics, *1:* 5–8, 1966.
47. Stoyva, J., and Kamiya, J. Electrophysiological studies of dreaming as the prototype of a new strategy in the study of consciousness. Psychol. Rev., *75:* 192–205, 1968.
48. Thurstone, L. L. The stimulus-response fallacy in psychology. Psychol. Rev., *30:* 354–369, 1923.
49. Wolf, S., and Hardy, J. D. Studies on pain: Observations on pain due to local cooling and on factors involved in the "cold pressor" effect. J. Clin. Invest., *20:* 521–533, 1941.

[7]

A Frontal Assault on Dissociated Control

Erik Z. Woody
Kenneth S. Bowers

In English literature, the most famous instance of dissociation is surely *The Strange Case of Dr. Jekyll and Mr. Hyde* (Stevenson, 1886/1967). The circumstances that surrounded the writing of this work are quite interesting. No stranger to dissociation himself, Stevenson described the process that led to some of his best writing as one in which the characters took on an independent life of their own and seemed to move about and speak for themselves, completely unaided. In addition, he was sometimes haunted by serial dreams in which he nightly played out a dreadful second life that seemed every bit as real as his daytime one. Indeed, the story of Jekyll and Hyde originated as a nightmare. At the point in the story at which Jekyll is first transformed into Hyde, Stevenson began screaming so loudly that his wife woke him up, whereupon he scolded her, saying that he had been dreaming "a fine bogey tale" (Pope-Hennessey, 1974).

He wrote down the story feverishly in the next 3 days, and then exultantly read it aloud to his wife. She, it turns out, was very unimpressed, and "finally blurted out that Louis had missed the point of his own story, and that it was an allegory that he should have written, and not a straight piece of sensationalism" (Pope-Hennessey, 1974, p. 180). After a furious argument, Stevenson threw the 40,000-word manuscript into the fire. Then he started over from the beginning, completely refashioning the story, particularly with regard to its central theme.

What had been a straightforward horror tale, in which a drug induces a pathology that produces a new and evil, second self, turned in the new version into something quite different. Stevenson's revised theme emerges clearly in the following statement from the chastened Jekyll: "Man is not truly one, but truly two. . . . I hazard the guess that man will be ultimately known for a mere polity of multifarious, incongruous and independent denizens" (Stevenson, 1886/1967, p. 68). In other words, the action of the drug in the story is simply to bring to light divisions that were *already* within: The action tendencies elicited in Hyde, horrific as they are to Jekyll, always lay dormant within Jekyll. The drug, rather than creating a second personality, weakens the integrative mechanisms by which the gaping cracks in a personality are papered over and normally hidden from view.

Accordingly, in the present chapter we contrast two psychological views of dissociation:

1. One view of dissociation starts with the assumption that mental processes normally represent some kind of unity. However, this unity may be uncharacteristically disrupted by an unusual and special mechanism (dissociation), in which mental processes become divided. (This might be dubbed the "bogey tale" view.)
2. The second view of dissociation begins with the assumption that some multiplicity of mental process is typical and normal, in the sense of coexisting levels of control that are usually well-coordinated by higher conscious functioning. Circumstances in which dissociation becomes evident, therefore, are ones in which this higher functioning is weakened, laying bare some of the underlying "multifarious" architecture of the mind. (This is, properly, the Stevensonian view.)

Our specific task will be to apply these conceptions of dissociation to an understanding of hypnosis. Hypnosis, for our present purposes, serves as a very useful arena in which dissociative processes are commonly assumed to be evident.

AMNESTIC BARRIERS AND PARALLEL PROCESSORS

The "bogey tale" view of dissociation has a long history in psychology. Interestingly, it originated in the same era as Stevenson's work, with Janet (1901, 1907/1965). For Janet, dissociation—the splitting off of various mental contents from consciousness—was something that occurred under stress, particularly to individuals who were congenitally predisposed to dissociate. The implication was that there was some particular kind of mental deficit or biological weak-mindedness in people disposed to dissociation.

Janet's biologizing has fallen out of favor. However, a strictly psychological view of dissociation is difficult to differentiate from the concept of repression. Indeed, Erdelyi (1985, 1990) has argued that there is no difference—in both cases, ideas or information have an unconscious status. However, historically, at least, repression has always implied that information was *motivated* into an unconscious status, whereas this was not necessarily the case for dissociation. Moreover, E. R. Hilgard 's neodissociation theory (1977), which was partially inspired by Janet's work, elaborated on the distinction between dissociation and repression by arguing that the repressed unconscious was dominated by primary-process thinking that made it unrealistic and illogical in nature. In contrast, he considered dissociation to pertain to a system of ideas that were disconnected from consciousness by an "amnestic barrier," but which maintained realistic, logical relations amongst themselves.

This amnestic-barrier conception of dissociation also has the implication that a "split" in consciousness can exist, such that two parallel streams of consciousness can coexist. The classic demonstration of this supposed splitting of consciousness in the sphere of hypnosis is E. R. Hilgard's (1973, 1977) "hidden observer" phenomena, in which a part of a person (the hidden observer) knows about the presence of pain that the other, conscious part of him or her knows nothing about. On a larger scale, this consciousness-splitting function of dissociation has long been invoked as the basis for multiple personality disorder (MPD). Specifically, dissociation is allegedly a likely defense mechanism against child abuse: the child who cannot escape physically from the abuse escapes psychologically, by imagining him- or herself elsewhere, perhaps as another person, while his or her body remains behind to receive the abuse unfeelingly. This conceptualization of dissociation as a defense mechanism clearly seems to presuppose that an amnestic barrier is central to its functioning (although here again the differentiation of dissociation from repression seems to become rather problematic).

The implication typically is that when one of the parallel streams is conscious the other is not. However, this is not always the case. For example, a secondary "personality" is often nonamnestic for a primary personality (though the reverse is not true), and, likewise, the hidden observer remains in touch with the hypnotized person (though, again, not the reverse).

The amnestic-barrier conception of dissociation has played an often tacit, but nevertheless pervasive role in the neodissociation conception of hypnotic responding. For example, it has commonly been assumed that the experiences of involuntariness and effortlessness that virtually define hypnotic responding are *entirely* illusory; that is, the subject enacting a hypnotic suggestion is thought to exert considerable effort and self-mediated control, which is, however, hidden from consciousness (e.g., Bowers & Brenneman, 1981).

A vigorous expression of this view appears in a very recent review essay on hypnosis by Kihlstrom (1992). He quotes approvingly a memorable statement by Shor (1979):

> Although the hypnotic subject may look as if he is no longer in control of his own volitional activities—for example, he may behave as if he is unable to bend his hypnotically stiffened elbow—that is only because at some deeper level than is operative within the bounds of consciousness, he is actively, deliberately, voluntarily keeping his elbow stiff while simultaneously orchestrating for himself the illusion that he is really trying his best to bend it. (p. 124)

Kihlstrom (1992) himself then goes on to explain in the language of neo-dissociation theory that

> when the cognitive control system that executes the response to a hypnotic suggestion is dissociated from conscious awareness, S will experience that response as automatic and nonvolitional . . . however, that experience is illusory—obviously, there is *some* executive control involved in hypnotic responding, even if the hypnotized S does not experience it as such. (p. 308)

Clearly the point expressed above is that hypnotic behavior is controlled and executed like any nonhypnotic behavior; however, the subject's *experience* of why the act occurred is incomplete and incorrect. Kihlstrom does not explicitly mention any kind of amnesia-like barrier behind which the cognitive control system hides. However, unless we presume such a mechanism, this explanation of the nature of hypnosis is virtually indistinguishable from the misattributional explanation of the social-psychological theorists (Spanos, 1986; Lynn, Rhue, & Weekes, 1990) that he is trying to argue against.

In any case, defining the essence of hypnosis in terms of such amnesia-like barriers and consequent distortions of experience is problematic. To see why, it is useful to distinguish between strong and weak senses of the notion of amnestic barrier.

In the strong sense of amnestic barrier, hypnotic performances may be viewed as requiring *spontaneous amnesia*, in which some information that should normally be available to consciousness is lost. For example, the fact that a subject cannot remember his or her *deliberate* failure to bend his or her arm may be seen as a mild instance of spontaneous amnesia for the events occurring during a hypnotic session. However, despite the strong association of hypnosis with spontaneous amnesia historically and in the popular imagination, such spontaneous amnesia is quite rare (E. R. Hilgard & Cooper, 1965); hence, we have the unappealing prospect of attempting to explain routine hypnotic behaviors in terms of a very rare one. More telling is the fact that such unsuggested amnesias would need to be arbitrarily selective. To illustrate, Bowers (1992) has pointed out that "the pain and cognitive effort involved to reduce it is hidden behind an amnestic barrier, but not the original suggestions for analgesia, nor the goal-directed fantasies that typically accompany the reductions in pain" (pp. 261–262). Finally, it may be pointed out that individual differences in hypnotically *suggested* amnesia seem to be only rather peripherally associated with the core of individual differences in hypnotic ability; for example, there are many subjects who show strong hypnotic performances of most other kinds, but little or no amnesia (e.g., Monteiro, Macdonald, & Hilgard, 1980). This pattern of association is, of course, not what we would expect if amnestic processes were at the root of other kinds of hypnotic tasks.

In the weak sense of amnestic barrier, it may be argued that we are only talking about temporary occlusions of some information that might have been available to consciousness—in other words, a process more like disattention than spontaneous amnesia. However, unless one assumes some kind of unity of mental process and accompanying transparency of consciousness, this more modest notion does not appear to tell us anything very interesting, and little about hypnosis per se. Consider that current conceptions of the mind (e.g., Baars, 1988) involve very numerous, distributed, specialized modules that work in parallel, are typically unconscious, and jointly have enormous information-processing capacity. In contrast, consciousness involves a single, serial flow of information of quite limited capacity. This might be likened to a televised event, in which a great variety of events are occurring simultaneously, but in which only one thing at a time may appear on the television screen, and the sequence of events is orchestrated so as to form a coherent narrative. Hence, even outside of hypnosis, there are virtually always many layers of "amnestic barrier" occurring in the performance of any reasonably complex behavior, in the sense parallel ongoing processes and materials are present that are necessarily deleted from the conscious accounting. Furthermore, the conscious experience of the causes of one's behavior is therefore necessarily incomplete and frequently incorrect, again, with or without hypnosis (cf. Nisbett & Wilson, 1977). In short, consciousness is such a narrow window on mental processes that we cannot rely on any notion of dissociated experience to explain its uncountable lacunae.

This tension between an unconscious mind of multiple, reasonably independent modules and a conscious mind that somehow integrates these diverse modules and makes them appear as one is of great importance. It harkens back to what we labeled as "the Stevensonian view"—that is, of the mind as a "mere polity of multifarious, incongruous and independent denizens" (Stevenson, 1886/1967, p. 68), whose apparent unity is, at least in part, an illusion of normal consciousness. Stevenson focused on the very high level of personal identity, but of course the notion of the mind as consisting of parallel modules applies even more readily and broadly to lower levels of functioning.

According to this view, the mind is already, in a sense, deeply divided (among many parallel modules), and higher conscious functioning somehow acts to bridge these gaps. As Baars (1991) has argued, the chief function of consciousness may be to "help integrate otherwise dissociated functions" (p. 440). Thus, if higher conscious functioning is weakened, the already-dissociated nature of mind, so to speak, should become more frankly evident.

It will come as no surprise that a hypnotic induction, with its typically relentless monotony and many allusions to sleep, may be thought of as releasing lower-level functions from the integration that is normally imposed on them by consciousness. In fact, a widely recognized effect of hypnosis is a reduced "general reality orientation" (Shor, 1959). Therefore, rather than viewing hypnotic responses as being due to the onset of a special amnestic barrier that *hides* control processes from consciousness, we may alternatively think of them as resulting from a partial loss of the higher integrative functioning normally associated with consciousness.

The notion that hypnosis weakens higher integrative functioning has an extremely important implication: hypnosis alters not just the experience of behavior, but how it is *controlled*. Let us refer one more time to the Stevenson story, as the metaphor is quite apt. The effect of the drug, which we may think of for present purposes as an analogue of hypnosis, is not simply to provide Jekyll with some novel experiences, but to release patterns of behavior that would have been entirely suppressed when in his normal state.

Perhaps partly due to the specter of its Jekyll–Hyde-like implications, there has long been considerable ambivalence in the hypnosis literature concerning the possibility that hypnosis can alter the control of behavior. With his highly influential neodissociation model of hypnosis, E. R. Hilgard (1977) made use of a current view in cognitive psychology that there is a hierarchy of levels of control involved in the generation of behavior. He proposed that hypnosis allows the bypassing of the highest level of control, an executive level associated with the willful planning, monitoring, and coordination of behavior. Thus, he argued, hypnotic suggestions may directly activate lower subsystems of control, such as those which enact specific behavior sequences. The hypnotic subject's experience of nonvolition and effortlessness, then, would accurately correspond to a genuine alteration in the usual hierarchy of control that governs behavior.

Nonetheless, in this and subsequent accounts of hypnotic phenomena, Hilgard has shown a consistent tendency to revert back to the older, amnestic-barrier account, in which no genuine alteration of control is implied. This tendency unfortunately obscures the fact that in crucial ways the amnestic-barrier and the altered-control accounts of hypnosis are quite inconsistent with each other, despite being lumped together under the protean term "dissociation." In addition, the cautiousness about admitting any genuine alterations of control in hypnosis has been widely influential, as is reflected in the very clear views of Shor and of Kihlstrom quoted earlier, as well as in the views, until fairly recently, of one of us (e.g., Bowers & Brenneman, 1981).

More recently, Bowers (1990, 1992) has advanced a modified version of Hilgard's neodissociation model of hypnosis, in which he rejects the amnestic-barrier concept of dissociation and emphasizes the altered-control concept. This modification, in effect, amputates the seemingly less viable part of Hilgard's theory—namely, the part that maintained the historically important link between hypnosis and amnesia-based dissociation—while retaining the more modern hierarchical-control model of the mind. Indeed, Bowers (1990) makes explicit that what remains is a theory of *dissociated control*, rather than one of *dissociated experience*. With regard to the latter, he points out that "dissociation is not intrinsically a matter of keeping things out of consciousness—whether by amnesia, or any other means" (Bowers, 1992, p. 267). Instead, with regard to dissociated control, Bowers (1992) has maintained Hilgard's original neodissociation language, as seen in the following definition of the theory: "Dissociation is primarily concerned with the fact that subsystems of control can be directly and automatically activated, instead of being governed by high level executive control" (p. 267). In other words, in hypnotic behavior what is "dissociated" is lower from higher, executive levels of control.

Despite what we, naturally enough, perceive to be its many strengths, this account of the altered-control theory can appear to have a number of potential shortcomings, including the following:

1. When applied to specific hypnotic behaviors, the language of *subsystems of control* can seem to strain credibility. For example, when Miller and Bowers (1993) argue that hypnotic analgesia is due to the direct activation of subsystems of control, one might wonder what sort of preexisting subsystem of control could be in place for the reduction of pain, and what sense it makes to refer to its being *directly* (vs. indirectly) activated. In a way, invoking dissociated control might just seem to postpone the problem of explaining hypnotic responding, rather than really solving it.

2. What specifically could it mean to "dissociate" lower levels of control from executive control? At present, this kind of dissociation seems to be defined chiefly in a dangerously circular manner. For example, Hilgard (1977) claims of a hypnotic response that the "less it is felt to be under the subject's control the more it has been dissociated from the normal executive functions" (p. 228). Nonetheless, in the passages quoted earlier from Shor and from Kihlstrom, it was held to be self-evident that there is some degree of higher executive control in any hypnotic behavior, irrespective of the subject's report.

3. What happens to amnesia in light of this theory? Certain classical

and widely recognized hypnotic phenomena involve suggested (rather than spontaneous) amnesia. Hence, surely these remain important to explain. How can a theory of dissociated control account for these hypnotically mediated amnestic phenomena?

We will attempt to address these questions in the rest of this chapter by relating the dissociated-control theory to some current cognitive and neuropsychological models of mental functioning. Our aims are both to substantiate the plausibility of such a theory, and in the process of fleshing it out, to suggest some novel directions for further work.

WILLED VERSUS AUTOMATIC CONTROL OF BEHAVIOR

In ordinary conditions when people do as they are told, we do not call their cooperativeness "hypnosis." The essence of hypnotic responding, as seen in the so-called "classic suggestion effect" (Weitzenhoffer, 1953), is that the subject's carrying out of the suggestion is experienced as involuntary. Hence, alterations in the experience of volition are perhaps the single most crucial thing to explain in understanding hypnosis.

The different ways in which an action may be experienced, from willed to automatic, has been a major concern, likewise, for some cognitive psychologists. A recent theory by Norman and Shallice (1986), for example, attempts to explain how these different ways of experiencing an action come about, and does so by relating them to differences in underlying control processes.

Let us briefly review Norman and Shallice's model. On the basis of a wide variety of findings in cognitive and neuropsychology (see Shallice, 1988), they argue that there are two complementary control systems for the initiation and control of action. The lower-level control system, which they term "contention scheduling," is decentralized and takes care of the routine selection of routine acts that do not require conscious or attentional control. Contention scheduling works through the competitive and cooperative activation of schemas. The activation level of a particular schema is affected partly by various environmental triggers and partly by other schemas, of both a supporting and conflicting nature, that are being activated at the same time. Once the activation level of a particular schema exceeds a threshold, the schema is selected and the corresponding action ensues. The essence of this process is conveyed well in the following quote: "For well-learned, habitual tasks an autonomous, self-sufficient strand of processing structures and procedures can usually carry out the required activities without the need for conscious or attentional control" (Norman & Shallice, 1986, p. 4).

However, in cases where the required action is novel or complex, or a strong habitual response must be overcome, the contention-scheduling system may fail to make appropriate schemas available. A second, higher-level control system, which Norman and Shallice term the "supervisory attentional system," assists with such nonroutine actions in a qualitatively different, and centralized way. The supervisory system not only can monitor processes taking place in the contention-scheduling system, but also has access to its own relatively unique information, including the individual's goals and intentions. Nonetheless, this higher-level control system is held to operate only indirectly, by modulating the lower-level control system, rather than by directly controlling behavior. Through the addition of extra activation and inhibition to particular schemas, the supervisory system biases the selection of schemas by the contention-scheduling system.

Because higher executive control is normally experienced as dominant (rather than supplementary), the indirect role that Norman and Shallice assign to the supervisory system can at first seem rather counterintuitive. However, the role of the supervisory system might be likened to that of a chief executive officer, who guides and redirects the activities in a company with memos and so forth. The CEO's function is not to directly execute any action (e.g., roll up his or her sleeves and shovel), but is mainly to manage the initiation and termination of actions, especially when some novel adjustment of usual operating procedures is required. In addition, despite the CEO's dominant role, workers will sometimes fail to carry out some directives successfully, and will sometimes act on their own in ways that may be inconsistent with the CEO's intentions.

Regarding the phenomenology of the individual from the perspective of this two-tier model of control, how an action is experienced depends on the nature of the involvement of the supervisory system. When the supervisory system is actively modulating the selection of schemas, we have the phenomenal experience of will, or deliberate conscious control. In contrast, when the supervisory system is neither modulating nor monitoring the contention-scheduling system, the action is experienced as automatic. Between these two extremes, a range of other states of awareness of an action is possible. For example, if the supervisory system is monitoring the contention-scheduling process but not actively modulating it, then the experience is one wherein the action immediately followed the idea of it in the mind—what William James (1890/1981) called an "ideo-motor act," to distinguish it from a genuinely willed act.

It is reasonably straightforward to apply this cognitive model to an understanding of the altered experience of volition in hypnosis. For reasonably highly hypnotizable subjects, hypnosis may be thought of as weakening the operation of the supervisory system; that is, hypnosis may partly disable the higher-level control system, associated with the phenomenal experience of will, by which the contention-scheduling system may normally be modulated. This weakening of the supervisory system, then, explains what we mean by "dissociating" lower levels of control from higher-level, executive control.

According to this conception, hypnosis results in a genuine change in the control of behavior—namely, the hypnotized individual is especially dependent on the contention-scheduling level of control, and this control can not be modulated readily in a willful manner. One should keep in mind that routine control of action can occur without the intervention of the supervisory system (the one weakened by hypnosis), for instance, with action that is triggered directly by environmental stimuli and coactive schemas. Control at the level of the contention-scheduling system, then, would be what is meant—in the language of the neodissociation theory of hypnosis—by "subsystems of control," which may be "directly activated."

It is important to point out that this increased dependence on the lower-level of control does not rule out a vast repertoire of possible behavior. Norman and Shallice (1986) argue that although well-learned action sequences and cognitive skills can be modulated by deliberate conscious control, they do not *require* this higher-level control system. In short, it is mainly an individual's capacity for novel or particularly complex behaviors that could be diminished under hypnosis, as well as, more generally, behavior that requires the exertion of his or her will.

Finally, while there may be unsolved mysteries about the nature of some of the subsystems of control referred to in neodissociation theory, the general notion that such systems lie outside of higher executive control is nevertheless quite unproblematic. Recall that the supervisory system is held to have only a relatively indirect influence on action—that is, through biasing the selection of schemas by the lower-level system. Thus, although the supervisory system may strongly affect the selection of actions, it does not have any direct role in carrying them out. Because the supervisory system (i.e., the one weakened by hypnosis) does not directly control any action, a system of control for virtually any action must lie elsewhere.

Thus, the dissociated-control theory of hypnosis can be seen to be highly consistent with the Norman and Shallice model of willed versus automatic control of behavior. In addition, the Norman and Shallice model can shed some interesting light on our understanding of various hypnotic phenomena, of which we here give a few examples.

First, if the effect of hypnosis is to weaken the supervisory system, we would expect hypnotized subjects to show two seemingly contradictory patterns of behavior: a behavioral rigidity characterized by a lack of spontaneous, self-generated action; and a tendency for thought and behavior to be triggered inappropriately by irrelevant stimuli and associations. Despite the preservation of the ability to carry out routine actions when specifically requested, a general impoverishment of spontaneous, self-generated behavior would be expected because spontaneous voluntary behavior requires an active supervisory system, whereas the responding to reasonably routine requests does not. That a paucity of spontaneous voluntary behavior characterizes hypnotized subjects will be evident to anyone who has ever conducted a group hypnosis scale—the spontaneously behaving subjects are almost certainly the ones who are not hypnotized. Another intriguing illustration of the impoverishment of spontaneous behavior in hypnosis comes from studies by Orne (1979), in which he compared the behavior of hypnotized subjects to that of simulators in response to a novel circumstance, such as an apparent power outage. Hypnotized subjects seemed to respond much more slowly to such altered circumstances, even though the conditions make the continuation of the experiment nonsensical.

A weakened supervisory system may also lead to disinhibition of control, and hence the eliciting of inappropriate or irrelevant associations and behavior (Shallice, 1988). When circumstances threaten to trigger an inappropriate or irrelevant schema, a major function of the supervisory system is ordinarily to inhibit this activation. Loss of supervisory control due to hypnosis, then, would be expected to disable such inhibition, so that peculiar associations and behavior might be activated if triggers are present. The hypnotic circumstance, however, at least in laboratory conditions, seems typically to present few such possible triggers. Hence, such disinhibition is infrequently reported, and the operative triggers are found to be quite idiosyncratic to particular subjects. J. R. Hilgard (1974) noted that people who had previously had bad experiences with drugs sometimes found themselves reexperiencing these events when being hypnotized. More generally, the phenomenon of sequelae—relatively rare, but sometimes striking effects of hypnosis that were not suggested by the hypnotist (Coe & Ryken, 1979; Crawford, Hilgard, & Macdonald, 1982; Reyher, 1967)—seems consistent with the theory that the disinhibition of tangential associations is due to a loss of supervisory control.

Second, the Norman and Shallice model seems to be quite helpful in disentangling what is going on in hypnotic performances of the easy to moderate range of difficulty. Particularly for the easiest kinds of suggestions traditionally associated with hypnosis, it is difficult to resist the impression that it does not take any special dissociative capacity to pass them. Instead, passing relatively easy hypnosis items would seem only to require some social-psychological influencibility or compliance-like attribute. Nonetheless, previous attempts to show a consistent relationship between such nonhypnotic variables and hypnotizability have not been successful (Bowers, 1976).

Accordingly, in a recent study, Woody, Oakman, and Drugovic (1992) took a new approach to devising a nonhypnotic measure of susceptibility. Borrowing a paradigm used in alcohol research to study expectancy effects, they asked subjects to consume two drinks that purportedly contained a moderate dose of alcohol, but were actually alcohol-free. Later, subjects rated the extent to which they had experienced each of 13 suggested effects, that is, alterations in sensation, perception, and thinking that might plausibly have ensued from the consumption of alcohol. These suggested effects paralleled those typically attributed to hypnosis—for example, checking for a "feeling of sluggishness or immobilization" in one's limbs, and producing a daydream to check for "more vivid or more fluid images than normal." Ratings on the 13 suggested effects showed high internal consistency and were summed to form an overall nonhypnotic suggestibility score.

This nonhypnotic suggestion measure showed a strongly differential pattern of correlation with the individual items of the Harvard Group Scale of Hypnotic Susceptibility, Form A (Shor & Orne, 1962). Namely, the easier the A-Scale item, the more strongly it correlated with the alcohol expectancy measure. Indeed, for the easiest A-Scale items, the correlations with the alcohol expectancy measure approached the items' corrected item-total correlations, indicating that these items tap little more than such expectancy effects. By contrast, the most difficult A-Scale items had virtually nothing to do with such expectancy effects.

More specifically, the great majority of items on the Harvard A-Scale consist of suggestions for motor behaviors, which are of two quite distinct types—direct motor items, which tend to be the easiest ones, and motor inhibition or challenge items, which tend to be somewhat harder to pass. The relationship of the alcohol-expectancy measure to each of the direct motor items was quite strong, whereas the measure's relationship to the challenge items was weaker and trailed toward zero as the challenge items became harder. Hence, the processes that underlie the ability to pass each type of item appear to be quite different.

The Norman and Shallice model provides an intriguing approach to understanding how direct motor and challenge items differ. To begin, consider that a direct motor suggestion can be carried out automatically and requires so little attentional effort that the role of the will is ambiguous or indeterminate. As Norman and Shallice (1986) specifically point out, "introspection fails in determining whether the will is involved in the voluntary lifting of the arm" (p. 15). Thus, the relevant characteristic of direct motor items in hypnosis appears to be this ambiguity, or indeterminacy, of the role of the will and attention. The hypnotic context, then, offers the subject a plausible hypothesis concerning the nature of this ambiguous experience—namely, the hypothesis that it is happening because of hypnosis (rather than one's own will). It is this attribution that makes the experience potentially impressive and conveys at least some sense of involuntariness. What is happening in the alcohol-expectancy measure, arguably, is very similar, except that the context offers the subject a somewhat different kind of plausible attribution—namely, that the ambiguous experience is happening due to alcohol. The connecting individual difference, then, would have to do with the propensity to interpret an ambiguous experience in terms of a plausible hypothesis offered by the context. Although some subjects high in hypnotic ability may well pass direct motor suggestions via a different mechanism from this, many subjects without much genuine hypnotic talent can probably pass such items in this nondissociative way.

It is worth reflecting for a moment on how different this explanation of passing a direct motor item is from the classic amnestic-barrier or "dissociated experience" explanation. According to the classic account, the suggested behavior is actually enacted by the subject voluntarily, but the activities of his or her higher-level control system are blocked from consciousness, and the act is therefore experienced as nonvolitional. However, according to the Norman and Shallice model, it is not necessary for the hypnotic subject to dissociate the fact of higher-level control from consciousness for such simple actions, due to the simple reason that no such higher-level control is necessary for the occurrence of the act.

Turning now to the motor inhibition or challenge suggestions, these typically consist of a simple motor suggestion followed by the instruction to *try* to oppose or overcome it. This circumstance is quite different from the direct motor suggestion, in that to carry out the instruction to try, the subject must attempt to exert will; in the language of the Norman and Shallice model, he or she must involve the supervisory system in activating the appropriate schema. Consider how different the instruction "Raise your arm" is from the instruction "*Try* to raise your arm"—in the latter case, attentional effort is unmistakable, and the role of volition unambiguous. Recall that according to the Norman and Shallice model, this phenomenal experience of will is the indicator that the supervisory system is making a bid to modulate schema selection.

It would appear that in response to a motor inhibition suggestion, some hypnotic subjects would still respond in the fashion described previously for direct motor items by remaining "role consistent" and not exerting effort to bend their arm, or whatever (e.g., the subject might think, "If I really try to bend my arm, it might spoil the effect"). If some subjects do not actually attempt to exert will, the ambiguity of the experience is maintained, so that they might look to the context for a reasonable explanation, as described earlier for direct motor suggestions. However, as soon as a subject genuinely *tries* to carry out the challenge suggestion, thereby invoking supervisory control, the process involved must be quite different. If we conceive of the "genuine" effect of hypnosis as the weakening of the supervisory system, it follows that when a hypnotized subject really tries to exert will, he or she might have the experience that such effortful attention is notably less effective—that is, less tied to action—than it normally is outside of hypnosis. In other words, compared to the lower, contention-scheduling level of control, which is evoked by suggestion, effects of the supervisory system, or executive level of control, are uncharacteristically weak. Of course, this is a very different explanation of the experience of nonvolition than the one we argued for with regard to direct motor items, and it is closely allied with what Bowers (1990, 1992) has termed the capacity for "dissociated control."

Finally, although the Norman and Shallice model and the remarks here have focused on the control of action, we may use the example of hypnotic analgesia to illustrate similar insights about the control of perception. Indeed, paralleling (and in fact antedating) the distinction between automatic and willed control of action is the distinction between "automatic" and "controlled" processing of perceptual inputs (Shiffrin & Schneider, 1977).

It is interesting in this regard to compare hypnotic analgesia with cognitive-behavioral approaches to the control of pain (Turk, Meichenbaum, & Genest, 1983). First, cognitive-behavioral interventions involve the maintenance of deliberate attentional control over the experience of a pain-evoking stimulus, using such strategies as actively diverting attention away from the stimulus, imaginatively transforming it, engaging in a counter-pain fantasy, and inhibiting negative thoughts. In terms of the model proposed by Norman and Shallice, these strategies require strong ongoing activation of the supervisory system, and the experiential equivalent for this state of high demand for attentional activation, as they point out, is *concentration* (rather than simply will). The hallmark of such a state is that a lapse in its effortful maintenance brings failure of the perceptual control. (Such control of perception is no different in kind from control of action—for example, in a sport or game, where a momentary lapse of concentration can bring about a highly inappropriate action.)

One view of hypnotic analgesia is that it, too, is basically a deliberate, effortful, strategic controlling of attention (e.g., Spanos, 1986; Wagstaff, 1991). Nonetheless, according to the conception of hypnosis proposed here, hypnotic analgesia and cognitive-behavioral pain control might better be characterized as opposites. If we view hypnosis as weakening the supervisory system, then its ultimate effect should be to *diminish* the capacity for initiating and maintaining a well-organized set of deliberate attentional strategies (i.e., strong activation of the supervisory system), not to increase it. In this sense, hypnosis and cognitive-behavioral strategies would seem to be antithetical; that is, hypnotized subjects should not be very good at self-generating attentional control strategies nor at effortfully maintaining them.

Indeed, several findings in a set of recent studies by Bowers and his colleagues indicate that hypnotic analgesia is quite unlike cognitive-behavioral pain control. In particular, subjects who show hypnotic analgesia do not typically report spontaneously using any deliberate cognitive strategies; and highly hypnotizable subjects tend to show substantially greater benefit from hypnotic analgesia than from a nonhypnotic cognitive-behavioral approach (Miller & Bowers, 1986; see Miller & Bowers, 1993, for a result to the contrary). Furthermore, unlike cognitive-behavioral pain reduction, hypnotic analgesia is not accompanied by signs of cognitive effort, as measured by impairment on a competing task (Miller & Bowers, 1993). Finally, Hargadon and Bowers (1992) have shown that hypnotic analgesia can be obtained in the absence of any deliberate cognitive strategies, such as engaging in counter-pain imagery. A completely unelaborated hypnotic suggestion for the reduction of pain seems sufficient to produce analgesia in highly hypnotizable subjects, and many of these subjects report no strategic embellishment or amplification of the suggestion at all.

Thus, deliberate attentional control does not appear to be the mechanism underlying hypnotic analgesia; but, then, what is? Miller and Bowers (1993) argued that such results are consistent with a dissociated-control model of hypnosis, in which "suggestive communications more or less directly activate subsystems of control and thereby minimize the influence of executive initiative and effort" (p. 37). For our present purposes, an attractive aspect of this proposal is that it is quite congruent with the notion that hypnosis weakens supervisory system functions, as advanced here. However, a somewhat unattractive aspect is that it appears to presume the existence of a subsystem of control over pain, one that somehow tends to remain unactivated under normal, nonhypnotic conditions. A potential criticism of Miller and Bowers's proposal, then, is that while it makes clear that hypnotic analgesia differs from effortful, nonhypnotic pain-control strategies, it does not quite succeed in advancing a specific alternative mechanism.

Once again, we turn to the Norman and Shallice model to sketch some intriguing, if as yet incomplete, possibilities. The important aspect of a pain stimulus is its peremptory quality. Even though unbidden, it hogs attentional resources in a fashion that is difficult to overturn (McCaul & Malott, 1984). In addition, this attention-grabbing characteristic of pain is closely linked to its distressing and unpleasant quality, whereas other aspects of a pain stimulus such as its sensory location appear to be mediated by other mechanisms (Pribram, 1991). Norman and Shallice discuss such automatically attention-demanding characteristics of some stimuli in terms of the computer-science notion of an *interrupt*. Specifically, in addition to whatever impact a triggering stimulus may have on schema activation, there are occasions when it also produces an interrupt in the supervisory system—loosely meaning, a "moment of emergency" that breaks in upon any ongoing deliberative activity.

In accordance with the idea that the effect of hypnosis is to weaken supervisory system functions, hypnotic analgesia could possibly result from the fact that hypnosis reduces the sensitivity of the supervisory system to interrupts. In other words, due to hypnosis, some kinds of triggers may have a diminished capacity to break in at the supervisory level. (Note that this idea is quite consistent with the notion of reduced spontaneous behavior in hypnosis, as discussed earlier.) Given that much of the disturbing aspect of pain results from interrupts, hypnosis would attenuate such discomfort. Indeed, hypnosis might make the pain unnoticeable because it no longer draws attention to itself. However, if attention were directed to the pain stimulus by an external agent, such as the hypnotist, it makes sense to assume that the supervisory system could still monitor the pain stimulus, as in the case of the hidden observer.

There is another interesting, if rather more tentative, implication of this interrupt concept of pain. The supervisory system operates in such a way as to allow some kinds of triggers to have more broadly distributed consequences than they might have without its presence; that is, via the supervisory system, a stimulus may come to have an impact on schema selection that it otherwise would not have had. For example, a pain stimulus, via supervisory functions, may come to have an inhibiting effect on a particular schema—say, a numerical cognitive operation—that would have been relatively easy to execute in the absence of supervisory input. The important point, then, is that by weakening supervisory functions, hypnosis may reduce such distributed consequences of a pain stimulus, making it easier for the subject to engage in concurrent, relatively routine behavior.

What this line of reasoning leaves unclear is the role of *suggestions* for pain reduction in hypnotic analgesia. Recent work by Hargadon and Bowers (1992) shows that such analgesic suggestions may be surprisingly simple and straightforward, and may not require any amplification by suggested imagery, as is commonly assumed. Yet the specific instruction for the subject to reduce the pain still seems to be important for obtaining hypnotic analgesia. In contrast, the present reasoning would appear to imply that hypnosis alone (unaccompanied by suggestions for pain reduction) might be sufficient for analgesia. One tentative proposal would be that to some degree all subjects have at their disposal a mechanism for the temporary suppression of pain (as seen, e.g., in emergency situations), but that this mechanism is ordinarily overturned fairly rapidly by the interrupt phenomenon described above. Hypnotic analgesia, then, might result from evoking this mechanism through suggesting a reduction of pain, and making the mechanism much more lastingly effective by inhibiting its being overturned by the supervisory system. This proposal at least has the merit of seeming broadly consistent with the basic theme of dissociated control—that is, of lower levels of control becoming decoupled from higher-level functions. It is, however, obviously speculative and somewhat incomplete.

A DISSOCIATED-CONTROL VIEW OF HYPNOTIC AMNESIA

One of the classic and most striking effects of hypnosis is suggested amnesia. Clearly, this phenomenon represents an alteration in *retrieval*, rather than in the encoding processes of memory (Kihlstrom, 1985). That is, after the suggestion for amnesia, the hypnotized subject fails to bring to mind some material, but this material returns to mind when the suggestion is canceled. Indeed, one likely reason for the persistence of the amnestic-barrier conception of hypnosis, discussed earlier, is that it is very appealing to view such reversible lapses in memory in terms of a temporary barrier that blocks material that would normally emerge easily into consciousness. It is at first much less clear how a dissociated-control model of hypnosis could account for such a phenomenon.

Nonetheless, Shallice (1988) has developed a model that will provide the bridge we need, which describes how the supervisory system affects memory processes. He argues that the well-known distinction between semantic and episodic memory (Tulving, 1972) reflects not just a difference in the kinds of information needed or in the subsystems where the information is stored, but a crucial difference in the retrieval procedures that are employed. Specifically, episodic memory tasks require the utilization of "*specialized retrieval procedures directable by only the supervisory system*," whereas semantic memory tasks simply involve "accessing the relevant information through the operation of the schemata that control routine processing" (Shallice, 1988, p. 372). Hence, for memory, as with action, the supervisory system is hypothesized to function as a higher-control system, one which, again as with action, enables the negotiation of nonroutine problems—that is, ones that cannot be handled by standard memory retrieval routines.

Shallice suggests that although most information would not be stored in the supervisory system, some features of memories may be specially stored there—namely, those aspects "necessary for effective integration of the memory into the overall structure of a person's life history" (1988, p. 372). However, the more important point about the supervisory system is *how* it approaches retrieval tasks. Drawing on a theory by Norman and Bobrow (1979), Shallice proposes that when confronted by a nonroutine problem, the supervisory system first formulates descriptions of what the relevant memory records might be like if they existed. Next these descriptions are matched with records, and then those candidate records that have been retrieved are checked to verify that they are indeed relevant.

The process of remembering, as directed by the supervisory system, would consist, then, of cycles of description, matching, and verification. This process might be likened to using CD-ROM resources to locate any psychological literature possibly relevant to a particular question—material about which one has as yet, or retains, only a rough idea. One might need to try a variety of descriptions of what is desired, and at various stages, the verification process may reveal that most or even all of the candidate records (which are sometimes maddeningly numerous!) are actually totally irrelevant. Naturally, there are many other times when desired records can be accessed much more directly and simply than this—using our analogy, these would be comparable to the use of standard semantic memory retrieval routines.

This theory of supervisory system memory functions can be quite readily, if as yet somewhat tentatively, applied to an understanding of memory alterations in hypnosis. If hypnosis weakens the supervisory system, as we have argued, then it should tend to interfere with control over some memory functions while leaving other functions unaffected. Specifically, we would expect hypnosis to affect both the description and verification phases in the cycles, as they are directed by the Supervisory System, leading to at least the following two sorts of effects.

First, there should be relatively poor access to memories that require the formulation of preliminary descriptions—for example, ones for which there is no overlearned access routine. One way this change would likely be evident is that cases of hypnotically reduced free-recall memory should be accompanied by relatively well-preserved cued-recall and recognition memory. Memory tasks that provide external cues should be relatively unaffected because to some extent they supply the needed description; thus the formulation of descriptions by the supervisory system would be less important or even unnecessary with such tasks. Indeed, the evidence on hypnotic amnesia is strikingly consistent with these implications: hypnotic amnesia selectively impairs free recall, rather than recognition and implicit-memory tasks such as word associations (Evans, 1979; Kihlstrom, 1980; Kihlstrom & Shor, 1978; McConkey & Sheehan, 1981; McConkey, Sheehan, & Cross, 1980; Spanos, Radtke, & Dubreuil, 1982).

Second, hypnotized subjects should show poor verification—that is, diminished ability to discriminate appropriate or correct records from inappropriate or incorrect ones. Specifically, they should mistake irrelevant and inappropriate associations for the required memories, and be incorrectly confident that these incorrect associations "match" with the required material. Indeed, such distorting effects of hypnosis on memory have been shown in a number of studies (Dywan & Bowers, 1983; Laurence & Perry, 1983; Orne, Whitehouse, Dinges, & Orne, 1988). One striking example of impoverished verification is the "discovery" made during hypnotic age-regression of elaborate previous lives, which obviously consist of a mish-mash of irrelevant memories and fantasies.

To summarize, the essential point is that a dissociated-control theory of hypnotic amnesia is possible, even if, admittedly, much work remains to be done. Such a theory emphasizes hypnotic alteration in the control over memory processes, such as the description and verification phases of supervisory system processing—rather than the erection of amnestic barriers.

THE HYPNOTIZED SUBJECT AS A FRONTAL LOBE PATIENT

That a dissociated-control theory of hypnosis would implicate change in frontal lobe functioning is almost obvious, since the essence of dissociated control is the bypassing of high-level executive control, and the frontal cortex is strongly believed to be the site of such executive control (e.g., Pribram, 1973). More specifically, the prefrontal cortex is thought to be the site of the highest level of control in the hierarchy of motor control, and is thought to provide a system for the overall organization, regulation, and verification of activity (Kolb & Whishaw, 1985).

Indeed, Norman and Shallice (1986) developed the conceptual framework of the supervisory system in large part to account for uniquely frontal functions. Furthermore, there is a very close parallel between how we have used this framework to explain hypnotic behavior and how Norman and Shallice use it to explain the behavior of patients with frontal lobe disorders. In particular, we have argued that hypnosis, in highly susceptible subjects, weakens the supervisory system and increases dependence on the contention-scheduling level of control. Similarly, Shallice (1988) points out that damage to the supervisory system, resulting in "reliance on contention scheduling alone," gives rise to "the symptoms classically associated with frontal lobe disorders" (p. 335).

Let us examine this parallel in greater detail. Bowers (1992) has recently illustrated the principle of dissociated control through examining the nonhypnotic example of a person being distracted and inadvertently dialing a familiar telephone number rather than the intended one. As in the case of hypnotic behavior, a controlled action sequence seems to have escaped from higher executive control. Interestingly, Shallice (1988) uses the same capture-error action lapses in distracted normal subjects as an illustration of what happens when action is unaided by the supervisory system, and hence as the normal analogue of pathological behavior that ensues from damage to the supervisory system:

> Depending on the pattern of trigger-schema relations, a system of contention scheduling without supervisory control may show one of two apparently contradictory types of behaviour. Behavioural rigidity (a tendency to perseverate) should occur in some situations; in others, a distractibility and a tendency to be side-tracked by irrelevant associations. (p. 339)

There are a number of specific ways in which the hypnotic phenomena we described earlier suggest the inhibition of frontal functions. First, the general impoverishment of spontaneous, self-generated behavior we noted in hypnotized subjects is also one of the classic hallmarks of patients with frontal lobe lesions (Kolb & Whishaw, 1985; Hécaen & Albert, 1975). Such patients, like hypnotized subjects, are capable of carrying out most any action when urged to do so, yet spontaneously initiate little activity. Similarly, the weakening of volitional control we noted in hypnotized subjects is also a classic hallmark of frontal lobe dysfunction. Indeed, one of the first systematic reviews of patients with frontal lobe lesions noted their peculiar "other-directedness" (Feuchtwanger, 1923, as cited in Teuber, 1964). Further, there is general agreement that such patients typically show an inability to select and execute self-mediated plans (Kolb & Whishaw, 1985).

The fact that the most distressing aspect of pain (as opposed to its sensory location aspect) is associated with the frontal lobes is of further relevance to hypnotic analgesia (Pribram, 1991). Indeed, in cases of intractable pain, removal of the frontal cortex ameliorates the distress (Bouckoms, 1989).

Finally, hypnotic amnesia may be likened to what Shallice (1988) has termed "frontal amnesia." Patients diagnosed with this are unable to distinguish true memories from irrelevant associations elicited by stimuli, are highly confident about their incorrect memories, and are prone to confabulation, especially when prompted by leading questions—all characteristics of hypnotically influenced memory, as well. Shallice (1988) contrasts frontal amnesia with classical amnesia as follows:

> *Frontal amnesia*, then, appears to be an impairment of that part of the Supervisory System concerned with formulating the description of any memories that might be required and of verifying that any candidate memories that have been retrieved are relevant. *Classical amnesia*, by contrast, would arise from an interruption of the flow of memory information from the processing systems to the Supervisory System. (p. 378)

This contrast provides an intriguing and fairly direct parallel to the distinction between a dissociated-control model of hypnotic amnesia, as presented here, and the classic amnestic-barrier model. According to the dissociated-control model, hypnosis alters high-level controls over memory functions, so that material is more difficult to retrieve under conditions that require the control system to generate preliminary descriptions, and verification of retrieved material is faulty. This model is in contrast to the view that hypnosis blocks access to memories in a barrierlike, comparatively all-or-nothing fashion.

In addition, Kolb and Whishaw (1985) argue that the best established effect on memory of frontal lobe damage is impaired memory for recency, or the temporal ordering of events. Correspondingly, there is quite a body of evidence to indicate that hypnotized subjects show a disorganization in the temporal or sequential organization of events in memory (e.g., Evans & Kihlstrom, 1973; Geiselman et al., 1983; Kihlstrom & Evans, 1979; Kihlstrom & Wilson, 1984; Spanos & Bodorik, 1977; Spanos, Radtke-Bodorik, & Stam, 1980; Tkachyk, Spanos, & Bertrand, 1985; Wilson & Kihlstrom, 1986).

In summary, it is quite attractive to link a dissociated-control theory of hypnosis to the inhibition of functions subserved by the prefrontal cortex. There remains, however, the question of how best to proceed in making something useful out of the hypothesis of such a brain–behavior relationship. One approach to take is to do neuropsychophysiological studies that examine regional specificities of brain function during hypnosis. This is the approach predominantly employed by Crawford and by Gruzelier (for a review, see Crawford & Gruzelier, 1992). Based on a rather complex hypothesis of changes in hemispheric laterality with hypnosis, these researchers and their colleagues, as well as others, have produced a maze of complex and sometimes conflicting findings, using a variety of procedures such as sophisticated EEG analyses and brain imaging techniques. Toward the end of the review, however, Crawford and Gruzelier (1992) seem to have pulled away somewhat from the complex shift-in-laterality position and moved toward a simpler position quite in line with what has been argued here. They write: "With hindsight, what may be more central to hypnosis is the inhibition of anterior frontal lobe functions" (p. 265).

Another approach to take is a more cognitive-functional one, which would emphasize the construction and evaluation of explanatory cognitive models, and deemphasize (due to its prematurity) the issues of regional specificity in the brain. There are many testable hypotheses about hypnosis that might emerge from comparing it to frontal lobe disorders, of which the following are some examples:

1. The notion that frontal functions are inhibited in hypnosis suggests that hypnotized subjects should show some of the problem-solving behaviors of frontal lobe patients: for example, the "stuck-in-set" perseveration

on such tasks as the Wisconsin Card-Sorting Task (Milner, 1963), the relatively poor performance on tasks that require a planning or self-organizing component (e.g., Milner, Petrides, & Smith, 1985), and the relatively high rate of bizarre answers on tasks that require thinking of a nonroutine approach and checking the plausibility of a potential response (e.g., Shallice & Evans, 1978; Smith & Milner, 1984). Such findings would be consistent with the general hypothesis that under hypnosis, subjects show a reduced capacity to overcome routine responses and cope with novel problem-solving demands (the principal contribution of the supervisory system).

2. The notion that the effects of hypnosis on memory processes are akin to frontal amnesia suggests that hypnotized subjects should have more difficulty with certain kinds of memory tasks—for example, with accurately retrieving events that are long past and therefore not part of any standard semantic-memory retrieval routine (e.g., Sanders & Warrington, 1971; Shallice, 1988). Such findings would be consistent with the general hypothesis that under hypnosis, subjects show less capacity to engage in the description and verification procedures subserved by the supervisory system.

CONCLUSION: WHAT SORT OF CONTROL IS DISSOCIATED CONTROL?

To return finally to an issue raised much earlier in this chapter, let us begin by citing Kihlstrom's (1992) assertion, "The experience of automaticity, like so much else about hypnosis, is illusory" (p. 308). In light of the present dissociated-control account of hypnosis, this statement is quite interesting because it appears to be wrong in one way, and right in another. It is wrong in the sense that alterations of control in hypnosis are quite like automatized actions, in that they both involve the minimizing of supervisory system functions. Rather than simply colluding in the construction of an illusion of nonvolition, the hypnotized subject, within the context of the present account, undergoes a real change in the control of behavior—simply put, a shift down in the hierarchy of control. One important implication of a genuine change in control, as opposed to a collusive illusion, is that a subject could act quite unlike his or her "usual self" under hypnosis, in conflict with consciously represented standards. Such discrepant acts would perhaps be particularly likely when the behavior in question is well-learned or "deeply ingrained," but the person (outside hypnosis) is typically exerting a high degree of deliberate attentional control to inhibit it (e.g., a bad habit).

However, Kihlstrom's statement is right in the sense that there is no reason to think a hypnotic induction could make a behavior automatized that was not ever automatized before; for example, hypnosis cannot substitute for learning or practice. Indeed, the present view of what happens in hypnosis to highly susceptible subjects may be regarded as far less flattering than some other views of hypnosis (e.g., Crawford, 1991), it suggests that, for the most part, hypnosis simply allows already routinized behaviors to be run off without the volitional level of control.

How, then, does the notion of dissociated control allow hypnosis to add anything new say of potential clinical utility to a subject's behavioral repertoire? Consider that despite its wonderful flexibility, deliberate attentional control, with its serial processing steps, hypnosis is slow, limited in capacity, and unwieldy. Hence, in circumstances as varied as performing music and managing social interactions, effortful control at the level of the supervisory system can become counterproductive and lead to maladaptive "overcontrol." As Norman and Shallice (1986) remark, "deliberate control of skilled performance leads to deterioration of performance" (p. 11). Thus, hypnosis may be viewed as a therapeutic opportunity to relinquish some kinds of control in order to further others—of a more parallel and less centralized sort. In addition, by exerting some outboard planning and control functions, the hypnotist may sometimes promote the eliciting of novel solutions and responses, ones for which the subject has not yet quite "put together the pieces" (e.g., Talmon, 1990).

Given the current interest in the likely relation between hypnotizability and multiple personality disorder (e.g., Bliss, 1984; Bowers, 1992), it is intriguing to speculate about whether a process of dissociated control could produce something as new and novel as a second personality. Consider that by inhibiting supervisory system functions, hypnosis should lead to some temporary loss of personality integration, in the sense of how well behavior is integrated with overarching goals, and events with an overall life structure. However, the result would seem to be a state of attenuation, in which the sense of personal identity is weakened, rather than that a "new" personality is created. Given the link we have drawn between supervisory functions and the frontal lobes, it is also worth recalling the classic case of Phineas Gage, which truly involves a real-life Jekyll-to-Hyde transformation. After an accident that damaged Gage's left frontal lobe, the dramatic change in his behavior was described in words that might have come straight out of Stevenson's story:

> The equilibrium or balance, so to speak, between his intellectual faculties and animal propensities seems to have been destroyed. He is fitful, irreverent, indulging at times in the grossest profanity, manifesting but little deference to his fellows, impatient of restraint or advice when it conflicts with his desires, at times pertinaciously obstinate, yet capricious and vacillating. (Harlow, 1868, cited in Blumer & Benson, 1975, p. 153)

Here, too, Gage's condition seems better described as a severe loss of personality integration than as involving the emergence of a well-organized new personality. In short, one might well be skeptical of the idea that the mechanism of dissociative control, with its weakening of high-level executive functions, would account for the development of a true second personality, as opposed to loosened personality integration.

However, that may not quite be the end of the story. Shallice (1988) has noted that the concept of the supervisory system parallels Johnson-Laird's (1983) notion of consciousness as the operating system of the mind. Pursuing this computer metaphor, it is an intriguing fact that nothing can prevent the possibility of two operating systems coexisting on the same hardware—for example, Windows and OS/2, either of which could be "brought up" during a particular session. (It is amusing in the present context to note that Windows and OS/2 began as the same operating system, and then split apart rather late in their development.) Returning to people, normally one good supervisory or operating system is all that is needed; but perhaps in rare cases, two alternative, coexisting executive control systems, each with its own memory-management processes and access to unique records, may develop. They should be distinguishable in terms of different implicit self-knowledge, and so on. Admittedly, such demonstrations have been extremely rare. Nonetheless, within the context of this speculative model, the essence of MPD would not involve the erection of amnestic barriers, nor poor personality integration expressed metaphorically as "multiple personalities," but the development of alternative executive-control systems, each of which operates independently.

REFERENCES

Baars, B. J. (1988). *A cognitive theory of consciousness*. Cambridge: Cambridge University Press.

Baars, B. J. (1991). Consciousness and modularity. *Behavioral and Brain Sciences, 14*, 440.

Bliss, E. L. (1986). *Multiple personality, allied disorders and hypnosis*. New York: Oxford University Press.

Blumer, D., & Benson, D. F. (1975). Personality changes with frontal and temporal lobe lesions. In D. F. Benson & D. Blumer (Eds.), *Psychiatric aspects of neurologic disease* (pp. 151–170). New York: Grune & Stratton.

Bouckoms, A. J. (1989). Psychosurgery for pain. In P. D. Wall & R. Melzack (Eds.), *Textbook of pain* (2nd ed., pp. 868–881). Edinburgh: Churchill Livingstone.

Bowers, K. S. (1976). *Hypnosis for the seriously curious*. Monterey, CA: Brooks/Cole.

Bowers, K. S. (1990). Unconscious influences and hypnosis. In J. L. Singer (Ed.), *Repression and dissociation: Implications for personality theory, psychopathology, and health* (pp. 143–178). Chicago: University of Chicago Press.

Bowers, K. S. (1992). Imagination and dissociation in hypnotic responding. *International Journal of Clinical and Experimental Hypnosis, 40*, 253–275.

Bowers, K. S., & Brenneman, H. A. (1981). Hypnotic dissociation, dichotic listening, and active versus passive modes of attention. *Journal of Abnormal Psychology, 90*, 55–67.

Coe, W. C., & Ryken, K. (1979). Hypnosis and risks to human subjects. *American Psychologist, 34*, 673–681.

Crawford, H. J. (1991, October). *The hypnotizable brain: Attentional and disattentional processes*. Presidential address delivered at the annual meeting of the Society for Clinical and Experimental Hypnosis, New Orleans.

Crawford, H. J., & Gruzelier, J. H. (1992). A midstream view of the neuropsychophysiology of hypnosis: Recent research and future directions. In E. Fromm & M. R. Nash (Eds.), *Contemporary hypnosis research* (pp. 227–266). New York: Guilford Press.

Crawford, H. J., Hilgard, J. R., & Macdonald, H. (1982). Transient experiences following hypnotic testing and special termination procedures. *International Journal of Clinical and Experimental Hypnosis, 30*, 117–126.

Dywan, J., & Bowers, K. S. (1983). The use of hypnosis to enhance recall. *Science, 222*, 184–185.

Erdelyi, M. H. (1985). *Psychoanalysis: Freud's cognitive psychology*. New York: W. H. Freeman.

Erdelyi, M. H. (1990). Repression, reconstruction, and defense: History and integration of the psychoanalytic and experimental frameworks. In J. L. Singer (Ed.), *Repression and dissociation: Implications for personality theory, psychopathology, and health* (pp. 1–31). Chicago: University of Chicago Press.

Evans, F. J. (1979). Contextual forgetting: Posthypnotic source amnesia. *Journal of Abnormal Psychology, 88*, 556–563.

Evans, F. J., & Kihlstrom, J. F. (1973). Posthypnotic amnesia as disrupted recall. *Journal of Abnormal Psychology, 82*, 317–323.

Geiselman, R. E., Fishman, D. L., Jaenicke, C., Larner, B. R., MacKinnon, D. P., Shoenberg, S., & Swartz, S. (1983). Mechanisms of hypnotic and nonhypnotic forgetting. *Journal of Experimental Psychology: Learning, Memory, and Cognition, 9*, 626–635.

Hargadon, R., & Bowers, K. S. (1992, October). *High hypnotizables and hypnotic analgesia: An examination of underlying mechanisms*. Paper presented at the annual meeting of the Society for Clinical and Experimental Hypnosis, Arlington, VA.

Hécaen, H., & Albert, M. L. (1975). Disorders of mental functioning related to frontal lobe pathology. In D. F. Benson & D. Blumer (Eds.), *Psychiatric aspects of neourologic disease*. New York: Grune & Stratton.

Hilgard, E. R. (1973). A neodissociation interpretation of pain reduction in hypnosis. *Psychological Review, 80*, 396–411.

Higard, E. R. (1977). *Divided consciousness: Multiple controls in human thought and action*. New York: Wiley-Interscience.

Hilgard, E. R., & Cooper, L. M. (1965). Spontaneous and suggested post-hypnotic amnesia. *International Journal of Clinical and Experimental Hypnosis, 13*, 261–273.

Hilgard, J. R. (1974). Sequelae to hypnosis. *International Journal of Clinical and Experimental Hypnosis, 22*, 138–156.

James, W. (1981). *The principles of psychology*. Cambridge, MA: Harvard University Press. (Original work published 1890)

Janet, P. (1901). *The mental state of hystericals*. New York: Putnam.

Janet, P. (1965). *The major symptoms of hysteria*. New York: Hafner. (Original work published 1907)

Johnson-Laird, P. N. (1983). *Mental models*. Cambridge, MA: Harvard University Press.

Kihlstrom, J. F. (1980). Posthypnotic amnesia for recently learned material: Interactions with "episodic" and "semantic" memory. *Cognitive Psychology, 12*, 227–251.

Kihlstrom, J. F. (1985). Hypnosis. *Annual Review of Psychology, 36*, 385–418.

Kihlstrom, J. F. (1992). Hypnosis: A sesquicentennial essay. *International Journal of Clinical and Experimental Hypnosis, 40*, 301–314.

Kihlstrom, J. F., & Evans, F. J. (1979). Memory retrieval processes during posthypnotic amnesia. In J. F. Kihlstrom & F. J. Evans (Eds.), *Functional disorders of memory* (pp. 179–218). Hillsdale, NJ: Lawrence Erlbaum.

Kihlstrom, J. F., & Shor, R. E. (1978). Recall and recognition during posthypnotic amnesia. *International Journal of Clinical and Experimental Hypnosis, 26*, 330–349.

Kihlstrom, J. F., & Wilson, L. (1984). Temporal organization of recall during posthypnotic amnesia. *Journal of Abnormal Psychology, 93*, 200–208.

Kolb, B., & Whishaw, I. Q. (1985). *Fundamentals of human neuropsychology* (2nd ed.). New York: W. H. Freeman.

Laurence, J.-R., & Perry, C. (1983). Hypnotically created memory among highly hypnotizable subjects. *Science, 222*, 523–524.

Lynn, S. J., Rhue, J. W., & Weekes, J. R. (1990). Hypnotic involuntariness: A social cognitive analysis. *Psychological Review, 97*, 169–184.

McCaul, K. D., & Malott, J. M. (1984). Distraction and coping with pain. *Psychological Bulletin, 95*, 516–533.

McConkey, K. M., & Sheehan, P. W. (1981). The impact of videotape playback of hypnotic events on hypnotic amnesia. *Journal of Abnormal Psychology, 90*, 46–54.

McConkey, K. M., Sheehan, P. W., & Cross, D. G. (1980). Posthypnotic amnesia: Seeing is not remembering. *British Journal of Social and Clinical Psychology, 19*, 99–107.

Miller, M. E., & Bowers, K. S. (1986). Hypnotic analgesia and stress inoculation in the reduction of pain. *Journal of Abnormal Psychology, 95*, 6–14.

Miller, M. E., & Bowers, K. S. (1993). Hypnotic analgesia: Dissociated experience or dissociated control? *Journal of Abnormal Psychology, 102*, 29–38.

Milner, B. (1963). Effects of different brain lesions on card-sorting. *Archives of Neurology, 9*, 90–100.

Milner, B., Petrides, M., & Smith, M. L. (1985). Frontal lobes and the temporal organization of memory. *Human Neurobiology, 4*, 137–142.

Monteiro, K. P., Macdonald, H., & Hilgard, E. R. (1980). Imagery, absorption, and hypnosis: A factorial study. *Journal of Mental Imagery, 4*, 63–81.

Nisbett, R., & Wilson, T. D. (1977). Telling more than we can know: Verbal reports on mental processes. *Psychological Review, 84*, 231–254.

Norman, D. A., & Bobrow, D. G. (1979). Descriptions: An intermediate stage in memory retrieval. *Cognitive Psychology, 11*, 107–123.

Norman, D. A., & Shallice, T. (1986). Attention to action: Willed and automatic control of behavior. In R. J. Davidson, G. E. Schwartz, & D. Shapiro (Eds.), *Consciousness and self-regulation* (Vol. 4, pp. 1–18). New York: Plenum Press.

Orne, M. T. (1979). On the simulating subject as a quasi-control group in hypnosis research: What, why, and how. In E. Fromm & R. E. Shor (Eds.), *Hypnosis: Developments in research and new perspectives* (pp. 519–565). Chicago: Aldine.

Orne, M. T., Whitehouse, W. G., Dinges, D. F., & Orne, E. C. (1988). Reconstructing memory through hypnosis: Forensic and clinical implications. In H. M. Pettinati (Ed.), *Hypnosis and memory* (pp. 21–63). New York: Guilford Press.

Pope-Hennessey, J. (1974). *Robert Louis Stevenson*. London: Jonathan Cape.

Pribram, K. H. (1973). The primate frontal cortex—executive of the brain. In K. H. Pribram & A. R. Luria (Eds.), *Psychophysiology of the frontal lobes* (pp. 293–314). New York: Academic Press.

Pribram, K. H. (1991). *Brain and perception: Holonomy and structure in figural processing*. Hillsdale, NJ: Lawrence Erlbaum.

Reyher, J. (1967). Hypnosis in research on psychopathology. In J. E. Gordon (Ed.), *Handbook of clinical and experimental hypnosis* (pp. 110–147). New York: Macmillan.

Sanders, H. I., & Warrington, E. K. (1971). Memory for remote events in amnestic patients. *Brain, 94*, 661–668.

Shallice, T. (1988). *From neuropsychology to mental structure*. Cambridge: Cambridge University Press.

Shallice, T., & Evans, M. E. (1978). The involvement of the frontal lobes in cognitive estimation. *Cortex, 14*, 294–303.

Shiffrin, R. M., & Schneider, W. (1977). Controlled and automatic human information processing: II. Perceptual learning, automatic attending, and a general theory. *Psychological Review, 84*, 127–190.

Shor, R. E. (1959). Hypnosis and the concept of the generalized reality-orientation. *American Journal of Psychotherapy, 13*, 582–602.

Shor, R. E. (1979). The fundamental problem in hypnosis research as viewed from historic perspectives. In E. Fromm & R. E. Shor (Eds.), *Hypnosis: Developments in research and new perspectives* (2nd ed., pp. 15–41). Chicago: Aldine.

Shor, R. E., & Orne, M. T. (1962). *Harvard Group Scale of Hypnotic Susceptibility, Form A*. Palo Alto, CA: Consulting Psychologists Press.

Smith, M. L., & Milner, B. (1984). Differential effects of frontal lobe lesions on cognitive estimation and spatial memory. *Neuropsychologia, 22*, 697–705.

Spanos, N. P. (1986). Hypnotic behavior: A social psychological interpretation of amnesia, analgesia, and "trance logic." *Behavioral and Brain Sciences, 9*, 449–467.

Spanos, N. P., & Bodorik, H. L. (1977). Suggested amnesia and disorganized recall in hypnotic and task-motivated subjects. *Journal of Abnormal Psychology, 86*, 295–305.

Spanos, N. P., Radtke, H. L., & Dubreuil, D. L. (1982). Episodic and semantic memory in posthypnotic amnesia: A reevaluation. *Journal of Personality and Social Psychology, 43*, 565–573.

Spanos, N. P., Radtke-Bodorik, H. L., & Stam, H. J. (1980). Disorganized recall during suggested amnesia: Fact not artifact. *Journal of Abnormal Psychology, 89*, 1–19.

Stevenson, R. L. (1967). *The strange case of Dr. Jekyll and Mr. Hyde*. New York: Franklin Watts. (Original work published 1886)

Talmon, M. (1990). *Single-session therapy: Maximizing the effect of the first (and often only) therapeutic encounter*. San Francisco: Jossey-Bass.

Tkachyk, M. E., Spanos, N. P., & Bertrand, L. D. (1985). Variables affecting subjective organization during posthypnotic amnesia. *Journal of Research in Personality, 19*, 95–108.

Teuber, H.-L. (1964). The riddle of frontal lobe function in man. In J. M. Warren & K. Akert (Eds.), *The frontal granular cortex and behavior*. New York: McGraw-Hill.

Tulving, E. (1972). Episodic and semantic memory. In E. Tulving & W. Donaldson (Eds.), *Organization of memory* (pp. 381–403). New York: Academic Press.

Turk, D., Meichenbaum, D. H., & Genest, M. (1983). *Pain and behavioral medicine: A cognitive-behavioral perspective*. New York: Guilford Press.

Wagstaff, B. F. (1991). Compliance, belief, and semantics in hypnosis: A nonstate, sociocognitive perspective. In S. J. Lynn & J. W. Rhue (Eds.), *Theories of hypnosis: Current models and perspectives* (pp. 362–396). New York: Guilford Press.

Weitzenhoffer, A. M. (1953). *Hypnotism: An objective study in suggestibility*. New York: John Wiley.

Wilson, L., & Kihlstrom, J. F. (1986). Subjective and categorical organization of recall during posthypnotic amnesia. *Journal of Abnormal Psychology, 95*, 264–273.

Woody, E. Z., Oakman, J. M., & Drugovic, M. (1992, October). *Fleshing out a two-component view of individual differences underlying hypnotic responsiveness*. Paper presented at the annual meeting of the Society for Clinical and Experimental Hypnosis, Arlington, VA.

Part III
Theories of Hypnosis: Divergence and Convergence

[8]

TOWARD A NEO-DISSOCIATION THEORY: MULTIPLE COGNITIVE CONTROLS IN HUMAN FUNCTIONING

*ERNEST R. HILGARD**

Below the surface-stream, shallow and light,
Of what we *say* we feel—below the stream,
As light of what we *think* we feel—there flows
With noiseless current strong, obscure and deep,
The central stream of what we *feel* indeed.
[MATTHEW ARNOLD, 1870]

. . . let not thy left hand know what thy right hand doeth.
[MATT. 6:3]

The mysteries of mind have recently been receiving renewed attention among both laymen and psychological scientists. For a time the advances in behavior theory and behavioral control techniques, largely under the influence of Pavlov and the American behaviorists from Watson to Skinner, seemed to remove most of the mystery of mind by showing how readily behavior comes under stimulus control through the contingencies of reinforcement. In recent years a substantial fraction of people, particularly the young, fed up with technology and contemporary society, have turned inward to discover the range of human potential in other ways. These other ways have included experimentation with psychedelic drugs, meditation, Eastern religions, ESP, and occultism. Much of this searching lies outside the scientific establishment, but it does not leave the scientists unmoved. In psychology there is a growing interest in what is loosely called humanistic psychology,

*Professor of psychology, emeritus, Stanford University, Stanford, California 94305.
The experimentation leading to this paper and its preparation have been aided by research grant MH-3859 from the National Institute of Mental Health.

unified (to the extent that any unity can be detected) around the theme that a responsible psychology must be concerned with human values and the deeper meaning of life. Laboratory psychologists, not identified with any of the extreme movements, also begin to take a new interest in the voluntary control of normally involuntary movements (as in biofeedback studies), they offer conjectures about different modes of consciousness associated with the right and left hemispheres, and they turn increasingly to study of sleep and dreams, of hypnosis, of imagination and creativity. What begins as an anti-intellectual movement in the counterculture gradually shifts the center of gravity within the academic and scientific culture as well. The scientists who retain their identity with the prevailing culture do not give up their naturalistic interests, but they focus some measure of their attention on new problems.

This is not the first time that such a shift of interest among psychologists and psychiatrists has come about through stirrings in the nonacademic community. In the latter half of the nineteenth century, spiritualism became a great fad. Mediums had not always been around, but they began to appear following the prominence of the Fox sisters in the United States; the wave of interest soon spread to England, Germany, and France, and then throughout the world. This was a partial answer to man's loss of dignity as a consequence of Darwin's teachings, for if evidence could be found for the soul's survival of bodily death man's unique place in nature would be firmly established. The essence of the movement was not anti-Darwinism any more than the essence of the counterculture today is antibehaviorism, but the parallels are instructive. The new science of parapsychology emerged as serious investigators such as F. W. H. Myers and Edmund Gurney in England attempted to investigate spiritualistic claims sympathetically but critically. They founded the London Society for Psychical Research in 1882, to be followed shortly by the American Society of Psychical Research, with the distinguished American psychologist, William James, as one of its leading enthusiasts.

The scientific establishment's reply to the spirtualists was to take a look at neglected phenomena, incorporating the findings in naturalistic accounts of them. Borrowing from the psychic investigators such methods as automatic writing, a number of psychologists and psychiatrists became impressed by the dual controls operating in human functioning, a "subconscious mind" along with a "conscious mind." The evidence came not only from the study of purported "mediums," but from hysterical personalities, with their losses of ordinary sensorimotor controls in functional paralysis, blindness, or other sensory defects, and, in some cases, the emergence of hidden secondary personalities. Pierre Janet (1859–1947) was a leader in this new direction for psychology. His first book, on psychological automatisms [1], introduced the notion that parts of the personality can operate relatively autonomously, split off from the main consciousness. He gradually developed his theory of dissociation or disaggregation to account for these phenomena. Janet's concept was picked up by Boris Sidis and Morton Prince in America and remained in quite general use early in the twentieth century. Related conceptions were quite widespread and were not by any means limited to Janet's followers. In Germany, for example, in 1890, only a year after Janet's book, the distinguished psychologist, Max Dessoir, wrote an influential book entitled *Das Doppel-Ich* [The double-ego] in which he identified the two main streams of mental activity as an "upper consciousness" and a "lower consciousness" [2]. The secondary consciousness he believed could be tapped in hypnosis.

Classical Dissociation Theory

The nature of the human mind has always been of interest to reflective men who raise questions and formulate their answers according to contemporary beliefs expressed in theology, philosophy, and science, or even as influenced by popular social movements. The metaphor of dissociation was derived from the prevalent doctrine of the association of ideas. If ordinary integration of mental activity is accounted for by association, what more natural way to describe a bifurcation of control than by its reversal—a disassociation, or simply, dissociation?

The theories of mental organization that emerged can be concisely classified into two main groups: the theory of *dipsychism* and that of *polypsychism* [3], implying either two "layers" of consciousness or more than two.

If there were two layers (dipsychism) the first was conceived as the normal waking consciousness, the second as usually hidden, but occasionally revealing itself in dreams, abnormal symptoms, in hypnosis, and occasionally in unusual and unexpected creative acts. The two layers of personality (or consciousness) were assigned different qualities, depending on the authorities describing them. In what Ellenberger calls the "closed" form of the theory the subconscious contains only tendencies and memories arising in the experience of the individual, but no longer available to the waking consciousness. According to Janet, who was the first to use the expression "subconscious," the unavailable ideas, as we have already noted, became "dissociated" or "disaggregated," so that they could not be synthesized into waking awareness; Freud, in his first concept of the unconscious believed that it consisted of "repressed" thoughts or wishes. Hence dissociation and repression described essentially the same facts of a closed subconscious layer.

In the "open" form of the theory, the subconscious layer is not only more extensive than the conscious layer, but it has access to some broader sets of experience that may never have been in the waking consciousness. Such a "subliminal self" was posited by Myers [4, 5] and was favorably supported by James in his *Varieties of Religious Experience* [6]. This general position has found more recent expression in Jung's collective unconscious and in his belief in universal archetypes and mandala symbols in dreams [7]. The issue is again of interest because of present-day romanticism about consciousness expansion and human potentiality. The iceberg analogy is often used, with consciousness merely the portion that is visible and the larger (and more important) portion beneath the surface.

Another distinction differentiates various views of the subconscious in the "closed" and "open" form. In one position, common to Janet and the early Freud, the subconscious (or unconscious) portion is somewhat debased as being fragmented, illogical, or impulse ridden (as in the seething cauldron picture of the unconscious associated with early psychoanalysis). The opposite view is that the subconscious (whether "closed" or "open") may be the source of morality, inspiration, or creativity. Oddly enough, the phenomenal observations are as contradictory as the theories explaining them.

The polypsychic theories accept the general notion of splits in the personality or ego but assert that the cleavages may result in more than two subordinate parts. Freud, for example, moved from his earlier dipsychism[1] to a tripsychism in proposing the division into id, ego, and superego: "The poor ego has a still harder time of it; it has to serve three harsh masters, and has to do its best to reconcile the claims and demands of all three. . . . The three tyrants are the external world, the superego and the id" [8, p. 108]. His later disciples have divided the ego into numerous apparatuses and substructures [9, 10].

How independent were conscious and subconscious processes? This was always a matter of some dispute. Obviously they were not totally independent because there were usually some derivatives of the subconscious present in consciousness. The true nature of the unconscious thoughts might be disguised, as in dreams or symptoms of illness. Morton Prince [11] preferred the term "co-conscious" precisely to avoid the connotation that the two consciousnesses were always isolated from each other.

In attempting to state a case for something like dissociation, the historical background is too muddled for a restatement to be a reaffirmation of the old doctrine. Hence I use the term "neo-dissociationism" to acknowledge historical roots without obligating myself to be faithful to the views of predecessors.

[1]I am ignoring the preconscious in Freud's earlier formulation because it consists largely of available memories not now in consciousness; hence, for purposes of this discussion it may be viewed as part of the conscious control mechanism. This is, to be sure, an oversimplification of Freud's theory.

I have attempted to account elsewhere for the rapid fading of the dissociation concept [12]. There were few attacks upon it. The main historical reasons for later neglect probably lay in the general disappearance of interest in hypnotic phenomena and the rise to prominence of psychoanalysis, whose followers seldom used the word at all.

Interacting Control Structures

As Thorndike once remarked, if we are trying to develop a science there is no point in merely standing in awe at the marvels and complexities of human functioning. Freud, too, felt that he was not ready to deal with some of the problems that a Dostoevsky could picture. As psychological scientists we have to begin to explore where we can, in the hope that our small endeavors may lead us to something eventually of greater significance. The particular processes that dissociation theories began to explore were simultaneous or near-simultaneous cognitive activities and structures that showed some measure of independence from each other.

Illustrations of simultaneous or near-simultaneous control structures abound in ordinary experience: homeostatic control systems that regulate heart rate, breathing, and body temperature, while we attend to other activities, whether violent or sedentary; skilled acts that serve their purposes while the cerebellar processes take care of the synergic subsystems that are brought into play; dreams that go on out of voluntary control, with some part of our cognitive apparatus serving as an amused or concerned spectator of the drama that some other cognitive part of us is staging; a complicated interchange of communications, public and private, that goes on in ordinary conversation; selective listening that permits us to attend primarily to one conversation in a crowded room of talkative people while eavesdropping occasionally on an adjoining conversation. All of this is so commonplace that it does not seem puzzling; only in recent years have these processes been recognized as providing occasions for experimentation.

An experimental setting sometimes helps to bring processes of this kind into sharper focus. Hypnosis provides such a setting, and it is the arrangement par excellence for the study of conflicting cognitive controls that can be characterized as dissociative.

Automatic Writing as Illustrative of Dissociated Control Systems

The puzzles of simultaneous cognitive activities are brought to the fore most impressively when the subject is required to perform two tasks at once, one in the ordinary state of waking consciousness, the other out of awareness owing to hypnotic suggestion.

Natural scientists are a little fearful of "guilt by assocation" if they pay attention to occult phenomena. It must be acknowledged, however, that the efforts of nineteenth-century spiritualists to communicate with departed spirits taught us some things about cognitive controls that could be turned to advantage in our purely naturalistic experiments. One of the favorite methods used with mediums was that of automatic writing. The "spirit" made use of the hands of an earthly being (medium) to deliver a message. The message could be written out by the pencil attached to a planchette (a small device supported by rolling wheels, on which one or more hands might be placed while writing), or the message could be spelled out by the planchette of a ouija board,[2] coming to rest pointing to one letter after another.

It was soon discovered that under these circumstances the hand might indeed produce sensible messages, often very much to the surprise of all concerned. From a naturalistic standpoint this means that it is occasionally possible to tap levels of memory and imagination, cognitively comprehensible, that are not in the ordinary waking awareness of the person whose cognitions become displayed.

A few extreme cases came to light, of which one of the most striking was that of "Patience Worth." Mrs. Curran, a Saint Louis housewife, began playing with the ouija board. She did not graduate from high school, and she showed no evidence of literary capabilities or pretensions. When the guiding hand of Patience Worth introduced herself on the ouija board, Mrs. Curran soon became a successful author with the help of Patience Worth. Five novels were published under the authorship of Patience Worth between 1917 and 1928; while they were not great, they were not without literary merit and received favorable reviews at the time. The ouija board was gradually displaced, and Patience Worth began dictating directly to Mrs. Curran. There were a number of poems in addition to the novels. The case is of sufficient interest to have been given a recent thorough review [13].

It was early found that hypnotic suggestion could be used to elicit automatic writing from ordinary people willing to serve in laboratory experiments. William James was among those who reported such investigations [14]. Without reviewing the extensive use of automatic writing by clinicians in recovering lost memories, I shall turn to our own studies now under way.

The first of these, modeled after an earlier one by Cass [15], required the subject to name colors from a chart before him while his hand, concealed from view and out of awareness, engaged in an arithmetical task such as simple counting or serial addition. In serial addition he was asked, for example, to start with a given number and then add

[2]It is amusing to note the source of the name of the ouija board: *oui* ("yes" in French); *ja* ("yes" in German).

7's to it successively. In his doctoral dissertation done in our laboratory, Stevenson [16] found that it was possible for selected hypnotic subjects to do these operations satisfactorily, but at some cost. The costs were of two kinds. First, performing the arithmetical task out of awareness proved to be more difficult than performing it with awareness, even without any competing task. That is, to maintain the amnesia so that one did not know what he was doing took some toll in the way of cognitive effort that decreased the efficiency of his performance. The second cost was paid when the color-naming task was added to the arithmetic task out of awareness; this drained more cognitive effort and interfered further with the tasks. The more difficult the task out of awareness, the greater the interference.

A follow-up experiment has confirmed Stevenson's findings and added some finer details on the nature of the interferences [17]. Even a very simple automatic task such as pressing two keys in alternation (three to the left, three to the right, and so on) may suffer interference by conscious color naming so that errors in number of presses are made, even though the task proceeds smoothly enough and out of the subject's awareness. There are, of course, individual differences in the amount of such interference.

Conventional dissociation theory would have asserted that there should be *less* interference between the tasks when one of them is out of awareness. That the facts turned out the opposite is no objection to a modern form of dissociation theory, here proposed as neo-dissociation theory, for a modernized theory must accept the fact that one of the tasks is indeed out of awareness and that the cognitive costs of keeping it so must be explained.

A Reference Experiment for Neo-Dissociation Theory

The exposition of a scientific theory often can be carried out by citing a reference experiment, sometimes an experiment that itself gave rise to the theory. One can think of the swinging pendulum as a reference experiment for Galileo, the moon and the tides for Newton, the tall and dwarf peas for Mendel, the rat in the box for Skinner. If the theory fits (explains) the reference experiment, then it reaches out to encompass related phenomena. If the theory proves to be of more general significance, it eventually embraces a much wider range of phenomena than those in the reference experiment.

An experimental investigation upon which we are now engaged provides a very useful reference experiment for neo-dissociation theory because the phenomenal findings are of the kind that gave rise to dissociation theory in the first place, but the context is that of modern experimental controls and measurement.

Following a procedure that had already been much used in our laboratory, we suggested that the hand would be analgesic to the pain of circulating ice water (the cold pressor test) [18, 19]. There is no doubt that this can be done successfully in the laboratory, and results from clinical experience with obstetrics, burns, tooth extraction, and terminal cancer are convincing that, for hypnotically susceptible persons, pain can be reduced and often eliminated entirely by hypnotic procedures. For the purposes of this experiment, we used only subjects who reported complete anesthesia of the arm, feeling neither cold nor pain when the hand and forearm were in the circulating ice water. Each one felt pain normally when not given suggestions to reduce pain. While the left hand and forearm were kept in the ice water without any discomfort, the right hand was placed in a box arranged for automatic writing or for reporting pain on a numerical scale through key pressing. The hypnotized subject was told that the hand would tell us what we ought to know, but the subject would pay no attention to this hand and would not know what it was communicating or even that it was doing anything at all. It takes highly susceptible subjects to follow such suggestions, but in a sample of university students inexperienced in hypnosis there will be 1 or 2 percent who can do it, especially with a little practice. Now what did we find? The first subject with whom we tried this procedure was a highly susceptible young woman who had had many hours of experience in hypnosis. She gave verbal reports at 5-second intervals while her hand was in the water indicating that she felt absolutely no pain, and she was entirely calm in this normally stressful experience. Simultaneously, the dissociated part of herself was reporting in automatic writing and assigning numerical values to the felt pain. The hand out of awareness reported that the pain was being felt *just as in the normal state.*

In subsequent tests with her and with other subjects, the more usual report has been that some pain is being recorded at a dissociated level, but the pain is not quite as severe as when tested in the normal hypnotic condition. Such a moderate reduction would be expected if for no other reason than that the analgesic state is a quiescent one [20].

It is important to note that this hidden experience of pain differs from a felt pain that is unreported in order to please the hypnotist, or held private out of some sort of heroic denial. A woman who has had one baby with the help of hypnosis commonly asks to have her next one that way, even though she has a new obstetrician and has only herself to please. Many of our subjects who have learned self-hypnosis have gained pain relief on their own. The buried pain is indeed hidden from awareness, unless some special methods are used for uncovering it.

Our experiments are the first, to my knowledge, in which systematic or quantitative comparisons have been made between the "subconscious" and the "conscious" experience of pain. In a search of the past literature we find some anticipations of our findings. Beginning with the one case of William James [14], there are three case studies of single subjects with hypnotically anesthetic arms who report the pain of pin pricks to that arm by way of automatic writing. The two other cases have been independently reported [21, p. 98; 22].

We are now carrying on further experiments to see if there are depths of hypnotic involvement in which neither the "word" consciousness nor the "hand" consciousness reports the pain. Too much must not be made of the specific technique of reporting, because we have in some instances substituted automatic talking for automatic writing. By instructing the subject that when the hypnotist's hand is placed on his shoulder he will tell what is going on in the secondary consciousness, but will not know that he is talking, results similar to automatic writing are obtained. The subject describes the pain that is felt by some part of himself, even though the ordinary waking consciousness is oblivious to the pain. When the hand is lifted he stops talking, though he may have noticed the hand on his shoulder and may inquire, "Did I talk to you?" Here, then, we have an additional dissociation that calls for explanation.

The pain and automatic writing experiment just discussed can serve initially as a reference experiment for neo-dissociation theory. The essential findings, raising problems for theory, are diagrammed in figure 1.

The left-hand box represents in simplified form the condition of the relevant cognitive systems when the hand is immersed in ice water in the normal state, a condition in which all channels are open. The normal response is of felt pain, and there is no barrier to reporting this as a communication to the experimenter or other witnesses. Associated with this report there are visible signs of discomfort owing to the cold water, as in grimacing or restless movements, and instruments will report reflex changes in heart rate, blood pressure, and other physiological indicators. Some of these changes in bodily processes are reflected in the cognitive states, but the arrows go both ways because memories and anticipations also affect the physiological indicators. The voluntary responses of grimacing, breath holding, and the like, are noted separately from the reflex responses, but there is no communication barrier between them.

Now we move to the compartmentalized box on the right, with the changes in control structures that result because of the hypnotic interventions and that follow the suggestion that the hand will feel no pain in the ice water. There has been a split between two cognitions, *Cognition A* and *Cognition B*, with some barriers around portions of them. *Cognition A* actually continues the normal consciousness of pain, but because there

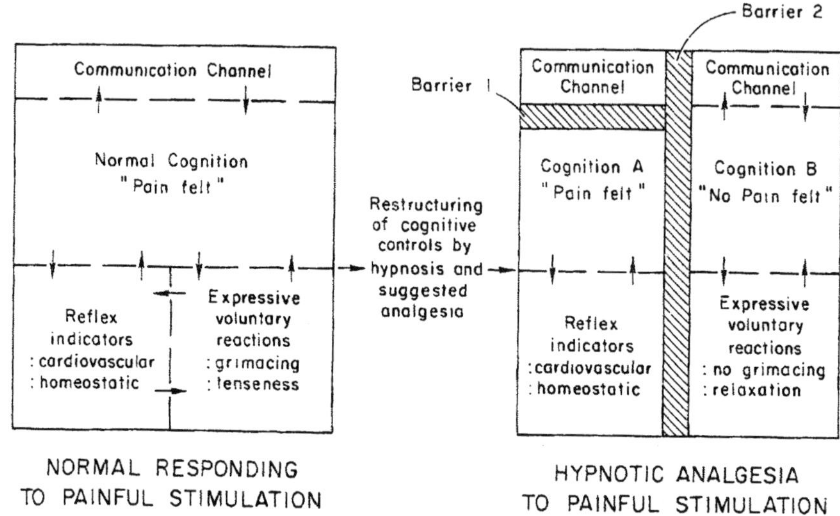

FIG. 1.—Restructuring of cognitive controls in hypnotic analgesia. The left-hand figure represents the normal controls, with all communication channels open. The right-hand figure represents the situation after hypnotic interaction has produced a cognitive restructuring. *Barrier 1* = the inability of the subject to report the pain felt in *Cognition A*. *Barrier 2* = the internal barrier that prevents *Cognition B*, which feels no pain, from knowing that *Cognition A* exists and feels pain. *Barrier 1* can be broken by automatic writing or automatic talking without affecting *Barrier 2*. The figure is reproduced from [23] by permission.

is a barrier to communication (*Barrier 1*) this cognition remains hidden until exposed by automatic writing or automatic talking. *Cognition A* remains in touch with the bodily processes that let it know it is being stressed, though it has lost contol of the voluntary movements that express stress, such as facial grimacing. In the diagram these have been moved to the other side of *Barrier 2*.

Cognition B, reporting no pain, remains open to external communication, but it is unaware that *Cognition A* continues to feel the pain and is out of touch with its own reflex bodily state of stress, although its awareness of the relaxation of voluntary musculature supports its sense of no pain.

Figure 1 is an incomplete diagram of what is happening in other respects and deals only with the immediate control systems affecting the physiological responses to the stressful stimulation that normally causes pain. It shows that one cognitive substructure (*Cognition A*) can still report the pain (but is normally concealed) while another one (*Cognition B*) now seems to be the ordinary waking cognition because its communication channels are open, although it has limited access to what is going on and reports no pain.

The task of constructing a neo-dissociation theory is to give a sensible account of the situation described in figure 1, and, of course, of related phenomena. I am working on such a theory, but additional data will be needed before it can be completed. The eventual theory cannot be a static one, for it must explain how the barriers illustrated are produced, what their nature is, and the conditions under which they become permeable. *Barrier 1,* preventing communication of something known to *Cognition A,* appears to be very much like familiar posthypnotic amnesia, in which an intact memory is unavailable for retrieval. However, it is not like amnesia in two respects. In the first place, the memories now hidden in amnesia were once in awareness, while the felt pain never reached the level of awareness; it is as though the felt pain was sealed in memory even while it was occuring. In the second place, the memory of the pain is less accessible than the memory hidden in posthypnotic amnesia. Hypnotic amnesia, if not relieved by the experimenter, often is relieved spontaneously, but our subjects in hypnotic analgesia experiments, although some of them have been around for years, have never reported to us that they now recall that they were really pained in the experiments in which they were not aware of pain. These, and other questions, are raised by the reference experiment just described.

The neurophysiological explanation of the dissociations sets further problems for theory. Most of the writers on dissociation have offered neurophysiological explanations, but these explanations have usually rested upon a kind of CNS that Skinner is fond of calling the Conceptual Nervous System. It may be that these explanations will have to wait until the phenomenal facts are in better order. We need to know, for example, if the physiological indicators of pain are modified in deeper states than those ordinarily experimented upon in the laboratory, perhaps of the kind reported by Indian yogis after years of practice. Only then can we really know where to look for the crucial junctures where normal neurophysiological controls are being interrupted.

Alternatives to a Dissociation Theory

The decline of classical dissociation theory did not mean that the problems to which the theory addressed itself were altogether neglected. The alternative theory that gained the widest support (and helped to divert interest from dissociation theory) was that of Freud. He and Jung and their associates made household words of unconscious processes, complexes, defenses, repression, and regression. Social psychologists with an objective social communication orientation have had their theories, too, of which Sarbin's role theory has been most directly related to the problems under discussion.

PSYCHOANALYTIC EGO PSYCHOLOGY

The later Freudians, in developing the psychoanalytic ego psychology, have modified the Freudian theory in a manner that corresponds somewhat to my proposal to revise Janet's. In addition to the familiar id, ego, and superego, they speak of various ego substructures (in addition to defenses), including a wide range of "ego-apparatuses" that serve the adjustment of the organization to the environment. They also favor a concept of partial and reversible regression called regression in the service of the ego, a concept that becomes central in the interpretation of hypnotic phenomena. In applying the ego theory to hypnosis, Gill and Brenman [24] considered the regression in hypnotic induction to result in a fractionation of the ego. As the hypnotic state becomes stabilized, the ego is restructured at a slightly primitive (regressed) level, as evidenced by its uncritical thought processes. A regnant ego remains, but somewhat in the background, observing what goes on and introducing some control. It is evident that this conceptualization permits a discussion of the relationships of my figure 1 in these terms.

There is an advantage in the Gill and Brenman theory that hypnosis is assimilated to a worked-out general theory, so that it does not appear to be as ad hoc as are many attempts to explain hypnotic phenomena. This embeddedness in psychoanalytic theory is an advantage for those convinced of the essential truth of psychoanalytic theory, but it is a burden to those who find the theory unclear or unacceptable. My preference at this point is not to argue either for the acceptance or rejection of the more general aspects of the psychoanalytic theory, but to note the relationship to the theory I am proposing of those features bearing on my reference experiment.

There are some conceptual differences between a regressive interpretation of hypnosis (the Gill and Brenman position) and the dissociative interpretation. The differences, schematic and oversimplified, are illustrated in figure 2. For simplicity purposes, the cognitive controls in psychoanalytic theory are represented by a classification into conscious and unconscious parts of the cognitive apparatus. Then the conscious represents chiefly the ego, with its reality orientation and conceptual thinking (secondary process thinking), while the unconscious part represents the id and whatever subsequent material has been repressed, characterized by impulsivity and irrationality (primary process thinking). (For simplicity of exposition I am ignoring the superego, which introduces some moral imperatives into the unconscious region.) Between conscious and unconscious there is some kind of barrier, across which interchanges take place as once-conscious material gets repressed or once-unconscious material produces its derivatives in consciousness. This is an oversimplification of psychoanalytic thinking, but is in essen-

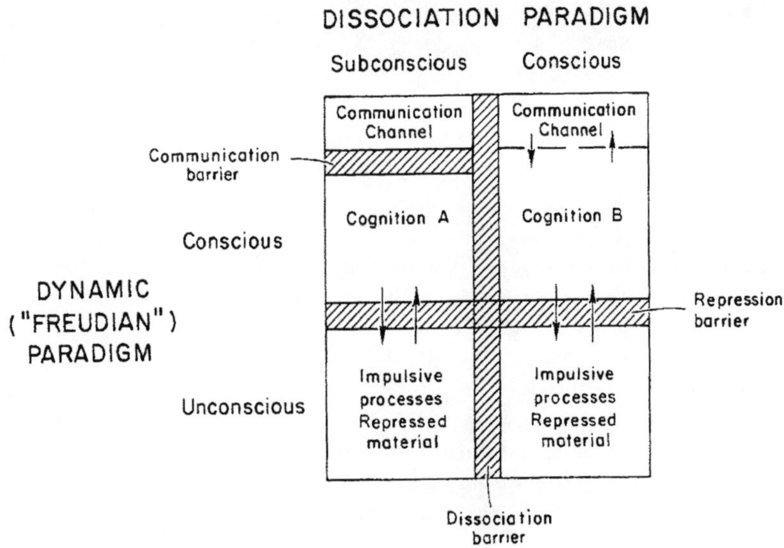

FIG. 2.—Conceptual differences between dissociative and psychoanalytic interpretations. The figure is schematic and simplified in order to indicate the differences between the dissociation barrier and the repression barrier. It is reproduced from [23] by permission.

tial agreement with its teachings. The subconscious and conscious splits that were characterized by my reference experiment are indicated as orthogonal to the psychoanalytic splits. *Cognition A* of figure 2 represents essentially a psychoanalytic normal ego, in touch with reality, with few intrusions of the reality distortions attributed to primary process. The fact that *Cognition A* is normally out of awareness does not fit the regressive concept of psychoanalysis, so that the dissociation barrier is indicated as at right angles to the repression barrier that separates the predominantly secondary process thinking from the (regressive) primary process thinking.

Cognition B of figure 2, the conscious part in the midst of the hypnotic analgesia experiment, is the one showing reality distortion, and it is therefore partly regressed in Gill and Brenman's terms. However, I have not shown it as extending below the repression barrier, because there is no evidence that it has more access to the (Freudian) unconscious than *Cognition A* has. It would be stretching things to say that the wish to feel no pain is an unconscious striving, and the fact that no pain is felt might mean that there is a special unconscious influence upon consciousness. The desire to feel no pain was fully conscious, a wish encouraged by the hypnotist.

Note that my diagram does not deny the Freudian unconscious, but it makes it largely irrelevant to the major splits within cognitive structures that are found in hypnosis. It may be recalled that Gill and Brenman [24] were able to carry out a normal psychoanalysis with the patient always in hypnosis within the analytic hour; dreams under hypnosis may serve as "projective techniques" similar to TAT cards in the waking state, revealing hidden aspects of the personality. Figure 2 permits these interplays between unconscious and conscious (in the Freudian sense) within the dissociative splits.

The main point of my analysis is that the dissociations in hypnotic experiments belong primarily to the conscious cognitive controls and have little to do with the "deeper" unconscious. Psychoanalytic ego psychology allows for this, because within the ego there are "conflict-free" spheres, not motivated by unconscious drives. Hence it is possible for those favoring psychoanalytic ego psychology to agree with my interpretations, without abandoning their own vocabulary. Which theory is ultimately to be preferred will depend on their respective clarities and the precision with which they fit empirical data.

ROLE THEORY

The role theory of Sarbin and Coe [25] is pertinent to the cognitive splits found in experiments revealing dissociation because it is a social communication theory that assumes a person may enact several roles, public and private, either simultaneously or in succession. It therefore provides a set of labels that can be used alternatively to the dissociation label for such divisions as those between *Cognitions A* and *B*. There are clearly many behaviors of the hypnotic subject that can be characterized as role enactments, and there are some correlations between hypnotic susceptibility and dramatic abilities [26].

Sarbin and Coe [25, p. 136] appear to believe that the hypnotically analgesic patient may feel the pain "privately," but because of his relationship to the hypnotist he denies the pain. If one concedes that the "private" experience of pain is so private that even the subject does not know he is feeling it, then dissociation and role theories converge. The role theorist uses a dimension of organismic involvement which, at the extreme, can cause psychic suicide, as in voodoo deaths. Then depth of involvement can be used to support role theory in the cases of genuine hypnotic analgesia.

Psychoanalysis and role theory are not the only alternatives to dissociation theory, but they are the ones that have most prominently discussed the problems as they emerge in hypnosis. Sears showed how a learning theory might be used to meet some of the problems [27]. A speculative model has been offered by Blum [28]. A fuller exposition will have to take these and other proposals into account.

Concluding Statement

I have described the theoretical problems posed by a puzzling experiment involving hypnotically induced analgesia to pain, in which a secondary report of the pain experience was made through automatic writing or automatic talking. This secondary report showed that the pain was being felt even while it was honestly being denied. By using this as a reference experiment, I have tried to show that the control mechanisms involved are not too dissimilar from those that Janet and his followers tried to encompass within his theory of dissociation.

Janet's theory needs to be modernized. Older theories can be learned from, without one becoming either a disciple or an opponent. By showing some differences in the major emphases of the dissociative and the psychoanalytic model, I believe I have succeeded in indicating the direction in which experimentation and theorizing might go.

I have set the groundwork for the theory, rather than developing the theory in this report. The theory is in process of elaboration and later accounts will be devoted to it.

REFERENCES

1. P. Janet. L'automatisme psychologique. Paris: Alcan, 1889.
2. M. Dessoir. Das Doppel-Ich. Leipzig: Günther, 1890.
3. H. F. Ellenberger. The discovery of the unconscious. New York: Basic, 1970.
4. F. W. H. Myers. Proc. Am. Soc. Psychic. Res., **3**:1, 1885.
5. ———. Human personality and its survival of bodily death. 2 vols. New York: Longmans, Green, 1903.
6. W. James. Varieties of religious experience. New York: Longmans, Green, 1902.
7. J. Jacobi. The psychology of C. G. Jung. 7th ed. New Haven, Conn.: Yale Univ. Press, 1968.
8. S. Freud. New introductory lectures on psychoanalysis. New York: Norton, 1933.
9. H. Hartmann. Ego psychology and the problem of adaptation. New York: International Universities Press, 1958.
10. D. Rapaport. *In* M. M. Gill (ed.). The collected papers of David Rapaport. New York: Basic, 1967.
11. M. Prince. J. Abnorm. Psychol., **3**:33, 1909.
12. E. R. Hilgard. *In* M. Henle, J. Jaynes, and J. Sullivan (eds.). Historical conceptions of psychology. New York: Springer, 1973.
13. I. Litvag. Singer in the shadows: the strange case of Patience Worth. New York: Macmillan, 1972.
14. W. James. Proc. Am. Soc. Psychic. Res., **1**:548, 1899.
15. W. A. Cass. An experimental investigation of the dissociation hypothesis, utilizing a posthypnotic technique. Unpublished M.A. thesis, Univ. Oregon, 1942.
16. J. H. Stevenson. The effect of hypnotic and posthypnotic dissociation on the performance of interfering tasks. Unpublished Ph.D. diss., Stanford Univ., 1972.

17. V. J. Knox, L. Crutchfield, and E. R. Hilgard. The nature of task interference in hypnotic dissociation. Paper presented at annual meeting, Soc. Clin. Exp. Hypn., Univ. California, Irvine, November 1973.
18. E. R. Hilgard. Proc. Nat. Acad. Sci. USA, **57,** 1581, 1969.
19. ———. Proc. Am. Philos. Soc., **115,** 470, 1971.
20. R. E. Shor. Int. J. Clin. Exp. Hypn., **10:**183, 1962.
21. G. H. Estabrooks. Hypnotism. Rev. ed. New York: Dutton, 1957.
22. E. A. Kaplan. Arch. Gen. Psychiatry, **2:**567, 1960.
23. E. R. Hilgard. *Psychol. Rev.*, **80,** 396, 1973.
24. M. M. Gill and M. Brenman. Hypnosis and related states: psychoanalytic studies in regression. New York: International Universities Press, 1959.
25. T. R. Sarbin and W. C. Coe. Hypnosis: a social psychological analysis of influence communication. New York: Holt, Rinehart & Winston, 1972.
26. T. R. Sarbin and D. T. Lim. Int. J. Clin. Exp. Hypn., **11:**98, 1963.
27. R. R. Sears. Psychol. Bull., **33:**229, 1936.
28. G. S. Blum. A model of the mind. New York: Wiley, 1961.

FORT GEORGE INLET

A beacon quickened on the eastern bank,
Glistening out its last light at the dawn.
The soft trees undulated overhead
Like restless children racing toward the shore.
Their silhouettes grew fundamental parts,
The great pines laced with limbs became alive,
Like dark green giants rising from the sand,
And marsh grass rustled, whistled with the wind.

A mile to east the mighty breakers rolled,
Rising with the tide upon the jetty rocks,
And breaking up the coral on the beach.
The solemn sun rose orange on the sea,
In momentary coolness like the moon,
And turned the once grey waters flaming red.

Jay Cohen

[9]

Hypnotic Behavior: A Cognitive, Social Psychological Perspective

Nicholas P. Spanos
Carleton University

Abstract

In this paper hypnotic responding is viewed as a contextually supported strategic enactment. According to this formulation, hypnotic behavior does not occur automatically, and like other social behavior it can be usefully described as goal-directed action. However, a central demand of the hypnotic situation is that subjects define their responses as involuntary "happenings" rather than self-initiated actions. The experience of involuntariness does not arise because strategic acts are transformed to automatic ones. Instead, it reflects an interpretation that subjects make about their own behavior. This interpretation, in turn, is fostered and legitimated by various aspects of the hypnotic situation; most importantly, by the wording of test suggestions. Thus, one important component of "becoming hypnotized" involves enacting situationally guided, goal-directed behaviors while interpreting these actions as involuntary happenings. Other components include heightened responsiveness following hypnotic versus nonhypnotic procedures, and, more recently, evidence of possessing a "hidden observer." Like experienced involuntariness, these other components can also be considered strategic enactments rather than the automatic results of hypnotic procedures.

Hypnosis has been traditionally conceptualized as an event that happens to people rather than as an enactment that people carry out. In this respect, hypnotic behavior has been viewed as differing fundamentally from everyday social behavior (Coe & Sarbin, 1977; Spanos, in press). Everyday behavior is typically described with adjectives like purposeful, goal-directed and voluntary. The actor is conceptualized, both by others and by himself, as one who initiates and moderates behavior in order to achieve a goal. On the other hand, responsive hypnotic subjects frequently describe their behavior as occurring effortlessly and involuntarily. Many investigators have taken subjects at their word and have posited a wide variety of hypothetical psychological and physiological processes to explain the "hypnotized" persons purported transformation from an "active doer" to a passive observer of his own automatically occurring behavior (e.g., Hilgard, 1979).

VOL. 7, NO. 2
1982

Research Communications in
Psychology, Psychiatry and Behavior

Social psychological formulations hold that the positing of special processes to account for hypnotic behavior is not only unnecessary, but also misleading. According to this perspective, hypnotic behavior is basically similar to other social behavior and, like other social behavior, can be usefully described as strategic and goal-directed (Barber, 1969; Coe & Sarbin, 1977; Spanos, in press). Responsive hypnotic subjects are conceptualized as sentient individuals who are aware of subtle variations in social context and motivated to define themselves in a manner consistent with their conceptions of what constitutes "being hypnotized" (Orne, 1959; Spanos, in press). Social psychological formulations acknowledge that subjects often define their hypnotic responses as occurring involuntarily (Spanos, Rivers, & Ross, 1977). According to these formulations, however, the experience of involuntariness is not a quality intrinsic to these responses. It does not result from special psychological processes that transform strategic acts into automatic ones. Instead, the experience of involuntariness reflects an interpretation made by subjects about their own behavior. Although the behaviors typically associated with hypnosis are strategic, hypnotic subjects often _interpret_ them as involuntary happenings rather than self-initiated actions (Spanos et al., 1977). In short, "becoming hypnotized" is a strategic enactment rather than a happening. A central component of this enactment, however, involves subjects coming to define their behaviors as happenings rather than actions.

Interpreting behavior as an action involves attributing causality to the self (e.g., I did it), while interpreting it as a happening requires that causality be attributed to sources other than the self (e.g., it happened to me). The first part of this paper examines structural factors in the hypnotic situation that determine subjects' attributions of nonvolition to their suggested behavior. Particular attention is given to the role of test suggestions in generating and legitimating such attributions.

Hypnotic enactments are, of course, multifaceted. Attributions of nonvolition are only one component, and test suggestions are only one of the sources of information that define the characteristics of the hypnotic role. For instance, hypnotic procedures often convey implicit expectations that heightened levels of responding are to follow an induction procedure. Moreover, hypnotic procedures have traditionally been credited with providing

VOL. 7, NO. 2
1982

Research Communications in
Psychology, Psychiatry and Behavior

access to unconscious or "hidden" facets of personality and mental functioning. The second part of the paper will briefly examine aspects of the hypnotic situation that communicate such expectations and that legitimate their translation into role validating enactments.

Hypnosis and Experienced Nonvolition

The hypnotic situation, particularly in experimental contexts, usually consists of two components, a hypnotic induction procedure and a series of test suggestions. From a social psychological perspective, hypnotic inductions are viewed as culturally meaningful rituals that define the situation as hypnosis and reinforce that definition by unfolding in a manner consistent with most subjects' conceptions of what hypnosis involves (e.g., instructions for relaxation and sleep, deepening instructions; Barber & DeMoor, 1972; Spanos, in press). Although inductions frequently begin with direct instructions (e.g., <u>relax</u> the muscles in your legs), these are gradually transformed to passively worded suggestions (e.g., your legs <u>feel</u> limp and heavy). In short, hypnotic inductions reinforce the general expectation that hypnosis involves a transformation of the subject from one who initiates actions to one who passively experiences automatic "happenings." More specific information concerning the nature of expected enactments is provided by the structure of test suggestions.

Responsiveness to test suggestions constitutes the major dependent variable in hypnosis research and is the criterion usually employed to determine the individual's "susceptibility to hypnotic influence" (Hilgard, 1965). It is surprising, therefore, that relatively little empirical work has focused on the structure of test suggestions and the effects of this structure on subjects' performance.

The Structure of Test Suggestions

The test suggestions used in hypnotic settings do not explicitly direct subjects to carry out overt behaviors. Instead, they invite them to adopt and temporarily treat as veridical a hypothetical (i.e., imaginary) definition of the situation. Thus, suggests invite subjects to temporarily convince themselves as well as the hypnotist that their arm is heavy, that they are unable to stand up from their chair, that they are unable to recall well-learned material, and so on. In short, suggestions implicitly ask subjects to temporarily suspend the tacit rules usually employed for differentiating imagined events from "real" situations and to define the ongoing situation in terms of the imaginary events they describe (Sarbin & Coe, 1972; Shor, 1970;

VOL. 7, NO. 2
1982

Research Communications in
Psychology, Psychiatry and Behavior

Spanos, 1971). The "moving hands" suggestion from the Stanford Hypnotic Susceptibility Scale, Form A (Weitzenhoffer & Hilgard, 1959) provides a typical example:

> Now I want you to imagine a force attracting your hands toward each other, pulling them together. As you think of this force pulling your hands together, they will move together...closer and closer together as though a force were acting on them...(pgs. 21-22).

This suggestion can be analysed in terms of two interrelated requests; a veiled request to move the arms and a more direct request to define this movement as occurring involuntarily (i.e., as a result of the imagined force). Thus, subjects are tacitly requested to both enact a response, and to disavow responsibility for the enactment. In short, to define the enactment as a "happening" rather than as an "action."

Subjects can respond to such a suggestion in at least three different ways. First, they may respond to neither of the requests and thereby fail the suggestion. This may occur either because they choose not to cooperate with the suggestion, or, because they miss the import of the veiled request. the latter case is exemplified by subjects who simply wait passively for their arms to "move together themselves." These subjects may be quite willing to cooperate, but have failed to understand that they must, in fact, initiate the arm movements that are to be defined as <u>not</u> self-initiated (i.e., involuntary).

A second pattern involves responding to the implicit request while deemphasizing the request for involuntariness; i.e., responding overtly in terms of the suggestion while defining the response as occurring voluntarily. This pattern of response is by no means uncommon. For example, Spanos et al. (1977) found that almost half of the subjects who responded to an arm rigidity suggestion defined their response as primarily a voluntary action. A third pattern involves responding to both requests and constitutes what most investigators mean by "genuine" hypnotic responding. Subjects enact the approiate overt response and define that response as an involuntary occurrence.

<u>Manipulations of suggestion structure</u>. Several studies (Spanos, 1971; Spanos & Barber, 1972; Spanos & Gorassini, 1981; Weitzenhoffer, 1974) have highlighted the role of suggestion structure in determining subjects' construal of their responses as an involuntary occurrence. For example, Spanos and

VOL. 7, NO. 2
1982

Research Communications in
Psychology, Psychiatry and Behavior

Gorassini (1981) administered suggestions for arm lowering, arms moving apart, and arm rising under one condition and direct instructions for the same behaviors under another condition. The instructions and suggestions were equal in length, but differed in terms of defining the target behavior either as an action (e.g., raise your arm) or as a happening (e.g., your arm is rising). Subjects were more likely to rate their overt responses as occurring involuntarily under the suggestion condition than under the instruction condition. Similar findings for suggested motor responses were obtained by Spanos and Barber (1972) and Weitzenhoffer (1974) and for suggested amnesia by Ham, Radtke, and Spanos (1981). In the latter study, half of the subjects were instructed to forget a previously learned word list by actively distracting themselves. The remaining half were informed that the words would go away as their attention passively shifted elswhere. Amnesics who had been given the passive suggestion rated their forgetting as significantly more involuntary than those given the active suggestion. In short, one important determinant of the attribution of involuntariness associated with hypnotic responding is the wording of test suggestions. These suggestions define the situation as one in which involuntary responding is required and thereby set subjects to interpret their overt behaviors as happenings rather than actions (Spanos et al., 1977).

The process of responding to suggestions often exposes subjects to information that either facilitates or contradicts the effects that the suggestion is designed to engender. For example, subjects given either an arm lightness or an arm heaviness suggestion usually hold an arm outstretched for several seconds while the suggestion is administered. During this period the arm is acted upon by gravity and, therefore, tends to feel heavy. Such feedback from an outstretched arm should make it particularly easy for subjects given an arm heaviness suggestion to define their arm lowering as occurring involuntarily. On the other hand, the same feedback should make an attribution of involuntariness particularly difficult in the case of an arm-lightness suggestion. If subjects are to experience their arm as lighter and define it as rising involuntarily, they must somehow ignore or reinterpret the contradictory feedback. Data obtained by Spanos and Gorassini (1981) were consistent with these ideas. Suggested responses that were congruent with naturally occurring feedback were defined as occurring more involuntarily than responses that contradicted such feedback.

VOL. 7, NO. 2
1982

Research Communications in
Psychology, Psychiatry and Behavior

Cognitive strategies and experienced involuntariness. Some test suggestions provide subjects with an imaginal strategy to aid them in defining their responses as involuntary occurrences. For instance, an arm lightness suggestion might instruct subjects to imagine a large helium balloon lifting their arm (Spanos & Barber, 1972), while an arm heaviness suggestion might ask them to imagine holding a billiard ball (Weitzenhoffer & Hilgard, 1959). Strategies of this kind that invite subjects to covertly construct an imaginary situation that is congruent with the involuntary occurrence of the suggested behavior have been labeled goal-directed fantasies (GDF's; Spanos, 1971). A number of studies have compared the efficacy of suggestions that do and do not contain GDF's. The results, however, have been inconsistent. Several studies (Coe, Allan, Krug, & Wurtzman, 1974; Spanos, 1971; Spanos, Spillane, & McPeake, 1976) have reported enhanced responding to GDF suggestions, while others (Buckner & Coe, 1977; Spanos & McPeake, 1977) found no enhancement. Although there are probably several reasons for these inconsistencies (see Spanos et al., 1977), one of the most important stems from the weak relationship between what subjects are asked to imagine and what they actually imagine. Post-experimental inquiries indicate that many subjects given GDF suggestions fail to carry out such fantasies. Moreover, subjects who have not been provided with a GDF sometimes spontaneously devise goal-directed fantasies of their own (Spanos & McPeake, 1977). Studies that postexperimentally assessed the strategies actually carried out, as well as those provided by the suggestions, have consistently found a relationship between reported goal-directed fantasy and degree of rated involuntariness. When given identical suggestions, subjects who reported goal-directed fantasy were more likely than those who did not to define their overt responses as occurring involuntarily (Spanos et al., 1976; Spanos & McPeake, 1977; Spanos et al., 1977).

It is important to emphasize that imaginal strategies are not conceptualized here as causing subjects' overt responses to suggestion. However, given that subjects enact the overt behavior tacitly requested by a suggestion their simultaneous generation of goal-directed fantasy may be a factor that aids them to interpret their behavior as an involuntary occurrence (Spanos et al., 1977).

Absorption in imaginings. Several studies have assessed the degree to which subjects become absorbed in imaginal strategies while responding

VOL. 7, NO. 2
1982

Research Communications in
Psychology, Psychiatry and Behavior

to suggestions (Spanos & McPeake, 1974; Spanos et al., 1977). The notion of absorption in imaginings refers to the degree of sustained attention that individuals invest in the imaginative process. While highly absorbed, individuals do not simultaneously attend to information that contradicts the status of their imaginings as "real" events (Spanos & Barber, 1974; Tellegen & Atkinson, 1974). For example, when given a suggestion that their arm is held in a cast, individuals who become highly absorbed in fostering that definition of the situation might be likely to imagine details of the cast, the sensations it would generate, and a context that would legitimate wearing a cast (e.g., a hospital emergency room). These individuals would be unlikely to simultaneously tell themselves that a real cast was not on their arm, that they were only imagining, or that there had been no cast on their arm when the experiment began (Spanos, 1971; Spanos et al., 1977). In several studies ratings of absorption in suggestion-related imaginings have correlated positively with the degree of involuntariness attributed to overt responding and the extent that the imagined events were experienced as "really happening" (Spanos & McPeake, 1974; Spanos et al., 1977; Spanos & Stam, 1979).

Thus far we have focused on individual test suggestions and have argued that responsiveness to such suggestions involves a willingness to temporarily adopt and act in accordance with the definition of the situation proffered by the suggestions. Hypnotic susceptibility simply refers to the number of standardized test suggestions out of a series that subjects enact during a hypnotic session. Therefore, it is not surprising to find that questionnaire measures of subjects' overall attitudes toward hypnosis, their willingness to cooperate with hypnotic procedures, and their expectations of becoming hypnotized correlate positively with hypnotic susceptibility (see reviews by Barber, Spanos, & Chaves, 1974; Spanos, in press). Interestingly, susceptibility also correlates with self-report measures that index a general tendency to become absorbed in a wide variety of imaginative activities outside of the hypnotic setting (Hilgard, 1974; Spanos & McPeake, 1975; Tellegen & Atkinson, 1974).

Taken together, these results indicate that subjects who score high on questionnaire measures of absorption in nonhypnotic imaginative activities are particularly proficient at engaging in the kind of fantasy activity encouraged by most suggestions. Therefore, given that they are willing to cooperate with the hypnotic procedures, they are particularly likely to

VOL. 7, NO. 2
1982

Research Communications in
Psychology, Psychiatry and Behavior

generate imaginings that enable them to experience suggested effects. This account, however, is incomplete. Questionnaire measures of cooperativeness and absorption in nonhypnotic imaginings, even in combination, account for only a moderate proportion of the variance in hypnotic susceptibility scores (e.g., Spanos & McPeake, 1975). One reason for the relatively low predictive abilities of these questionnaires may stem from the ambiguity that characterizes most test suggestions. For instance, a typical suggestion for arm rigidity informs subjects that their arm is stiff and will not bend until the experimenter cancels the stiffness. Before presentation of the cancellation cue, subjects are challenged to try to bend their arm. This suggestion contains at least two elements of ambiguity. First, it may be unclear to subjects whether they are required to participate in stiffening their arm, or whether they are to do nothing and simply wait for the suggested effect to happen. Second, the meaning of the challenge to try to bend their arm may be unclear to subjects. For instance, are they to stop whatever they might be doing to define their arm as unable to bend and, instead, simply bend it? Are they to try to bend it while simultaneously attempting to define it as stiff? Or are they to simply ignore the challenge altogether and focus on defining it as unable to bend?

These considerations indicate that the definition of the situation provided by test suggestions is a complex matter. Subjects may not adopt a definition of the situation that enables them to pass such suggestions for a number of reasons. For instance, some may be willing to "give the suggestions a try" while simultaneously focusing on such thoughts as "no suggestion can make me see what isn't really there" (Spanos et al., 1977). Some may not possess the imaginal abilities that facilitate defining hypothetical situations as "really" happening, and others may possess such abilities but fail to exercise them consistently because they interpret suggested effects as having to happen automatically or interpret challenges as requests to stop engaging in suggestion-related imaginings. Recent work dealing with the structure of amnesia suggestions (reviewed by Spanos & Radtke in press) indicate that preliminary information aimed at clarifying the ambiguities in test suggestions can produce large effects on subjects' responsiveness. Nevertheless, more work exploring the relationships among subjects' interpretations of specific test suggestions and their general levels of cooperativeness and absorptive ability remains to be done in order to accurately

VOL. 7, NO. 2
1982

Research Communications in
Psychology, Psychiatry and Behavior

predict hypnotic susceptibility.

Nonsuggested Communications and Expectations

The discussion thus far has focused on communications transmitted by the structure of test suggestions. However, information about hypnotic role enactments is also transmitted by other means. For instance, in a lecture about hypnosis Orne (1959) informed one group of students that arm catalepsy occurred spontaneously during the induction of hypnosis. Control subjects heard a similar lecture but were told nothing about arm catalepsy. Later, subjects from both groups were administered hypnotic procedures by someone other than the lecturer. Some of the experimental subjects, but none of the controls, exhibited "spontaneous" arm catalepsy. In short, subjects geared their hypnotic enactments in terms of their preconceptions even when the specific behavior enacted was not called for by the hypnotic test situation.

Earlier, hypnotic inductions were described as cultural rituals. According to this perspective, these procedures do not contain intrinsic qualities that in some automatic way facilitate responsiveness to suggestions. Nevertheless, by defining the situation as hypnosis they convey information about the level of performance expected. These considerations are illustrated by studies (reviewed by Spanos & Radtke, in press) that compared how hypnotic and motivated control subjects rated the intensity of their visual imagery. When these studies assigned different subjects to hypnotic and control treatments, they invariably found that the two groups rated their imagery in equivalent fashion. However, in studies where the same subjects rated their imagery under both a hypnotic and a nonhypnotic condition, imagery was usually rated as more intense under the hypnotic condition. These findings indicate that hypnotic procedures convey the expectation that hypnotic performance should be enhanced relative to nonhypnotic performance. In studies that assigned different subjects to hypnotic and nonhypnotic groups, the hypnotic subjects had no objective baseline against which to measure an improvement, and, as a result, they performed in the same manner as controls. However, when the same subjects were tested under both conditions they employed their own nonhypnotic performance as a yardstick against which to demonstrate the enhanced performance implied by the definition of the situation as hypnosis. These studies, of course, provide no support for the proposition that hypnotic procedures enhance the intensity of visual imagery. They do, however, indicate

VOL. 7, NO. 2
1982

Research Communications in
Psychology, Psychiatry and Behavior

that hypnotic subjects are attuned to implicit contextual demands and moderate their enactments strategically in order to meet those demands.

Similar findings have been reported in recent research on hypnotic analgesia. Moreover, this research highlights the differences in theoretical approach that characterize traditional and social-psychological accounts of hypnotic phenomena.

Expectations and hypnotic analgesia. As was the case with imagery research, equivalent degrees of suggested analgesia in hypnotic and non-hypnotic subjects have been found consistently in studies that assigned different subjects to these two treatments. On the other hand, studies that assigned the same subjects to both hypnotic and waking analgesia treatments have just as consistently found greater reductions in reported pain with hypnosis (see review by Spanos, Radtke-Bodorik, Ferguson, & Jones, 1979). Hilgard (1979) has interpreted the results of these "same-subjects" experiments to mean that hypnotic analgesia is intrinsically more effective than waking analgesia. In fact, he has argued that hypnotic analgesia, unlike waking analgesia, involves a dissociation of pain from conscious awareness. Purportedly, the hypnotically analgesic subject continues to experience pain at an unconscious level. However, this unconscious pain is "hidden" from awareness by an "amnesic barrier." Nonhypnotic subjects achieve some analgesia by using conscious strategies like self-distraction. However, because these subjects do not undergo dissociation they supposedly do not experience the more profound pain reductions that characterize hypnotic analgesia.

Hilgard's (1979) dissociation hypothesis cannot account for the equivalent reductions in reported pain found in studies that assigned different subjects to hypnotic and nonhypnotic conditions. On the other hand, the superiority of hypnotic to waking analgesia found in "same-subjects" studies can be accounted for parsimoniously, and without recourse to the notion of dissociation, when due consideration is given to the strategic nature of hypnotic responding.

As mentioned above, individuals who obtain high scores on tests of hypnotic susceptibility have a strong investment in presenting themselves in the experimental setting as good hypnotic subjects (Spanos, in press). When these individuals are tested under both waking and hypnotic analgesia conditions, they are aware that the two treatments are being compared, and therefore they become invested in demonstrating the superiority of the

VOL. 7, NO. 2
1982

Research Communications in
Psychology, Psychiatry and Behavior

hypnotic treatment. Stam and Spanos (1980) obtained support for this hypothesis in a study that dealt with cold pressor pain (i.e., pain produced by limb immersion in ice water). All of their subjects had previously obtained high scores on hypnotic susceptibility, and all received three cold pressor trials. However, the order in which treatments were administered differed between groups. In some groups subjects underwent waking analgesia while believing that they could be later tested with hypnosis. In other groups they received waking analgesia with no expectation of hypnosis.

When subjects were tested under waking analgesia while expecting hypnotic analgesia to follow, they reported greater pain reduction in the hypnotic than in the waking condition. However, if they were tested under waking analgesia, with no expectation for subsequent hypnosis, reported pain reductions were equally large in hypnotic and waking analgesia conditions. In other words, subjects performed less than optimally under waking analgesia in order to "leave room" for optimal performance under hypnosis. These findings belie the notion of an intrinsic superiority for hypnotic as compared to waking analgesia, and once again, underscore the strategic nature of hypnotic responding. Subjects in the Stam and Spanos experiment were obviously motivated to present themselves in the experimental setting as hypnotized. Implicit in this self-definition is the expectation that hypnotic performance transcends waking performance. Therefore, when subjects knew that their performance under both conditions would be compared, they reduced their responsiveness under the waking condition in order to legitimize their later self-presentation as hypnotized.

Experimental instructions and the "hidden observer." In traditional accounts, hypnotic inductions and other instructions administered within the hypnotic setting are often seen as providing a context that allows the intrinsic qualities of hypnotic phenomena to become manifest. Therefore, when unusual behavior occurs in this setting it tends to be attributed to the essential nature of hypnosis rather than to subjects' interpretations of the communications they receive. Hilgard's (1979) theoretical account of the "hidden observer" experiments carried out in his laboratory serves as an example of traditional thinking in this area. Hilgard (1979) contents that during hypnotic analgesia intense pain continues to be felt unconsciously, but remains hidden from consciousness behind an amnesic barrier. He further contents that the experimenter can communicate with this "hidden part" of the

VOL. 7, NO. 2
1982

Research Communications in
Psychology, Psychiatry and Behavior

person and obtain estimates of pain intensity from "it" (i.e., hidden pain estimates). At the same time, the hypnotically analgesic person can estimate the degree of pain that he/she consciously feels (i.e., overt pain estimates).

In a typical hidden observer experiment (see reviews by Hilgard, 1979 and Spanos & Hewitt, 1980) subjects who previously scored high on hypnotic susceptibility estimate their pain intensity during a baseline cold pressor trial. Later they are administered a hypnotic induction and informed that a hidden part of them is aware of experiences that their hypnotized part is unaware of. These instructions are quite explicit and clearly convey the expectations that (a) subjects are to define themselves as having both a conscious and a dissociated part and (b) during hypnotic analgesia the conscious part is to feel and report little pain while the dissociated part feels and reports intense pain. Subjects in hidden observer experiments have frequently behaved in terms of these communications. During cold pressor trials under hypnotic analgesia they reported low levels of overt pain (i.e., from their analgesic part) and high levels of hidden pain.

Hilgard (1979) interprets reports of hidden pain as reflecting the intrinsic characteristics of a dissociated level of consciousness. He views the explicit "hidden observer" instructions employed in his experiments as creating a setting in which these intrinsic characteristics can come to light. He does not view them as communications that teach subjects to behave as though they had hidden parts.

In contrast to Hilgard, Spanos and Hewitt (1980) argued that hidden reports were part of a strategic role enactment engendered and shaped by the communications transmitted in hidden observer experiments. To test this hypothesis they divided highly responsive hypnotic subjects into two groups. Subjects in both groups were informed that they possessed a hidden part. Instructions given to one group (modeled after those used in Hilgard's studies) implied that subjects' hidden parts would feel more pain than their analgesic parts. However, those in the second group received instructions implying that their hidden part would feel even less pain that their analgesic part. Subjects in the two groups behaved as though they had hidden observers with opposite characteristics; high sensitivity to pain in one case, greatly reduced sensitivity to pain in the other. These findings clearly indicate that the instructions employed in hidden observer experiments do something quite different from simply "setting the stage" for the emergence of preexisting

VOL. 7, NO. 2
1982

Research Communications in
Psychology, Psychiatry and Behavior

dissociated mental events. They provide willing subjects with information that enables them to enact a "dissociated subject role;" a role in which they are encouraged to construe and describe their experiences in terms of dissociated parts that have well defined characteristics.

Overview

In 1941 White advanced two reasons for thinking that hypnotic behavior reflected an altered state of consciousness. First, "hypnotized" subjects could purportedly carry out behaviors that transcended normal volitional capacities. Second, the suggested responses of these subjects were experienced as nonvolitional occurrences. A great deal of research conducted since the publication of White's (1941) article contradicts his first proposition; there is no convincing evidence that hypnotic procedures enable subjects to carry out "transcendent feats" (see review by Barber, 1972). Moreover, modern social-psychological formulations indicate that the attribution of nonvolition that characterizes hypnotic responding can also be understood without recourse to notions like "hypnotic state" or "automatic dissociation." These formulations suggest that hypnotic responding can be usefully conceptualized as strategic social enactment. Like other social enactments, the form taken by hypnotic enactments is dependent upon the actor's preconceptions, motivations and abilities, as well as the contextual demands that guide and legitimate both his/her behavior and his/her interpretation of that behavior.

References

Barber, T.X. Hypnosis: A scientific approach. Princeton, N.J.: Van Nostrand-Reinhold, 1969.

Barber, T.X. Suggested ("hypnotic") behavior: The trance paradigm versus an alternative paradigm. In E. Fromm & R.E. Shor (Eds.) _Hypnosis: Research developments and perspectives_. Chicago: Aldine-Atherton, 1972, 115-182.

Barber, T.X., & DeMoor, W. A theory of hypnotic induction procedures. _Amer. J. of Clin. Hyp._, 1972, _15_, 112-135.

Barber, T.S., Spanos, N.P., & Chaves, J.F. _Hypnosis, imagination and human potentialities_. New York: Pergamon, 1974.

Buckner, L.G., & Coe, W.C. Imaginative skill, wording of suggestions and hypnotic susceptibility. _Inter. J. Clin. Exper. Hyp._, 1977, _25_, 27-36.

Coe, W.C., Allan, J.L., Krug, W.M., & Wurzman, A.G. Goal-directed fantasy in hypnotic responsiveness: Skill item, wording, or both? _Inter. J. Clin. Exper. Hyp._, 1974, _22_, 157-166.

VOL. 7, NO. 2
1982

Research Communications in
Psychology, Psychiatry and Behavior

Coe, W.C., & Sarbin, T.R. Hypnosis from the standpoint of a contextualist. Annals of the New York Academy of Sciences, 1977, 296, 2-13.

Ham, M.L., Radtke, H.L., & Spanos, N.P. The effects of suggestion type and the experience of involuntariness on the breaching of hypnotic amnesia. Unpublished Manuscript, Department of Psychology, Carleton University.

Hilgard, E.R. Hypnotic susceptibility. New York: Harcourt, 1965.

Hilgard, E.R. Divided consciousness in hypnosis: The implications of the hidden observer. In E. Fromm & R.E. Shor (Eds.) Hypnosis: Developments in research and new perspectives, 2nd ed. New York: Aldine, 1979, 45-79.

Hilgard, E.R. Imaginative involvement: Some characteristics of the highly hypnotizable and the non-hypnotizable. Inter. J. Clin. Exper. Hyp., 1974, 22, 138-156.

Orne, M.T. The nature of hypnosis: Artifact and essence. J. Ab. Soc. Psych. 1959, 58, 277-299.

Sarbin, T.R., & Coe, W.C. Hypnotic behavior: The psychology of influence communication. New York: Holt, 1972.

Shor, R.E. The three factor theory of hypnosis as applied to the book reading fantasy. Inter. J. Clin. Exper. Hyp., 1970, 18, 89-98.

Spanos, N.P. A social-psychological approach to hypnotic behavior. In G. Weary & H.L. Mirels (Eds.). Integrations of clinical and social psychology. New York: Oxford, in press.

Spanos, N.P. Goal-directed fantasy and the performance of hypnotic test suggestions. Psychiatry, 1971, 34, 86-96.

Spanos, N.P., & Barber, T.X. Cognitive activity during hypnotic suggestion: Goal-directed fantasy and the experience of non-volition. J. Pers., 1972, 40, 510-524.

Spanos, N.P., & Barber, T.X. Toward a convergence in hypnosis research. Amer. Psycho., 1974, 29, 500-511.

Spanos, N.P., & Gorassini, D. Suggestion structure and the experience of non-volition. Unpublished manuscript, Depart. Psychol., Carleton University.

Spanos, N.P., & McPeake, J.D. Involvement in suggestion-related imaginings, experienced involuntariness, and credibility assigned to imaginings in hypnotic subjects. J. Ab. Psychol., 1974, 83, 687-690.

Spanos, N.P., & McPeake, J.D. Involvement in everyday imaginative activities, attitudes toward hypnosis and hypnotic suggestibility. J. Person. Soc. Psychol. 1975, 31, 584-598.

Spanos, N.P., & McPeake, J.D. Cognitive strategies, reported goal-directed fantasy, and response to suggestion in hypnotic subjects. Am. J. Clin. Hyp., 1977, 114-123.

VOL. 7, NO. 2
1982

Research Communications in
Psychology, Psychiatry and Behavior

Spanos, N.P., & Hewitt, E.C. The hidden observer in hypnotic analgesia: Discovery or experimental creation? J. Person. Soc. Psychol., 1980, 39, 1201-1214.

Spanos, N.P., & Radtke, H.L. Hypnotic visual hallucinations as imaginings: A cognitive social psychological perspective. Imag. Cog. Pers., in press.

Spanos, N.P., & Radtle, H.L. Hypnotic amnesia as strategic enactment: A cognitive social psychological perspective. This Volume.

Spanos, N.P., Rivers, S.M., & Ross, S. Experienced involuntariness and response to hypnotic suggestions. Ann. N. Y. Acad. Scien., 1977, 296, 208-221.

Spanos, N.P., Radtke-Bodorik, H.L., Ferguson, J., & Jones, B. The effects of hypnotic susceptibility, suggestions for analgesia and the utilization of cognitive strategies on the reduction of pain. Journal of Abnormal Psychology, 1979, 88, 282-292.

Spanos, N.P., Spillane, J., & McPeake, J.D. Cognitive strategies and response to suggestion in hypnotic and task-motivated subjects. American Journal of Clinical Hypnosis, 1976, 18, 252-262.

Spanos, N.P., & Stam, H.J. The elicitation of visual hallucinations via brief instructions in a normal sample. Journal of Nervous and Mental Disease, 1979, 167, 488-494.

Stam, H.J., & Spanos, N.P. Experimental designs, expectancy effects and hypnotic analgesia. Journal of Abnormal Psychology, 1980, 89, 751-762.

Tellegen, A., & Atkinson, G. Openness to absorbing and self-altering experiences ("absorption"), a trait related to hypnotic susceptibility. Journal of Abnormal Psychology, 1974, 83, 268-277.

Weitzenhoffer, A.M. When is an "instruction" an "instruction"? International Journal of Clinical and Experimental Hypnosis, 1974, 22, 258-269.

Weitzenhoffer, A.M., & Hilgard, E.R. Stanford Hypnotic Susceptibility Scale, Forms A and B. Palo Alto, Calif.: Consulting Psychologists Press, 1959.

White, R.W. A preface to a theory of hypnotism. Journal of Abnormal and Social Psychology, 1941, 36, 477-505.

[10]

Response Expectancy as a Determinant of Experience and Behavior

Irving Kirsch *University of Connecticut*

ABSTRACT: Response expectancies, defined as expectancies of the occurrence of nonvolitional responses, have generally been ignored in theories of learning. Research on placebos, hypnosis, and fear reduction indicates that response expectancies generate corresponding subjective experiences. In many cases, the genuineness of these self-reported effects has been substantiated by corresponding changes in behavior and physiological function. The means by which response expectancies affect experience, physiology, and behavior are hypothesized to vary as a function of response mode. The generation of changes in subjective experience by corresponding response expectancies is hypothesized to be a basic psychological mechanism. Physiological effects are accounted for by the mind–body identity assumption that is common to all nondualist philosophies of psychology. The effects of response expectancies on volitional behavior are due to the reinforcing properties of many nonvolitional responses. Classical conditioning appears to be one method by which response expectancies are acquired, but response expectancy effects that are inconsistent with a conditioning hypothesis are also documented.

Expectancy is a central construct in a number of influential theories of learning (Bolles, 1972; Rotter, 1954; Tolman, 1932). Bolles (1972) classified expectancy constructs into two types. *R–S* expectancies are beliefs about the relation between behavior and environmental consequences. *S–S* expectancies are beliefs that certain stimulus events or cues predict the occurrence of other stimulus events. The purpose of this article is to draw attention to a type of expectancy that has demonstrable effects on experience, behavior, and physiological function but that has not been considered in previous learning theories. *Response expectancies* are expectancies of the occurrence of nonvolitional responses, either as a function of behavior (R–R expectancies) or as a function of specific stimuli (S–R expectancies). In Rotter's (1954) social learning theory, the occurrence of a response is hypothesized to be a function of the expectancy that the behavior will be reinforced and of the value of the expected reinforcement. However, Rotter's theory is limited to the prediction of voluntary behavior. The response expectancy hypothesis described in this article extends social learning theory in two ways. It defines a construct that predicts the occurrence of nonvolitional responses, and it considers the effect of nonvolitional response expectancies on voluntary behavior.

Nonvolitional responses are responses that are experienced as occurring automatically, that is, without volitional effort (cf. Beck, 1976). They include emotional reactions (e.g., fear, sadness, elation), sexual arousal, conversion symptoms, pain, and so forth. Because nonvolitional responses have positive and negative reinforcement value, expectancies of their occurrence affect the probability that a person will engage in particular voluntary behaviors. For example, agoraphobics avoid a wide variety of situations because of their expectancy that entering those situations will result in the occurrence of panic attacks (Goldstein & Chambless, 1978). In addition, a considerable body of data indicates that nonvolitional responses are elicited and/or enhanced by the expectancy of their occurrence. These data are drawn from three areas of investigation: placebo effects, fear reduction, and hypnosis.

Placebo Effects

Placebos are substances that are administered in the guise of active drugs but that do not in fact have the pharmacological properties attributed to them. Placebos can reduce clinical pain, increase arousal to erotic stimuli, reduce generalized anxiety and depression, cause or reduce feelings of nausea, and induce feelings of alertness, tension, relaxation, or drowsiness. These subjective responses are frequently accompanied by corresponding physiological changes, for example, changes in pulse rate, blood pressure, galvanic skin response, gastric function, penile tumescence, skin conditions, and possibly endorphin activity in the brain (Barber, 1978; Marlatt & Rohsenow, 1980; Ross & Olson, 1982; Ross & Buckalew, 1983).

Placebo effects generally correspond to people's knowledge or beliefs about the kind of drug they believe they are receiving, and for that reason, a causal relation between expectancy and placebo reaction has generally been assumed. However, classical conditioning has been proposed as an alternative to the idea that placebo effects are due to expectancies (Gliedman, Gantt, & Teitelbaum, 1957; Herrnstein, 1962; Knowles, 1963; Wickramasekera, 1980). According to these formulations, administrations of active treatment constitute conditioning trials, during which treatment effects are associated with a variety of concurrent and antecedent stimuli including the pill, capsule, or syringe in which the medication was administered. Rather than being viewed as an alternative to expectancy, classical conditioning can be understood as one method by which expectancies are formed (Bolles, 1972; Reiss, 1980). However, if the data on placebo effects could be accounted for solely in terms of conditioning, then the concept of response expectancy would be redundant. Therefore, the data reviewed in this section are evaluated with respect to three questions: (a) Do classical conditioning trials contribute to the elicitation of placebo responses? (b) Are there placebo responses that cannot be accounted for in terms of conditioning? (c) What are the effects of expectancies of responses that are the opposite of those that would be predicted on the basis of previous conditioning trials?

Conditioned Placebo Responses

Support for the classical conditioning hypothesis has been drawn from early reports on the use of drugs (e.g., morphine) as unconditioned stimuli in conditioning experiments with laboratory animals (Pavlov, 1927/1960). More recently, "placebo effects" have been elicited in rats by means of classical conditioning procedures (Herrnstein, 1962; Ross & Schnitzer, 1963). In these studies, injections of inert solutions, or simply the insertion of a needle, produced responses similar to those produced by a previously administered drug. Pihl and Altman (1971) replicated this phenomenon using amphetamine as the unconditioned stimulus but found a "reverse" placebo effect when saline was substituted for a tranquilizer. Although chlorpromazine produced a decrease in activity from baseline activity, subsequent administration of a saline solution resulted in a significant increase over baseline activity levels. The authors concluded that "the applicability of the conditioning model may be relative to the nature of the active substance utilized" (p. 94).

Two studies have purported to demonstrate the acquisition of a placebo response in human beings by means of conditioning trials. Lang and Rand (1969) obtained increases in heart rate of at least 15 beats per minute as an unconditioned response to glyceryl trinitrate in three women. Substitution of a placebo after numerous additional conditioning trials elicited pronounced tachycardia in two of these subjects but a much lesser heart-rate increase in the third, who "stated that she knew she had been given a placebo" (p. 913). Although generalization from the behavior of only three subjects is difficult at best, the failure to obtain a clear conditioned response from the subject who suspected that a placebo had been substituted for the active drug fits a conditioned expectancy model better than it does a conditioned response model.

In the other study claiming to demonstrate a conditioned placebo response in human subjects (Knowles, 1963), the reaction time of six habitual coffee drinkers was assessed following the ingestion of regular or decaffeinated (placebo) coffee and also in a no-liquid control condition. Although the ingestion of both caffeinated and decaffeinated coffee produced a decrease in reaction time, the design of the study was such that conditioning could not have occurred during the course of the experiment for four of the six subjects. Subjects were assigned in pairs to three experimental groups. Each group experienced one of the following orders of treatment administration: (a) placebo, caffeine, control; (b) control, placebo, caffeine; or (c) caffeine, control, placebo. Because the placebo was administered prior to the caffeine in orders (a) and (b), for these four subjects the effects of decaffeinated coffee could not have been due to a conditioning trial within the experimental period. The claim that conditioning had taken place rests on the fact that all six subjects were habitual coffee drinkers. However, the assumption that similar effects would not have occurred in subjects who were not coffee drinkers was not tested.

Consistent with the results of Pihl and Altman's (1971) study on laboratory rats, the effects of conditioning trials on human response to a placebo appear to vary as a function of the drug used as an unconditioned stimulus. Prior experience with the active drug enhances the effects of placebo marijuana (Carlin, Post, Cornelis, Bakker, & Halpern, 1974; Jones, 1971) and placebo analgesia (Batterman & Lower, 1968). Also, pain relief with placebo analgesia is greater when it is administered after a more potent drug than it is following a less potent drug (Kantor, Sunshine, Laska, Meisner, & Hopper, 1966). In contrast, prior experience inhibits the effects of placebo tranquilizers (Meath, Feldberg, Rosenthal, & Frank, 1956; Rickels, Lipman, & Raab, 1966; Segal & Shapiro, 1959; Zukin, Arnold, & Kessler, 1959). Furthermore, with placebo tranquilizers, there is an inverse relation between the strength of the presumed unconditioned stimulus (UCS) and the magnitude of the presumed conditioned response (*CR;* Rickels et al., 1966). These data support the hypothesis that conditioning trials enhance the effects of placebo marijuana and analgesia, but they disconfirm con-

I thank Julian B. Rotter, James R. Council, Christine Winter, Reuben Baron, Laurie Pearlman, and Robert Neiss for their helpful comments on earlier drafts.

Requests for reprints should be sent to Irving Kirsch, Department of Psychology, U-20, University of Connecticut, Storrs, CT 06268.

ditioning hypotheses as explanations of the effects of placebo tranquilizers.

Unconditioned Placebo Effects

In the previous section, it was assumed that due to stimulus generalization from experience with other medications, some placebo effects might be found in subjects who had not had prior exposure to the specific medication under study. In this section, studies are considered in which the placebo response is either unrelated or in a direction opposite to that of the presumed UCS. As noted by Wickramasekera (1980), "there can be no *CR* if there were no *UCS* (active ingredients)" (p. 14). Therefore, placebo responses that are unrelated to the pharmacological effects of a drug cannot be accounted for by conditioning models.

Although the design of Knowles's (1963) study precluded the possibility of demonstrating that the obtained effect was due to conditioning, it did provide evidence that the effect was *not* due to conditioning. Mean reaction times in the caffeine and placebo conditions were shortest immediately after ingestion and increased with each subsequent assessment. At 60 minutes after ingestion, reaction times for all three conditions were virtually identical. At 90 minutes, reaction times under caffeine and placebo conditions were slower than under control conditions. However, Knowles cited earlier data indicating that effective blood levels of caffeine are not likely to be reached for at least one hour following oral ingestion. The fact that caffeine did not result in shorter reaction times one hour or more after administration suggests that it is not an unconditioned stimulus for decreased reaction time. If this is true, the decreased reaction times observed immediately following ingestion of the caffeinated and decaffeinated coffee could not have been due to conditioning. Thus, Knowles demonstrated a placebo effect in humans in the absence of the conditions that are necessary for classical conditioning to occur.

A similar conclusion can be drawn from a case report of a placebo-induced conversion reaction (Levy & Jankovic, 1983). Phenytoin (Dilantin) produced a variety of idiosyncratic reactions in a patient, including speech distortions; visual, auditory, and tactile hallucinations; and muscle spasms. Neuropsychological testing following the administration of saline in the guise of phenytoin revealed a number of dose-dependent effects, including loss of consciousness, unresponsiveness to intense pain stimuli, disappearance of corneal reflexes, and convulsive seizures. However, administration of phenytoin in the guise of a neutral substance failed to elicit any abnormalities. Because phenytoin did not elicit the placebo-induced responses when it was given in disguised form, it could not have served as an unconditioned stimulus for those responses.

Research on expectancy effects has resulted in the development of the *balanced placebo design* (Marlatt & Rohsenow, 1980). The balanced placebo design yields a 2 × 2 matrix comprising the following four conditions in which subjects are (a) told they will get a drug/receive drug, (b) told they will get a drug/receive placebo, (c) told there will be no drug/receive drug, (d) told there will be no drug/receive no drug. This design allows independent evaluation of pharmacological and expectancy effects and has led to the discovery of placebo alcohol effects that are unrelated to or inconsistent with its pharmacological effects. For example, the pharmacological effect of alcohol is to decrease sexual arousal (Farkas & Rosen, 1976; Rubin & Henson, 1976). However, consistent with common expectations (Brown, Goldman, Inn, & Anderson, 1980), the belief that one has consumed alcohol results in *increased* sexual arousal to erotic stimuli (Bridell et al., 1978; Wilson & Lawson, 1976a, 1976b). Placebo alcohol also produces increased aggressive behavior (Lang, Goeckner, Adesso, & Marlatt, 1975) and increased craving for and consumption of alcohol (Engle & Williams, 1972; Marlatt, Demming, & Reid, 1973). Because the administration of alcohol in disguised form failed to produce these effects, they cannot be accounted for by a conditioning hypothesis. In anxiety-eliciting heterosexual situations, the belief that one has consumed alcohol is associated with decreased heart rate in males (Wilson & Abrams, 1977) and increased heart rate in females (Abrams & Wilson, 1979). It seems highly unlikely that alcohol as an unconditioned stimulus would have opposite pharmacological effects on male and female heart rates.

Marlatt and Rohsenow (1980) maintain that these placebo phenomena are consistent with a conditioning model, suggesting that the "conditioned response is a compensatory reaction, one that is in the opposite direction to the unconditioned response" (p. 192). Although this is consistent with the data on sexual arousal, it is inconsistent with the data on alcohol craving, aggression, and social anxiety, in which cases no unconditioned responses were observed. It is also inconsistent with most placebo effects, which correspond to the pharmacological effects of the drug under investigation. Thus, if conditioning accounts for placebo alcohol effects on sexual arousal, it cannot account for other placebo effects. Conversely, if most placebo effects are due to conditioning, then the effect of placebo alcohol on sexual arousal is an anomaly.[1]

[1] Since writing this article, Siegel's (1983) work on classically conditioned drug tolerance has come to my attention. Siegel and his colleagues have convincingly demonstrated that classical conditioning produces compensatory conditioned responses (i.e., a CR that is opposite in direction to the UCR) for some responses (those for which tolerance develops) to some drugs. This phenomenon

Strength of the Placebo Response

Placebo and drug effects are widely assumed to be additive. For example, Lasagna, Mosteller, von Felsinger, and Beecher (1954) found that morphine elicited a mean pain relief rating of 95% among patients who consistently reported relief from placebos (placebo reactors) as compared to 54% among consistent nonreactors to placebos. The 41% difference between placebo reactors and placebo nonreactors in pain relief following morphine administration is presumably due to the placebo effect of having been given medication. In other words, "the response to any *UCS* will include two components. The first component will be a *CR* (placebo response) and the second component a *UCR* (e.g., specific effect of a drug)" (Wickramasekera, 1980, p. 8). On the basis of his classical conditioning model, Wickramasekera predicted that, as a fractional component of the *UCR,* the placebo component ought to be weaker than the pharmacological effect. I have located three studies in which the placebo and pharmacological components of stimulant or depressant medications have been experimentally isolated (Frankenhaeuser, Post, Hagdahl, & Wrangsjoe, 1964; Lyerly, Ross, Krugman, & Clyde, 1964; Ross, Krugman, Lyerly, & Clyde, 1962). The results of these three studies reveal expectancy effects that are of a magnitude equal to or greater than the pure pharmacological effects of stimulant and tranquilizing drugs. Because these placebo effects are more than fractional components of the corresponding pharmacological effects, they constitute disconfirmatory evidence for Wickramasekera's conditioning model.

Summary

Classical conditioning procedures can produce a placebo response in animals with some drugs but produce a reverse placebo response with tranquilizers. Similarly, studies with human subjects have reported results that were consistent with conditioning theory when analgesia or marijuana was the unconditioned stimulus but have resulted in disconfirmatory results with tranquilizers. Although placebo responses generally mimic the effects of the active drug, when people have response expectancies that are contrary to the pharmacological effects of the active drug, their response to placebo is consistent with their expectations rather than with the drug's pharmacological effects. Finally, the placebo component of drug administration can be as powerful as or more powerful than the pharmacological component of drug effects. These data suggest that classical conditioning may be one method by which response expectancies are formed but that the effects of conditioning trials are mediated by expectancy.

Expectancy and Fear

People fear and avoid situations in which they expect aversive consequences (Beck, 1976; Rotter, 1954). However, expectations of harm cannot account for the degree of fear that is experienced by phobic individuals, because fear is defined as phobic only if it is "recognized by the individual as excessive or unreasonable in proportion to the actual dangerousness of the object, activity or situation" (American Psychiatric Association, 1980, p. 225). A number of investigators have proposed that the expectation of intense fear is a cause of this excessive fear and avoidance (Goldstein & Chambless, 1978; Kirsch, Tennen, Wickless, Saccone, & Cody, 1983; Reiss, 1980, Reiss & McNally, in press). Because the experience of intense fear is extremely aversive, the expectancy of its occurrence provides strong motivation for avoidance. For example, people with severe snake phobias avoid looking at pictures of snakes because of the unpleasant feelings that the pictures provoke. Similarly, agoraphobics are less afraid of supermarkets, shopping malls, and all the other situations that they avoid than they are of the panic attacks they fear might occur.

Evidence of the role of fear expectancies in phobias is provided by therapy outcome studies in which "placebo" control procedures have been employed. These procedures are designed to induce an expectancy of improvement, and it is generally assumed that their effectiveness is due to the same underlying mechanisms governing the effectiveness of placebo drugs. However, attempts at defining the term *placebo* in a way that is appropriate to both pharmacological and psychological contexts have not been successful (Critelli & Neumann, 1984; Kirsch, 1978; Kirsch, 1985a). Therefore, "placebo" psychotherapy procedures will be termed *expectancy modification procedures.* Expectancy modification is a specific active psychological mechanism that can be an effective therapeutic component of psychological treatment.

Expectancy Modification and Fear Reduction

The seminal study in which an expectancy modification procedure was used to control for "placebo" effects in the evaluation of a psychological treatment was Paul's (1966) research on systematic desensiti-

may account for the effects of placebo alcohol on sexual arousal and more certainly explains the negative placebo effect that Pihl and Altman (1971) obtained with chlorpromazine. However, because the conditioned response to morphine is hyperalgesia (Siegel, 1983), the positive analgesic response to placebo morphine (Evans, 1974) cannot be due to conditioning. Similarly, if the CR to tranquilizers is increased activity (Pihl & Altman, 1971), then the decreased activity produced by placebo tranquilizers (Frankenhaeuser et al., 1963, 1964) is not due to conditioning. The role of conditioned tolerance in the inhibitory effects of prior experience with placebo tranquilizers is unclear (Meath et al., 1956; Rickels et al., 1966; Segal & Shapiro, 1959; Zukin et al., 1959). However, even if these are due to compensatory CRs, the positive effects of placebo tranquilizers on self-reported psychiatric symptoms cannot be due to conditioning.

zation. Paul's expectancy modification procedure was more effective than a no-treatment control, indicating that expectancy modification can produce a significant reduction in anxiety. Although most studies comparing desensitization to expectancy modification procedures have reported greater fear reduction for desensitization (Kazdin & Wilcoxon, 1976), Borkovec and Nau (1972) demonstrated that many expectancy modification procedures are perceived as less credible than systematic desensitization. Independently, McReynolds, Barnes, Brooks, & Rehagen (1973) demonstrated that a more compelling expectancy modification procedure was as effective as desensitization and more effective than Paul's (1966) "attention placebo" in reducing fear of snakes.

To date, at least 11 studies have shown that credible expectancy modification procedures are capable of producing as great a reduction in fear as that produced by systematic desensitization (Gatchel, Hatch, Maynard, Turns, & Taunton-Blackwood, 1979; Kirsch & Henry, 1977; Kirsch et al., 1983; Lick, 1975; Marcia, Rubin, & Efran, 1969; McGlynn, 1971; McGlynn, Gaynor, & Puhr, 1972; McGlynn, Reynolds, & Linder, 1971; McReynolds et al., 1973; Slutsky & Allen, 1978; Tori & Worell, 1973). In addition, Gelder et al. (1973) found an expectancy modification procedure to be as effective as desensitization in treating animal and tissue damage phobias. Although desensitization was more effective than expectancy modification in the treatment of agoraphobia and social fear, Gelder et al.'s expectancy modification treatment failed to elicit outcome expectancies comparable to those elicited by desensitization. Expectancy modification treatments also have been reported to be as effective as cue-controlled relaxation, relaxation as an active coping skill, and heart-rate biofeedback (Gatchel et al., 1979; Gatchel, Hatch, Watson, Smith, & Gaas, 1977; Russel & Lent, 1982).

Many of the causal mechanisms that have been hypothesized as explanations of the effects of desensitization have been based on classical conditioning models. These hypothesized mechanisms include reciprocal inhibition (Wolpe, 1958), counterconditioning (Davison, 1968) and extinction (O'Leary & Wilson, 1975). In a test of conditioning hypotheses, Kirsch and Henry (1977) compared the effects of systematic desensitization and two credible expectancy modification procedures. One of these procedures was specifically designed to rule out conditioning hypotheses. In an "operant desensitization" condition, visualizations of anxiety-related scenes were paired with painful electric shocks, which subjects were told would "punish the anxiety." Both expectancy modification procedures were as effective as standard systematic desensitization in reducing public-speaking fear. Because aversive stimuli are assumed to be the unconditioned stimuli leading to the acquisition of fear as a conditioned response, the substantial degree of fear reduction produced by "operant desensitization" cannot be accounted for by extinction or counterconditioning. Furthermore, because the addition of the electric shock was the only procedural difference between "operant" and traditional desensitization, it is reasonable to suspect that the effects of the two procedures were due to a common causal mechanism. Substantial correlations between pretreatment ratings of treatment credibility and treatment outcome measures suggest that expectancy modification was the common causal agent.

In a subsequent study (Kirsch et al., 1983), 46 snake-phobic adults were assigned to either systematic desensitization, a credible expectancy modification treatment, or a delayed-treatment control condition. Anxiety expectancies were assessed by having subjects rate the degree of fear they thought they would experience at each step of a behavioral approach test. These ratings accounted for more than 50% of the variance in pre- and posttreatment approach behavior. In addition, immediately after the treatment was described, but before it was initiated, subjects were asked to predict their posttreatment fear. Within-cell correlations indicated that these predictions were especially accurate for desensitization subjects, accounting for about 60% of the variance in posttreatment approach behavior. These data can be interpreted most parsimoniously as indicating that systematic desensitization is an effective procedure for modifying fear expectancies, which in turn alter experienced fear.

Response Expectancy and Self-Efficacy

As defined by Bandura (1977), self-efficacy is the belief that one is able to execute a behavior upon which reinforcement is contingent. Defined in this manner, self-efficacy is conceptually distinct from response expectancy, whch refers to the occurrence of nonvolitional responses. Bandura has hypothesized that alterations in efficacy judgments are central to the effects of all psychotherapies and has supported this contention with reports of high correlations between responses to snake-approach self-efficacy questionnaires and posttreatment approach to a previously feared snake. However, recent data raise serious questions about the construct validity of snake-approach self-efficacy questionnaires.

Kirsch (1982) asked snake-fearful students to complete two self-efficacy questionnaires, one pertaining to approaching a live snake, the other to tossing a wad of paper into a basket from various distances. Subjects were then asked if increasing levels of hypothetical incentives would enable them to perform snake-approach and paper-toss tasks that they had previously rated as beyond their ability. Whereas hypothetical incentives as low as $20 were sufficient to alter most subjects' efficacy judgments for approaching a snake, such incentives as one million dollars and saving one's own life or the life of another failed to alter most subjects' efficacy judgments for the paper-toss task. When asked to explain this discrepancy, subjects expressed certainty of their ability to approach a snake if it were necessary to do so. Kirsch (1982) concluded that efficacy questionnaires measured subjects' *willingness* to approach a snake given their expected fear and the incentives for approach.

In another study (Kirsch et al., 1983), efficacy ratings and fear response expectancies had virtually identical power in predicting behavioral approach and ratings of experienced fear. In addition, the two expectancy measures were highly correlated during pretreatment ($r = -.75$) and posttreatment ($r = -.90$) assessment periods. When two measures are that highly correlated and have virtually identical predictive power, it is reasonable to suspect that they are measuring the same construct. Examination of the items on the two scales suggests that both measure expected fear. The anxiety expectancy scale asks people to predict their level of fear at each step of the approach test. Efficacy scales ask them to predict the number of steps they will accomplish. If behavior on an approach test is a measure of fear, then predicted approach (i.e., efficacy ratings) is a measure of expected fear.

Although self-efficacy and response expectancy are conceptually distinct, when measured in fear-provoking situations there is considerable overlap between them. This is because fear-related efficacy questionnaires do not measure people's self-efficacy. Instead, they measure people's willingness to approach a feared stimulus. Social learning theory predicts volitional behavior as a function of expected reinforcement. In the absence of sufficient incentive, people are unwilling to engage in behavior that they believe will lead to intense fear. Thus, when external consequences are held constant, high correlations are obtained between fear response expectancies and supposed measures of self-efficacy (cf. Kirsch, 1985b).

Summary

Subjective and behavioral manifestations of specific fears can be predicted by procedures designed to modify response expectancies. More credible expectancy modification procedures produce greater alterations in expectancy and fear, and procedures that are as credible as systematic desensitization are generally as effective in reducing fear. The effects of these procedures cannot be accounted for by classical conditioning but are highly correlated with changes in response expectancies. These data support Reiss's (1980) hypothesis that the experience of fear is in part a function of the expectancy of its occurrence and the hypothesis that fear reduction can be brought about by altering the expectancy of its occurrence. In addition, Emmelkamp (1982) has hypothesized that the effects of in vivo exposure treatments are mediated by expectancy. According to Emmelkamp, the self-observed habituation that occurs during in vivo exposure is interpreted as evidence of improvement, thereby altering subjects' expectancies.

Hypnosis

There are three kinds of cognitions that ought to affect response expectancies in hypnotic situations: (a) perceptions of the situation as more or less appropriate for the occurrence of hypnotic responses; (b) perceptions of the response as being appropriate to the role of a hypnotized subject (Sarbin, 1950; Sarbin & Coe, 1972), and (c) judgments of one's hypnotizability. If response expectancies affect hypnotic responses, then hypnotic responses ought to be affected by each of these variables. More specifically, the probability of occurrence of a particular response ought to vary as a function of the degree to which subjects perceive the situation as hypnotic, perceive the response as characteristic of the experience and behavior of good hypnotic subjects, and judge themselves to be good subjects (cf. Barber, Spanos, & Chaves, 1974).

Situational Perceptions

In the 18th century, a variety of procedures were used by mesmerists to induce "crises." These included stroking or making "passes" over the patient barehanded or with a magnet, having patients sit around a bucket of water containing iron filings, having the subject stand by a "magnetized" tree or drink "magnetized" water, and having the person sit with his or (more frequently) her knees pressed between the thighs of the mesmerist who applied pressure to the hypochondria (the area between the rib cage and the navel) or the ovarium. In modern placebo terminology, 18th-century induction procedures were nonspecific in the sense that no particular components were necessary for successful induction of a crisis. Experiments conducted by the French Royal Commission established to investigate mesmerism concluded that belief in the appropriateness of the situation was sufficient to elicit crises in susceptible subjects. For example, crises could be elicited by falsely informing people that they were being magnetized through a closed door (Franklin et al., 1784/1965; Franklin et al., 1785/1970).

Although there is still variety in induction procedures, most hypnotic inductions involve suggestions for deep relaxation. However, equivalent degrees of response enhancement have been produced by task motivational instructions (Barber, 1969), brief training in the use of imaginative strategies (Council, Kirsch, Vickery, & Carlson, 1983; Katz, 1978, 1979; Vickery, Kirsch, Council, & Sirkin, 1985), and a variety of expectancy modification procedures (Council et al., 1983; Glass & Barber, 1961; Wilson, 1967). The only component that is common to these methods of enhancing suggestibility is the credibility of the enhancement procedure. As had the French Royal Commission two centuries earlier, Sheehan & Perry (1976) have concluded that "it is not the procedural conditions per se that are important but whether or not the subject perceives them as part of a context that is 'appropriate' for displaying hypnotic behavior" (p. 72).

Role Perceptions

During the 18th and early 19th centuries, the behavior of magnetized subjects was as variable as the induction rituals that were employed to bring that behavior about. Some people coughed; others laughed. Some markedly increased their breath rates; others became very relaxed. Feelings of warmth and of cold were reported, as were sensations of pain or numbness. Sensitivity to stimulation might be heightened or lowered, sometimes heightened and then lowered. Many, but by no means all, magnetized subjects exhibited convulsive seizures (Deleuze, 1825/1965; d'Eslon, 1784/1965; Franklin et al., 1785/1970).

Just as hypnotic procedures have become standardized over the course of time, so too has the role of hypnotic subject. The hypnotized subject typically sits passively with eyes closed, shows little or no spontaneous speech or movement, and speaks slowly and softly in response to questions. Sarbin (1950) hypothesized that the behavior of hypnotized subjects is in part a function of their expectations of how a good subject ought to behave. Subsequent data support this hypothesis. For example, people who are informed that hypnotized subjects exhibit dominant arm catalepsy are likely to do so when hypnotized (Orne, 1959; Sheehan, 1971); being informed that spontaneous amnesia is a characteristic of hypnosis substantially increases the likelihood of its occurrence (Young & Cooper, 1972); and information about the difficulty of responding to suggestions affects subsequent responses (Barber & Calverley, 1964; Botto, Fisher, & Soucy, 1977; Klinger, 1970).

Role perceptions also affect self-reports of the experience of "trance." Henry (1985) constructed a questionnaire consisting of opposing subjective experiences that might be associated with hypnosis. The criterion for item inclusion was an endorsement rate of not more than 60% in either direction by subjects who had not previously experienced hypnosis. In general, subjects' experience of trance matched their preconceptions. Depending on their preconceived notions, good hypnotic subjects experienced "trance" as a state in which time passed either more slowly or more quickly than usual, logical thought was either more or less difficult than normal, the hypnotist's voice sounded closer or farther away than before, sounds were experienced as muffled or more clear than usual, the subject felt more or less involved than usual, and so on.

Expectancy Ratings and Responsiveness

Self-reported expectancies of naive subjects typically account for about 10% of the variance in hypnotizability (Melei & Hilgard, 1964; Saavedra & Miller, 1983; Shor, 1971; Wadden, 1983). However, correlations between expectancy and response account for approximately 25% of the variance when trance induction is replaced with brief training in goal-directed imagining (Kirsch, Council, & Vickery, 1984). Similarly, Barber and Calverley (1969) reported that expectancy was more highly correlated with responsiveness when subjects were instructed to place themselves in hypnosis than when a formal trance induction was used.

Council and Kirsch (1983) assessed response expectancies prior to administering a traditional trance induction and again after the induction but prior to administration of dependent variable suggestions. They also obtained subjective reports of trance depth immediately after the trance induction. Responsiveness to suggestions was significantly correlated with both pre- and postinduction expectancies, but the correlation between responsiveness and postinduction expectancies was significantly greater than that between responsiveness and preinduction expectancies. Although trance depth reports were also correlated with responsiveness, regression analyses revealed that only postinduction response expectancies contributed unique variance to the prediction of responsivity. A path analysis supported the hypothesis that hypnotic inductions enhance responsiveness by altering response expectancies.

Modification of Hypnotic Response Expectancies

Procedures designed to modify subjects' expectancies of hypnotic responding have been shown to affect responses to suggestions. For example, Vickery and Kirsch (1985) told subjects that repeated testing resulted in increased, decreased, or unchanged levels of hypnotic response, and found that responsiveness varied as a function of that information. Similarly, manipulating expectancies by providing bogus feedback from "personality scales" affects responsiveness (Gregory & Diamond, 1973; Saavedra & Miller, 1983). Wilson (1967) increased subjects' response expectancies by providing them with experiences designed to convince them that they were experiencing a variety of imagined perceptual phenomena. For example, while suggesting that subjects imagine that the room was red, Wilson imparted a red tinge to the room by means of a small hidden light bulb. These subjects were later tested for responsiveness to standard hypnotic suggestions, without mention of "hypnosis" or the use of a hypnotic induction procedure. Not only did the experimental subjects achieve significantly higher scores than control subjects, but their scores were such that none would be classified as "low hypnotizables" as that term is typically defined (e.g., Weitzenhoffer & Hilgard, 1962).

Imaginative Involvement and Response Expectancy

The idea that hypnotic experiences are a function of imagination dates back to the 18th century (Franklin et al., 1785/1970). The modern counterpart to this notion, the concept of absorption in imaginative activities (Tellegen & Atkinson, 1974), has provided a point of convergence for state and nonstate theorists (Barber et al., 1974; E. Hilgard, 1965; J. Hilgard, 1979; Sarbin & Coe, 1972). However, recent data suggest that the relation between absorption and hypnotic responsiveness is mediated by expectancy. For example, Council et al. (1983) reported that although Tellegen and Atkinson's (1974) absorption scale predicted subjects' responses to hypnotic suggestions, it was more highly correlated with response expectancies, which in turn were even more highly correlated with responsiveness. Furthermore, when variance associated with expectancy was statistically controlled, the relation between absorption and hypnotizability was nonsignificant.

As noted above, bogus feedback from personality tests can alter subjects' responsiveness to hypnotic suggestions. Because items on the absorption scale are face obvious, Council and Kirsch (1983) hypothesized that administering it in the context of an experiment on hypnosis might be a way of indirectly providing subjects with bogus feedback. Thus, the association between absorption and responsiveness might be an artifact of the scale's effect on subjects' response expectancies. In a test of that hypothesis, they administered the scale to 64 subjects in the context of a hypnosis experiment and to an additional 64 subjects in a context that was unrelated to hypnosis. Regression analyses revealed a significant interaction between scores on the absorption scale and the context in which the scale was administered. Absorption was significantly correlated with responsivity and expectancy only when the scale was administered in a context that was clearly associated with a subsequent hypnotic experience.

Barber et al. (1974) hypothesized that positive attitudes, motivations, and expectancies lead subjects to engage in goal-directed fantasies, which in turn generate suggested behaviors and experiences. However, when instructed to do so, good hypnotic subjects are able to respond to suggestions while imagining conflicting events (Spanos, Weekes, & de Groh, 1984; Zamansky, 1977). In addition, Council and Kirsch (1984) demonstrated that the effects of intentionally imagining along with hypnotic suggestions (parallel imagery) and the effects of imagining events that were incompatible with suggestions (counter imagery) varied as a function of the instructional set that was provided to subjects. Parallel imagery enhanced responding among subjects who were provided with a convincing rationale indicating that this would be its effect, but it inhibited responsiveness among subjects given a negative instructional set. Similarly, counter imagery inhibited responsiveness only among subjects who were given a response-inhibition rationale.

High test–retest correlations across a wide variety of hypnotic inductions, training procedures, and measures of responsiveness have led to the conclusion that hypnotizability is a relatively stable trait (Perry, 1977). However, having given subjects information designed to elicit conflicting expectancies, Council and Kirsch (1984) obtained test–retest correlations accounting for only 10% of the variance in hypnotic responsiveness. In contrast, their expectancy manipulation accounted for approximately 46% of the variance, suggesting that previously reported correlations reflected stable response expectancies rather than the presence of an underlying personality trait (cf. Spanos, 1982).

Summary

The data reviewed above reveal that "hypnosis" refers to a wide variety of procedures by means of which many people's response expectancies can be temporarily altered. Both the efficacy of the procedure and the nature of the response depend primarily on subjects' beliefs and expectancies. Similarly, the degree of responsiveness varies as a function of expectancy. Although hypnotizability has been viewed as a relatively stable trait, in at least some situations conflicting expectancy instructions can account for more variance than "trait hypnotizability," suggesting that high test–retest correlations on measures of hypnotic response may be due to the presence of relatively stable response expectancies. It is possible that, with sufficiently strong response expectancies, *all* individuals would show high levels of hypnotic response.

Causal Mechanisms

A number of intervening variables have been hypothesized to mediate expectancy effects on particular responses. For example, Frank (1973) proposed that placebos engender feelings of hopefulness associated with faith in improvement, feelings that in turn reduce generalized depression and anxiety in psychiatric outpatients. Hopefulness has also been hypothesized to promote physical healing (Frank, 1973), possibly by enhancing immunologic function (Simonton, Mathews-Simonton, & Creighton, 1978). Similarly, placebo-induced pain reduction may be mediated by decreased anxiety (Evans, 1974) or the release of endorphins in the brain (Fields & Levine, 1981).

Each of these hypothesized mechanisms is specific to particular types of response. Although some of them may be related to other response expectancy effects (e.g., anxiety reduction may be an important factor in hypnotic pain reduction), the wide range of nonvolitional responses that are affected by expectancy and the similarly wide range of situations in which these effects occur suggest the heuristic value of a more general response expectancy hypothesis. For example, endorphin activity does not appear to be related to hypnotic pain reduction (Spiegel & Albert, 1983). Furthermore, because one cannot feel hopeful and hopeless at the same time, it is difficult to imagine how the hopefulness hypothesis might account for placebo-induced side effects in patients who also experience positive effects from the same placebo. Nor can it easily explain the opposing effects of stimulant and tranquilizer placebos on healthy, nonpatient volunteers for a drug experiment (e.g., Frankenhaeuser, Jarpe, Svan, & Wrangsjö, 1963). Because these subjects are not being treated for a disorder, the concept of faith in improvement is not applicable. Similarly, the fact that simple instructions about the effects of repeated testing produce opposing alterations in the probability of responding to standard hypnotic suggestions (e.g., hand lowering, taste hallucination, posthypnotic amnesia) cannot be readily explained by any of these hypothesized mediating mechanisms.

The response expectancy hypothesis is not intended to replace the mechanisms described above. There is ample evidence that hopefulness produces symptomatic relief in psychiatric outpatients (e.g., Frank, Nash, Stone, & Imber, 1963; Shapiro, Struening, & Shapiro, 1980), and although the evidence is scant (Hall, 1984; Jemmott & Locke, 1984), the hypothesis that positive emotional states enhance immunologic function is intriguing and merits further investigation. Similarly, data linking placebo pain relief to endorphin release are extremely important, although they pose the question of how placebos produce an increase in endorphin activity. Endorphin release may be more profitably viewed as one of the effects of placebos, rather than as the cause of placebo effects. The purpose of the response-expectancy hypothesis is to supplement previous hypotheses in order to account for expectancy effects on a wider range of responses.

Response expectancies affect subjective experience, overt behavior, and physiological function. The mechanisms by which these effects are produced can best be understood by separate consideration of each of these response systems. In brief, I propose that (a) there is an unmediated causal relation between response expectancy and subsequent experience, (b) some of the physiological changes that are associated with response expectancies can be accounted for by the *identity assumption* that is logically required of all nondualist philosophies of mind, and (c) volitional behavior is affected by response expectancies because of the reinforcement value of nonvolitional responses.

Response Expectancy and Subjective Experience

In critiquing the introspective methods of prebehaviorist experimental psychology, Dodge (1912) introduced the idea that an expectancy can produce a corresponding conscious experience. Since that time, response expectancy effects have been viewed as artifacts to be controlled for in psychological research. However, given the data reviewed above, it seems reasonable to view those effects as evidence of a basic psychological mechanism that is capable of affecting a wide range of responses. As a basic psychological mechanism, response expectancies generate corresponding subjective experiences without additional intervening mechanisms. In this respect, the response expectancy hypothesis is not different from other hypothesized causal relations between cognitions and subsequent experience. Beck (1976), for example, proposed that sadness is caused by thoughts of loss, anger by the belief that one has been wronged, fear by expected harm or loss, and anticipatory excitement by expectations of positive reinforcement. The response expectancy hypothesis asserts that the expectancy of a subjective experience has a direct (i.e., unmediated) corresponding effect on experience.

Response Expectancy and Physiological Function

Part of the difficulty in understanding the apparent causal relation between response expectancies and physiological function results from the assumption of mind–body dualism that is implicit in the formulation of the question. All monist solutions to the mind–body issue involve some form of identity thesis. For example, double-aspect or neutral monist positions view mental and physical descriptions as different aspects of a single underlying reality. Similarly, materialist philosophies hold that mental events do not cause physical events; rather, they are identical to physical events in the same way that water is identical to H_2O. Water does not cause nor is it caused by H_2O; it *is* H_2O. The common factor in these views is the implication of physical counterparts to any subjectively described event.

The only logical alternative to the identity assumption is to allow the existence of mental events without physical correlates, which implies a dualist mind–body position. However, if cognitions do not correspond to physical processes, either they do not affect behavior or physiological function, which is inconsistent with considerable data, or the law of conservation of energy is invalid. In contrast, the identity thesis implies an isomorphic relation between mental and physical causality. If mental events correspond to physical events, then a statement that one mental event (e.g., expectancy) causes another mental state (e.g., fear) is equivalent to a statement that the physiological state corresponding to the first mental state causes the physiological state corresponding to the second mental state. In other words, physiological changes accompany changes in mental states because any particular mental state corresponds to some particular physical state. Physiological changes are not generated by the expectancy of their occurrence but by the expectancy of corresponding subjective experiences. Changes in pulse rate, for example, are not brought about by the expectancy of their occurrence but by expectancies of alterations in subjectively experienced arousal levels.

The identity thesis does not imply totally dissimilar patterns of physiological response for different psychological states. For example, increased arousal is associated with a variety of affective states (Reisenzein, 1983; Schacter & Singer, 1962). Conversely, because a single subjective term (e.g., anxiety) can be used to describe a variety of experiences, different instances in which the same label is used may correspond to different states of the nervous system (e.g., Tyrer & Lader, 1974). The identity thesis merely asserts that any particular instance of a subjective experience is associated with some specific state of the organism. The principle of causal isomorphism adds that any pattern of causal relations between psychological variables implies a similar causal relation among corresponding physiological variables.

At the psychological level, the problem is to establish the causal relations between specific cognitive states (e.g., irrational thoughts, images, response expectancies) and subsequent subjective experiences (e.g., alterations in mood or pain perception). At the physiological level, the problem is to identify the central and peripheral concomitants of each of these states. Although the physiological concomitants of expectancies are not known, some of the physiological concomitants of resulting experiences have been identified. Expectancy-induced changes in fear and subjective arousal levels are frequently accompanied by corresponding changes in pulse or heart rate, skin conductance, and blood pressure (Beiman, 1976; Blackwell, Bloomfield, & Buncher, 1972; Brodeur, 1965; Frankenhaeuser, Jarpe, Svan, & Wrangsjö, 1963; Frankenhaeuser, Post, Hagdahl, & Wrangsjoe, 1964; Grayson & Borkovec, 1978; Kirsch & Henry, 1979; Lick, 1975). Expectancy-induced changes in male sexual arousal are accompanied by increases in penile tumescence (Briddell et al., 1978; Wilson & Lawson, 1976a). Expectancy-induced pain reduction may be accompanied by increased endorphin activity in the brain (Fields & Levine, 1981) and by reduced respiratory and electromyographic responses (Barber & Hahn, 1962). However, the most difficult problem in identifying complete causal sequences involves the discovery of central state correlates of cognitions and other subjective experiences.

Response Expectancy and Volitional Behavior

According to Rotter (1954), the probability of a behavioral response is a function of the expectancy that the response will lead to reinforcement and of the subjective value of the reinforcement. Because many nonvolitional experiences (e.g., pain, fear, sexual arousal) have obvious positive or negative reinforcement value, they are among the reinforcements determining the probability of behavior upon which they are believed to be contingent. Thus, alcohol consumption is partially determined by expectancies that it will lead to enhanced social and physical pleasure, enhanced sexual performance, increased confidence, shorter sleep-onset latencies, pain reduction, and reduced tension (Brown et al., 1980).

Reiss and McNally's (in press) expectancy model of phobias is generally consistent with Rotter's social learning theory and with the response expectancy hypothesis proposed in this article. According to their model, phobic avoidance can be predicted as a function of expected harm (a reinforcement expectancy), expected fear (a response expectancy), and the degree to which fear is experienced as aversive (i.e., the reinforcement value of the anticipated fear). Similarly, response expectancies and their reinforcement values affect the likelihood of initiating sexual contact, ingesting medication or other drugs, volunteering to be an hypnotic subject, and so forth.

Response Expectancy and Social Learning

By way of summary, the following propositions integrate the response expectancy hypothesis presented in this article with some of the hypotheses proposed by other cognitive theorists.

1. The probability of a volitional response is a function of the expectancy that the response will lead to reinforcement and of the value of the expected reinforcement (Rotter, 1954). These expectancies have been termed R–S expectancies by Bolles (1972). Operant conditioning procedures are one means by which R–S expectancies are acquired.

2. Certain stimuli have primary or unlearned reinforcement value (Rotter, 1982). In addition, stimuli can acquire reinforcement value through their association with other reinforcing stimuli. The secondary reinforcement value of a stimulus is determined by the expectancy that it will lead to other reinforcements (Rotter, 1954). Classical conditioning is one means by which these S–S expectancies are formed (Bolles, 1972).

3. From propositions 1 and 2, it can be deduced that the probability of a volitional response is determined by the sum total of expected reinforcements

and of their primary reinforcement values (Kirsch, 1985b).

4. Nonvolitional responses can be elicited by unconditioned stimuli. In addition, some cognitions (e.g., perceptions of loss and of having been wronged, and expectancies of harm and of positive reinforcement) function as unconditioned stimuli for specific emotional states (sadness, anger, fear, and anticipatory excitement; Beck, 1976).

5. Nonvolitional responses can also be elicited by the expectancy of their occurrence, either as a function of specific stimuli (S–R expectancies) or as a function of voluntary responses (R–R expectancies). Classical conditioning is one means by which response expectancies are acquired (Reiss, 1980). In addition, verbal persuasion, attributional processes, modeling, and self-observation are involved in the acquisition and modification of response expectancies.

6. The effects of unconditioned stimuli and response expectancies are additive. Therefore, response expectancies can enhance, inhibit, or reverse the effects of unconditioned stimuli (Frankenhaeuser, Post, Hagdahl, & Wrangsjoe, 1964; Lyerly et al., 1964; Ross et al., 1962; Wolf, 1950).

7. The probability of occurrence of a nonvolitional response varies directly with the strength of the expectancy of its occurrence and inversely with the magnitude or difficulty of the expected response. Therefore, a weak expectancy for a large change in subjective response is likely to be disconfirmed, whereas a strong expectancy for a small change is likely to be confirmed, thereby strengthening the expectancy and initiating a cycle for continued change.

8. Nonvolitional responses have reinforcement value. The reinforcement value of some nonvolitional responses may be due to expectancies of further subsequent reinforcement. Other nonvolitional responses (e.g., the experience of pain, sadness, or fear) function as primary reinforcers, in that they have reinforcement value that is independent of expectancies of subsequent additional reinforcement. It should be noted, however, that even these may acquire secondary reinforcement value if followed by social reinforcement (e.g., sympathy).

9. Because nonvolitional responses have reinforcement value, they are among the reinforcers that determine volitional behavior. Specifically, the probability of a volitional response is a function of the sum total of expected stimuli and nonvolitional responses and of the primary reinforcement value of those stimuli and responses.

REFERENCES

Abrams, D. B., & Wilson, G. T. (1979). Effects of alcohol on social anxiety in women: Cognitive versus physiological processes. *Journal of Abnormal Psychology, 88,* 161–173.

American Psychiatric Association. (1980). *Diagnostic and statistical manual of mental disorders* (3rd ed.). Washington, DC: Author.

Bandura, A. (1977). Self-efficacy: Toward a unifying theory of behavioral change. *Psychological Review, 84,* 191–215.

Barber, T. X. (1969). *Hypnosis: A scientific approach.* New York: Van Nostrand Reinhold.

Barber, T. X. (1978). Hypnosis, suggestions, and psychosomatic phenomena: A new look from the standpoint of recent experimental studies. *The American Journal of Clinical Hypnosis, 21,* 13–27.

Barber, T. X., & Calverley, D. S. (1964). Toward a theory of hypnotic behavior: Effects on suggestibility of defining the situation as hypnosis and defining response to suggestions as easy. *Journal of Abnormal and Social Psychology, 68,* 585–592.

Barber, T. X., & Calverley, D. S. (1969). Multidimensional analysis of "hypnotic" behavior. *Journal of Abnormal Psychology, 74,* 209–220.

Barber, T. X., & Hahn, K. W. (1962). Physiological and subjective responses to pain-producing stimulation under hypnotically-suggested and waking-imagined "analgesia." *Journal of Abnormal and Social Psychology, 65,* 222–228.

Barber, T. X., Spanos, N. P., & Chaves, J. F. (1974). *Hypnosis, imagination, and human potentialities.* New York: Pergamon Press.

Batterman, R. C., & Lower, W. R. (1968). Placebo-responsiveness—The influence of previous therapy. *Current Therapeutic Research, 10,* 136–143.

Beck, A. T. (1976). *Cognitive therapy and the emotional disorders.* New York: International Universities Press.

Beiman, I. (1976). The effects of instructional set on physiological response to stressful imagery. *Behaviour Research and Therapy, 14,* 175–180.

Blackwell, B., Bloomfield, S. S., & Buncher, C. R. (1972). Demonstration to medical students of placebo responses and non-drug factors. *The Lancet, 19,* 1279–1282.

Bolles, R. C. (1972). Reinforcement, expectancy, and learning. *Psychological Review, 79,* 394–409.

Borkovec, T. D., & Nau, S. D. (1972). Credibility of analogue therapy rationales. *Journal of Behavior Therapy and Experimental Psychiatry, 3,* 257–260.

Botto, R. W., Fisher, S., & Soucy, G. P. (1977). The effect of a good and a poor model on hypnotic susceptibility in a low demand situation. *International Journal of Clinical and Experimental Hypnosis, 25,* 175–183.

Bridell, D. W., Rimm, D. C., Caddy, G. W., Krawitz, G., Sholis, D., & Wunderlin, R. J. (1978). The effects of alcohol and cognitive set on sexual arousal to deviant stimuli. *Journal of Abnormal Psychology, 87,* 418–430.

Brodeur, D. W. (1965). The effects of stimulant and tranquilizer placebos on healthy subjects in a real-life situation. *Psychopharmacologia, 7,* 444–452.

Brown, S. A., Goldman, M. S., Inn, A., & Anderson, L. R. (1980). Expectations of reinforcement from alcohol: Their domain and relation to drinking patterns. *Journal of Consulting and Clinical Psychology, 48,* 419–426.

Carlin, A. S., Post, R. D., Cornelis, B., Bakker, C. B., & Halpern, L. M. (1974). The role of modeling and previous experience in the facilitation of marijuana intoxication. *Journal of Nervous and Mental Disease, 159,* 275–281.

Council, J. R., & Kirsch, I. (1983, August). *"Absorption": Personality construct or expectancy-mediated artifact?* Paper presented at the meeting of the American Psychological Association, Anaheim, CA.

Council, J. R., & Kirsch, I. (1984, August). *Imaginative involvement and hypnotic responding: The effects of discrepant rationales.* Paper presented at the meeting of the American Psychological Association, Toronto, Canada.

Council, J. R., Kirsch, I., Vickery, A. R., & Carlson, D. (1983). "Trance" vs. "skill" hypnotic inductions: The effects of credibility, expectancy, and experimenter modeling. *Journal of Consulting and Clinical Psychology, 51,* 432–440.

Critelli, J. W., & Neumann, F. K. (1984). The placebo: Conceptual analysis of a construct in transition. *American Psychologist, 39,* 32–39.

Davison, G. C. (1968). Systematic desensitization as a counterconditioning process. *Journal of Abnormal Psychology, 73,* 91–99.

Deleuze, J. P. F. (1965). Rules of magnetizing. In R. E. Shor & M. T. Orne (Eds.), *The nature of hypnosis: Selected basic readings* (pp. 24–29). New York: Holt, Rinehart & Winston. (Reprinted from T. C. Hartshorn, Trans., *Practical instructions in animal magnetism: Part I,* 1837. French original published 1825)

D'Eslon, C. (1965). Observations on the two reports of the commissioners named by the king to investigate animal magnetism. In R. E. Shor & M. T. Orne (Eds.), *The nature of hypnosis: Selected basic readings* (pp. 8–20). New York: Holt, Rinehart & Winston. (French original published 1784. D. Chval, Trans.)

Dodge, R. (1912). The theory and limitations of introspection. *American Journal of Psychology, 23,* 214–229.

Emmelkamp, P. M. G. (1982). *Phobic and obsessive-compulsive disorders: Theory, research, and practice.* New York: Plenum Press.

Engle, K. B., & Williams, T. K. (1972). Effect of an ounce of vodka on alcoholics' desire for alcohol. *Quarterly Journal of Studies on Alcohol, 33,* 1099–1105.

Evans, F. J. (1974). The placebo response in pain reduction. *Advances in Neurology, 4,* 289–296.

Farkas, G. M., & Rosen, R. C. (1976). Effect of alcohol on elicited male sexual response. *Journal of Studies on Alcohol, 37,* 265–272.

Fields, H. L., & Levine, J. D. (1981). Biology of placebo analgesia. *American Journal of Medicine, 70,* 745–746.

Frank, J. D. (1973). *Persuasion and healing* (Rev. ed.). Baltimore: Johns Hopkins University Press.

Frank, J. D., Nash, E. H., Stone, A. R., & Imber, S. D. (1963). Immediate and long-term symptomatic course of psychiatric outpatients. *American Journal of Psychiatry, 120,* 429–439.

Frankenhaeuser, M., Jarpe, G., Svan, H., & Wrangsjö, B. (1963). Physiological reactions to two different placebo treatments. *Scandinavian Journal of Psychology, 4,* 245–250.

Frankenhaeuser, M., Post, B., Hagdahl, R., & Wrangsjoe, B. (1964). Effects of a depressant drug as modified experimentally-induced expectation. *Perceptual and Motor Skills, 18,* 513–522.

Franklin, B., Bory, Lavoisier, Bailly, Majault, Sallin, d'Arcet, Guillotin, & Le Roy. (1965). Secret report on mesmerism, or animal magnetism. In R. E. Shor & M. T. Orne (Eds.), *The nature of hypnosis: Selected basic readings* (pp. 3–7). New York: Holt, Rinehart & Winston. (Original work published 1784)

Franklin, B., Majault, LeRoy, Sallin, Bailly, D'Arcet, De Borie, Guillotin, & Lavoisier. (1970). Report on animal magnetism. In M. M. Tinterow (Ed.), *Foundations of hypnosis: From Mesmer to Freud* (pp. 82–128). Springfield, IL: Charles C Thomas. (Original work dated 1785)

Gatchel, R. J., Hatch, J. P., Maynard, A., Turns, R., & Taunton-Blackwood, A. (1979). Comparison of heart rate biofeedback and systematic desensitization in reducing speech anxiety: Short- and long-term effectiveness. *Journal of Consulting and Clinical Psychology, 47,* 620–622.

Gatchel, R. J., Hatch, J. P., Watson, P. J., Smith, D., & Gaas, E. (1977). Comparative effectiveness of voluntary heart rate control and muscular relaxation as active coping skills for reducing speech anxiety. *Journal of Consulting and Clinical Psychology, 45,* 1093–1100.

Gelder, M. G., Bancroft, J. H., Gath, D. H., Johnston, D. W., Mathews, A. M., & Shaw, P. M. (1973). Specific and non-specific factors in behaviour therapy. *British Journal of Psychiatry, 123,* 445–462.

Glass, L. B., & Barber, T. X. (1961). A note on hypnotic behavior, the definition of the situation, and the placebo effect. *Journal of Nervous and Mental Diseases, 132,* 539–541.

Gliedman, L. H., Gantt, W. H., & Teitelbaum, H. A. (1957). Some implications of conditional reflex studies for placebo research. *American Journal of Psychiatry, 113,* 1103–1107.

Goldstein, A. J., & Chambless, D. L. (1978). A reanalysis of agoraphobia. *Behavior Therapy, 9,* 47–59.

Grayson, J. B., & Borkovec, T. D. (1978). The effects of expectancy and imagined response to phobic stimuli on fear reduction. *Cognitive Therapy and Research, 2,* 11–24.

Gregory, J., & Diamond, M. J. (1973). Increasing hypnotic susceptibility by means of positive expectancies and written instructions. *Journal of Abnormal Psychology, 82,* 363–367.

Hall, H. (1984). Imagery and cancer. In A. A. Sheikh (Ed.), *Imagination and healing* (pp. 159–170). Farmingdale, NY: Baywood.

Henry, D. (1985). *Subjects' expectancies and subjective experience of hypnosis.* Unpublished doctoral dissertation, University of Connecticut.

Herrnstein, R. (1962). Placebo effect in the rat. *Science, 138,* 677–678.

Hilgard, E. R. (1965). *Hypnotic susceptibility.* New York: Harcourt, Brace & World.

Hilgard, J. R. (1979). *Personality and hypnosis: A study of imaginative involvement* (2nd ed.). Chicago: University of Chicago Press.

Jemmott, J. B., & Locke, S. E. (1984). Psychosocial factors, immunologic mediation, and human susceptibility to infectious diseases: How much do we know? *Psychological Bulletin, 95,* 78–108.

Jones, R. T. (1971). Marijuana-induced "high": Influence of expectation, setting, and previous drug experience. *Pharmacological Review, 23,* 359–369.

Kantor, T. G., Sunshine, A., Laska, E., Meisner, M., & Hopper, M. (1966). Oral analgesic studies: Pentazocine, hydrochloride, codeine, aspirin, and placebo and their influence on response to placebo. *Clinical Pharmacology and Therapeutics, 7,* 447–454.

Katz, N. (1978). Hypnotic inductions as training in self-control. *Cognitive Therapy and Research, 2,* 365–369.

Katz, N. (1979). Comparative efficacy of behavioral training, training plus relaxation, and a sleep/trance induction in increasing hypnotic susceptibility. *Journal of Consulting and Clinical Psychology, 47,* 119–127.

Kazdin, A. E., & Wilcoxon, L. A. (1976). Systematic desensitization and nonspecific treatment effects: A methodological evaluation. *Psychological Bulletin, 83,* 729–758.

Kirsch, I. (1978). The placebo effect and the cognitive-behavioral revolution. *Cognitive Therapy and Research, 2,* 255–264.

Kirsch, I. (1982). Efficacy expectations or response predictions: The meaning of efficacy ratings as a function of task characteristics. *Journal of Personality and Social Psychology, 42,* 132–136.

Kirsch, I. (1985a). The logical consequences of the common-factor definition of the term *placebo. American Psychologist, 40,* 237–238.

Kirsch, I. (1985b). Self-efficacy and expectancy: Old wine with new labels. *Journal of Personality and Social Psychology, 49,* 824–830.

Kirsch, I., Council, J. R., & Vickery, A. R. (1984). The role of expectancy in eliciting hypnotic responses as a function of type of induction. *Journal of Consulting and Clinical Psychology, 52,* 708–709.

Kirsch, I., & Henry, D. (1977). Extinction vs. credibility in the desensitization of speech anxiety. *Journal of Consulting and Clinical Psychology, 45,* 1052–1059.

Kirsch, I., & Henry, D. (1979). Self-desensitization and meditation in the treatment of public speaking anxiety. *Journal of Consulting and Clinical Psychology, 47,* 536–541.

Kirsch, I., Tennen, H., Wickless, C., Saccone, A. J., & Cody, S. (1983). The role of expectancy in fear reduction. *Behavior Therapy, 14,* 520–533.

Klinger, B. I. (1970). Effect of peer model responsiveness and length of induction procedure on hypnotic responsiveness. *Journal of Abnormal Psychology, 75,* 15–18.

Knowles, J. B. (1963). Conditioning and the placebo effects of decaffeinated coffee on simple reaction time in habitual coffee drinkers. *Behaviour Research and Therapy, 1,* 151–157.

Lang, A. R., Goeckner, D. J., Adesso, V. J., & Marlatt, G. A. (1975). Effects of alcohol on aggression in male social drinkers. *Journal of Abnormal Psychology, 84,* 508–518.

Lang, W. J., & Rand, M. J. (1969). A placebo response as a conditional reflex to glyceryl trinitrate. *Medical Journal of Australia, 1,* 912–914.

Lasagna, I., Mosteller, F., von Felsinger, J. M., & Beecher, H. K. (1954). A study of the placebo response. *American Journal of Medicine, 16,* 770–779.

Levy, R. S., & Jankovic, J. (1983). Placebo-induced conversion reaction: A neurobehavioral and EEG study of hysterical aphasia, seizure, and coma. *Journal of Abnormal Psychology, 92,* 243–249.

Lick, J. (1975). Expectancy, false galvanic skin response feedback, and systematic desensitization in the modification of phobic anxiety. *Journal of Consulting and Clinical Psychology, 43,* 557–567.

Lyerly, S. B., Ross, S., Krugman, A. D., & Clyde, D. J. (1964). Drugs and placebos: The effects of instructions upon performance and mood under amphetamine sulphate and chloral hydrate. *American of Abnormal and Social Psychology, 68,* 321–327.

Marcia, J. E., Rubin, B. M., & Efran, J. S. (1969). Systematic desensitization: Expectancy change or counter-conditioning? *Journal of Abnormal Psychology, 74,* 382–387.

Marlatt, G. A., Demming, B., & Reid, J. B. (1973). Loss of control drinking in alcoholics: An experimental analogue. *Journal of Abnormal Psychology, 81,* 233–241.

Marlatt, G. A., & Rohsenow, D. J. (1980). Cognitive processes in alcohol use: Expectancy and the balanced placebo design. In N. K. Mello (Ed.), *Advances in substance abuse: Behavioral and biological research* (pp. 159–199). Greenwich, CT: JAI Press.

McGlynn, F. D. (1971). Experimental desensitization following three types of instructions. *Behaviour Research and Therapy, 9,* 367–369.

McGlynn, F. D., Gaynor, R., & Puhr, J. (1972). Experimental desensitization of snake-avoidance after an instructional manipulation. *Journal of Clinical Psychology, 28,* 224–227.

McGlynn, F. D., Reynolds, E. J., & Linder, L. H. (1971). Experimental desensitization following therapeutically oriented and physiologically oriented instructions. *Journal of Behavior Therapy and Experimental Psychiatry, 2,* 13–18.

McReynolds, W. T., Barnes, A. R., Brooks, S., & Rehagen, N. J. (1973). The role of attention-placebo influences in the efficacy of systematic desensitization. *Journal of Consulting and Clinical Psychology, 41,* 86–92.

Meath, J. A., Feldberg, T. M., Rosenthal, D., & Frank, J. D. (1956). Comparison of reserpine and placebo in treatment of psychiatric outpatients. *AMA Archives of Neurology and Psychiatry, 76,* 207–214.

Melei, J. P., & Hilgard, E. R. (1964). Attitudes toward hypnosis, self-predictions, and hypnotic susceptibility. *International Journal of Clinical and Experimental Hypnosis, 12,* 99–108.

O'Leary, K. D., & Wilson, G. T. (1975). *Behavior therapy: Application and outcome.* Englewood Cliffs, NJ: Prentice-Hall.

Orne, M. T. (1959). The nature of hypnosis: Artifact and essence. *Journal of Abnormal and Social Psychology, 58,* 277–299.

Paul, G. L. (1966). *Insight vs. desensitization in psychotherapy.* Stanford, CA: Stanford University Press.

Pavlov, I. P. (1960). *Conditioned reflexes.* New York: Dover. (Original work published 1927)

Perry, C. (1977). Is hypnotizability modifiable? *International Journal of Clinical and Experimental Hypnosis, 25,* 125–146.

Pihl, R. O., & Altman, J. (1971). An experimental analysis of the placebo effect. *Journal of Clinical Pharmacology, 11,* 91–95.

Reisenzein, R. (1983). The Schachter theory of emotion: Two decades later. *Psychological Bulletin, 94,* 239–264.

Reiss, S. (1980). Pavlovian conditioning and human fear: An expectancy model. *Behavior Therapy, 11,* 380–396.

Reiss, S., & McNally, R. J. (in press). The expectancy model of fear. In S. Reiss & R. R. Bootzin (Eds.), *Theoretical issues in behavior therapy.* New York: Academic Press.

Rickels, K., Lipman, R., & Raab, E. (1966). Previous medication, duration of illness, and placebo response. *Journal of Nervous and Mental Disease, 142,* 548–554.

Ross, M., & Olson, J. M. (1982). Placebo effects in medical research and practice. In J. R. Eiser (Ed.), *Social psychology and behavioral medicine* (pp. 441–458). New York: Wiley.

Ross, S., & Buckalew, L. W. (1983). The placebo as an agent in behavioral manipulation: A review of problems, issues, and affected measures. *Clinical Psychology Review, 3,* 457–471.

Ross, S., Krugman, A. D., Lyerly, S. B., & Clyde, D. J. (1962). Drugs and placebos: A model design. *Psychological Reports, 10,* 383–392.

Ross, S., & Schnitzer, S. B. (1963). Further support for a placebo effect in the rat. *Psychological Reports, 13,* 461–462.

Rotter, J. B. (1954). *Social learning and clinical psychology.* Englewood Cliffs, NJ: Prentice-Hall.

Rotter, J. B. (1982). *The development and application of social learning theory: Selected papers.* New York: Praeger.

Rubin, H. B., & Henson, D. E. (1976). Effects of alcohol on male sexual responding. *Psychopharmacology, 47,* 123–134.

Russell, R. K., & Lent, R. W. (1982). Cue-controlled relaxation and systematic desensitization versus nonspecific factors in treating test anxiety. *Journal of Consulting and Clinical Psychology, 29,* 100–103.

Saavedra, R. L., & Miller, R. J. (1983). The influence of experimentally induced expectations on responses to the Harvard Group Scale of Hypnotic Susceptibility, Form A. *International Journal of Clinical and Experimental Hypnosis, 31,* 37–46.

Sarbin, T. R. (1950). Contributions to role-taking theory: I. Hypnotic behavior. *Psychological Review, 57,* 225–270.

Sarbin, T. R., & Coe, W. C. (1972). *Hypnosis: A social psychological analysis of influence communication.* New York: Holt, Rinehart & Winston.

Schachter, S., & Singer, J. E. (1962). Cognitive, social, and physiological determinants of emotional states. *Psychological Review, 69,* 379–399.

Segal, M., & Shapiro, K. L. (1959). A clinical comparison study of the effects of reserpine and placebo on anxiety. *Archives of Neurology and Psychiatry, 81,* 392–398.

Shapiro, A. K., Struening, E., & Shapiro, E. (1980). The reliability and validity of a placebo test. *Journal of Psychiatric Research, 15,* 253–290.

Sheehan, P. W. (1971). Countering preconceptions about hypnosis: An objective index of involvement with the hypnotist [monograph]. *Journal of Abnormal Psychology, 78,* 299–322.

Sheehan, P. W., & Perry, C. W. (1976). *Methodologies of hypnosis.* Hillsdale, NJ: Erlbaum.

Shor, R. E. (1971). Expectations of being influenced and hypnotic performance. *International Journal of Clinical and Experimental Hypnosis, 19,* 154–166.

Siegel, S. (1983). Classical conditioning, drug tolerance, and drug dependence. In Y. Israel, F. B. Glaser, H. Kalant, R. E. Popham, W. Schmidt, & R. G. Smart (Eds.), *Research advances in alcohol and drug problems* (Vol. 7). New York: Plenum Press.

Simonton, O. C., Mathews-Simonton, S., & Creighton, J. L. (1978). *Getting well again.* Toronto, Canada: Bantam Books.

Slutsky, J. M., & Allen, G. J. (1978). Influence of contextual cues on the efficacy of desensitization and a credible placebo in alleviating public speaking anxiety. *Journal of Consulting and Clinical Psychology, 46,* 119–125.

Spanos, N. P. (1982). A social psychological approach to hypnotic behavior. In G. Weary & H. L. Mirels (Eds.), *Integrations of clinical and social psychology* (pp. 231–271). New York: Oxford University Press.

Spanos, N. P., Weekes, J. R., & de Groh, M. (1984). The "involuntary" countering of suggested requests: A test of the ideomotor hypothesis of hypnotic responsiveness. *British Journal of Experimental and Clinical Hypnosis, 1,* 3–11.

Spiegel, D., & Albert, L. H. (1983). Naloxone fails to reverse hypnotic alleviation of chronic pain. *Psychopharmacology, 81,* 140–143.

Tellegen, A., & Atkinson, G. (1964). Openness to absorbing and self-altering experiences ("absorption"), a trait related to hypnotic susceptibility. *Journal of Abnormal Psychology, 83,* 268–277.

Tolman, E. C. (1932). *Purposive behavior in animals and men.* New York: Appleton-Century-Crofts.

Tori, C., & Worell, L. (1973). Reduction of human avoidance behavior: A comparison of counterconditioning, expectancy, and cognitive information approaches. *Journal of Consulting and Clinical Psychology, 41,* 269–278.

Tyrer, P., & Lader, M. H. (1974). Response to propanolol and diazepam in somatic and psychic anxiety. *British Medical Journal, 2,* 14–16.

Vickery, A. R., & Kirsch, I. (1985, August). *Expectancy and skill-training in the modification of hypnotizability.* Paper presented at the meeting of the American Psychological Association, Los Angeles, CA.

Vickery, A. R., Kirsch, I., Council, J. R., & Sirkin, M. I. (1985). Cognitive skill and traditional trance hypnotic inductions: A within-subject comparison. *Journal of Consulting and Clinical Psychology, 53,* 131–133.

Wadden, T. A. (1983, August). *Self-prediction of hypnotic susceptibility.* Paper presented at the meeting of the American Psychological Association, Anaheim, CA.

Weitzenhoffer, A. M., & Hilgard, E. R. (1962). *Stanford hypnotic susceptibility scale: Form C.* Palo Alto, CA: Consulting Psychologist Press.

Wickramasekera, I. (1980). A conditioned response model of the placebo effect: Predictions from the model. *Biofeedback and Self-Regulation, 5,* 5–18.

Wilson, D. L. (1967). The role of confirmation of expectancies in hypnotic induction. *Dissertation Abstracts, 28,* 4787-B. (University Microfilms No. 66-6781)

Wilson, G. T., & Abrams, D. (1977). Effects of alcohol on social anxiety and physiological arousal: Cognitive versus pharmacological processes. *Cognitive Therapy and Research, 1,* 195–210.

Wilson, G. T., & Lawson, D. M. (1976a). Expectancies, alcohol, and sexual arousal in male social drinkers. *Journal of Abnormal Psychology, 85,* 587–594.

Wilson, G. T., & Lawson, D. M. (1976b). Effects of alcohol on sexual arousal in women. *Journal of Abnormal Psychology, 85,* 489–497.

Wolf, S. (1950). Effects of suggestion and conditioning on the action of chemical agents in human subjects—The pharmacology of placebos. *Journal of Clinical Investigation, 29,* 100–109.

Wolpe, J. (1958). *Psychotherapy by reciprocal inhibition.* Stanford, CA: Stanford University Press.

Young, J., & Cooper, L. M. (1972). Hypnotic recall amnesia as a function of manipulated expectancy. *Proceedings of the 80th Annual Convention of the American Psychological Association, 7,* 857–858.

Zamansky, H. S. (1977). Suggestion and countersuggestion in hypnotic behavior. *Journal of Abnormal Psychology, 86,* 346–351.

Zukin, P., Arnold, D. G., & Kessler, C. (1959). Comparative effects of phenaglycodol and meprobromate on anxiety reactions. *Journal of Nervous and Mental Disease, 129,* 193–195.

Part IV
Individual Differences in Hypnotic Suggestibility

[11]

THE HERITABILITY OF HYPNOTIC SUSCEPTIBILITY IN TWINS

ARLENE H. MORGAN

Stanford University

A sample of 140 pairs of twins and their families was tested on the Stanford Hypnotic Susceptibility Scale, Form A. A significant heritability index for the scores of the twin pairs and a significant correlation between the midparent score and the mean child score supported a genetic component in hypnotizability. However, a statistically significant interaction between parent hypnotizability and the child's hypnotizability, conditional upon the resemblance of the child to the like-sexed parent in personality, was interpreted as a consequence of environmental influence, either through social learning or identification.

Hypnotic susceptibility has been shown to be a relatively stable characteristic when measured by standardized instruments such as the Stanford Hypnotic Susceptibility Scale (Weitzenhoffer & Hilgard, 1959). Reliability coefficients between Form A of the Stanford scale and its parallel, Form B, based on intervals of one day to a few weeks, are generally in the .80's (E. R. Hilgard, 1965). A recent study retested 85 subjects on Form A after a 10-year period and found a correlation of .60 between the two sessions (Morgan, Johnson, & Hilgard, in preparation).[3]

Attempts to explain these stable differences have been less successful, however. The hypnotizable person tends to be one whose attitude toward hypnosis is favorable (London, Cooper, & Johnson, 1962; Melei & Hilgard, 1964), who has a tolerance for unusual experiences, as measured by experience inventories (O'Hara & Munger, 1962; Lee-Teng, 1965; Shor, 1960), and who has a high capacity for fantasy and imagined experiences (Evans, 1963; J. R. Hilgard, 1970; Sutcliffe, 1962). Further, the hypnotizable person is more likely to have a history of strict parental discipline and deep early imaginative involvements in such activities as fiction reading, listening to music, or noncompetitive sports (J. R. Hilgard, 1970). The relationship between any of these variables and hypnotizability is not strong; correlations are generally of the magnitude of .30, leaving most of the variance unexplained.

Children are consistently found to be more hypnotizable, overall, than adults (e.g., Barber & Calverley, 1963; London & Cooper, 1969). Thus it is possible that all people are born hypnotizable, but that the demands of reality on the maturing personality discourage the freedom of imagination which our society encourages only in children. Yet *all* children are not hypnotizable, and *some* adults retain their hypnotic abilities despite maturing influences. This suggests that there may be predispositional factors which determine the degree to which the individual develops his hypnotic abilities within his own particular environment. Such a predisposition may be in part genetic.

It was this perspective—that the stable individual differences in hypnotic susceptibility might in part be inherent—that led to a study of the hypnotizability of twins and their families from a behavior genetics approach. A preliminary report of earlier data from this study has already appeared (Morgan, Hilgard, & Davert, 1970). The present report is based on a much larger sample and a more detailed analysis of relationships within the data.

[1] This research was supported by Grant MH-03859 from the National Institute of Mental Health to Ernest R. Hilgard, Hypnosis Research Program, Department of Psychology, Stanford University. The help of Hilgard and the entire laboratory staff is sincerely appreciated. Special thanks are extended to Luigi L. Cavalli-Sforza of the Department of Genetics, Stanford University, School of Medicine, for his assistance in the genetic interpretations of this study.

[2] Requests for reprints should be directed to Arlene H. Morgan, Department of Psychology, Stanford University, Stanford, California 94305.

[3] A. H. Morgan, D. L. Johnson, and E. R. Hilgard, The stability of hypnotic susceptibility: A longitudinal study.

THE TWIN METHOD

Behavior genetics research on man has been conducted primarily on samples of twins. Monozygotic twins are assumed to be genetically identical, so that any differences between them are attributable to environmental factors. Dizygotic twins, on the other hand, have only 50% (on the average) of their genes in common, so that differences between them are the result of both environmental and genetic factors.

Classification of Zygosity

Of basic importance, then, is the determination of the zygosity of the twin pairs. Various indicators have been used: placental examination, blood grouping, fingerprint analysis, anthropometric measurements, and a simple appraisal of how much the twins are like each other. Cederlöf, Frieberg, Jonson, and Kaij (1961) asked their 400 adult twin subjects: "When you were growing up, were you alike as two peas, or was there only a family likeness?" Answers to this question correctly identified 95% of the sample which had been classified on the basis of blood grouping. The World Health Organization (1966) has reported similar success with a "similarity index" which rates the similarity of physical characteristics, such as color of eyes, hair, skin, size and shape of ears, shape and texture of teeth, etc. The consensus currently seems to be that such a diagnosis is as good a single criterion as any other.

In the present study, the zygosity of the twin pairs was based primarily on the mother's report. As a check on the accuracy of such reports, a similarity index was derived from that described above.[4] Two members of the hypnotist team independently completed the similarity index for a subsample of 20 pairs of twins prior to having knowledge of the mother's report.

As a further objective check, close-up color photographs were made, one full-face and one profile view of each twin. These photographs were subsequently rated by three independent observers as to the degree of similarity between the twin pairs. The overall ratings made by these five observers agreed with the mother's report in all but one case. The raters classified this pair as monozygotic, while the mother considered them dizygotic. The mother's report was accepted. In general, the 95% agreement with the mother's report in this subsample (19 or 20 cases) compares favorably with the accuracy predictions of the best recommended methods of zygosity determination.[5]

Statistical Treatment of Twin Data

The statistic usually employed to estimate the genetic contribution to the variance in twin data is the heritability index h^2, first proposed by Holzinger in 1929 as "a measure of the relative effects of nature and nurture factors upon the differences found between members of twin pairs reared within a family [p. 244]." Holzinger himself proposed two formulas for computing h^2 (see Vandenberg, 1966), and researchers in the field have proposed various others (e.g., Mittler, 1971, p. 169). All of them yield slightly different results. Cavalli-Sforza and Bodmer (1971) concluded that a significant h^2 value is

> likely to be an indication of enough genetic polymorphism with respect to genes affecting the character in question to give rise to variation between dizygous twins (that is, sibs) which is significant, relative to the observed environmental variation between monozygous twins [p. 579].

The heritability index tells us nothing about the number of such polymorphic genes or their relative dominance, however; further, most researchers agree that little meaning should be attached to the absolute size of h^2, though its statistical significance can be determined on the basis of an F ratio as described in Vandenberg (1966, p. 334) in which $h^2 = 1 - 1/F$.

Heritability indices for intelligence and other ability tests typically range from .70 to .90. For personality and interest measures, such as responses on the California Personality Inventory, Minnesota Multiphasic Personality Inventory, introversion–extraversion scales, or Cattell's Junior Personality Quiz, the highest h^2 that is consistently reported is around .40 (based on the intraclass correlations for

[4] Copies of this index, with a complete report of the results, are available from the author.

[5] The author expresses appreciation to Aleda Lynton and David L. Johnson, who rated the twins in person; and to Ernest R. Hilgard, Josephine R. Hilgard, and Martha F. Newman, who rated the photographs.

monozygotic and dizygotic twins summarized in Lindzey, Loehlin, Manosevitz, and Rosenzweig, 1971).

THE HERITABILITY OF HYNPOTIC SUSCEPTIBILITY

There is little theoretical agreement on *what* hypnosis is, although most researchers in the field agree that the people who experience hypnotic phenomena do so through some *ability* in this area. E. R. Hilgard (1965), for example, spoke of an ability component and an attitude component. The attitude component presumably reflects influences of the social environment on our motivation to be hypnotized, while the ability component determines the degree to which we can be hypnotized if we want to. It would seem necessary that both of these components be present in the highly hypnotizable subject.

Although there is some evidence that hypnotic ability can be improved with training (Diamond, 1972; Kinney, 1969; Sachs & Anderson, 1967), responses on the standard scales tend to remain quite stable over time if no intervening training is given. The question relevant to the present study is whether the ability to be hypnotized is in part inherent or whether it is completely determined by developmental factors interacting to produce a favorable attitude and the concomitant *learning* of a skill which is potentially accessible to all individuals.

METHOD

Procedure

A sample of 140 pairs of twins was obtained through the cooperation of the National Organization of the Mothers of Twins Clubs. Individual chapters were invited to participate in the project for a small honorarium. Testing was arranged in facilities convenient to the participating members.

Families were included if any part of its membership volunteered. For example, a number of families came whose twins were younger than the minimum testing age of 4 years. Frequently, the father did not participate. On the average, approximately 50% of the club membership are represented by at least a part of the family. In addition, 31 families were included who had no twins, for the purpose of increasing the samples for parent–child comparisons.

A team of hypnotists administered the Stanford Hypnotic Susceptibility Scale, Form A (SHSS:A) in individual sessions, and both members of a twin pair were hypnotized simultaneously (in separate rooms) to avoid communication between the twins or experimenter bias.

In addition, the parents were asked to complete a Similarity of Child to Parents form[6] on each child who was tested, rating the child as "high" or "low" and indicating which parent the child was "most like" on 11 personality variables: sensitivity to criticism, sense of humor, curiosity, competitiveness, cautiousness, self-control, adventuresomeness, compliance, imagination, strives for perfection, and fearfulness. These personality variables were selected on the basis of relationships reported by J. R. Hilgard (1970) in which, for example, the curious, adventuresome, imaginative person tends to be more hypnotizable than the competitive, controlled, fearful one.

TABLE 1

COMPOSITION AND HYPNOTIC SUSCEPTIBILITY OF THE TOTAL SAMPLE

Sample	N	Age		Hypnotic susceptibility[a]	
		$\bar{X}$	SD	$\bar{X}$	SD
Fathers	131	36.7	7.2	4.8	3.5
Mothers	178	34.4	6.5	6.7	3.5
Sons	278	10.3	3.9	6.8	2.9
Daughters	250	8.9	3.7	7.4	3.3

Note. For fathers versus mothers, $t = -4.70$, $df = 307$, $p = .001$; for sons versus daughters, $t = -2.21$, $df = 526$, $p = .05$.

[a] Maximum score = 12 on the SHSS: A.

RESULTS

The composition of the total sample, with mean age and mean hypnotic susceptibility scores, is given in Table 1. Mothers are significantly more hypnotizable than fathers in this sample, and daughters more hypnotizable than sons (see Table 1). Further, mothers show a significant negative correlation between age and susceptibility ($r = -.43$, $n = 178$, $p < .001$), while the fathers do not. Because of these inconsistencies as a function of sex and age in this sample, SHSS:A scores were converted to z scores based on the mean and standard deviation of the sex and age group to which that score belonged. These corrected scores were subsequently used in the correlational analysis.

Intraclass Correlations for the Twin Pairs

Intraclass correlations were computed for the twin and sibling pairs using the analysis of

[6] Copies of the form are available from the author on request.

TABLE 2

INTRACLASS CORRELATIONS FOR HYPNOTIC SUSCEPTIBILITY SCORES OF TWIN AND SIBLING PAIRS

Sample	No. pairs	Intra-class r
Monozygotic twins		
Male	30	.54***
Female	28	.49**
Total monozygotic pairs	58	.52***
Dizygotic twins		
Male	30	.24
Female	23	.08
Total like sex	53	.18
Unlike-sex dizygotic	29	.15
Total dizygotic	82	.17
Sibling nontwin pairs		
Male	40	.25
Female	48	.19
Unlike sex	44	.10
Total sibling pairs	132	.19*
Total, excluding monozygotic pairs	214	.18**

Note. Scores are corrected for age.
* $p < .05$.
** $p < .01$.
*** $p < .001$.

variance formula described in Snedecor and Cochran (1967, p. 294):

$$r_I = \frac{s^2_B - s^2_W}{s^2_B + s^2_W}.$$

These results are given in Table 2. The sibling-pair sample derives from those families in which scores were available for two nontwin siblings. If there were more than two, those two nearest in age were selected as a pair. The intraclass correlations for these sibling pairs are comparable to those for dizygotic twin pairs.

Most interest centers upon the correlations between monozygotic pairs, which turn out to be .54 for male pairs, .49 for female pairs, and .52 for total monozygotic pairs. As shown in Table 2, these are all highly significant. Because these correlations are to be contrasted with those for like-sexed dizygotic twins, it is important that they be shown to be statistically higher than those for dizygotic pairs. Using the r to z transformation, the r_I of .52 for all monozygotic pairs is significantly higher than the r_I of .18 for dizygotic pairs ($z = 2.02$, $p < .05$). These correlations are comparable to those reported by Rawlings (1972), based on a study conducted in Australia.

A heritability index was computed for males, for females, and for the total group of monozygotic (MZ) versus like-sexed dizygotic (DZ) pairs, according to Holzinger's formula:

$$h^2 = \frac{\sigma W^2_{DZ} - \sigma W_{MZ}}{\sigma^2 W_{DZ}}.$$

These h^2 values are given in Table 3. The overall heritability index of .64 falls between those usually reported for personality measures (around .40) and for ability measures (.70–.90). If we accept this h^2 of .64 as evidence for some genetic contribution to hypnotic susceptibility, then we would expect some relationship between parents and children as well, regardless of twinning. Such relationships are examined next.

Correlations of Hypnotic Susceptibility Scores for Parent–Child Combinations

The results of the comparisons between parent and child are given in Table 4. The correlations between parents and sons are significant for both fathers and mothers, while those with daughters are not significant for either. Parent–son correlations are only moderate, however, and in neither the father–child correlations nor the mother–child correlations is there a significant *difference* between the correlation with sons and the correlation with daughters. Thus, the most useful correlation for estimating the "true" parent–child correlation is that of .22 between the midparent and the mean child (see Table 4). This is approximately the correlation we would expect on the basis of the observed correlations between monozygotic twins and nonmonozygotic siblings, assuming there is no effect of assortive mating between the parents and that there is no interaction between genotype and environ-

TABLE 3

HERITABILITY INDEX h^2 FOR THE TWIN SAMPLE

Pairs	$\sigma^2 W_{DZ}$	$\sigma^2 W_{MZ}$	h^2	F^a	df	p
Male	.92	.40	.57	2.32	29,29	.05
Female	1.16	.31	.73	3.70	27,22	.01
All like-sexed	1.02	.37	.64	2.78	57,52	.01

Note. DZ = dizygotic; MZ = monozygotic.

[a] $F = \frac{1}{1 - h^2}$ (Vandenberg, 1966).

TABLE 4

CORRELATIONS OF STANFORD HYPNOTIC SUSCEPTIBILITY SCALE, FORM A SCORES FOR PARENT–CHILD COMBINATIONS

Mean child group[b]	Parent score								
	Father			Mother			Midparent[a]		
	N	*r*	*p*	*N*	*r*	*p*	*N*	*r*	*p*
Sons (total of 259 represented)	94	.29	.01	123	.20	.05	91	.26	.02
Daughters (total of 233 represented)	86	.01	*ns*	120	.10	*ns*	84	.06	*ns*
Mean child	116	.16	.10	160	.12	*ns*	113	.22	.05

Note. Scores are corrected for age.
[a] Average of father and mother.
[b] The average of all children tested in the family.

ment. The first assumption is a safe one, since the correlation between the hypnotizability scores of father and mother was not different from zero. The second assumption is not so safe and constitutes a serious limitation to all studies of human genetics (Cavalli-Sforza & Bodmer, 1971, p. 533). In spite of this limitation, however, the heritability findings suggest that a heredity contribution to hypnotizability should not be rejected.

Resemblances in Hypnotizability and Personality of Parents and Children

The Similarity of Child to Parents rating scale yielded two scores: (*a*) a personality score, based on whether the child was high or low in the personality variables proposed to be related to hypnotizability; and (*b*) a similarity-to-parent score, based on the number of variables in which the child was rated to be *most*

TABLE 5

MEAN STANFORD HYPNOTIC SUSCEPTIBILITY SCALE, FORM A (SHSS: A) SCORES OF CHILDREN BASED ON PERSONALITY RESEMBLANCE TO PARENT AND THE PARENT'S LEVEL OF HYPNOTIZABILITY

Item	Mean SHSS: A of children of:				Significance of difference between means			Significance of interaction between personality resemblance and parent hypnotizability		
	More hypnotizable parent[a]		Less hypnotizable parent[b]							
	N	Mean SHSS: A	*N*	Mean SHSS: A	*t*	*df*	*p*	*F*	*df*	*p*
Sons who resemble father	50	7.9	33	5.1	4.99	81	.01	18.52	1/128	.001
Sons who do not resemble father	19	6.4	30	7.9	−1.76	47	*ns*			
Sons who resemble mother	33	6.5	31	6.6	.07	62	*ns*	.03	1/128	*ns*
Sons who do not resemble mother	35	6.8	33	6.8	.00	66	*ns*			
Daughters who resemble father	27	7.2	23	7.7	−.58	48	*ns*	1.01	1/110	*ns*
Daughters who do not resemble father	25	7.5	39	7.2	.34	62	*ns*			
Daughters who resemble mother	18	7.9	33	7.2	1.02	49	*ns*	3.98	1/110	.05
Daughters who do not resemble mother	42	6.9	21	8.2	−1.86	61	.10			

[a] For father, $\bar{X}$ = 8.4; for mother, $\bar{X}$ = 9.3.
[b] For father, $\bar{X}$ = 2.4; for mother, $\bar{X}$ = 4.3.

like father or *most like* mother. The personality score showed no correlation with hypnotic susceptibility, owing perhaps to the unreliability of the personality measures on an absolute scale. Parents estimated the personalities of themselves and their children; hence, one set of parents may have used criteria different from those of another. This would lead to incommensurability. However, if the same criteria are used for parent and child, similarity-to-parent scores may have some validity, despite discrepant criteria for the items as rated by other parents.

A personality resemblance score was therefore computed as the total number of variables on which the child was rated as being like the parent. This personality resemblance score was then correlated with the parent–child SHSS:A score *difference*. This comparison resulted in a significant correlation for fathers and sons ($r = -.30$, $n = 132$, $p < .01$); that is, the more the son is like the father in personality, the less is their difference in hypnotizability. This led to a further analysis of parent–child SHSS:A scores on the basis of whether or not the child resembled the parent. These results are given in Table 5. Personality resemblance was a significant factor only for fathers and sons, although a significant interaction was demonstrated between personality resemblance and hypnotizability scores for either sexed child and the *like-sexed parent*. Figures 1 and 2 illustrate this interaction for father–son and mother–daughter pairs, respectively. Because no such interaction existed between the child and the opposite-sexed parent, these results suggest an environmental contribution to hypnotizability. That is, environmental factors lead to identification with the like-sexed parent, with subsequent modeling of that parent's behavior, whether the parent is high or low in the characteristics associated with hypnotizability. Such identification with the like-sexed parent is not universal, but when it does occur the parent–child similarity in hypnotizability is greater.

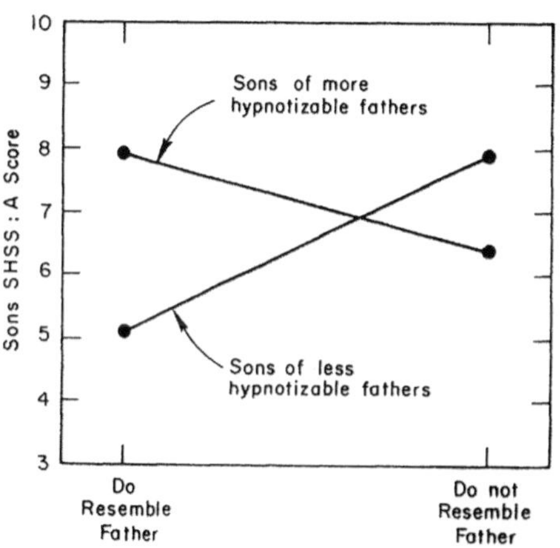

FIG. 1. Resemblance in hypnotizability of sons to fathers, as related to their resemblance in personality.

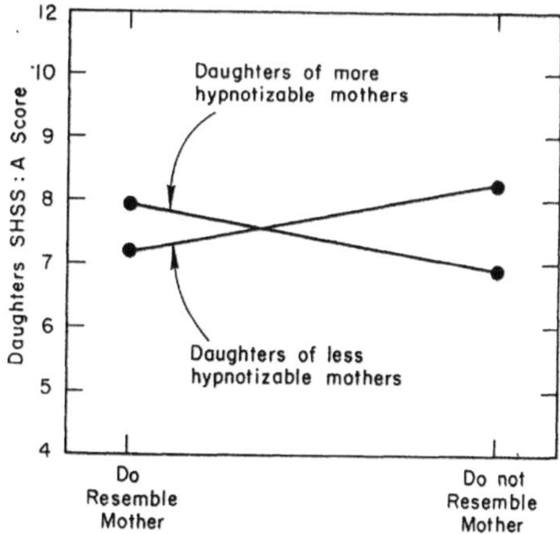

FIG. 2. Resemblance in hypnotizability of daughters to mothers, as related to their resemblance in personality.

CONCLUSION

In conclusion, the significantly different intraclass correlations for monozygotic and dizygotic twins provide evidence for a genetic contribution to hypnotic susceptibility, leading to a heritability index of .64. The low but statistically significant correlation between midparent and mean child susceptibility is consistent with a genetic contribution. The influence of environment is best demonstrated by an interaction between personality resemblance and the hypnotic scores of parents and their like-sexed children, as might best be explained by identification as an environmental consequence of social learning.

Hypnotizability thus appears to be the product of both a genetic predisposition and subsequent environmental influences, as well as their interaction. Such an interaction is expected of course in complex human behavior.

REFERENCES

Ås, A., O'HARA, J. W., & MUNGER, M. P. The measurement of subjective experiences presumably related to hypnotic susceptibility. *Scandinavian Journal of Psychology*, 1962, **3**, 47–64.

BARBER, T. X., & CALVERLEY, D. S. "Hypnotic-like" suggestibility in children and adults. *Journal of Abnormal and Social Psychology*, 1963, **66**, 589–597.

CAVALLI-SFORZA, L. L., & BODMER, W. F. *The genetics of human populations*. San Francisco: Freeman, 1971.

CEDERLÖF, R., FRIEBERG, L., JONSON, E., KAIJ, L. Studies of similarity diagnosis in twins, with the aid of mailed questionnaires. *Acta Genetica*, 1961, **11**, 338–362.

DIAMOND, M. J. The use of observationally presented information to modify hypnotic susceptibility. *Journal of Abnormal Psychology*, 1972, **79**, 174–180.

EVANS, F. J. The structure of hypnosis: A factor analytic investigation. Unpublished doctoral dissertation, University of Sydney, Australia, 1963.

HILGARD, E. R. *Hypnotic susceptibility*. New York: Harcourt Brace Jovanovich, 1965.

HILGARD, J. R. *Personality and hypnosis: A study of imaginative involvement*. Chicago: University of Chicago Press, 1970.

HOLZINGER, K. J. The relative effect of nature and nurture influences on twin differences. *Journal of Educational Psychology*, 1929, **20**, 245–248.

KINNEY, J. M. The modification of hypnotic susceptibility. Unpublished doctoral dissertation, Stanford University, 1969.

LEE-TENG, E. Trance susceptibility, induction susceptibility, and acquiescence as factors in hypnotic performance. *Journal of Abnormal Psychology*, 1965, **70**, 383–389.

LINDZEY, G., LOEHLIN, J., MANOSEVITZ, M., & THIESSEN, D. Behavioral genetics. *Annual Review of Psychology*, 1971, **22**, 39–94.

LONDON, P., & COOPER, L. M. Norms of hypnotic susceptibility in children. *Developmental Psychology*, 1969, **1**, 113–124.

LONDON, P., COOPER, L. M., & JOHNSON, H. J. Subject characteristics in hypnosis research. *International Journal of Clinical and Experimental Hypnosis*, 1962, **10**, 13–21.

MELEI, J. P., & HILGARD, E. R. Attitudes toward hypnosis, self-predictions, and hypnotic susceptibility. *International Journal of Clinical and Experimental Hypnosis*, 1964, **12**, 99–108.

MITTLER, P. *The study of twins*. Middlesex, England: Penguin Books, 1971.

MORGAN, A. H., HILGARD, E. R., & DAVERT, E. C. The heritability of hypnotic susceptibility of twins: A preliminary report. *Behavior Genetics*, 1970, **1**, 213–224.

RAWLINGS, R. M. The inheritance of hypnotic amnesia. Paper presented at the 44th Congress of the Australian and New Zealand Society for the Advancement of Science, July 1972.

SACHS, L. B., & ANDERSON, W. L. Modification of hypnotic susceptibility. *International Journal of Clinical and Experimental Hypnosis*, 1967, **15**, 172–180.

SHOR, R. E. The frequency of naturally occurring "hypnotic-like" experiences in the normal college population. *International Journal of Clinical and Experimental Hypnosis*, 1960, **8**, 151–163.

SNEDECOR, G. W., & COCHRAN, W. G. *Statistical methods*. Ames, Iowa: Iowa State University Press, 1967.

SUTCLIFFE, J. P. The relation of imagery and fantasy to hypnosis. (Progress Report on National Institute of Mental Health. Project M-3950) Sydney, Australia: University of Sydney, 1962. (Mimeo)

VANDENBERG, S. G. Contributions of twin research to psychology. *Psychological Bulletin*, 1966, **66**, 327–352.

WEITZENHOFFER, A. M., & HILGARD, E. R. *The Stanford Hypnotic Susceptibility Scale, Forms A and B*. Palo Alto, Calif.: Consulting Psychologists Press, 1959.

WORLD HEALTH ORGANIZATION. The use of twins in epidemiological studies. *Acta Genetica Medica Gemellogica*, 1966, **15**, 109–128.

(Received October 12, 1972)

[12]

OPENNESS TO ABSORBING AND SELF-ALTERING EXPERIENCES ("ABSORPTION"), A TRAIT RELATED TO HYPNOTIC SUSCEPTIBILITY [1]

AUKE TELLEGEN [2]
University of Minnesota

GILBERT ATKINSON
Youngstown State University

A questionnaire containing items of varied content believed to be related to hypnotizability was administered to 481 female subjects. Two subsamples of 142 and 171 subjects, respectively, also completed Block's Ego Resiliency and Ego Control questionnaire scales and measures of hypnotic susceptibility. Analysis of the combined questionnaire data yielded three replicated higher order factors: the familiar dimensions of Stability and Introversion and a third factor, Absorption. Absorption is interpreted as a disposition for having episodes of "total" attention that fully engage one's representational (i.e., perceptual, enactive, imaginative, and ideational) resources. This kind of attentional functioning is believed to result in a heightened sense of the reality of the attentional object, imperviousness to distracting events, and an altered sense of reality in general, including an empathically altered sense of self. Only Absorption was consistently correlated with hypnotizability. Absorption appears to be of interest for the study of hypnosis and personality.

One of the most important advances in the study of hypnosis has been the development of standardized and reliable measures of individual differences in hypnotic susceptibility. Scales of this kind, for example, the Stanford Hypnotic Susceptibility Scales (Weitzenhoffer & Hilgard, 1959, 1962), are direct measures of a subject's responsiveness to a series of specific suggestions. It is not surprising that psychologists have wanted to clarify the nature of hypnosis by investigating possible relations between these relatively stable but highly specific and circumscribed measures of susceptibility and broader dimensions of personality. Several such studies have appeared and have been reviewed fairly recently by Barber (1969)and Hilgard (1965).

For the present purpose, these past studies can be divided into two groups. In one group of studies existing inventories were used, on the whole with negative results. Scales from inventories such as the California Personality Inventory, the 16 Personality Factor Scale, Guilford-Zimmerman, Minnesota Multiphasic Personality Inventory, and the Maudsley Personality Inventory failed to show appreciable and consistent relations to hypnotic susceptibility. As Hilgard pointed out, the results of these studies suggest the possibility that these inventories do not adequately sample content areas that are related to susceptibility. In fact, there is growing evidence that purportedly multidimensional inventories, such as those just mentioned, are primarily saturated with two major dimensions (Block, 1965; Eysenck & Eysenck, 1969; Nichols & Schnell, 1963; Sells, Demaree, & Wills, 1971). Eysenck has labeled these two dimensions Stability versus Neuroticism and Introversion versus Extraversion. It appears, then, that hypnotic susceptibility might not be strongly related to either Stability or Introversion.

The second group of studies is more promising. In these studies special inventories were constructed consisting of items describing "hypnotic-like" experiences that occur in daily life or attitudes and tendencies that were thought to be specifically related to hypnotic "talent." The initial work was done by Shor (Shor, 1960; Shor, Orne, & O'Connell, 1962) and was followed up and extended by Ernest Hilgard's associates (e.g., Ås, 1963; Ås & Lauer, 1962; Ås, O'Hara, & Munger, 1962; Lee-Teng, 1965) and by others (e.g., Roberts & Tellegen, 1973). The

[1] This research was supported in part by National Institute of Mental Health Grant MH 18856-03.

[2] Requests for reprints should be sent to Auke Tellegen, Department of Psychology, Elliott Hall, University of Minnesota, Minneapolis, Minnesota 55455.

measures in question were analyzed on the level of either items or scales, and in several of these studies the relation to measures of susceptibility was directly investigated. The results were generally positive, if not without exception (Barber & Calverley, 1965).

As a result of these investigations, valuable information was obtained regarding characteristics related to hypnotizability. However, the findings resulting from these studies remain tentative and are for several reasons in need of further clarification. For example, the analyses were not conducted within the context of known major personality dimensions as reference variables. Each of the studies in question is also subject to several of the following limitations: a restricted item pool, a small number of subjects, reliance on a priori scales rather than on scales derived from an empirical dimensional analysis of the items, inclusion in the same dimensional analysis of variables representing different methods (producing results dominated by method dimensions), and failure to cross-validate.

These considerations suggested that a further investigation should address itself to the following three interrelated questions: First, how many and what kind of primary dimensions are present in a pool of items thought to be related to hypnotic susceptibility and representing a broad range of content? Second, how are these primary dimensions related to already established major or higher order dimensions of personality: Will the former be subsumed by the latter, or will one or more new major dimensions emerge? Third, having confirmed a final set of major dimensions, what is the relation between each of these and hypnotic susceptibility?

METHOD

Measures

***Research questionnaire** (Q3)*. A 71-item, self-report questionnaire was assembled (which will be referred to as Q3) covering a wide range of content. Thirty of the items were taken from Lee-Teng (Lee, 1963; Lee-Teng, 1965), who had borrowed many of her items from Shor (1960) and Ås (e.g., Ås, O'Hara, & Munger, 1962). The selected items had either been found to be related individually to hypnotic susceptibility (Ås, 1963) or to belong to scales showing that relationship (Lee-Teng, 1965). To conform to the format of Q3, these 30 items were reworded from "you" questions into declarative "I" statements. Several items were further changed so as to refer to a *disposition* (as did most of the other Q3 items) rather than to a particular *incident* in the subject's past. Some items were also shortened. Another 18 items were chosen from a previously constructed "Trust Rating Scale" (Roberts & Tellegen, 1973) on the basis of individual correlations with hypnotic susceptibility. These 18 items are the only ones written in the form of an adjective followed by a parenthetical defining sentence, for example, "ALOOF (maintains distance between self and others)." The remaining 23 items were new.

Q3 was considered to represent at least the following five content areas: Absorption, Dissociation, Trust, Impulsiveness, and Relaxation. Any item, however, that seemed promising was included whether or not it could be assigned unequivocally to a particular category. Q3, then, was not designed to measure a fixed set of a priori dimensions. On the contrary, its internal structure was to be an object of exploratory analysis. The results of this analysis are presented in the Results section of this paper, at which point the content of the questionnaire is presented in more detail.

Measures of stability–neuroticism and introversion–extroversion. Recently, Block (1965) published what is probably the most intensive validation study in this country of measures of the stability and introversion dimensions which he renamed Ego Resiliency and Ego Control, respectively. Twenty items were selected from Block's pool of Ego Resiliency items to form a Stability–Neuroticism scale. Items with extreme endorsement frequencies or with content likely to elicit objections (Butcher & Tellegen, 1966) were avoided.

In two samples to be reported in the present paper the Ego Resiliency scale had alpha reliability coefficients of .58 and .59, respectively. A 20-item Ego Control or Introversion–Extraversion scale was assembled in the same way, and its reliability in the same two samples was .78 and .71, respectively. These reliabilities, while rather low for individual measurement, were satisfactory for purposes of dimensional analysis.

Group Scales of Hypnotic Susceptibility (GSHS and GSHS-A). The GSHS is a modified version of the Harvard Group Scale of Hypnotic Susceptibility (Shor & Orne, 1962) and is described in detail by Roberts and Tellegen (1973). The GSHS, like the Harvard Scale, is a standard hypnotic induction procedure which may be administered to several individuals simultaneously (between 20 and 40 in the present investigation). The GSHS was used in one of the samples, while the GSHS-A (Atkinson, 1971) was used in another sample. The total scores derived from these two scales had identical compositions, with the exception that one of the GSHS motoric items was replaced in the GSHS-A by two hypnotic dream items. A further difference was the use of a tape-recorded induction with the GSHS-A, whereas the GSHS induction was done in person.

The alpha coefficients of the total score were .89 and .88, respectively, for the GSHS and GSHS-A. In a subsample of 40 subjects a correlation of .80 was obtained between GSHS total score and scores based on behavior ratings made by an independent observer during administration of the scale.

Measure of hypnotic depth. Field (1965) developed a self-report Hypnotic Depth Scale which allows the subject to itemize in detail the subjective changes that took place during a preceding hypnotic session. The scale consists of those 38 items, out of an initial 300-item pool, which correlated highest with hypnotic susceptibility.

While a subsequent factor analysis of the 38 items (Field & Palmer, 1969) suggested that four factors could be distinguished, the same data also indicated the presence of a substantial general factor. The Field scale was administered to one of our subsamples. The correlations among the four factor scales were all high (about .60) and were, therefore, combined in one overall Hypnotic Depth score. Only the overall score, which had an alpha coefficient of .92, is reported.

Subjects

The subjects were female undergraduate college students enrolled in the introductory psychology course who volunteered to participate for course credits. A total of 481 subjects took part in the studies to be reported.

For purposes of analysis and presentation, different groups of subjects must be distinguished to whom different sets of measures were administered. All 481 subjects completed Q3, and they are referred to as the total sample. One subgroup of 142 subjects, to be called Sample 1, completed in addition to Q3 the Ego Resiliency and Ego Control scales, the GSHS, and the Hypnotic Depth Scale. A second subgroup of 171 subjects, Sample 2, were given Q3, the Ego Resiliency and Ego Control scales, and the GSHS-A.

RESULTS

Identification of Primary Factors in Q3: Construction of Factor Scales

The first analysis was conducted in order to replace the original 71 items of Q3 by a smaller number of homogeneous scales, each representing an empirically defined "primary factor." The 71 items were factor analyzed in the total sample by the method of principal axes, using squared multiple correlations as communality estimates. The first 13 principal axes, which accounted for 99% of the common variance, were rotated to a normal varimax solution. An alternative set of 13 rotated varimax factors was obtained using unities in the diagonal. This set proved to be very similar to the first set but could be subsumed slightly better under the five a priori categories and was adopted for purposes of constructing the primary factor scales.

The primary factor scales consisted of unweighted items assembled by assigning each item to one factor scale according to its highest loading, provided that this loading exceeded .30. Two of the resulting scales were discarded, one because its content defied interpretation, the other because it consisted of only two items. The 11 remaining primary factor scales had coherent and distinct contents and acceptable internal consistencies. The alpha reliability coefficients ranging between .48 and .74 in Sample 1 and between .53 and .80 in Sample 2 are shown in Table 1.

Before reporting their use in subsequent analyses, all scales are identified, and at least one item from each scale is reproduced. The 11 factor scales obviously represent a more detailed breakdown of the content of Q3 than the one provided by the five a priori categories. The classifications are nevertheless related, and each a priori category is used as a heading for the scale or scales that primarily emerged from its items.

Absorption

Scale 1: Reality Absorption (a tendency to become immersed in movies, acting, nature, voices, past events, etc.):

The sound of a voice can be so fascinating to me that I can just go on listening to it.

While acting in a play, I have sometimes really felt the emotions of the character and have "become" him (her) for the time being, forgetting, as it were, both myself and the audience.

I can sometimes recollect certain past experiences in my life with such clarity and vividness that it is like living them again or almost so.

Scale 2: Fantasy Absorption:

If I wish, I can imagine (or daydream) some things so vividly that they hold my attention in the way a good movie or story does.

I can tell a story with elaborations to make it sound better and then have the elaboration seem as real to me as the actual incident, or almost so.

I am sometimes able to forget about my present self and get absorbed in a fantasy that I am someone else.

Dissociation

Scale 3: Dissociation:

If I wish, I can imagine that my body is so heavy that I could not move it if I wanted to.

Scale 4: Sleep Automatism:

I know that at some time I have walked in my sleep.

Trust

Scale 5: Openness to Experience:

I enjoy—or would enjoy—getting beyond the world of logic and reason to experience something new and different.

Scale 6: Devotion and Trust:

It gives me—or would give me—deep satisfaction to devote myself to someone I care about.

TRUSTING (generally believes in other people's good intentions; is not afraid of having to depend upon others).

Scale 7: Autonomy-Skepticism. (Items decribe an opposite of "Trust.")

I would much rather stick to my own ideas than be guided by others.

SKEPTICAL (tends to have persistent intellectual doubts about claims and assertions made by others).

Scale 8: Optimism-Placidity:

OPTIMISTIC (has faith in the future).

Regardless of what happens around me, I stay and feel pretty much the same.

Scale 9: Aloofness-Reserve (another opposite of "Trust."):

I prefer not to "open up" much, not even to friends, but to maintain a certain distance.

Impulsiveness versus Control

Scale 10: Caution vs. Impulsiveness:

When faced with a decision I usually ponder and weigh all aspects carefully.

Relaxation

Scale 11: Relaxation:

When I want to take a nap during the day I can make myself go to sleep in very little time.

Identification of Major Factors in Q3

The purpose of the next analysis was to identify the more inclusive or higher order dimensions of our questionnaire by means of a factor analysis of the 13 scales now available, that is, the 11 primary factor scales and the Ego Resiliency and Ego Control scales. (It may be useful to point out that the 11 primary factor scales, while derived from orthogonal factor analysis, are not necessarily uncorrelated. While each item was assigned to a scale representing a particular primary factor because its highest loading was on that factor, it was allowed to have nontrivial secondary loadings on other factors as well. Consistent patterns of secondary loadings could give rise to substantial correlations between primary factor scales and thus reveal a higher order structure.)

The 13 scales were analyzed separately in Samples 1 and 2. Using squared multiple correlations as communality estimates, three principal axes were found to account for approximately 100% of the common variance in both samples. Normal varimax rotations were carried out and the results are presented in Table 1. The table shows that the rotated factors are highly similar in the two samples. The factor tables, moreover, exhibit an almost ideal simple structure, with each variable having a high loading on one factor only.

As for the interpretation of the three factors, two are familiar ones. One, the second one listed in Table 1, shows salient loadings on Block's Ego Resiliency scale as well as on the Optimism and Relaxation scales and clearly represents the Stability dimension. The third factor in Table 1 is characterized by salient loadings on Block's Ego Control scale and on the Aloofness and Caution scales, identifying it as the Introversion dimension. Inclusion of the Ego Resiliency and Ego Control scales as markers enabled us, therefore, to subsume 4 of the 11 Q3 scales under familiar constructs.

The remaining Q3 scales identify a third major factor, the largest one in the present analysis and appearing first in Table 1. The scales with the highest loadings in both samples on this factor are Reality Absorption, Fantasy Absorption, Dissociation, and Openness to Experience, with Devotion-Trust and Autonomy-Criticality showing somewhat lower salient loadings. We labeled this factor "Openness to Absorbing and Self-Altering Experiences" or "Absorption."

TABLE 1

VARIMAX FACTOR MATRICES BASED ON THIRTEEN BASIC SCALES ANALYZED SEPARATELY IN TWO SAMPLES

Scale	Factors in Sample 1					Factors in Sample 2				
	I	II	III	h^2	alpha	I	II	III	h^2	alpha
1. Reality Absorption	75	—	—	60	67	73	—	—	54	69
2. Fantasy Absorption	69	—	—	50	68	62	—	—	47	67
3. Dissociation	58	—	—	34	66	56	—	—	31	48
5. Openness to Experience	57	—	—	50	63	51	—	—	44	74
6. Devotion-Trust	41	—	—	19	48	52	—	—	29	62
7. Autonomy-Criticality	45	—	—	22	51	38	—	—	18	51
4. Sleep Automatism	—	—	—	11	56	37	—	—	15	68
8. Optimism-Placidity	—	66	—	46	63	—	65	—	43	66
11. Relaxation	—	50	—	27	58	—	48	—	25	51
Ego Resilience	—	56	—	48	58	—	62	—	43	59
9. Aloofness-Reserve	—	—	64	43	79	—	—	62	42	72
10. Caution vs. Impulsiveness	—	—	54	30	70	—	—	55	31	68
Ego Control	—	—	64	53	78	—	—	64	52	71
Factor Contribution	2.34	1.22	1.36	4.91		2.12	1.31	1.32	4.75	

Note. Decimals are omitted from factor loadings and communalities. Loadings smaller than .35 in absolute value are not listed. Alpha = alpha coefficient of reliability. *N* for Sample 1 = 142; *N* for Sample 2 = 171.

RELATIONS BETWEEN *Q3* AND HYPNOTIC SUSCEPTIBILITY

The relations between the three major questionnaire factors and hypnotic susceptibility were analyzed. Factor scores were computed for each of the three major factors by means of multiple regression estimates which combined the 13 questionnaire scales in appropriately weighted composites. Separate sets of regression formulas were derived from Samples 1 and 2.

For purposes of comparison, we also present results obtained with criterion-based or "empirical" questionnaire predictors of hypnotizability. These measures were developed in two ways. One approach involved a traditional item analysis. Q3 items correlating .20 or higher with hypnotic susceptibility were combined without special weights into a scale. Separate scales were developed in Samples 1 and 2. The second method involved developing multiple regression equations predicting hypnotic susceptibility from the 11 primary factor scales. Again, two formulas were derived separately in the two samples. All factorial and empirical measures were correlated with hypnotic susceptibility in both samples. In other words, factor scores and scores on the criterion-based measures were not only computed and correlated with hypnotizability in the derivation sample but were also cross-validated in the other sample.

The results are presented in Table 2. The table shows correlations with the hypnotic susceptibility scales in Samples 1 and 2 and with Field's Hypnotic Depth Inventory in Sample 1. The correlations show a clear pattern. Of the three factor scores, only Absorption shows positive correlations (of .27, .42 and .43, respectively) with indicators of hypnotizability.

Interestingly, the two kinds of criterion-based measures, which were specifically designed to predict hypnotic susceptibility, were on cross-validation *not* superior to the Absorption factor measure. The possibility still existed that the criterion-based measures predicted a component of hypnotic susceptibility *differing* from the one predicted by Absorption. This possibility was investigated by computing from the available cross-validation results partial correlations between the two-criterion based measures and all three measures of hypnotizability, with the contribution of Absorption partialed out. The mean partial correlation in the two samples was .02. Thus the unique contribution of the criterion-based measures proved negligible and Absorption, by the same token, proved sufficient for representing those individual differences tapped by

Q3 that were related to hypnotic susceptibility. It may also be noted that the correlations involving the criterion-based measures show the expected shrinkage relative to the correlations in the derivation samples. Since the factor estimates, on the other hand, are not criterion based, they do not show such correlational shrinkage.

Finally, two 20-item scales (about the same length as the empirical scales) were constructed using items which did not belong to the Absorption group and which were all keyed in the affirmative direction. In both samples the two scales were correlated with the hypnotizability measures. The mean correlation was .11, showing that the relationship between responses to Q3 items and hypnotic susceptibility cannot be attributed simply to variations in "acquiescence," that is, a general and relatively indiscriminate tendency to endorse items of varied content.

Conclusions and Discussion

Relative to the investigations referred to earlier (e.g., Ås & Lauer, 1962; Ås, O'Hara, & Munger, 1962; Lee-Teng, 1965), the present findings appear to provide an extension and clarification. For example, in Lee-Teng's study, it was found that three out of five a priori scales correlated significantly with hypnotic susceptibility. Items belonging to these scales were incorporated in our questionnaire; thus it could be determined that Lee-Teng's Role-Playing, Trancelike Experiences, and Impulsivity scales contained several items representing aspects of Absorption. Lee-Teng's Impulsivity scale, on the other hand, also contained a number of Caution versus Impulsiveness items, now identified as belonging to the Introversion dimension.

It is of particular interest that our questionnaire, while covering a wide range of content drawn from various sources, yielded, nevertheless, only one major dimension other than Stability and Introversion. This dimension, Absorption, encompasses a substantial portion of Q3's varied content; it exemplifies the combination of *substantive divergence* and *structural convergence* that is suggestive of a major dimension or, in Eysenck's terms, a "combinatorial" trait (Eysenck & Eysenck, 1969).

How should the Absorption factor be interpreted? Some tentative notions are here proposed which we hope will have some heuristic value and which are based on the item content of scales with salient Absorption loadings. Our working assumption is that item responses often represent essentially correct self-descriptions; the status of this assumption appears to have improved of late (e.g.,

TABLE 2

Correlations of Factor Measures and Criterion-Based Measures with Hypnotizability

Item	Sample 1		Sample 2
	Hypnotic Susceptibility	Hypnotic Depth	Hypnotic Susceptibility
Factor measures			
I: Absorption	27*	42**	43**
	(27)	(41)	(42)
II: Stability	13	16	−02
	(16)	(20)	(−05)
III: Introversion	−14	−03	−18
	(−14)	(−06)	(−16)
Criterion-based measures			
Item composite	29**	39**	37**
	(51)	(55)	(51)
Scale composite	29**	39**	35**
	(42)	(48)	(49)

Note. Decimals are omitted from the correlation coefficients. The correlations observed in the derivation sample are listed in parentheses underneath the correlations in the cross-validation sample. N for Sample 1 = 142; N for Sample 2 = 171.
* $p < .01$.
** $p < .001$.

Hase & Goldberg, 1967; Jackson, 1971; Payne & Wiggins, 1972).

Our point of departure is the frequent reference of Absorption items to episodes of a special attentional object relationship which can be described by such terms as "absorption" and "fascination." These terms suggest a state of "total attention" during which the available representational apparatus seems to be entirely dedicated to experiencing and modeling the attentional object, be it a landscape, a human being, a sound, a remembered incident, or an aspect of one's self.

Phenomena of this kind, while apparently overlooked by contemporary academic treatments of attention, perception, and memory, have been described and discussed widely in literature on meditation, expanded awareness, peak experiences, mysticism, esthetic experience, regression in the serivce of the ego, altered states of consciousness, and in the literature on drug effects. For example, Maslow (1968) spoke of the "fascination" and "complete absorption" that characterize peak experiences. Schachtel (1959), to whom Maslow refers, described the "allocentric" perceptual mode as involving "totality of interest [p. 221]," and openness to the object in all its aspects with all one's senses, including one's kinesthetic experience. We suggest, in a similar vein, that the attention described in Absorption items is a "total" attention, involving a *full commitment of available perceptual, motoric, imaginative and ideational resources to a unified representation of the attentional object.*

If we consider this kind of attentional process to be at the core of Absorption, then the following phenomena might be seen as inherent correlates:

A Heightened Sense of the Reality of the Attentional Object

Even when the attentional object is constructed from memory, it is experienced as present and real. It is assumed that an already fully engaged representational system cannot, in addition to representations of the focal object, maintain salient qualifying "meta-cognitions," that is, thoughts *about* the primary representation, such as "this is only my imagination" or "this is not really happening."

Imperviousness to Normally Distracting Events

The absorbed individual often seems not to notice external events that would normally draw attention. This too could be seen as inherent to having an already fully committed representational system.

An Altered Sense of Reality in General and of the Self in Particular

Absorbed attention is highly "centered" (in a roughly Piagetian sense) and amplifies greatly the experience of one part of reality, while other aspects recede from awareness. Consequently, the vivid subjective reality experienced during episodes of absorbed attention may well, in retrospect, during more "decentered" normal states of wakefulness, impress one as "altered," "unreal," or "imaginary."

It should, perhaps, be noted that in at least one interpretation of imagination, namely Sartre's classical phenomenological study (Sartre, 1940; see also Spiegelberg, 1969, v. II) the element of unreality is treated as a core feature. According to Sartre the imaginative attitude poses its object under a negative aspect, as, for example, *not* here or *not* existing, or, using the word that later became central in his philosophy, as a "nothing." Thus the imaginative attitude as defined by Sartre involves precisely those negating metacognitions that are incompatible with absorbed attention, even if it is directed to a memory object. It would seem, then, that Sartre's concept of imagination has more in common with a retrospective sense of altered reality of the kind just described than with absorbed imagination.

If some aspect of the *self,* for example, one's breathing or the weight of one's hand, happened to be the object of immersed attention, then an *alteration of self* could take place and be experienced as such in retrospect. (Here and throughout we are referring to the "self-as-object," a region of one's constructed reality, rather than to the "self-as-process" [cf. Hall & Lindzey, 1970].) If there is a marked discontinuity between the usual self and the self during an episode of absorbed concentration on some aspect of the self, then we may, indeed, speak of a "dissociative experience" of the kind suggested by several of the Fantasy Absorption and Dissociation items.

Absorbed attention can also result in an altered self when the attentional object is *someone else*. Full representation of someone else's activities and experiences often involves the enactive or "body-english" component of absorbed attention. The resulting kinesthetic feedback enhances empathic participation and an experience of equivalence of the attentional object and one's self. This identification with the object, in turn, implies a temporary alteration of one's usual self of the kind described in some Reality Absorption and Fantasy Absorption items.

One might add that self-altering identifications appear to be possible with a very wide range of animate and inanimate things and that their occurrence may not be entirely dependent on enactive representation. Objects of absorbed attention acquire an importance and intimacy that are normally reserved for the self and may, therefore, acquire a temporary self-like quality. These object identifications have mystical overtones. And, indeed, one would expect high-absorption persons to have an affinity for mystical experience, even if true *unio mystica* is, itself, a rare attainment.

These varied phenomena are seen as *state*-like manifestations of the cognitive-motivational *trait* Absorption. The *cognitive* component of this trait appears to include the ability to operate diverse representational modalities synergistically so that a full but unified experience is realized. This imaginative and integrative aspect is, perhaps, captured by the term "syngnosia," (analogous to "synesthesia" which may be one of its components). It is reminiscent of the Freudian mechanism of "condensation" and may be an important ingredient of creativity, particularly image-oriented, artistic creativity.

Another cognitive aspect involves the empathic quality and versatility of the representations of high-Absorption persons. It seems plausible that this ability to realize diverse states of being could be cultivated and elaborated into role-playing skills in the more specific interpersonal and theatrical sense.

The *motivational-affective* component would seem to consist in a sentient and tolerant "openness to experience" (Fitzgerald, 1966), a desire and readiness for object relationships, temporary or lasting, that permit experiences of deep involvement. The content of several Absorption markers, including the Openness to Experience and Devotion-Trust scales, is suggestive in this respect.

While absorbed attention is in itself unreserved and "wholehearted," Absorption also reflects a distinctive cognitive style and may generate unconventional and idiosyncratic appraisals. For this reason, high-Absorption persons may feel the need for cognitive independence that is reflected in one other variable with low but consistent Absorption loadings, the Autonomy-Skepticism scale.

Finally, a valid conception of Absorption cannot contradict its independence of Stability (or Ego Resiliency) and Introversion (or Ego Control). Whether endowed with much or little Absorption, a person may either show the adaptability of Block's Ego Resilient subjects or the vulnerability to stress associated with low Resiliency. Similarly, he may exhibit the restraint and reflectiveness characteristic of high Ego Control or the impulsiveness Block found associated with low Ego Control (Block, 1965).

Of the three dimensions, Stability, Introversion, and Absorption, only Absorption is consistently associated with hypnotic susceptibility. The strength of this association is only modest and would of course have been greater had the present Absorption measure and the hypnotic susceptibility scales only reflected the capacity for absorbed attention. However, method factors undoubtedly affect both kinds of measures and attenuate the relations between them (e.g., Lee-Teng, 1965). The assessment of Absorption can undoubtedly be improved by developing additional methods. Efforts in that direction are presently underway. As for measures of hypnotic susceptibility, these indicators, too, surely reflect more than a capacity for absorbed attention. In the case of the usual hypnotic phenomena the hypnotic "essence" is, according to Orne (1959), partially obscured by various "artifacts" such as the response to demand characteristics. The influence of such factors has also been documented by Barber and his co-workers (e.g., Barber, 1969). Even if Absorption belongs to the essence of hypnotic susceptibility, nonhypnotic artifacts would attenuate the relationship between the present measures of the two.

The present data are, nevertheless, clear enough to indicate that hypnotic performance, in part, reflects the trait Absorption. To some extent, then, it is possible to view hypnotic phenomena as experiential and behavioral manifestations of a certain kind of thought process, namely, the imaginative, enactive, and self-altering representation of an attentional object. For example, the immobilization of an arm following a suggestion that it is stiff and rigid or chasing a fly in response to the suggestion that one is buzzing around annoyingly could be explained as the observable manifestations of an imaginative and enactive thought process by which the subject fully immerses himself in the representation of a rigid arm or of his annoyance over a bothersome insect. In these cases, at least to the extent that they are expressions of Absorption, there is no direct compliance with explicit or implicit demands to act in a certain way; there is compliance only with respect to the choice of attentional object.

Thus we conclude that Absorption, interpreted as a capacity for absorbed and self-altering attention, represents an essential component of hypnotic susceptibility. The literature on hypnosis, in fact, often refers to hypnotic characteristics which have an affinity with aspects of Absorption. A few illustrative examples are cited briefly. White has elaborated Braid's concept of mono-ideism (see Sarbin, 1950), a concept reminiscent of the centering of attention which we have associated with Absorption. Hilgard (1965) has assigned a central role to dissociation in the explanation of hypnosis, and, as suggested earlier, some such concept appears also to be intrinsic to Absorption. Sarbin's interpretation of hypnosis in terms of imaginative skills or capacity for organismic involvement (e.g., Sarbin, 1950; Sarbin & Coe, 1972) again refers to an important aspect of Absorption. Recently, Barber and DeMoor (1972) and Spanos (1971) have likewise emphasized goal-motivated fantasy as an important aspect of hypnosis. Shor's (1962) concepts of depth of role-taking involvement, depth of trance, and depth of archaic involvement would seem to have approximate counterparts in the Absorption facets of, respectively, enactive representation, heightened sense of reality, and devotion-trust.

Most directly pertinent to the present findings, however, is the intensive interview study by Josephine Hilgard (1970). Hilgard documented the occurrence among her subjects of deep involvements in a variety of experiences and activities and advances the concept of "imaginative involvement." The nature of the involvements of Hilgard's subjects corresponds to the content of the Absorption factor, particularly that of its two strongest markers, the Reality Absorption and Fantasy Absorption scales. Hilgard, furthermore, found the frequency of involvements to be related to hypnotic susceptibility, just as we found to be the case for Absorption. Her findings, then, are clearly supported by the present trait-oriented psychometric investigation.

In general, the manifestations of Absorption appear to encompass in one covariational structure several of the features emphasized in different conceptions relating to hypnosis. Continued study of this trait should prove fruitful for the study of both personality and hypnosis.

REFERENCES

Ås, A. Hypnotizability as a function of nonhypnotic experiences. *Journal of Abnormal and Social Psychology,* 1963, **66**, 142–150.

Ås, A., & Lauer, L. W. A factor analytic study of hypnotizability and related personal experiences. *International Journal of Clinical and Experimental Hypnosis,* 1962, **10**, 169–181.

Ås, A., O'Hara, J. W., & Munger, M. P. The measurement of subjective experiences presumably related to hypnotic susceptibility. *Scandinavian Journal of Psychology,* 1962, **3**, 47–64.

Atkinson, G. A. Personality and hypnotic cognition. Unpublished doctoral dissertation, University of Minnesota, 1971.

Barber, T. X. *Hypnosis: A scientific approach.* New York: Van Nostrand Reinhold, 1969.

Barber, T. X., & Calverley, D. S. Hypnotizability, suggestibility, and personality. II. Assessment of previous imaginative-fantasy experiences by the Ås, Barber-Glass, and Shor questionnaires. *Journal of Clinical Psychology,* 1965, **21**, 57–58.

Barber, T. X., & DeMoor, W. A theory of hypnotic induction procedures. *American Journal of Clinical Hypnosis,* 1972, **15**, 112–135.

Block, J. *The challenge of response sets.* New York: Appleton-Century-Crofts, 1965.

Butcher, J. N., & Tellegen, A. Objections to MMPI items. *Journal of Consulting Psychology,* 1966, **30**, 527–534.

Eysenck, H. J., & Eysenck, S. B. G. *Personality structure and measurement.* San Diego, Calif.: Knapp, 1969.

Field, P. B. An inventory scale of hypnotic depth. *International Journal of Clinical and Experimental Hypnosis,* 1965, **13**, 238–249.

Field, P. B., & Palmer, R. D. Factor analysis: Hypnosis inventory. *International Journal of Clinical and Experimental Hypnosis,* 1969, **17**, 50–61.

Fitzgerald, E. T. Measurement of openness to experience; a study of regression in the service of the ego. *Journal of Personality and Social Psychology,* 1966, **4**, 655–663.

Hall, C. S., & Lindzey, G. *Theories of personality.* New York: Wiley, 1970.

Hase, H. D., & Goldberg, L. R. The comparative validity of different strategies of deriving personality inventory scales. *Psychological Bulletin,* 1967, **67**, 231–248.

Hilgard, E. R. *Hypnotic susceptibility.* New York: Harcourt, Brace & World, 1965.

Hilgard, J. R. *Personality and hypnosis: A study of imaginative involvement.* Chicago: University of Chicago Press, 1970.

Jackson, D. N. The dynamics of structured personality tests: 1971. *Psychological Review,* 1971, **78**, 229–248.

Lee, E. M. A questionnaire measure of hypnotic characteristics and their relationship to hypnotizability. Unpublished doctoral dissertation, Stanford University, 1963.

Lee-Teng, E. Trance-susceptibility, induction-susceptibility, and acquiescence as factors in hypnotic performance. *Journal of Abnormal Psychology,* 1965, **70**, 383–389.

Maslow, A. H. *Toward a psychology of being.* (2nd ed.) Princeton: Van Nostrand, 1968.

Nichols, R. C., & Schnell, R. R. Factor scales for the California Psychological Inventory. *Journal of Consulting Psychology,* 1963, **27**, 228–235.

Orne, M. T. The nature of hypnosis: Artifact and essence. *Journal of Abnormal and Social Psychology,* 1959, **58**, 277–299.

Payne, F. D., & Wiggins, J. S. MMPI profile types and the self-report of psychiatric patients. *Journal of Abnormal Psychology,* 1972, **79**, 1–8.

Roberts, A. H., & Tellegen, A. Ratings of "trust" and hypnotic susceptibility. *International Journal of Clinical and Experimental Hypnosis,* 1973, **21**, 289–297.

Sarbin, T. R. Contributions to role-taking theory: I. Hypnotic behavior. *Psychological Review,* 1950, **57**, 255–270.

Sarbin, T. R., & Coe, W. C. *Hypnosis: A social psychological analysis of influence communication.* New York: Holt, Rinehart & Winston, 1972.

Sartre, J-P. *L'imaginaire.* Paris: Gallimard, 1940.

Schachtel, E. G. *Metamorphosis: On the development of affect, perception, attention, and memory.* New York: Basic Books, 1959.

Sells, S. B., Demaree, R. G., & Wills, D. P., Jr. Dimensions of personality: II. Separate factor structures in Guilford and Cattell Trait Markers. *Multivariate Behavioral Research,* 1971, **6**, 135–185.

Shor, R. E. The frequency of naturally occurring "hypnotic-like" experiences in the normal college population. *International Journal of Clinical and Experimental Hypnosis,* 1960, **8**, 151–163.

Shor, R. E. Three dimensions of hypnotic depth. *International Journal of Clinical and Experimental Hypnosis,* 1962, **10**, 23–28.

Shor, R. E., & Orne, E. C. Harvard Group Scale of Hypnotic Susceptibility. Palo Alto, Calif.: Consulting Psychologists Press, 1962.

Shor, R. E., Orne, M. T., O'Connell, D. N. Validation and cross-validation of a scale of self-reported personal experiences which predict hypnotizability. *Journal of Psychology,* 1962, **53**, 55–75.

Spanos, N. P. Goal-directed fantasy and the performance of hypnotic test suggestions. *Psychiatry,* 1971, **34**, 86–96.

Spiegelberg, H. *The phenomenological movement: A historical introduction.* (2nd ed.) The Hague: Martinus Nyhoff, 1969.

Weitzenhoffer, A. M., & Hilgard, E. R. *Stanford Hypnotic Susceptibility Scale, Forms A and B.* Palo Alto, Calif.: Consulting Psychologists Press, 1959.

Weitzenhoffer, A. M., & Hilgard, E. R. *Stanford Hypnotic Susceptibility Scale, Form C.* Palo Alto, Calif.: Consulting Psychologists Press, 1962.

(Received September 12, 1973)

[13]

A Social-Cognitive Skills Approach to the Successful Modification of Hypnotic Susceptibility

Donald R. Gorassini and Nicholas P. Spanos
Carleton University

Subjects low and medium in hypnotic susceptibility were administered cognitive strategy and instructional set information and also practiced responding to test suggestions in order to enhance susceptibility. Those in one modification treatment received this information both from the experimenter and by observing a videotaped female model who responded successfully to suggestions and reported on the cognitive strategies she used to do so. Those in a second modification treatment received the information and practice but were not exposed to the model. Low and medium susceptibles in a third condition (practice alone) received a hypnotic induction procedure and practice suggestions but neither modification information nor modeling. No-treatment controls performed a filler task. All subjects were posttested on two different susceptibility scales. Information plus modeling produced significantly greater increments on all objective and subjective indices of susceptibility on both posttests than did practice-alone or control treatments. Susceptibility increments in the information without model treatment always fell between those of the model and practice-alone treatments. In the modeling treatment, over half of the initial low susceptibles and over two thirds of the initial medium susceptibles scored as high susceptibles on both posttests. These findings provide strong support for a social-cognitive skill formulation of hypnotic susceptibility.

Hypnotic susceptibility is conceptualized by some investigators as a relatively stable traitlike attribute (Bowers, 1976; Hilgard, 1975; Perry, 1977) and by others as involving a relatively modifiable interrelated set of social-cognitive skills and attitudes (Barber, 1969; Barber, Spanos, & Chaves, 1974; Diamond, 1972, 1974, 1977a; Katz, 1979; Sachs, 1971; Sarbin & Coe, 1972; Spanos, 1982). Both groups of investigators have attempted to buttress their respective theoretical positions by variously interpreting the findings of the same studies. These studies indicate that hypnotic susceptibility can be enhanced to a statistically significant degree by a wide variety of social psychological manipulations (Comins, Fullam, & Barber, 1975; Cooper, Branford, Schubot, & Tart, 1967; Council, Kirsch, Vickery, & Carlson, 1983; Cronin, Spanos, & Barber, 1971; Diamond, 1972; Diamond, Steadman, Harada, & Rosenthal, 1975; Katz, 1979; Kinney & Sachs, 1974; Sachs & Anderson, 1967; Sanders & Reyher, 1969; Springer, Sachs, & Morrow, 1977; Tart, 1970).

Trait theorists who make reference to these studies emphasize that the obtained increments in susceptibility, although statistically significant, are frequently rather small (Bowers, 1976; Perry, 1977). Typically, these theorists (e.g., Perry, 1977) contend that susceptibility involves both a modifiable attitude component and a largely unmodifiable aptitude component. From this perspective, successful modification studies have enhanced subject's attitudes and, thereby, have allowed for a fuller expression of their aptitudes. Nevertheless, because hypnotic aptitude is, itself, largely unmodifiable, the gains produced by enhancing attitude have been (and necessarily will be) small.

For social-cognitive skill theorists, on the other hand, cognitiv strategies mediating responsiveness to suggestion, cognitive se concerning how suggestions are to be interpreted, and attitude about hypnotic responding are all modifiable as well as inte dependent (Barber et al., 1974; Diamond, 1977b). As pointe out by Diamond (1977a), modification studies that produce only small increments in susceptibility rarely focused directl on inculcating effective cognitive strategies, or even on changir hypnosis specific attitudes and expectations. Instead, they pr vided subjects with repeated individualized hypnotic testing e periences (As, Hilgard, & Weitzenhoffer, 1963; Cooper et al 1967), "personal growth" training (Tart, 1970), EEG biofeedbac (London, Cooper, & Engstron, 1974), and the like. From a co nitive skill perspective, it is not surprising that such trainir procedures were relatively ineffective. They were simply n aimed at directly influencing the most important determinan of hypnotic susceptibility. On the other hand, modification studi that focused on inculcating effective cognitive strategies and i terpretational sets as well as on positive attitudes and expectatic often produced rather substantial increments in susceptibili (Diamond, 1972; Kinney & Sachs, 1974; Sachs & Anderso 1967). Modification procedures were particularly effective wh they provided exposure to models who verbalized the strategi they used to respond successfully, and when they provided o portunities for practicing newly acquired cognitive skills (Di mond, 1972; Kinney & Sachs, 1974).[1]

This research was supported by a grant from the Social Sciences and Humanities Research Council of Canada. We thank Lorne D. Bertrand for critical comments on earlier versions of the article.

Correspondence concerning this article should be addressed to Nicholas P. Spanos, Department of Psychology, Carleton University, Ottawa, Ontario, Canada, K1S 5B6.

[1] Several studies (Simon & Salzberg, 1981; Wickramasekaera, 197 reported that electromyographic (EMG) feedback training for relaxati produced substantial increments in hypnotic susceptibility. Unfortunate other studies (Radtke, Spanos, Armstrong, Dillman, & Boisvenue, 19

The present study assessed the effectiveness of two cognitive behavior modification "treatment packages" for enhancing hypnotic susceptibility in subjects who pretested as either low or medium on this variable. As in previous successful modification studies, one component of these packages involved presenting positive information and allaying misconceptions about hypnosis. A second component emphasized the importance of becoming absorbed in imagining the "make-believe" situations described in suggestions (Spanos & Barber, 1974). These treatment packages also contained a third component that has not been strongly emphasized in previous modification studies: detailed information concerning how to interpret specific types of suggestions coupled with practicing responses to such suggestions. For subjects assigned to one of the treatment packages (i.e., no-model package), information concerning appropriate interpretations and appropriate cognitive strategies was provided by the experimenter. In the second treatment package condition, subjects received the same information from the experimenter and, in addition, were shown a videotaped female model who (a) responded to suggestions appropriately, (b) verbalized appropriate suggestion-related experiences as she responded and in a postexperimental videotaped interview, (c) reiterated her interpretation of suggested communications.

Interpretation information (or information plus model) was given immediately before the administration of each of four practice test suggestions. The suggestions called for arm levitation, arm rigidity, visual hallucination, and amnesia, and the information provided to subjects was specifically tailored to each type of suggestion. Following their response to the last practice suggestion, subjects were encouraged to generalize what they had just learned by responding without further information to four new practice suggestions. Following their treatment session (Session 2) subjects were administered two hypnotic susceptibility posttest sessions (Sessions 3 & 4). The effectiveness of the model and no-model modification packages were compared against two control treatments. During Session 2, subjects in a practice-alone treatment were administered an hypnotic induction procedure and eight practice suggestions, but no information aimed at changing their attitudes or their cognitive responses to suggestions. No-treatment control subjects simply filled out personality questionnaires during Session 2. Practice-alone and no-treatment control subjects were posttested in the same manner as those in the treatment package groups.

Our rationale for building detailed and explicit interpretational set information into the treatment packages was based on theorizing that emphasizes the complex and sometimes inconsistent nature of the communications that constitute test suggestions (Haley, 1958; Spanos, 1982; Spanos & Gorassini, 1984). Spanos (1982) argued that test suggestions are often ambiguous, and that differential response to them may, in part, reflect different ways of interpreting the communications they contain. For instance, the wording of many suggestions implies both (a) that the subject should do something to bring about the requisite effects (e.g., "try to forget") and (b) that the requisite effects will happen automatically without the subject's efforts (e.g., "the words will be gone, gone completely from your mind"). Thus, the same suggestion may be interpreted by subjects to mean either that they must actively bring about suggested effects (e.g., "do things to avoid remembering") or that no such activity is required (e.g., "don't do anything to forget, just wait passively for amnesia to happen"). Both interpretations are consistent with holding positive attitudes and expectations about hypnosis. Nevertheless, the two interpretations are likely to be associated with very different levels of amnesia.

In the present study the interpretations conveyed to subjects in the two treatment packages groups emphasized that responses to suggestion never "just happen," they must be enacted (Coe & Sarbin, 1977; Spanos, 1982). On the other hand, subjects were informed that enacted responses can be made to feel involuntary by becoming highly and consistently absorbed in "make-believe" situations that imply involuntariness (e.g., imagining that the arm is hollow and pumped up with helium; Spanos, 1971; Spanos, 1982). Subjects were further informed that challenges to counter suggested effects were not to be interpreted as requests to terminate absorption in the "make-believe" situation. Instead, the challenge was to be incorporated into and to reinforce the make-believe situation (e.g., to imagine that an iron lock keeps the arm stiff and, when challenged to bend it, to imagine that the lock is so strong that no amount of effort can break it).

Some modification studies (e.g., Cooper et al., 1967) have reported data only for overt suggestibility. However, a number of recent studies (Spanos, Radtke, Hodgins, Stam, & Bertrand, 1983c; Spanos, Rivers, & Ross, 1977) indicate that discrepancies between overt and subjective responses to suggestion are quite common. For this reason we assessed subjective as well as objective response to suggestion during pre- and posttesting.

Method

Subjects

One hundred and twenty Carleton University undergraduates (ages 18–25), who in group pretesting scored in the low (0–2) or medium (3–4) range on the objective dimension of the Carleton University Responsiveness to Suggestion Scale (CURSS:O; Spanos et al., 1983c), volunteered to participate in three additional testing sessions involving hypnosis. All subjects received course credit for their participation.

Procedure

Following the pretest session, subjects were randomly assigned to four conditions with the restriction of an equal number of initially low susceptibles ($N = 15$) and initially medium susceptibles in each condition. The four conditions were (a) behavior change information plus practice, (b) behavior change information and modeling plus practice, (c) practice alone, (d) no-treatment control. All treatments were administered individually by the same male experimenter in a single 1-hour session (Session 2).

Behavior change information plus practice. Following initial greetings, the subject was presented with tape-recorded information aimed at removing misconceptions about hypnosis and providing positive attitudes, motivations, and expectancies about hypnotic performance (e.g., hypnosis involves interesting and valuable cognitive skills). The positive information used was similar to that used by Cronin et al. (1971) and Diamond (1972). Interspersed with the positive information, hypnosis was depicted as in-

Spanos & Bertrand, 1985) have been unable to replicate these findings. Studies that used progressive relaxation training procedures in place of EMG biofeedback have consistently failed to find large increments in susceptibility (Radtke et al., 1983; Simon & Salzberg, 1981; Springer, Sachs, & Morrow, 1977).

volving the ability to absorb one's self deeply in make-believe, and absorption was described as a valuable skill that was rewarding to practice and to master.

In the next phase of their treatment, subjects were informed that they would practice responding to several test suggestions, the first of which was a suggestion for arm levitation. Before receiving this suggestion, however, they were given explicit information concerning how it was to be interpreted. For example:

> [The suggestion] will specifically tell you that your arm is like a hollow balloon being pumped up with helium . . . and that it's rising into the air by itself. In response . . . you must do everything that is required of someone making believe such a thing. You must lift your arm up and you must imagine that the arm is really a hollow balloon that is being pumped full of helium, rising by itself . . . You must become very deeply involved in the make-belive and actually make it seem real . . . Rivet your attention on the hollow arm, the lightness, the fact it's going up by itself and so on. Don't imagine anything or pay attention to anything that is unrelated to the make-believe situation. . . .

Following these instructions, subjects were administered the arm levitation suggestion. Each of the next three practice test suggestions was also preceded by interpretation information appropriate to it. Following their response to the fourth test suggestion, subjects completed two subjective experience questionnaires. The first questionnaire assessed the degree to which subjects had the subjective experiences called for by each suggestion (e.g., for arm levitation, the extent to which the arm felt light), and the second questionnaire assessed the extent to which the response called for was experienced as involuntary.

In the final phase, subjects were administered four new practice suggestions (arms moving apart, head heaviness, auditory hallucination, amnesia for previous suggestions). Overt and subjective responses to these were scored in the same manner as previously, but these suggestions were not preceded by interpretation information or followed by feedback. However, they were preceded by encouragement to generalize what had been previously learned.

Behavior change information, modeling, plus practice. The only difference between this treatment and the previous one was the addition of a videotaped model that subjects observed immediately before each of their first four practice suggestions. The model (a female in her early twenties) was described to subjects as someone who had been initially unresponsive to test suggestions, but who had learned the cognitive skills required to respond successfully. Each of the four videotaped segments was divided into two phases. During the first phase, the model responded to the practice suggestion the subject was about to receive. The model verbalized suggestion appropriate sensations and imaginings as she responded (e.g., "I can see the pump, I can feel the arm being pumped up. It's really light . . ."). During the second phase, the model was being interviewed postexperimentally about her experiences. The interview focused on and reinforced the model's appropriate interpretation of suggested requirements and the importance of her absorption in make-believe as a vehicle for experiencing suggested effects.

Practice-alone subjects. These subjects were administered a hypnotic induction procedure equated for length with the information presented to subjects in the behavior change groups. They were then administered the first four practice suggestions with interspersed "sleepy–drowsy" instructions, and were then administered the second four practice suggestions. After the last suggestion, subjects again responded to the two subjective experience questionnaires.

No-treatment control. Subjects in this group spent an hour responding to standardized personality inventories. They were informed that the study involved assessing relations between hypnotic susceptibility and personality.

Subjects in all conditions received their first posttest (Session 3) within one week of their treatment manipulation (Session 2). The last posttest (Session 4) was administered within one week of the first posttest. Subjects were pretested and posttested by experimenters other than the one who administered the treatment, and these experimenters were blind to subjects' treatment condition. The susceptibility scales used for pre- and posttesting were administered via tape recording to subjects in small groups.

Susceptibility Measures

On the pretest and also on the first of two posttests, hypnotic susceptibility was assessed with the Carleton University Responsiveness to Suggestion Scale (CURSS; Spanos et al., 1983c). The CURSS is a seven item scale that contains motor (e.g., arm levitation), challenge (e.g., arm rigidity), and cognitive (e.g., visual hallucination) suggestions. Test–retest stability for the CURSS is high (Spanos, Radtke, Hodgins, Bertrand, Stam, & Dubreuil, 1983a), and it correlates substantially with other standardized measures of hypnotic susceptibility (Spanos, Radtke, Hodgins, Bertrand, Stam, & Moretti, 1983b).

Following their response to all seven suggestions, subjects rated several aspects of their response to each suggestion. On the basis of these ratings, three CURSS suggestibility scores were derived for each subject. CURSS:O (objective) scores reflected the number of suggestions to which subjects made the appropriate overt response, and ranged from 0 (no suggestions "passed") to 7 (all suggestions "passed"). This dimension is self-scored in the same manner as the Harvard Group Scale of Hypnotic Susceptibility (HGSHS; Shor & Orne, 1962). CURSS:S (subjective) scores reflected the extent to which subjects had the subjective experiences called for by each suggestion. Each suggestion is associated with a four item subscale. For instance, the subscale for the arm levitation suggestion is as follows: During the suggestion my arm felt light: (a) not at all, (b) to a slight degree, (c) to a moderate degree, (d) to a great degree. Alternatives a through d are scored 0 through 3, respectively, and scores on the seven subscales are summed to yield a CURSS:S score that can range from 0 to 21.

After completing the CURSS:S response dimension, subjects rated the extent to which their response to each suggestion felt involuntary, for example, "During the suggestion my arm felt like it rose in the air by itself. I experienced this: (a) not at all, (b) to a slight degree, (c) to a moderate degree, (d) to a great degree." A CURSS:O-I (objective–involuntariness) score was obtained for each subject by combining objective and involuntariness ratings. Thus, a subject who "passed" a suggestion objectively *and* who chose Alternatives c or d on the above involuntariness subscale received one point on the CURSS:O-I scale. A subject who did not "pass" the suggestion using the objective criterion received a 0 for that suggestion on the O-I dimension regardless of his or her involuntariness ratings. Similarly, a subject who chose Alternatives a or b on the involuntariness scale received a zero O-I for that suggestion regardless of objective performance. In short, CURSS:O-I scores reflect the number of suggestions that were objectively "passed" *and* experienced as at least moderately involuntary. These scores range from 0 to 7.

For their second posttest session, subjects were administered a 10 item version of the Stanford Hypnotic Susceptibility Scale, Form C (SHSS:C; Weitzenhoffer & Hilgard, 1962) modified for group administration. On the modified scale the anosmia and negative hallucination items from the full 12 item version of the SHSS:C were dropped, and several items (age regression, dream, auditory hallucination, and amnesia) were altered to allow subjects to write rather than speak their answers. Following their response to the 10 test suggestions subjects scored the objective, subjective, and involuntariness aspects of their response to each suggestion using the subscale format just described for the CURSS. Thus, SHSS:C/O, SHSS:C/S, and SHSS:C/O-I scores were obtained for each subject.

Attitude Measure

Prior to the susceptibility pretest and again prior to each susceptibility posttest, subjects were administered a 14 item attitudes toward

Table 1

Means for Treatments × Pre/Posttest Interactions for the Objective (O), the Objective-Involuntariness (O–I), and the Subjective (S) Scales of the Carlton University Responsiveness to Suggestion Scale (CURSS)

Treatment	CURSS:O Pre	CURSS:O Post	CURSS:S Pre	CURSS:S Post	CURSS:O–I Pre	CURSS:O–I Post
Control						
M	2.17_a	1.47_a	5.73_a	5.53_a	$.83_a$	1.23_a
SD	1.34	1.61	2.94	4.20	1.05	1.48
Practice alone						
M	2.23_a	2.20_b	6.27_a	5.53_a	1.00_a	1.23_a
SD	1.41	1.63	2.94	4.26	1.17	1.57
Information no model						
M	2.40_a	4.40_c	7.37_a	9.37_b	1.47_a	1.73_a
SD	1.22	1.85	3.66	4.66	1.38	1.80
Information + Model						
M	2.30_a	5.27_d	6.17_a	11.20_b	$.90_a$	3.20_b
SD	1.32	1.71	3.91	6.21	1.09	2.70

Note. Within columns means sharing the same subscript fail to differ significantly at $\alpha = .05$.

hypnosis questionnaire. Each item was scored on a 7-point Likert-type subscale so that relatively high scores always indicated relatively more positive attitudes. A single attitude score was obtained for each subject by summing across the items.

Results

Pretest to Posttest 1 Changes

Changes from Pretest to Posttest 1 on CURSS:O scores for the four treatments were assessed with a 4 × 2 × 2 split plot analysis of variance (ANOVA). The four treatments and low/medium initial susceptibility were between-subjects factors, and the pre/posttest was a within-subjects factor. The Treatments × Pre/Posttest interaction was highly significant, $F(3, 112) = 33.60$, $p < .001$; and analyses of simple effects were conducted. The relevant means are shown in Table 1. The simple main effect of pre/posttest was significant in the model treatment, $F(1, 112) = 100.67$, $p < .001$, and in the information without model treatment, $F(1, 112) = 45.67$, $p < .001$. In both of these conditions, subjects showed much higher CURSS:O scores after the treatment than before it. The main effect of pre/posttest was nonsignificant in the practice-alone condition, but significant in the control condition, $F(1, 112) = 5.61$, $p < .05$. Practice-alone subjects showed no significant pretest to posttest change in CURSS:O scores, whereas controls showed a slight but significant decrease in these scores from pretest to posttest.

The simple main effect for treatments at the pretest did not approach significance, $F < 1$. However, the main effect for treatments on the posttest was highly significant, $F(3, 112) = 47.75$, $p < .001$. As indicated in Table 1, all four means differed significantly from one another. Subjects in the model treatment obtained the highest CURSS:O scores and controls obtained the lowest.

On the CURSS:O, high susceptibility is conventionally defined as a score of 5 or above (Spanos et al., 1983c). Table 2 shows the number of subjects in each treatment that scored as high susceptibles on Posttest 1. Only one initially low control subject and none of the initially low practice-alone subjects scored in the high susceptibility range on this posttest. On the other hand, the majority of initially low information plus model subjects scored as high susceptibles on Posttest 1.

A 4 × 2 × 2 ANOVA with the same independent variables as above was conducted on CURSS:S scores. The Treatment × Pre/Posttest interaction was again significant, and analyses of simple main effects were conducted. The relevant means are given in Table 1. Subjects given modeling, $F(1, 112) = 47.93$, $p < .001$, and those given information without modeling, $F(1, 112) = 7.57$, $p < .05$, showed significant pretest to posttest increments in CURSS:S scores. Practice-alone subjects and controls showed no significant pretest to posttest CURSS:S changes.

The simple main effect for treatments was not significant at the pretest, $F < 1$, but was highly significant at the posttest, $F(3, 112) = 10.30$, $p < .01$. Post hoc comparisons on the posttest means indicated that the model and information without model treatments failed to differ significantly from one another. However, both of these conditions showed significantly higher CURSS:S scores than did the practice-alone or control treatments. Subjects in the latter two treatments failed to differ from one another on CURSS:S scores.

A 4 × 2 × 2 ANOVA on CURSS:O-I scores also yielded a significant Treatment × Pre/Posttest interaction, $F(3, 112) = 9.79$, $p < .001$, and the relevant means are given in Table 1. Analyses of simple effects indicated that only the model treatment showed a significant increment on CURSS:O-I scores from pretest to posttest, $F(1, 112) = 51.53$, $p < .001$. Once again, the simple main effect for treatments was nonsignificant at the pretest, $F < 1$, but significant at the posttest, $F(3, 112) = 8.65$, $p < .01$. Subjects in the model treatment had significantly higher CURSS:O-I posttest scores than did those in the remaining three treatments. The means for the remaining treatments did not differ significantly from one another.

Treatment Differences at Posttest 2

Separate 4 × 2 (Treatments × Initial Susceptibility) between-subjects ANOVAS yielded significant treatment effects for the SHSS:C/O, $F(3, 112) = 15.34$, $p < .001$, for the SHSS:C/S, $F(3, 112) = 5.67$, $p < .01$, and for the SHSS:C/O-I, $F(3, 112) = 3.56$,

Table 2
Number of Initially Low and Initially Medium Susceptible "Created Highs" on Posttest 1 and on Both Posttests 1 and 2

	Information + Model		Information no model		Practice alone		Control	
Condition	*n*	% *n*	*n*	% *n*	*n*	% *n*	*n*	% *n*
Posttest 1								
Initial lows	10	67	6	40	0	0	1	7
Initial mediums	11	73	8	53	2	13	2	13
Posttests 1 & 2								
Initial lows	8	53	6	40	0	0	0	0
Initial mediums	10	67	6	40	2	13	2	13

Note. % *n* = percentage of subjects in each treatment.

$p < .05$. The relevant means are shown in Table 3. Mean magnitudes were ordered in the same direction in the case of each dependent variable: No-treatment control < practice-alone subjects < information subjects < modeling subjects. Post hoc comparisons indicated no significant differences between controls and practice-alone subjects on any of the dependent measures. Moreover, controls and practice-alone subjects had significantly lower scores than modeling subjects on each of the dependent measures. Information subjects did not differ significantly from modeling subjects on any of the dependent variables. However, on the SHSS:C/S information subjects also failed to differ from practice-alone subjects, and on the SHSS:C/O-I information subjects failed to differ from either controls or practice-alone subjects.[2]

On the SHSS:C, high susceptibility is conventionally defined as a score of 8 or above (Weitzenhoffer & Hilgard, 1962). Table 2 shows the number of initially low and medium susceptible subjects in each treatment who scored as high susceptibles on *both* the CURSS:O and the SHSS:C/O posttests. The information plus modeling treatment transformed over half the initial low susceptibles and more than two thirds of the initial medium susceptibles into high susceptibles on both scales. In the control and practice-alone treatments, none of the initial low susceptibles and very few of the initial mediums were transformed into high susceptibles.

Novel SHSS:C Items

Our modification of the SHSS:C contained four test suggestions that were rather different from those on which subjects had practiced (hypnotic dream, age regression, taste hallucination, and posthypnotic amnesia). In order to insure that treatment effects had generalized to novel items, susceptibility scores were calculated for each subject using only those four suggestions. Separate 2 × 4 (Initial Susceptibility × Treatments) ANOVAS on O, S, and O-I scores yielded a significant treatment effect in each case; O, scores, $F(3, 112) = 8.09$, $p < .001$; S scores, $F(3, 112) = 4.83$, $p < .01$; O-I scores, $F(3, 112) = 2.66$, $p = .051$; the relevant means are given in Table 4. As in earlier analyses, information plus modeling led to significantly higher scores on each dependent variable than did the control or practice-alone treatments, and the information without modeling treatment always fell between the modeling and practice-alone treatments.

Created Versus "Natural" High Susceptibles

Table 1 shows that even after training, CURSS:O scores were substantially higher than CURSS:O-I scores. In other words, subjects who obtained high overt response scores as a result of training (i.e., created highs) did not necessarily experience their responses as occurring involuntarily. However, higher CURSS:O than CURSS:O-I scores are also characteristic of high susceptibles who obtained their high CURSS:O scores without training (i.e., natural highs; Spanos et al., 1983c). In order to determine whether created and natural highs differed on subjective aspects of response, we selected those initially low and medium susceptibles from the information and information plus modeling treatments who obtained CURSS:O scores of 5 or above on Posttest 1 and SHSS:C/O scores of 8 or above on Posttest 2. The 16 initially medium susceptible subjects who met this criterion were matched on the basis of CURSS:O scores with natural highs who had been routinely pretested in our laboratory during the same academic year for participation in a wide variety of hypnosis experiments. Separate one-way ANOVAS indicated no significant differences among the three groups on CURSS:S scores, but a significant difference on CURSS:O-I scores, $F(2, 43) = 3.66$, $p < .05$. The relevant means are given in Table 5. Post hoc comparisons indicated that natural highs failed to differ significantly from either initially low or initially medium created highs on the CURSS:O-I. However, initially medium created highs obtained higher CURSS:O-I scores than did initially low created highs.[3]

[2] Analyses of variance involving the Carlton University Responsiveness to Suggestion Scale and the Sanford Hypnotic Susceptibility Scale, Form C scores as dependent variables usually yielded a significant main effect for the low/medium initial susceptibility factor, but never yielded a significant interaction between low/medium initial susceptibility and other factors. These significant main effects indicated that initial medium susceptibles obtained higher posttest susceptibility scores than initial low susceptibles. A more extensive description of these effects is omitted here because correlations between initial susceptibility and posttested susceptibility are provided in Table 6.

[3] The natural high susceptibles that formed the comparison group were all Carleton University undergraduates tested during the same academic terms and under the same group testing procedures as the subjects in the present experiment. Natural highs were selected from a file that included only an identification number, date of the Carlton University Responsiveness to Suggestion Scale (CURSS) testing, and CURSS:O (objective)

Table 3
Treatment Means for the Objective (O), the Subjective (S), and the Objective-Involuntariness (O–I) Scales of the Stanford Hypnotic Susceptibility Scale, Form C (SHSS:C)

Scale	Information + Model	Information no model	Practice alone	Control
SHSS:C/O				
M	7.56_a	6.43_a	4.10_b	3.60_b
SD	2.31	2.80	2.81	2.75
SHSS/CS				
M	15.20_a	13.57_{ab}	10.30_{bc}	8.78_c
SD	7.26	7.17	6.23	7.24
SHSS:C/O–I				
M	4.13_a	3.43_{ab}	2.23_b	2.13_b
SD	3.42	2.89	2.50	2.86

Note. Within rows means sharing the same subscript fail to differ significantly at $\alpha = .05$.

Attitudes

Subjects' attitudes about hypnosis were assessed before the pretest and again before each posttest. A 4 × 2 (Treatments × Initial Susceptibility) ANOVA on attitudes prior to the pretest indicated no significant effect for treatments. Our major interest was in the degree of attitude change induced by treatments. Therefore, two attitude difference scores were obtained for each subject by subtracting pretest attitude scores from attitudes scores at Posttest 1 and at Posttest 2, respectively. The larger the difference score, the greater the increment in positive attitudes from pretest to posttest. A 4 × 2 (Treatments × Posttest 1/2) ANOVA on these difference scores yielded a main effect for treatments, $F(3, 116) = 6.04$, $p < .001$, and a main effect for posttests, $F(1, 116) = 5.32$, $p < .05$. Post hoc comparisons on the treatment means indicated that subjects given modeling, $M = 9.58$, and those given information without modeling, $M = 8.43$, showed equivalent pretest to posttest increments in positive attitudes. The increments in both of these groups were significantly greater than the increments shown by the practice-alone subjects, $M = 3.73$, or the control subjects, $M = 2.52$. The latter two groups failed to differ significantly from one another. The posttests main effect indicated that the increment in positive attitudes from Pretest to Posttest 2, $M = 6.65$, was significantly larger than the increment from Pretest to Posttest 1, $M = 5.48$.

Correlations

Treatments were collapsed and correlation coefficients were computed on O, S, and O-I scores among and between the pretest and two posttest susceptibility scales. Within each session correlations among O, S, and O-I scores were always highly significant. These ranged in magnitude from $r = .60$ to $r = .92$ with a mean magnitude of $r = .77$. Between-sessions correlations for each susceptibility dimension are shown in the upper portion of Table 6. As this table indicates, the correlations between pretest scores and corresponding posttest scores, although significant, were only moderate in magnitude. On the other hand, correlations between the CURSS and SHSS:C posttest dimensions were uniformly high. As shown in the lower portion of Table 6, a similar pattern emerged when correlations were computed separately within each treatment. In each case, correlations between posttest scores were higher than correlations between pretest and posttest scores. Moreover, correlations between subjective scores were consistently higher than correlations between objective scores. The relatively low pretest to posttest correlations in all treatments probably reflect the truncation in range produced by our initial selection criterion (i.e., pretest CURSS:O scores below 5). According to this interpretation, correlations between subjective scores were higher than those between objective scores because pretest subjective scores were not a selection criterion and thereby exhibited more variability than objective scores. By this same token, correlations between posttests were higher than those between pretest and posttest because both posttests were associated with a wider range of scores than was the pretest.

score. CURSS:S (subjective) and CURSS:O-I (objective-involuntariness) scores for these subjects were obtained from their original data booklets only after matching and been completed.

Discussion

Compared to retest and practice-alone controls, subjects in the information plus modeling treatment showed large and statistically significant increments on both objective and subjective aspects of hypnotic susceptibility. The objective and subjective susceptibility posttest scores for subjects given information without modeling always fell between those of the modeling and practice-alone subjects. In most cases, posttested susceptibility in the information without modeling treatment more closely resembled that of the modeling treatment than that of the practice-alone condition. These findings replicate and extend those of several other studies (Diamond, 1972; Kinney & Sachs, 1974; Sachs & Anderson, 1967) which found that various combinations of favorable information, strategy modeling, and practice of new skills produced substantial increments on objective and subjective components of hypnotic susceptibility. Like Diamond (1972) and Kinney and Sachs (1974) we also found that treatment induced gains in susceptibility were maintained on two different susceptibility scales and generalized to items that had not been practiced during training. Subjects who initially scored low in susceptibility and those who initially scored in the medium range, achieved treatment gains of equivalent magnitude on both objective and subjective aspects of response. Similar results have been obtained by most modification studies that provided extensive and concrete information about the cognitive strategies required for successful responding (Diamond, 1977a).

Table 4
Treatment Means for the Novel Items on the O, S, and O–I, Dimensions of the Stanford Hypnotic Susceptibility Scale, Form C (SHSS:C)

SHSS:C dimension	Information + Model	Information no model	Practice alone	Control
O				
M	2.63_b	2.23_b	1.47_a	1.20_a
SD	1.30	1.31	1.31	1.19
S				
M	5.26_b	4.33_{ab}	3.71_a	2.68_a
SD	2.97	3.10	2.35	2.69
O–I				
M	1.27_b	1.00_{ab}	$.60_a$	$.53_a$
SD	1.39	1.05	.97	1.22

Note. Within rows means sharing the same subscript fail to differ significantly at $\alpha = .05$.

The present findings are also consistent with the results of studies that were aimed at enhancing performance on individual test suggestions. For instance, in two recent studies (Spanos, Kennedy, & Gwynn, 1984; Spanos, Voorneveld, & Gwynn, 1984) brief instructions aimed at changing attitudes and expectancies were given to low susceptible subjects who attempted to cognitively control pain. Following their instructions these subjects exhibited substantial decreases in rated pain and increases in pain tolerance. In fact, the pain reductions exhibited by these low susceptibles were as large as those shown by natural highs given hypnotic suggestions for analgesia. Spanos, Stam, D'Eon, Pawlak, and Radtke-Bodorik (1980) found that the provision of an appropriate interpretational set substantially enhanced degree of hypnotic amnesia. Relatedly, Spanos and de Groh (1984) found that nonhypnotic low susceptibles given explicit and unambiguous information concerning strategy usage reduced their recall of a previously learned categorized word list to the same degree as natural high susceptibles given hypnotic amnesia suggestions. Importantly, Spanos and de Groh's (1984) nonhypnotic instruction subjects were as likely as hypnotic amnesics to show disorganized clustering; a nonsuggested aspect of amnesia that characterizes the performance of natural highs (e.g., Spanos et al., 1980). Recently, Spanos, de Groh, and de Groot (in press) again found that information plus modeling produced substantial increments on objective and subjective aspects of susceptibility. In a final posttest session, subjects were tested on an amnesia task that was quite different from the one on which they had been trained. Created highs exhibited even more amnesia than the natural highs against whom they had been matched. Moreover, the created highs were as likely as the natural highs to report that their amnesia felt involuntary.

Trait theorists acknowledge that cognitive behavior modification procedures produce statistically significant enhancements in susceptibility. Nevertheless, they have argued that these enhancements are relatively small, and that such procedures have failed to transform low susceptibles into high susceptibles (Hilgard, 1975; Perry, 1977). However, our findings demonstrate just such a transformation in a substantial proportion of low susceptibles. Somewhat more than half of the low susceptibles who

Table 5
The Carlton University Responsiveness to Suggestion Scale (CURSS) Posttest 2 CURSS:S (Subjective) and CURSS:O–I (Objective-Involuntariness) Scores for Created Highs and CURSS:S and CURSS:O–I Scores for Matched Natural Highs

Scale	Initial low susceptibles	Initial medium susceptibles	Natural high susceptibles
CURSS:S			
M	12.14	15.44	13.25
SD	4.75	3.93	2.62
n	14	16	16
CURSS:O–I			
M	3.00_a	4.81_b	3.44_{ab}
SD	2.29	2.01	1.46
n	14	16	16

Note. Means sharing the same subscript fail to differ significantly at $\alpha = .05$.

Table 6
Correlations Between Pretest and Posttest Susceptibility Dimensions Across Treatments and Within Treatments

Dimension	Pre–Post 1	Pre–Post 2	Post 1–Post 1
Treatments collapsed			
O	.31*	.34*	.79*
S	.56*	.57*	.86*
O–I	.40*	.41*	.79*
Information & modeling			
O	.29	.29	.84*
S	.67*	.72*	.90*
O–I	.62*	.58*	.82*
Information – No model			
O	.23	.42*	.70*
S	.55*	.66*	.78*
O–I	.47*	.54*	.74*
Practice alone			
O	.60*	.34*	.58*
S	.55*	.44*	.71*
O–I	.45*	.41*	.82*
Control			
O	.35*	.43*	.71*
S	.59*	.45*	.85*
O–I	.34*	.10	.77*

* $p < .05$.

were administered the modeling treatment performed as high susceptibles on both posttests. Results were even more dramatic for initially medium susceptibles given the modeling treatment. More than two thirds of these subjects scored as high susceptibles on both posttests. None of the initially low susceptibles in either the control or practice-alone groups scored as high susceptible on both posttests. Importantly, both the initially low and initially medium "created highs" failed to differ significantly from a comparison group of natural high susceptibles on subjective aspects of susceptibility.

The high test–retest correlations that characterize standarized susceptibility scales are frequently cited by trait theorists in support of their theoretical position (Bowers, 1976; Perry, 1977). Therefore, it is worth noting that this finding is equally consistent with a social psychological perspective on susceptibility. For most experimental subjects, hypnotic susceptibility testing is a rare occurrence that has little relevance to how they lead their lives. Between testings (even testings widely separated in time), very few subjects are likely to expose themselves to information that will have a significant impact on their attitudes and interpretational sets toward hypnotic responding. In short, high test–retest reliabilities for susceptibility may reflect stable situation specific attitudes and interpretations rather than a largely unmodifiable trait (Diamond, 1977a; Spanos, 1982). The present results are consistent with these ideas. Thus, our control and practice-alone subjects failed to show increments in susceptibility across three testing sessions, and they showed only relatively small changes in their attitudes toward hypnosis. On the other hand, subjects in our modeling treatment showed substantial pretest to posttest increments in positive attitudes towards hypnosis as well as in susceptibility. Across the two posttests, however, both their newly modified attitudes and their susceptibility remained highly stable.[4]

Implications and Conclusions

Despite its overall effectiveness, even the modeling group contained some recalcetrant individuals who obtained low posttest scores on susceptibility dimensions (particularly on O-I dimensions) and on the attitudes questionnaire. However, it is important to keep in mind that our training procedures were relatively brief and highly standardized. Future studies might profitably focus on such recalcetrant subjects and expose them to further and more individualized training and practice. Subjects who remain recalcetrant despite further training could be compared to both created and natural high susceptibles on a variety of cognitive style variables (e.g., absorption, imagery vividness, daydreaming frequency) as well as on attitudes toward hypnosis. There may, in fact, be stable individual differences in attitudinal and cognitive style variables that limit the degree of susceptibility that subjects can attain. If so, these limitations are likely to be seen most clearly in subjects who have failed to show susceptibility gains even after extensive and individualized training and practice.

Future research might also be aimed at more extensively examining the generalizability of treatment induced susceptibility increments. High susceptibility is associated with a number of discrete phenomena that are not routinely assessed on standardized susceptibility scales. For example, these include transparent visual hallucinations (Orne, 1959; Spanos, Bridgeman, Stam, Gwynn, & Saad, 1983) and "hidden observer" responding during hypnotic analgesia (Hilgard, Morgan, & Macdonald, 1975; Spanos & Hewitt, 1980). It would be of interest to compare the frequencies with which created and natural high susceptibles enacted such responses. It would also be of interest to compare the responses of both trained subjects and natural highs to the responses of low susceptibles who were explicitly instructed to fake hypnosis (Orne, 1959).

In summary, the present findings along with those of Diamond (1972, 1977a) and Sachs (Kinney & Sachs, 1974; Sachs & Anderson, 1967; Springer et al., 1977) are consistent with a social-cognitive skills account of hypnotic responding. Hypnotic susceptibility appears to be a good deal more maliable than trait theory indicates. A substantial number of low susceptible subjects can be transformed into high susceptibles, and training induced susceptibility increments are maintained across time and on novel test times. Determining the limits to which susceptibility is modifiable awaits further research conducted on recalcetrant low susceptible subjects.

[4] The correlations between attitudes at Posttest 1 and attitudes at Posttest 2 were statistically significant and high in all treatments. They ranged in magnitude from $r = .71$ to $r = .87$. Positive attitudes toward hypnosis probably constitute a precondition for high hypnotic susceptibility. In and of themselves, however, positive attitudes do not appear to produce high susceptibility (Spanos, 1982). We anticipate that treatment packages aimed only at inculcating positive attitudes toward hypnosis will be much less successful at enhancing susceptibility than treatment packages aimed both at inculcating positive attitudes and inculcating the appropriate (i.e., active) interpretational set.

References

As, A., Hilgard, E. R., & Weitzenhoffer, A. M. (1963). An attempt at experimental modification of hypnotizability through repeated individualized hypnotic experiences. *Scandinavian Journal of Psychology, 4,* 81–89.

Barber, T. X. (1969). *Hypnosis: A scientific approach.* New York: Van Nostrand Reinhold.

Barber, T. X., Spanos, N. P., & Chaves, J. F. (1974). *Hypnosis, imagination and human potentialities.* Elmsford, NJ, Pergamon.

Bowers, K. S. (1976). *Hypnosis for the seriously curious.* Monterey, CA: Brooks/Cole.

Coe, W. C., & Sarbin, T. R. (1977). Hypnosis from the standpoint of a contextualist. *Annals of the New York Academy of Sciences, 296,* 2–13.

Comins, J. R., Fullam, F., & Barber, T. X. (1975). Effects of experimenter modeling, demands for honesty, and initial level of suggestibility on response to "hypnotic" suggestions. *Journal of Consulting and Clinical Psychology, 43,* 668–675.

Cooper, L. M., Branford, S. A., Schubot, E., & Tart, C. T. (1967). A further attempt to modify hypnotic susceptibility through repeated individualized experience. *International Journal of Clinical and Experimental Hypnosis, 15,* 118–124.

Council, J. R., Kirsch, I., Vickery, A. R., & Carlson, D. (1983). "Trance" versus "skill" hypnotic inductions: The effects of credibility, expectancy, and experimenter modeling. *Journal of Consulting and Clinical Psychology, 51,* 432–440.

Cronin, D. M., Spanos, N. P., & Barber, T. X. (1971). Augmenting hypnotic suggestibility by providing favorable information about hypnosis. *American Journal of Clinical Hypnosis, 13,* 259–264.

Diamond, M. J. (1972). The use of observationally presented information to modify hypnotic susceptibility. *Journal of Abnormal Psychology, 79,* 174–180.

Diamond, M. J. (1974). Modification of hypnotizability: A review. *Psychological Bulletin, 81,* 180–198.

Diamond, M. J. (1977a). Hypnotizability is modifiable. *International Journal of Clinical and Experimental Hypnosis, 25,* 147–165.

Diamond, M. J. (1977b). Issues and methods for modifying responsivity to hypnosis. *Annals of the New York Academy of Sciences, 296,* 119–128.

Diamond, M. J., Steadman, C., Harada, D., & Rosenthal, J. (1975). The use of direct instructions to modify hypnotic performance: The effects of programmed learning procedures. *Journal of Abnormal Psychology, 84,* 109–113.

Haley, J. (1958). An interactional explanation of hypnosis. *American Journal of Clinical Hypnosis, 1,* 41–57.

Hilgard, E. R. (1975). Hypnosis. *Annual Review of Psychology, 26,* 19–44.

Hilgard, E. R., Morgan, A. H., & Macdonald, H. (1975). Pain and dissociation in the cold pressor test: A study of hypnotic analgesia with "hidden reports" through automatic key-pressing and automatic talking. *Journal of Abnormal Psychology, 84,* 280–289.

Katz, N. W. (1979). Comparative efficacy of behavioral training, training plus relaxation, and a sleep/trance hypnotic induction in increasing hypnotic susceptibility. *Journal of Consulting and Clinical Psychology, 47,* 119–127.

Kinney, J. M., & Sachs, L. B. (1974). Increasing hypnotic susceptibility. *Journal of Abnormal Psychology, 83,* 145–150.

London, P., Cooper, L. M., & Engstrom, D. R. (1974). Increasing hypnotic susceptibility by brain wave feedback. *Journal of Abnormal Psychology, 83,* 554–560.

Orne, M. T. (1959). The nature of hypnosis: Artifact and essence. *Journal of Abnormal and Social Psychology, 58,* 277–299.

Perry, C. (1977). Is hypnotizability modifiable? *International Journal of Clinical and Experimental Hypnosis, 25,* 125–146.

Radtke, H. L., Spanos, N. P., Armstrong, L. A., Dillman, N., & Boisvenue, M. E. (1983). Effects of electromyographic feedback and progressive relaxation on hypnotic susceptibility: Disconfirming results. *International Journal of Clinical and Experimental Hypnosis, 31,* 98–106.

Sachs, L. B. (1971). Construing hypnosis as modifiable behavior. In A. B. Jacobs & L. B. Sachs (Eds.), *Psychology of private events* (pp. 61–75). New York: Academic Press.

Sachs, L. B., & Anderson, W. L. (1967). Modification of hypnotic susceptibility. *International Journal of Clinical and Experimental Hypnosis, 15,* 172–180.

Sanders, R. S., Jr., & Reyher, J. (1969). Sensory deprivation and the enhancement of hypnotic susceptibility. *Journal of Abnormal Psychology, 74,* 375–381.

Sarbin, T. R., & Coe, W. C. (1972). *Hypnosis: A social psychological analysis of influence communication.* New York: Holt, Rinehart & Winston.

Shor, R. E., & Orne, E. C. (1962). *The Harvard Group Scale of Hypnotic Susceptibility Form A.* Palo Alto, CA: Consulting Psychologists Press.

Simon, M. J., & Salzberg, H. (1981). Electromyographic feedback and taped relaxation instructions to modify hypnotic susceptibility and amnesia. *American Journal of Clinical Hypnosis, 24,* 14–21.

Spanos, N. P. (1971). Goal-directed fantasy and the performance of hypnotic test suggestions. *Psychiatry, 34,* 86–96.

Spanos, N. P. (1982). A social psychological approach to hypnotic behavior. In G. Weary & H. L. Mirels (Eds.), *Integrations of clinical and social psychology* (pp. 231–271). New York: Oxford University Press.

Spanos, N. P., & Barber, T. X. (1974). Toward a convergence in hypnosis research. *American Psychologist, 29,* 500–511.

Spanos, N. P., & Bertrand, L. D. (1985). EMG biofeedback, attained relaxation and hypnotic susceptibility: Is there a relationship? *American Journal of Clinical Hypnosis, 27,* 219–225.

Spanos, N. P., Bridgeman, M., Stam, H. J., Gwynn, M., & Saad, C. L. (1983). When seeing is not believing: The effects of contextual variables on the reports of hypnotic hallucinators. *Imagination, Cognition and Personality, 2,* 195–209.

Spanos, N. P., & de Groh, M. (1984). *Effects of active and passive wording on response to hypnotic and nonhypnotic instructions for complete and selective forgetting.* Unpublished manuscript, Carleton University.

Spanos, N. P., de Groh, M., & de Groot, H. (in press). Social cognitive skills training for modifying hypnotic susceptibility: Response generalization to a novel amnesia item. *British Journal of Experimental and Clinical Hypnosis.*

Spanos, N. P., & Gorassini, D. R. (1984). The structure of hypnotic test suggestions and attributions of responding involuntarily. *Journal of Personality and Social Psychology, 46,* 688–696.

Spanos, N. P., & Hewitt, E. G. (1980). The hidden observer in hypnotic analgesia: Discovery of experimental creation? *Journal of Personality and Social Psychology, 39,* 1201–1214.

Spanos, N. P., Kennedy, S. D., & Gwynn, M. I. (1984). Moderating effects of contextual variables on the relationship between hypnotic susceptibility and hypnotic analgesia. *Journal of Abnormal Psychology, 93,* 285–294.

Spanos, N. P., Radtke, H. L., Hodgins, D. C., Bertrand, L. D., Stam, H. J., & Dubreuil, D. L. (1983a). The Carleton University Responsiveness to Suggestion Scale: Stability, reliability, and relationships with expectancy and hypnotic experiences. *Psychological Reports, 53,* 555, 563.

Spanos, N. P., Radtke, H. L., Hodgins, D. C., Bertrand, L. D., Stam, H. J., & Moretti, P. (1983b). The Carleton University Responsiveness to Suggestion Scale: Relationship with other measures of hypnotic susceptibility, expectancies, and absorption. *Psychological Reports, 53,* 723–734.

Spanos, N. P., Radtke, H. L., Hodgins, D. C., Stam, H. J., & Bertrand, L. D. (1983c). The Carleton University Responsiveness to Suggestion Scale: Normative data and psychometric properties. *Psychological Reports, 53,* 523–535.

Spanos, N. P., Rivers, S. M., & Ross, S. (1977). Experienced involuntariness and response to hypnotic suggestions. *Annals of the New York Academy of Sciences, 296,* 208–221.

Spanos, N. P., Stam, H. J., D'Eon, J. L., Pawlak, A. E., & Radtke-Bodorik, H. L. (1980). The effects of social psychological variables on hypnotic amnesia. *Journal of Personality and Social Psychology, 39,* 737–750.

Spanos, N. P., Voorneveld, P., & Gwynn, M. I. (1984). *The mediating effects of expectation on hypnotic and nonhypnotic pain reduction.* Unpublished manuscript, Carleton University.

Springer, C. J., Sachs, L. B., & Morrow, J. E. (1977). Group methods of increasing hypnotic susceptibility. *International Journal of Clinical and Experimental Hypnosis, 25,* 184–191.

Tart, C. T. (1970). Increases in hypnotizability resulting from a prolonged program for enhancing personal growth. *Journal of Abnormal Psychology, 75,* 260–266.

Weitzenhoffer, A. M., & Hilgard, E. R. (1962). *The Stanford Hypnotic Susceptibility Scale, Form C.* Palo Alto, CA: Consulting Psychologists Press.

Wickramasekaera, I. (1973). Effects of electromyographic feedback on hypnotic susceptibility: More preliminary data. *Journal of Abnormal Psychology, 82,* 74–77.

Received April 29, 1985
Revision received September 9, 1985 ■

[14]

Fantasy Proneness

Hypnosis, Developmental Antecedents, and Psychopathology

Steven Jay Lynn *Ohio University*
Judith W. Rhue *University of Toledo*

ABSTRACT: This article presents a summary of the findings of our ongoing research program on the fantasy-prone person. In seven studies, nearly 6,000 college students were screened in order to obtain five samples of 156 fantasy-prone subjects. Fantasy-prone subjects (fantasizers) were selected from the upper 2%–4% of the college population on a measure of imaginative involvement and contrasted with nonfantasizers (lower 2%–4%), and medium fantasy-prone subjects (middle range). General support was secured for Wilson and Barber's construct of fantasy proneness: Fantasizers were found to differ from nonfantasizers, and in many cases also from medium-range subjects, on measures of hypnotizability, imagination, waking suggestibility, hallucinatory ability, creativity, psychopathology, and childhood experiences. Differences in hypnotizability were most reliable when subjects participated in a multisession study and were screened not only with the screening inventory, but also with an interview that substantiated their fantasy-prone status. However, our findings indicated that less correspondence between fantasy proneness and hypnotizability exists than Wilson and Barber suggested. Hypnotic responsiveness is possible even in the absence of well-developed imaginative abilities, and not all fantasizers were highly hypnotizable. Fantasizers recollected being physically abused and punished to a greater degree than other subjects did and reported experiencing greater loneliness and isolation as children. Many fantasizers appeared to be relatively well-adjusted; however, a subset of fantasizers were clearly maladjusted based on self-report, Minnesota Multiphasic Personality Inventory (MMPI), and Rorschach test data. Because of the diversity inherent in the fantasy-prone population, it is misleading to think of individuals at the extreme end of the fantasy-proneness continuum as conforming to a unitary personality type.

In a series of fascinating articles, Wilson and Barber (1981, 1983) described their serendipitous discovery of a group of individuals whom they alternately termed "fantasy addicts," "fantasy-prone personalities," and "fantasizers." These terms captured the essence of their subjects' defining characteristic—a unique constellation of personality traits and experiences that coalesced around a deep, profound, and long-standing involvement in fantasy and imagination. Wilson and Barber discovered fantasizers in the context of an intensive-interview study of excellent hypnotic subjects. The authors contended that fantasizers' intense imaginal involvements represent manifestations of adaptive fantasy abilities at the extreme end of the continuum of the trait of fantasy proneness. Estimated to be evident in as much as 4% of the population, but heretofore unrecognized as a unitary entity, the fantasy-prone syndrome was believed to have important implications for understanding such diverse phenomena as hypnosis; out-of-body, religious, visionary, parapsychological, and near-death experiences; mind–body relations; and creativity.

In delineating the construct of fantasy proneness, Wilson and Barber noted that, with one exception, their 27 excellent hypnotic subjects reported the following experiences with greater frequency than did the 25 nonexcellent (poor, medium, and medium-high susceptible) hypnotic subjects with whom they were compared: (a) fantasizing much of their waking life; (b) the ability to hallucinate objects and fully experience what they fantasize "as real as real," including rich and vivid hypnagogic imagery, achievement of orgasm in the absence of physical stimulation, physical manifestations and concomitants of observed violence on television (e.g., nausea, anxiety), and vivid recall of personal experiences; (c) psychic and out-of-body experiences; (d) occasional difficulty in differentiating fantasized events and persons from nonfantasized ones; (e) the belief in their ability to heal (e.g., "they feel a natural tendency to move toward injured or sick individuals while empathizing with them and touching them" [Wilson & Barber, 1983, p. 363]); and (f) a sense of social awareness along with a sensitivity to social norms that resulted in a secret fantasy life to which few were privy.

Wilson and Barber's contention that fantasy-prone persons are overrepresented in groups of hypnotically responsive subjects is corroborated by an abundance of data. In fact, Wilson and Barber were not the first to hypothesize a link between hypnotizability, adult imaginative involvements, and gratifying fantasy-related activities that have their origin in childhood. Indeed, the concept of "fantasy proneness" is largely derivative of and encompasses the construct Josephine Hilgard (1965, 1970, 1974, 1979) first elaborated—"imaginative involvement." Wilson and Barber's work followed in the path of Hilgard's ground-breaking intensive-interview and rating research at Stanford University, in which she attempted to predict hypnotic susceptibility in advance of hypnosis. Thought to represent a central dimension underlying hypnotic responsiveness, the capacity for imaginative involvement was believed to facilitate a temporary absorption in satisfying experiences in which fantasy played a prominent role. Consistent with this assumption, Hilgard found that hypnotizable subjects were more likely than less hypnotizable subjects to report long-standing imaginative involvements in sensory experiences, dramatic arts, reading, and religious and creative experiences.

Allied to the concepts of fantasy proneness and imaginative involvement is the construct of "absorption" (Tellegen & Atkinson, 1974). Absorption refers to the capacity for absorbed and self-altering attention, which is presumed to represent an essential component of hypnotizability. Indeed, hypnotic suggestions invite subjects to focus directly on the hypnotist's communications and to engage in fantasy and give free rein to the imagination in accord with suggested experiences. Research supportive of the dual constructs of absorption and imaginative involvement derives from early studies using inventories that documented an association between hypnotic susceptibility and imaginative involvements characterized by deep absorption and concentration, pleasure, and loss of awareness of external reality (As, O'Hara, & Munger, 1962; Barber & Glass, 1962; Lee-Teng, 1965; Shor, 1960; Shor, Orne, & O'Connell, 1962). More recent studies using scales specifically designed to measure absorption have also provided confirmatory data (for reviews, see Council, Kirsch, & Hafner, 1986; Spanos, 1982). These studies have documented a modest association (r = .25–.4) between hypnotic susceptibility and absorption (Tellegen, 1976; Tellegen & Atkinson, 1974). For the most part, measures of absorption correlate more highly with hypnotizability than with personality traits measured by multidimensional personality inventories such as the Minnesota Multiphasic Personality Inventory (MMPI) and the California Personality Inventory (CPI; Kihlstrom, 1985). The studies cited suggest that excellent hypnotic subjects are able to fantasize and imagine in accordance with hypnotic suggestions as well as in response to nonhypnotic activities that require a temporary diminution of rational, reality-bound analytical thinking.

As our review suggests, the constructs of fantasy proneness, imaginative involvement, and absorption are not truly discriminable; they converge in their emphasis on cognitive abilities related to imagination and fantasy that bridge hypnotic and nonhypnotic contexts. We have, however, adopted the terms *fantasy proneness* and *fantasy-prone person* because Wilson and Barber's major contribution rests on their claim to have identified a heretofore unrecognized personality syndrome. If fantasizers share the tendency to "live much of the time in a world of their own making—in a world of imagery, imagination, and fantasy" (Wilson & Barber, 1981, p. 31), then the intensive study of such individuals has the potential to address important questions that extend beyond the domain of hypnosis to the childhood antecedents of adult imaginative involvements and to the relation between psychopathology and profound fantasy involvement.

We would like to thank Hal Arkes, John Brentar, Bruce Carlson, Wendi Cross, David Kucharski, John Weekes, Michael Zoborowski, and anonymous reviewers for their helpful comments on earlier versions of this article.

Correspondence concerning this article should be addressed to Steven Jay Lynn, Department of Psychology, Ohio University, Athens, OH 45701.

Despite the intriguing and heuristic contribution of Wilson and Barber's study, it should be regarded as exploratory and their findings preliminary. The conclusions drawn by Wilson and Barber are limited, owing to the select nature of their sample (e.g., their subjects were women and largely postgraduate professionals); the selection procedures used (e.g., the majority of subjects were recruited from the ranks of participants in workshops the authors conducted and from personal or professional relationships, such as therapy clients); the failure to clearly standardize the nature and administration of hypnotic suggestions and to report the precise hypnotizability level of their subjects on the basis of widely used scales for assessing hypnotizability; the lack of objective and empirically validated measures of imagination, fantasy, creativity, psychopathology, and developmental experiences; the failure to use interviewers who were unaware of the subjects' hypnotizability status; and the absence of a comparison group of subjects who were truly low in hypnotizability or fantasy proneness. Given these limitations, further research is needed to determine whether subjects at the extreme end of the continuum of imaginative/fantasy involvements can be characterized by a unique constellation of personality attributes (Lynn & Rhue, 1986).

This article presents a summary of our research studies on fantasy-prone persons (Lynn & Dudley, 1987; Lynn & Rhue, 1986, 1987; Rhue & Lynn, 1987a, 1987b; Rhue & Lynn, 1987b, in press). We initiated this series of studies in an attempt to elaborate the construct validity of fantasy proneness and to redress some of the shortcomings of previous research. Over the past six years, we screened nearly 6,000 college students in order to obtain five samples of 156 fantasy-prone subjects. At the heart of our research was the question whether fantasizers' personality attributes and developmental histories could be distinguished from those of less fantasy-prone subjects. Three general areas were targeted for investigation, based on Wilson and Barber's description of the syndrome of fantasy proneness, and on the broader literature on fantasy, imagination, and hypnotizability: (a) hypnosis, imagination, and creativity; (b) developmental antecedents of fantasy proneness; and (c) fantasy proneness and psychopathology.

Hypnosis, Imagination, and Creativity

The conjoining of hypnotizability and imaginative tendencies figures prominently in the elaboration of the construct of fantasy proneness. For this reason, we evaluated the relation between fantasy proneness and measures presumed to be related to hypnotizability, imagination, and the creative, adaptive concomitants of fantasy.

In our first study (Lynn & Rhue, 1986), subjects were screened with the Inventory of Childhood Memories and Imaginings (ICMI), a 52-item instrument developed by Wilson and Barber (1981) with adequate reliability and validity (see Lynn & Rhue, 1986; Rhue & Lynn,

1985). This dichotomous, paper-and-pencil questionnaire was adapted from Wilson and Barber's (1981) 103-item Memory, Imagining, and Creativity Interview Schedule, which was used in their study of fantasy proneness. In this and our other studies, fantasy-prone persons were identified by a score falling in the upper 2% to 4% of the population, nonfantasizers in the lower 2% to 4%, and medium fantasy-prone subjects in the range between the scores of the fantasy-prone subjects and the nonfantasizers. In each of our studies, three levels of fantasy proneness (high, medium, and low) were contrasted.

In our initial study, an intensive interview yielded data pertinent not only to hypnotizability, but also to psychopathology and the developmental antecedents of fantasy proneness. However, our research departed from Wilson and Barber's in a number of ways. First, we used multiple quantitative measures of hypnotizability, imagination, personality, and play and punishment history. Second, interviewers were not aware of the subjects' status. Finally, rather than using hypnotizability level as a selection factor, group designation was determined by a score on the screening inventory and later corroborated in an interview. In the interview, fantasy proneness was defined in accord with Wilson and Barber's (1983) definition of being able to "set the theme, and then an imaginative scenario unfolds that has some of the characteristics of a dream and some of a motion picture" (p. 342).

Subjects were screened in groups for fantasy proneness with the ICMI. They were informed that the questionnaire related to an ongoing research project dealing with personality and early life experiences. Subjects who were invited to participate were informed that the 8–10-hour "study of personality" would be divided into five sessions. No set sequence of sessions was adhered to. In the first session, prior to being hypnotized, (Harvard Group Scale of Hypnotic Susceptibility, Form A [HGSHS: A]; Shor & Orne, 1962), subjects completed the following measures: the Tellegen Absorption Scale (Tellegen, 1976), a second ICMI, and a measure of the tendency to respond in a socially desirable manner (Crowne & Marlowe, 1960), which was used as a statistical covariate. Subjects also received an MMPI test booklet and answer sheet to complete and return at a subsequent test session. As a means of gauging the subjects' ability to function in an academic environment, subjects' official grade-point averages were obtained from the registrar.

In the second session, a measure of response to waking suggestion (Creative Imagination Scale; Wilson & Barber, 1978) was administered, along with a measure of creativity (the Barron–Welsh Revised Art Scale; Barron & Welsh, 1952) and a vividness-of-mental-imagery scale (Sheehan, 1967). In the third session, subjects received a Rorschach test. In the fourth session, they participated in a semistructured interview for 1–5 hours; subjects were asked to be objective about both past and present events, and strong demands for honesty were made. In the fifth session, subjects participated in a reading-absorption task (Baum & Lynn, 1981).

Our first study (Lynn & Rhue, 1986) provided support for the construct validity of fantasy proneness. Fantasizers differed from less-fantasy-prone subjects on measures of hypnotizability, absorption, vividness of mental imagery, response to waking suggestion, and creativity. However, fantasy proneness was not a perfect predictor of hypnotizability. Our data indicated that hypnotic responsiveness is possible even in the absence of well-developed imaginative abilities: More than a third of the nonfantasizers scored as high hypnotizables, and nonfantasizers were just as hypnotizable as medium fantasy-prone subjects. Yet subjects classified as fantasizers were likely to score as high hypnotizables—nearly 80% of fantasizers scored in the high-susceptible range. These results are compatible with the findings of Hilgard (1965, 1970, 1974) and Wilson and Barber (1981, 1983), and with Shor et al.'s (1962) findings that scores on an inventory of naturally occurring "hypnotic-like" experiences predicted hypnotizability, especially in the "deeper" region of the hypnotizability continuum.

In our second study (Rhue & Lynn, 1987a), we examined the robustness of our findings by varying the subject-selection procedures and the conditions of testing. Although the ICMI screening measure proved to be an excellent device in our first study, volunteers who participate in a multisession (8–10 hour) hypnosis experiment may have a particular interest in experiencing hypnosis and exhibit a high level of motivation and willingness to cooperate—factors shown to influence hypnotic responsivity in their own right (Barber, 1981; Spanos, 1982). Furthermore, extensive testing procedures that involve the joint administration of measures of imagination and hypnotizability might generate context-based expectancies and demands (Council et al., 1986) that promote correspondent responding to these measures.

Subjects in our second study were not interviewed but were classified according to fantasy-proneness level on the basis of their scores on the ICMI screening instrument. Furthermore, rather than participating in an extensive testing program, subjects participated in a single-session hypnosis experiment. In this session, the Harvard Group Scale of Hypnotic Susceptibility, Form A (Shor & Orne, 1962) and the Tellegen Absorption Scale (Tellegen, 1976) were administered to high (N = 56), medium (N = 62), and low (N = 50) fantasy-prone persons.

We were successful in partially replicating the findings of our initial investigation. As in our first study, we found that fantasizers were more hypnotizable than nonfantasizers and that fantasizers differed from less-fantasy-prone subjects on the measure of absorption. The latter finding is understandable: In both studies, high correlations between the measures of absorption and fantasy proneness ($r > .70$) were found, confirming the high degree of correspondence between these measures and constructs.

Our second study did not support the hypothesis that fantasy proneness is an aptitudinal measure that is a reliable predictor or alternative measure of hypnotizability. We found that fantasy-prone subjects were no more hypnotizable than medium fantasy-prone subjects,

Table 1
Comparison of Fantasy-Proneness and Hypnotizability Levels in Percentages

Variable	High Study 1	High Study 2	Low Study 1	Low Study 2
	Hypnotizability			
Fantasy Proneness				
High	78.26	51.79	0.00	3.57
Low	35.29	32.00	0.00	18.00
	Fantasy Proneness			
Hypnotizability				
High	54.55	37.66	18.18	20.78
Low	0.00	18.75	0.00	37.50

and nonfantasizers emerged as the group distinctly lower in hypnotizability. Using identical instruments, Huff and Council (1987) recently replicated this pattern of results. Table 1 shows that a majority of fantasizers can be classified as high hypnotizables. Furthermore, although low hypnotizables infrequently score as fantasizers, about a third of the nonfantasizers can be classified as high hypnotizables. Testing subjects for hypnotizability with scales that are particularly useful for discriminating subjects with high levels of hypnotic ability (e.g., Stanford Profile Scales; Weitzenhoffer & Hilgard, 1963) might have produced a greater differentiation among the groups of subjects tested. However, our results indicate that less correspondence between fantasy proneness and hypnotizability exists than Wilson and Barber's (1983) and Hilgard's (1970, 1974) earlier research suggested.

Taken together, our findings indicate that the relation between scores on the measure of fantasy proneness and hypnotizability is not robust and that fantasy proneness and hypnotizability are only modestly related. Although the majority of fantasizers in both studies scored as high susceptibles, level of fantasy proneness was not a reliable predictor of hypnotizability level. Both Hilgard (1979) and Wilson and Barber (1981) were careful to note that attitudinal and motivational factors may moderate the relation between hypnotizability and measures of fantasy and imagination.

A decrement in hypnotizability scores across the two studies is apparent when we examine the responses of fantasizers. An inspection of the means in Table 2 reveals that in our second study, fantasizers scored a point lower on the hypnotizability scale than did fantasizers in our first investigation. Perhaps our first study's extensive testing program both ensured that the sample of fantasizers was particularly cooperative and positively motivated to experience hypnosis and conveyed strong demands for responding to hypnotic suggestions. Subjects might also have formed more definite impressions of themselves as fantasy prone and behaved in accordance with their self-perceptions.

Factors other than fantasy proneness contribute significant variance to hypnotizability scores. Our research is consistent with a sizable body of literature indicating that attribute measures of imagination and fantasy do not consistently predict hypnotizability (see Council et al., 1986; Spanos, 1982). A number of cognitive, interpersonal, and situational factors in addition to imaginative involvement have been shown to augment hypnotic responding: positive attitudes, beliefs, and motivation to participate fully in the events of hypnosis (Cronin, Spanos, & Barber, 1971); correct interpretation of hypnotic suggestions (e.g., Diamond, 1972, 1982; Spanos, 1982); and comfort and rapport with the hypnotist (e.g., Gfeller, Lynn, & Pribble, 1986; Sheehan, 1980). In contrast, negative attitudes toward hypnosis, lack of motivation, atypical interpretation of suggestions, and poor rapport with the hypnotist may dampen responding in even highly imaginative subjects (Lynn & Rhue, 1986, 1987). Although expectancies appear to exert a more potent influence on hypnotic responding than sustained and vivid suggestion-related imaginings do (Kirsch, Council, & Mobayed, 1987; Lynn, Snodgrass, Rhue, & Hardaway,

Table 2
Means of Hypnotizability, Absorption, and ICMI Screening Scores Across Studies

Scale	Fantasy proneness: High Study 1	High Study 2	Medium Study 1	Medium Study 2	Low Study 1	Low Study 2
Harvard Group Scale of Hypnotic Susceptibility[a]	9.78	8.74	7.98	8.93	7.58	7.00
Tellegen Absorption Scale[b]	33.43	30.30	21.64	24.39	11.41	12.59
Screening instrument (ICMI)[c]	42.39	40.12	23.45	24.63	7.47	10.40

Note. ICMI = Inventory of Childhood Memories and Imaginings. For Study 1 (Lynn & Rhue, 1986), differences among dependent measures were as follows: (a) high > medium ($p < .05$); high > low ($p < .01$); (b) high > medium > low ($p < .01$); (c) high > medium > low ($p < .01$). For study 2 (Rhue & Lynn, 1987a), differences among dependent measures were as follows: (a) high > low ($p < .01$); medium > low ($p < .01$); (b) high > medium > low ($p < .01$); (c) high > medium > low ($p < .01$).

[a] Harvard range = 0–12. [b] Tellegen Absorption range = 0–37. [c] ICMI range = 0–52.

in press; Spanos, Cobb, & Gorassini, in press; Spanos, Weekes, & de Groh, 1984; Zamansky, 1977), just how these and other variables presumed to be related to hypnotic responding interact has yet to be fully elaborated. A multifactorial model that encompasses and integrates aptitudinal and contextual factors may well provide the most durable account of hypnotic phenomena and their relation to fantasy and imagination.

Our third study (Rhue & Lynn, in press) evaluated Wilson and Barber's (1983) contention that fantasizers are able to have compelling fantasy experiences that attain hallucinatory intensities. Wilson and Barber maintained that nearly two thirds of their fantasizers typically experienced their fantasies "as real as real" in all sensory modalities and that they could achieve such vivid hallucinatory experiences with their eyes closed or open. To examine this possibility, we recruited a sample of high ($N = 23$), medium ($N = 24$), and low ($N = 20$) fantasy-prone subjects. Of the fantasizers, 9 were participants in our first study and 14 were recruited for participation from our ongoing efforts to screen fantasy-prone persons. Subjects were required to hallucinate a second cup beside an actual Styrofoam cup (see Stanley, Lynn, & Nash, 1986). In addition to comparing fantasizers and less-fantasy-prone subjects on the frequency of their reporting seeing the second cup, we used subjects' reports of the image to gauge its lifelikeness, transparency, stability, and detail.

When asked to hallucinate an object on demand, most of the fantasizers (86.96%) reported that they could visualize a second cup beside the actual Styrofoam cup. In contrast, less than half of the medium-range subjects and only about a fifth of the nonfantasizers reported being able to visualize the cup. However, contrary to Wilson and Barber's observations, fantasizers do not hallucinate "as real as real," at least when the object to be hallucinated is suggested by another individual. Even when fantasizers who were also high hypnotic responders were considered, incomplete and imperfect hallucinatory experiences were characteristic. As a rule, hallucinated images were not lifelike, stable, or characterized by the elaboration of detail. Indeed, only a quarter of the fantasizers who could visualize a second cup said that their image of the cup was lifelike. It could be argued that the incidence of reports of lifelike hallucinations might have been enhanced by a hypnotic induction, with its attendant buildup of expectations and implicit demands for veridical hallucinations. However, our findings are consistent with those of a large number of studies (see Spanos, 1986; Stanley et al., 1986) showing that the great majority of hypnotized and nonhypnotized subjects describe suggested visual hallucinations as lacking lifelike properties (e.g., ghost image, blurry, fuzzy, vague).

One explanation for fantasizers' high frequency of scoring positively on the cup hallucination is that they adopt a relatively lax criterion for acknowledging that they can see the cup. Given fantasizers' self-perceptions as imaginative persons, as well as demands that convey the expectation that acknowledging the presence of the cup is appropriate for imaginative subjects, fantasizers may be more inclined to report that they can see the hallucinated image, even though it lacks lifelike properties. It will be necessary for future investigations to determine whether fantasizers have more realistic and elaborated hallucinatory experiences in response to self-directed fantasies that are intrinsically gratifying, reduce anxiety, or have some compensatory function (Rhue & Lynn, in press).

Our research illuminates the diversity of fantasizers' hypnotic and hallucinatory responses and abilities. Although the majority of individuals who exhibit a long-standing history of fantasy-related involvements score as high hypnotizables and report the ability to hallucinate on demand, fantasy proneness in no way guarantees success at hypnotic tasks or the ability to hallucinate "as real as real." Perhaps certain facets of fantasy proneness, such as a history of unusually intense fantasy experiences, subjected to cognitive controls, will be found to be better predictors of adult hypnotic and imaginative abilities. However, our research suggests that it would be a mistake to equate hypnotic abilities and fantasy proneness, and to minimize the contribution of variables other than fantasy proneness to hypnotic responding, such as attitudes, motivation, rapport, and the hypnotic context.

Developmental Antecedents

Hilgard's (1970, 1974) and Wilson and Barber's (1983) research converged in their identification of two major childhood developmental pathways to extreme hypnotic susceptibility and fantasy proneness in later life: (a) encouragement to fantasize from a significant adult and (b) fantasizing and involvement in imaginative activities as a means of coping with loneliness and isolation, and as an escape from an aversive early life environment.

With regard to the first pathway, the adult who provided encouragement was frequently a parent, grandparent, teacher, or friend who reinforced the child's fantasies, diverse imaginal activities, and make-believe play experiences. "Encouraging" adults frequently read their children fairy tales and treated the child's dolls and stuffed animals "as if they were alive." Numerous studies (e.g., Bandura, Ross, & Ross, 1961; Freyberg, 1973; Jalongo, 1984; Klinger, 1969; Manosevitz, Prentice, & Wilson, 1973; Singer, 1973) have underscored the importance of imitative play and reinforcement and exposure to an adult model in facilitating the expression of fantasy.

Another way that parents can encourage the expression of fantasy is by exposing children to such activities as ballet, piano, and dramatics. More than a third of the fantasizers in Wilson and Barber's study (1983) reported involvement in one or more of these activities as children. Unfortunately, there is a paucity of research that examines the relation between adult imaginative involvements and special life situations in childhood, although a number of researchers (Hilgard, 1970; Lee-Teng, 1965; Sarbin & Lim, 1963; Shor, 1960) have noted that involvement in dramatic arts and role-taking ability describe more high-hypnotizable subjects than low-hypnotizable subjects.

Fantasizing due to loneliness and isolation, and as an escape from an aversive environment, has received substantially more research attention. Indeed, fantasy appears to serve an adaptive and defensive function for some children who experience significant failure or frustration or limited contact with other children or adults (e.g., Fraiberg, 1968; Singer, 1973; Tower, 1983). The majority of fantasizers studied by Wilson and Barber (1983) perceived themselves as having been lonely and isolated as children and reported that fantasy helped them to cope with their isolation and provided companionship and entertainment. A number of the women reported stressful childhood histories that included physical abuse and a parent who either deserted the family or had severe emotional problems. Fantasy served as a means of achieving an emotional haven or respite from an unremittingly harsh environment. Wilson and Barber's observations are consistent with Hilgard's (1970, 1974) findings that hypnotic susceptibility was positively correlated with severity of punishment during childhood, and with the finding from our laboratory that the majority of subjects who reported being physically abused as children scored as high-susceptible hypnotic subjects as adults (Nash & Lynn, 1986; Nash, Lynn, & Givens, 1984). In a recent study (Rhue, Lynn, Henry, Buhk, & Boyd, 1987), students who reported a history of abuse were no more hypnotizable than nonabused subjects. However, those students who reported a history of being both physically and sexually abused as children were more fantasy prone than nonabused respondents who either had experienced the death of a parent before age 10 or were from an intact family.

To examine the developmental antecedents of fantasy proneness, and the question of whether fantasizers' developmental history diverges from that of less-fantasy-prone subjects, we examined fantasizers' reports of childhood play activities, punishment, loneliness, and parental encouragement to fantasize (Rhue & Lynn, 1987c). Data were secured from the semistructured interviews with the subject sample described in our initial study (Lynn & Rhue, 1986). Interviewers were advanced clinical psychology graduate students who were naive with respect to subjects' group designation.

Not only did fantasizers and less-fantasy-prone subjects diverge in their reports of early life experiences, but several relatively distinct pathways to fantasy proneness emerged. Whereas 6 of 21 fantasizers reported being severely physically abused as children (e.g., bruises, bleeding, or broken bones), none of the other subjects reported comparable punishment. Furthermore, fantasizers' reported frequency and severity of physical punishment across all age ranges exceeded that of the comparison samples. Although fantasizers reported a greater use of imagination to cope with pain and had more thoughts of revenge toward the punisher, they did not differ from other subjects in their ratings of the positivity of their early home environment. Imaginative abilities may serve a functional role in minimizing physical and psychic pain and in preserving a relatively positive view of the abusive environment. Other evidence that imaginative tendencies serve an adaptive and perhaps compensatory function derives from fantasizers' reports of greater loneliness, greater enjoyment of imaginary games, and greater enjoyment of solitary play and less enjoyment of playing with friends in comparison with their less-fantasy-prone counterparts. On balance, our findings are consistent with our earlier research (Nash & Lynn, 1986; Nash et al., 1984) supportive of a relation between the report of physical abuse and hypnotizability, and one between abuse and fantasy proneness (Rhue et al., 1987), as well as with the more anecdotal findings of Wilson and Barber (1981) and the research of Hilgard (1974).

Of the measures of parental encouragement to fantasize (e.g., direct encouragement to imagine and to read stories; parents' reading of stories, poems, or fairy tales) or special life situations presumed to foster extensive fantasy involvement (e.g., music, art, dance, acting lessons), only one discriminated fantasizers from less-fantasy-prone subjects: Fantasizers reported more parental encouragement to read stories. Despite this generally negative finding, some subjects did report an extensive history of parental encouragement and involvement in imaginative activities.

Are parental encouragement and severe punishment largely independent antecedents of fantasy proneness? Some overlap existed, but encouragement and punishment constituted essentially separate pathways to fantasy proneness. Of the 21 fantasizers, 8 reported being encouraged by a parent to imagine; however, only 2 of the "encouraged" fantasizers reported abusive punishment. Conversely, of the 6 fantasizers who reported abuse, only 2 reported being encouraged to imagine.

A number of interpersonal and situational factors not directly assessed in our research might have an impact on the emergence of fantasy involvements in childhood. For example, the level of adult-determined activity (Carpenter & Huston-Stein, 1980) and the security of early attachments (Stroufe, 1979) might be important mediators of imaginative tendencies in abused and nonabused populations. Council (1987) recently argued that adopting a vigilant style of coping with a harsh environment might discourage childhood fantasy involvements. The absence of parental discouragement of fantasy probably has an impact on the development of imaginative tendencies. Indeed, the interviewers were as impressed by the nonfantasizers' emphasis on logical, rational, and analytic thought processes and on embracing a realistic attitude toward life goals as they were by the fantasizers' depictions of the profound role of fantasy in their lives (Rhue & Lynn, 1987b).

Fantasy Proneness and Psychopathology

Despite fantasizers' reports of occasional difficulties in differentiating fantasy from reality, their reports of hallucinatory and paranormal experiences, and their endorsement of a variety of other unusual experiences, Wilson and Barber (1983) argued that fantasizers' colorful fantasy lives did not represent an autistic retreat into a fantasy world born of an inability to cope with the rigors of everyday life. Indeed, only a small minority of fantasizers were described as psychologically maladjusted, and many were high-functioning professionals with postgraduate degrees.

Despite the healthy emotional functioning attributed to fantasy-prone persons, the adaptiveness of pervasive fantasy involvement is questionable. For example, in describing the primary symptoms of "pseudoneurotic schizophrenia," Hoch and Cattell (1959) used the term *dereistic thinking* to characterize a mode of thought marked by the increasing predominance of the individual's fantasy life to the extent that difficulties in distinguishing fantasy from reality and problems in living ensue. Indeed, fantasizers' reports of vivid hallucinatory experiences, a preference for spending as much as half of their free time fantasizing, and the occasional inability to distinguish fantasy from reality all suggest the potential for fantasy to represent a retreat from the constraints of reality.

Although Wilson and Barber (1983) cast fantasizers' experience in positive terms, they noted that fantasizers exhibit qualities characteristic of hysterics. The authors speculated that many individuals diagnosed as hysteric during the 19th century may have been fantasizers. In support of a parallel between fantasy proneness and hysterical tendencies, Wilson and Barber's fantasizers reported false pregnancies and physical concomitants associated with vivid fantasies and memories.

We conducted three studies to profile fantasizers' affect, ideation, and symptom report. The first study (Experiment 1; Rhue & Lynn, 1987b) was based on our initial sample of fantasizers who received the Rorschach and MMPI tests in the context of our intensive-interview study. As expected, fantasizers scored higher than comparison subjects on measures of ideation presumed to be associated with fantasy proneness. Construct validity for fantasy proneness was evidenced in fantasizers' high scores on the MMPI Schizophrenia scale ($T = 83.80$) and Frequency (F) scale ($T = 71.42$). Fantasizers' willingness to report hallucinatory and paranormal experiences, along with their report of occasional problems in differentiating fantasy from reality, are consistent with their self-presentation on the MMPI, and with Wilson and Barber's (1981, 1983) observations of fantasy-prone subjects. Productivity of ideation, as measured by Rorschach data, was consistent with fantasizers' reports of an intense and rich fantasy life.

The clinical elevations on the Schizophrenia and Hypomania ($T = 77.95$) scales produced a modal MMPI profile with an 8/9 code type. Unfortunately, a paucity of data exists regarding the 8/9 code type with reference groups of relatively normally functioning college students, rendering so-called cookbook interpretations of limited value. However, given the demographics of our sample, the elevations on Scales 8 and 9 can conservatively be interpreted as reflecting ideational productivity, unconventional and peculiar thinking, and perhaps greater alienation and preoccupation with an internal world of fantasy. Fantasizers' life histories of intense and gratifying fantasy involvements apparently come to be associated with a heightened tolerance for unusual or atypical perceptions, experiences, and ideation. Indeed, impressionistic interview data suggested that fantasy played a pivotal role in the self-concept and identity of many of our fantasizers: Fantasizers perceived themselves as unique, creative individuals whose ideas and perceptions did not necessarily conform to mainstream beliefs and social tendencies.

Although fantasizers' ideation was distinctive in certain respects, it was not accompanied by a dysphoria syndrome of depression and anxiety, nor was fantasy proneness related to hysterical tendencies. Thus, whereas the hysterics described by Janet (1901) and Charcot (1889) may have been so-called fantasy-prone personalities, as Wilson and Barber (1981) suggested, our findings do not imply that fantasizers are aptly characterized as having hysterical qualities. Rorschach test data revealed that fantasizers displayed adequate reality testing and a rich affective and cognitive life, were in touch with social norms, and evidenced cognitive and emotional versatility that reflected an adequate balance between their inner life and the constraints of reality.

Our findings are consistent with the hypothesis that fantasy may serve an adaptive and perhaps compensatory function in relatively nondefensive individuals. As we have noted, instances of child abuse and lonely childhoods were overrepresented among the fantasizers. In addition to scoring higher than other subjects on an index of projected hostility, fantasizers reported using fantasy as an escape, as an outlet for anger, and as a means of regulating their internal life. Our results are consistent with Kris's (1952) concept of adaptive regression and his hypothesis that some individuals (e.g., those who are fantasy prone) may evidence pronounced tendencies to use fantasy adaptively to modulate and channel ego-dystonic impulses, using imagination and fantasy as an integral part of their everyday functioning.

Our second study (Experiment 2; Rhue & Lynn, 1987b) delineated aspects of the functioning of a separate sample of 50 high, 46 medium, and 33 low fantasy-prone persons who received questionnaires regarding their history of psychiatric hospitalizations, the use of psychotropic medications and contacts about psychological problems with persons in helping roles, and their perceptions of adjustment, self-concept, and ability to differentiate fantasy from reality.

Evidence that fantasizers cope adequately in the social realm derives from the finding that fantasy-prone subjects reported having as many close friends as did subjects in the comparison groups. The majority of fantasizers appeared to be successfully negotiating the demands of college life and had grade-point averages indistinguishable from those of less-fantasy-prone subjects. Although fantasizers reported more problems, most fantasizers rated themselves in the range of extremely to moderately well-adjusted and believed that others would rate them similarly. Furthermore, fantasizers' self-concepts were just as positive as those of their less fantasy-prone peers. Fantasizers are apparently able to incorporate the perception of having relatively more problems into their broader self-concept and identity as fantasy-prone persons. Indeed, fantasy proneness is adaptive in the sense that it may promote and preserve a positive self-concept. Further evidence of adequate psychological functioning derives from the finding that fantasizers did not differ from others in having sought professional help for psychological problems.

As a counterpoint to this picture of positive adjustment, evidence suggests that adaptive imaginative tendencies and more pathological autistic ideational functioning overlap, at least in a subset of fantasizers. For example, three fantasizers reported a history of psychiatric hospitalizations, and a fourth rated himself as having "many psychological problems/poorly adjusted," whereas none of the subjects in the comparison groups reported such problems. Furthermore, 5 of the 23 fantasizers in the first study produced MMPI profiles that conformed to the criteria of severe psychopathology delineated by Newmark and his colleagues (Newmark, Gentry, Simpson, & Jones, 1978). The common thread that runs through these fantasizers' backgrounds is a reported history of harsh childhood punishment and a frequency of physical punishment that averaged from 13 to 25 instances per month. What these findings suggest is that a history of abuse combined with fantasy proneness may predispose fantasizers to severe adjustment problems in adult life. In support of this possibility, Huff and Council (1987) recently found that fantasizers not only evidenced greater personality pathology, including being more likely to exhibit schizoid or borderline personality organization, but also reported more traumatic experiences during childhood. Female fantasizers reported more childhood sexual abuse from nonfamily members than did either male fantasizers or medium or low fantasy-prone subjects.

Our third study in this series (Lynn & Dudley, 1987) provided additional evidence that a subset of fantasizers are more maladjusted than the general population. We administered the ICMI screening instrument, the short-form MMPI (MMPI-168), the Magical Ideation Scale (Eckblad & Chapman, 1983), and the Perceptual Aberration Scale (Chapman, Chapman, & Raulin, 1976) to nearly 300 students. The latter scales are measures of hypothetical psychosis proneness or schizotypy, where magical ideation is defined as the belief in conventionally invalid forms of causation, and perceptual aberration encompasses five kinds of schizophrenic body-image aberration.

Of the 13 fantasizers identified in our sample, 5 scored more than two standard deviations above the mean on the combined Perceptual Aberration/Magical Ideation (PERMAG) scale of schizotypy or hypothetical psychosis proneness. Furthermore, the scale of fantasy proneness and the PERMAG scale were found to share approximately 30% of their variance. Finally, the scale of fantasy proneness was a better predictor of scores on the measure of schizotypy than any of the scales of the MMPI-168 that were administered. Thus, some degree of overlap exists between relatively healthy imaginative tendencies and pathological ideational processes (Lynn & Dudley, 1987; Rhue & Lynn, 1987b) in the fantasy-prone population. Our data suggest that a sizable minority of fantasy-prone persons—we estimate between 20% and 35%—exhibit significant signs of maladjustment, psychopathology, or deviant ideation, and perhaps a smaller proportion of fantasizers can be aptly characterized as schizotypal or borderline personalities.

Conclusion

It is important to note a number of limitations in the present research that suggest lines of future inquiry. A variety of variables moderate the relation between scales that tap imaginative involvement and variables hypothetically related to fantasy proneness. Scales that measure absorption and fantasy proneness rely on subjects' interpretations of their experiences and abilities, and self-reports are notoriously sensitive to social-desirability biases, demand characteristics, and context and expectancy effects (Lynn & Rhue, 1987). For example, recent studies (Council et al., 1986; deGroot, Gwynn, & Spanos, in press) found that hypnotic susceptibility and absorption correlated significantly only when the scales were administered in the same testing context. When subjects filled out the absorption questionnaire in a nonhypnotic context, with no knowledge that they would later be hypnotized, the correlations were not significant. Thus, situationally induced expectancies may account for disparate findings across studies.

Fantasy-related experiences that occur with a low base rate in the population may be perceived as reflecting deviance or psychopathology. If fantasy-prone subjects are aware of social norms yet vary in the degree of secrecy they maintain about their fantasy lives (Wilson & Barber, 1981), the report of fantasy-related experiences and the correlation of fantasy proneness with hypnotizability may well vary as a function of situational variables that legitimize or suppress the endorsement of unusual or fantasy-based experiences. Questions can be raised about the representativeness of the population of fantasy-prone subjects who participate in experimental research. Fantasizers screened in studies like ours might adopt a more liberal criterion for endorsing items that other subjects, concerned with portraying a more conventional image, are reluctant to endorse (e.g., child abuse). Furthermore, the consistencies observed across measures such as hypnotizability, absorption, and creativity may reflect subjects' strivings to maintain a consistent self-presentation as imaginative in response to measures perceived to be related to imaginative abilities. Evaluating the robustness of the relation between fantasy proneness and its hypothetical correlates should be undertaken in studies that vary the experimental context (e.g., tests administered in the context versus outside the context of hypnosis) and the demand characteristics for presenting oneself as fantasy prone.

Like other research in this area, the reliability of the

developmental data is limited by the retrospective nature of the study. It can also be argued that the reports of fantasizers are less reliable because their fantasy proneness is conducive to distortions and elaborations of their experiences (Rhue & Lynn, 1987c). This is a distinct possibility that should be evaluated in future research. However, it is noteworthy in the current research program that the interviewers placed strong demands for honesty and objective reporting on all subjects, that fantasizers did not differ from other subjects on a measure of social desirability, and that subjects were generally unable to identify the specific hypotheses of the study. In addition, many of our findings are consonant with those of other studies in this research area and have a high degree of internal consistency. Moreover, there is no reason to assume that fantasy-prone subjects would be motivated to present themselves as suffering greater punishment, for example (Rhue & Lynn, 1987b). However, studies that investigate the imaginative abilities of abused and nonabused children who differ in their degree of fantasy proneness are needed to address questions pertinent to the reliability of our findings. Indeed, we are in the process of studying populations of abused and nonabused children in order to explore the potential of imagery-based therapeutic approaches for enhancing childrens' adaptive capacities and abilities. We are also studying the effects of moderator variables (e.g., intelligence, supportive relationships) on the relation between developmental experiences, fantasy, and its concomitants across the entire life span.

It is important to resist the temptation to generalize the present results beyond the population tested. Fantasy-prone college students may represent a particularly well-adapted group of individuals who manifest an extensive history of imaginative involvements yet retain a measure of cognitive control of their fantasy lives. The development and role of fantasy in psychological disorders that appear to be related to a chaotic, unregulated, or overly rigid and inflexible use of fantasy are worthy of investigation. In certain psychological conditions (e.g., multiple personality disorder, schizophrenia, and obsessive-compulsive disorder), fantasy may minimize anxiety while perpetuating symptomatology by fostering an avoidant style of conflict and problem resolution. Indeed, it may be possible to isolate developmental experiences and personality attributes associated with the recreational, ego-abetting use of fantasy from fantasy that ultimately diminishes the individual by restricting involvement in developmentally appropriate experiences and coping with the demands of everyday life.

If one conclusion can be drawn from our research, it is that individuals at the extreme end of the continuum of fantasy proneness do not necessarily conform to a unitary personality type. Although we launched our research with the intent of studying a particular type of person, as we progressed, we were increasingly impressed by the diversity exhibited by the fantasizers we studied. We identified commonalities in the backgrounds and response patterns of so-called fantasy-prone persons, and we found that fantasizers diverged from less fantasy-prone individuals on measures presumed to be related to fantasy proneness. However, the term *fantasy-prone person* is misleading if used to denote a unified syndrome of affective, cognitive, and behavioral attributes. Fantasizers vary widely in their hypnotizability level, hallucinatory ability, developmental history, and psychological adjustment. Whereas some fantasizers are highly hypnotizable, others are not; whereas some fantasizers can hallucinate an object "as real as real," others are not able to generate convincing hallucinations; whereas some fantasizers report being abused as children, others paint a rosy picture of their childhood family environments; and whereas some fantasizers appear to be exemplars of healthy adjustment, other fantasizers' adjustment can be described as only marginal at best. Acknowledgment of the heterogeneous nature of fantasy-prone persons will broaden and deepen our understanding of the robustness and possible vicissitudes of fantasy proneness.

REFERENCES

As, A., O'Hara, J., & Munger, M. (1962). The measurement of subjective experiences presumably related to hypnotic susceptibility. *Scandinavian Journal of Psychology, 66,* 142–150.

Bandura, A., Ross, D., & Ross, S. (1961). Transmission of aggression through imitation of aggressive models. *Journal of Abnormal and Social Psychology, 63,* 575–582.

Barber, T. X. (1981). *Hypnosis: A scientific approach.* South Orange, N.J.: Power Publishers.

Barber, T. X., & Glass, L. (1962). Significant factors in hypnotic behavior. *Journal of Abnormal and Social Psychology, 64,* 222–228.

Barron, F., & Welsh, G. (1952). Artistic perception as a possible factor in personality style: Its measurement by a figure preference test. *Journal of Psychology, 33,* 199–203.

Baum, D., & Lynn, S. J. (1981). Hypnotic susceptibility level and reading involvement. *International Journal of Clinical and Experimental Hypnosis, 29,* 366–374.

Carpenter, C., & Huston-Stein, A. (1980). Activity structure and sex-typed behavior in preschool children. *Child Development, 51,* 862–872.

Chapman, L. J., Chapman, J. P., & Raulin, M. L. (1976). Scales for physical and social anhedonia. *Journal of Abnormal Psychology, 85,* 374–382.

Charcot, J. (1889). *Clinical lectures on the diseases of the nervous system, III.* London: New Sydenham Society.

Council, J. R. (1987, August). *Patterns of fantasy arising from childhood sexual abuse.* Paper presented at the meeting of the American Psychological Association, New York.

Council, J. R., Kirsch, I., & Hafner, L. (1986). Expectancy versus absorption in the prediction of hypnotic responding. *Journal of Personality and Social Psychology, 50,* 182–189.

Cronin, D. M., Spanos, N. P., & Barber, T. X. (1971). Augmenting hypnotic suggestibility by providing favorable information about hypnosis. *American Journal of Clinical Hypnosis, 13,* 259–264.

Crowne, D., & Marlowe, D. (1960). A new scale of social desirability independent of psychopathology. *Journal of Consulting Psychology, 4,* 349–354.

deGroot, H., Gwynn, M., & Spanos, N. P. (in press). The effects of contextual information and gender on the prediction of hypnotic susceptibility. *Journal of Personality and Social Psychology.*

Diamond, M. J. (1972). The use of observationally presented information to modify hypnotic susceptibility. *Journal of Abnormal Psychology, 79,* 174–180.

Diamond, M. J. (1982). Modifying hypnotic experience by means of indirect hypnosis and hypnotic skill training: An update (1981). *Research Communications in Psychology, Psychiatry and Behavior, 7,* 233–239.

Eckblad, M., & Chapman, L. J. (1983). Magical ideation as an indicator of schizotypy. *Journal of Consulting and Clinical Psychology, 51,* 215–225.

Fraiberg, S. (1968). *The magic years.* New York: Scribner's.

Freyberg, J. (1973). Increasing the imaginative play of urban disadvantaged kindergarten children through systematic training. In J. L. Singer (Ed.), *Child's world of make-believe.* New York: Academic Press.

Gfeller, J., Lynn, S. J., & Pribble, W. (1986). Enhancing hypnotic susceptibility: Interpersonal and rapport factors. *Journal of Personality and Social Psychology, 52,* 586–595.

Hilgard, J. R. (1965). Personality and hypnotizability: Inferences from case studies. In E. R. Hilgard, *Hypnotic susceptibility.* New York: Harcourt, Brace & World.

Hilgard, J. R. (1970). *Personality and hypnosis: A study of imaginative involvement.* Chicago: University of Chicago Press.

Hilgard, J. R. (1974). Imaginative involvement: Some characteristics of the highly hypnotizable and nonhypnotizable. *International Journal of Clinical and Experimental Hypnosis, 22,* 138–156.

Hilgard, J. R. (1979). Imaginative and sensory-affective involvements: In everyday life and hypnosis. In E. Fromm & R. Shor (Eds.), *Hypnosis: Developments in research and new perspectives.* New York: Aldine.

Hoch, P. H., & Cattell, J. P. (1959). The diagnosis of pseudoneurotic schizophrenia. *Psychiatric Quarterly, 33,* 17–43.

Huff, K., & Council, J. (1987, August). *Fantasy proneness and psychological coping.* Paper presented at the meeting of the American Psychological Association, New York.

Jalongo, M. (1984). Imaginary companions in children's lives and literature. *Childhood Education, 8,* 166–171.

Janet, P. (1901). *The mental state of hystericals.* New York: Putnam.

Kihlstrom, J. (1985). Hypnosis. In *Annual Review of Psychology, 36,* 385–418.

Kirsch, I., Council, J. R., & Mobayed, C. (1987). Imagery and response expectancy as determinants of hypnotic behavior. *British Journal of Experimental and Clinical Hypnosis, 4,* 25–31.

Klinger, E. (1969). Development of imaginative behavior: Implications of play for a theory of fantasy. *Psychological Bulletin, 72,* 277–298.

Kris, E. (1952). *Psychoanalytic explorations in art.* New York: International Universities Press.

Lee-Teng, E. (1965). Trance-susceptibility, induction susceptibility, and acquiescence as factors in hypnotic performance. *Journal of Abnormal Psychology, 7,* 383–389.

Lynn, S. J., & Dudley, K. (1987). *Magical ideation: A construct validation study.* Unpublished manuscript, Ohio University.

Lynn, S. J., & Rhue, J. W. (1986). The fantasy prone person: Hypnosis, imagination, and creativity. *Journal of Personality and Social Psychology, 51,* 404–408.

Lynn, S. J., & Rhue, J. W. (1987). Hypnosis, imagination, and fantasy. *Journal of Mental Imagery, 11,* 101–112.

Lynn, S. J., Snodgrass, M., Rhue, J., & Hardaway, R. (in press). Goal-directed fantasies, hypnotic susceptibility, and expectancies. *Journal of Personality and Social Psychology.*

Manosevitz, M., Prentice, N., & Wilson, F. (1973). Individual and family correlates of imaginary companions in preschool children. *Developmental Psychology, 8,* 72–79.

Nash, M. R., & Lynn, S. J. (1986). Child abuse and hypnotic ability. *Imagination, Cognition, and Personality, 5,* 211–218.

Nash, M. R., Lynn, S. J., & Givens, D. (1984). Adult hypnotic susceptibility, childhood punishment, and child abuse. *International Journal of Clinical and Experimental Hypnosis, 32,* 14–18.

Newmark, C. S., Gentry, L., Simpson, M., & Jones, T. (1978). MMPI criteria for diagnosing schizophrenia. *Journal of Personality Assessment, 42,* 366–373.

Rhue, J. W., & Lynn, S. J. (1985, July). *Correlates of fantasy proneness.* Paper presented at the meeting of the Midwest Psychological Association, Chicago.

Rhue, J. W., & Lynn, S. J. (1987a). *Fantasy proneness, absorption, and hypnosis: A re-examination.* Manuscript submitted for publication.

Rhue, J. W., & Lynn, S. J. (1987b). Fantasy proneness and psychopathology. *Journal of Personality and Social Psychology, 53,* 327–336.

Rhue, J. W., & Lynn, S. J. (1987c). Fantasy proneness: Developmental antecedents. *Journal of Personality, 55,* 121–137.

Rhue, J. W., & Lynn, S. J. (in press). Fantasy proneness: The ability to hallucinate "as real as real." *British Journal of Experimental and Clinical Hypnosis.*

Rhue, J. W., Lynn, S. J., Henry, S., Buhk, K., & Boyd, P. (1987, July). *Hypnosis, imagination, and child abuse.* Paper presented at the meeting of the Fourth European Congress of Hypnosis and Psychosomatic Medicine, Oxford, England.

Sarbin, R. T., & Lim, D. T. (1963). Some evidence in support of the role-taking hypothesis. *International Journal of Clinical and Experimental Hypnosis, 11,* 98–103.

Sheehan, P. W. (1967). A shortened form of Bett's Questionnaire Upon Mental Imagery. *Journal of Clinical Psychology, 23,* 386–389.

Sheehan, P. W. (1980). Factors influencing rapport in hypnosis. *Journal of Abnormal Psychology, 89,* 263–281.

Shor, R. E. (1960). The frequency of naturally occurring "hypnotic-like" experiences in the normal college population. *International Journal of Clinical and Experimental Hypnosis, 8,* 151–163.

Shor, R. E., & Orne, M. T. (1962). *Harvard Group Scale of Hypnotic Susceptibility, Form A.* Palo Alto, CA: Consulting Psychologists Press.

Shor, R. E., Orne, M. T., & O'Connell, D. N. (1962). Validation and cross-validation of a scale of self-reported personal experiences which predicts hypnotizability. *Journal of Psychology, 53,* 55–75.

Singer, J. (Ed.). (1973). *The child's world of make-believe.* New York: Academic Press.

Spanos, N. P. (1982). A social-psychological approach to hypnotic behavior. In G. Weary & H. L. Mirels (Eds.), *Integration of clinical and social psychology* (pp. 231–271). Oxford University Press.

Spanos, N. P. (1986). Hypnotic behavior: A social-psychological interpretation of amnesia, analgesia, and "trance logic." *The Behavioral and Brain Sciences, 9,* 449–502.

Spanos, N. P. (in press). Hypnosis, nonvolitional responding, and multiple personality: A social psychological perspective. In B. Maher (Ed.), *Progress in experimental personality research* (Vol. 14). New York: Academic Press.

Spanos, N. P., Cobb, P. N., & Gorassini, D. R. (in press). Failing to resist hypnotic suggestions: A strategy for self-presenting as deeply hypnotized. *Psychiatry.*

Spanos, N. P., Weekes, J., & deGroh, M. (1984). The "involuntary" countering of suggested requests: A test of the ideomotor hypothesis of hypnotic responsiveness. *British Journal of Experimental and Clinical Hypnosis, 1,* 3–11.

Stanley, S. M., Lynn, S. J., & Nash, M. R. (1986). Trance logic, susceptibility screening, and the transparency response. *Journal of Personality and Social Psychology, 50,* 447–454.

Stroufe, L. A. (1979). The coherence of individual development: Early care, attachment, and subsequent development. *American Psychologist, 34,* 834–841.

Tellegen, A. (1976). *Differential Personality Questionnaire.* Minneapolis: University of Minnesota.

Tellegen, A., & Atkinson, G. (1974). Openness to absorbing and self-altering experiences ("absorption"), a trait related to hypnotic susceptibility. *Journal of Abnormal Psychology, 83,* 268–277.

Tower, R. B. (1983). Imagery: Its role in development. In A. A. Sheikh (Ed.), *Imagery: Current theory, research, and application* (pp. 222–251). New York: Wiley.

Weitzenhoffer, A. M., & Hilgard, E. R. (1963). *Stanford Profile Scales of Hypnotic Susceptibility, Forms I & II.* Palo Alto, CA: Consulting Psychologists Press.

Wilson, S. C., & Barber, T. X. (1978). The Creative Imagination Scale as a measure of hypnotic responsiveness: Applications to experimental and clinical hypnosis. *American Journal of Clinical Hypnosis, 20,* 235–249.

Wilson, S. C., & Barber, T. X. (1981). Vivid fantasy and hallucinatory abilities in the life histories of excellent hypnotic subjects ("somnambules"): Preliminary report with female subjects. In E. Klinger (Ed.), *Imagery: Vol. 2. Concepts, results, and applications* (pp. 133–149). New York: Plenum.

Wilson, S. C., & Barber, T. X. (1983). The fantasy-prone personality: Implications for understanding imagery, hypnosis, and parapsychological phenomena. In A. A. Sheikh (Ed.), *Imagery: Current theory, research, and application* (pp. 340–390). New York: Wiley.

Zamansky, H. S. (1977). Suggestion and countersuggestion in hypnotic behavior. *Journal of Abnormal Psychology, 86,* 346–351.

[15]

On the Degree of Stability of Measured Hypnotizability Over a 25-Year Period

Carlo Piccione, Ernest R. Hilgard, and Philip G. Zimbardo
Stanford University

Conducted a longitudinal study of hypnotizability, as measured by the Stanford Hypnotic Susceptibility Scale, Form A, that yielded a relatively high degree of stability in hypnotic responsiveness over repeated testings spanning a 25-year period. The 50 Ss were retested in 1985, after tests when they were students, between 1958–1962 and again in 1970. The statistically significant stability coefficients were .64 (10-year retest), .82 (15-year retest), and .71 (25-year retest). The means did not change significantly, and the median change in the scores of individuals was only 1 point on the 12-item scale. A set of score measures and their intercorrelations are insufficient to resolve the issue of why stability occurs. The stability of hypnotizability over time compares favorably with that of other measures of individual differences.

In this article, we examine the degree of stability of scores on the Stanford Hypnotic Susceptibility Scale, Form A (SHSS:A; Weitzenhoffer & Hilgard, 1959) over a 25-year period. The study began in the fall of 1957 when the Stanford Laboratory of Hypnosis Research began the first phase of collaborative research examining individual differences in measured hypnotic susceptibility (E. R. Hilgard, 1965). The data on the relative stability of scores on a standardized hypnotic responsiveness scale, in this case over a period spanning a quarter of a century, bear importantly on varied investigations designed to understand hypnotic processes.

Domain of Hypnosis and Scale Construction

Tests attempting to measure hypnotizability appraise what has been variously called suggestibility, susceptibility, or hypnotic responsiveness. All of these descriptors can be considered synonyms of a person's measured talent or ability to produce behaviors and experiences falling within the complex domain of hypnosis (E. R. Hilgard, 1973).

The construction of a scale for the measurement of hypnotic responsiveness begins by selecting types of behavior and experiences characteristic of hypnosis. The items representing these types of experiences are then tried out on a large number of people inexperienced with hypnosis. Following an attempted induction of hypnosis by some standard method, the person is tested by being given the opportunity to respond to the various suggestions as a hypnotized person would. The test is but a sample of the broad range of possible hypnotic behaviors and experiences. The more of these suggestions the person "passes," the more hypnotizable that person is judged to be. Norms are derived through this empirical method. The method works because it is found that the various items (quite different in their surface structure) intercorrelate positively, and therefore represent a common phenomena.

The SHSS:A serves as one of the reference standards of measured hypnotic responsiveness. The SHSS:A is essentially a restandardization of the earlier Friedlander–Sarbin Scale (Friedlander & Sarbin, 1938), with some modifications in the wording and scoring of the items. Numerous other scales exist that sample other aspects of the domain (see E. R. Hilgard, 1979). The common factor in all of these scales is so prominent that Form A, although limited in the behaviors and experiences sampled, remains a test of hypnotizability whose scores correlate substantially with those from other adequately constructed scales.

Stanford Hypnotic Susceptibility Scale

The SHSS:A is a 12-item test, individually administered according to a standardized procedure. The eye-closure method of hypnotic induction used, as well as the verbal form of the suggestions used in other scored items, have been criticized as being somewhat directive (Wilson & Barber, 1978), but there is little evidence that this has affected the distribution of individual differences in scores as compared with tests using more permissive wording (Hilgard, 1978/1979). Some items on the SHSS:A permit the person to respond to direct suggestions, for example, the arm lowering item. Other items test for a loss or inhibition of motor control, as in the arm rigidity item. The participant is asked to extend his or her arm out and to make a tight fist, after which suggestions that the arm will become "as stiff as an iron bar which you can not bend" are given. The participant is then asked to test the stiffness and try to bend the outstretched arm. Additional items include a hallucination suggestion, amnesia, and a response to posthypnotic suggestion.

Each of the 12 items is scored pass–fail in terms of objective behavioral criteria. Passing an item adds 1 point, so the total

Portions of the results were presented in 1987 at the meeting of the Society for Clinical and Experimental Hypnosis in Los Angeles.

We gratefully acknowledge Joseph Barber, Jean Holroyd, and Anthony Piccione for the use of their offices and Richard Gonzalez for his statistical assistance.

Correspondence concerning this article should be addressed to Philip G. Zimbardo, Department of Psychology, Stanford University, Stanford, California 94305.

score on the SHSS:A can range from 0 to 12. Revised norms, serving as a standardization sample, were based on the scores of 533 Stanford University students. For this sample, the mean total score was 5.62, with a standard deviation of 3.27 (E. R. Hilgard, 1965).

The coefficients of reliability for the SHSS:A have been found to be satisfactory. The internal consistency of the SHSS:A was estimated for the standardization sample to be .83 (K–R 20). Furthermore, the analysis of the responses obtained from a subsample of this larger group yielded correlations (between the individual item and the total score minus that item) ranging from .38 to .83 (N = 124). Retesting on the next day with a parallel form, the Stanford Hypnotic Susceptibility Scale, Form B (SHSS:B; Weitzenhoffer & Hilgard, 1959), produced correlation coefficients of .83 and .90 (Ns = 124 and 96, respectively).

Retest Study of Hypnotizability Over Time

The present study of SHSS:A scores over a 25-year period sheds light on the stability or instability of such scores over time when no special effort has been made to modify the scores by special procedures.

The 10-Year Retest Study

The design of the sample relies on later participation by the same subjects who engaged in an earlier study of a retest over many years, as reported by Morgan, Johnson, & Hilgard (1974). During 1970, members of the Stanford Hypnosis Laboratory retested a total of 85 Stanford alumni who had been tested as undergraduates with the SHSS:A or SHSS:B (parallel forms) between 1958 and 1962. For convenience, this is referred to as a 10-year retest, although the actual interval varied between 8 and 12 years. The mean age of the respondents was 19.5 years at the time of the initial test and 29.8 years at the 10-year test in 1970. The earlier study found a significant test–retest correlation coefficient of .60 over a 10-year period.

The 25-Year Retest

In the present study, we retested a subsample of the subjects from the first retest using the same measuring instrument, the SHSS:A. The subjects now had three complete protocols on this scale: the initial testing, Test 1, conducted while a Stanford University student in the early 1960s; the 10-year retest, Test 2, in 1970; and Test 3 when approximately 45 years of age in 1985. Our goal was to measure the retest stability or instability of hypnotizability, as measured by the SHSS:A, over a 25-year period.

Method

Subjects

A list of names and subject numbers of the 85 respondents in the 10-year retest was compiled by an assistant unaware of this research's purpose. We obtained the addresses of 77 potential participants from the Stanford Office of the Registrar, and letters of invitation were sent to the 62 individuals residing in the greater San Francisco and Los Angeles areas. All were informed that they would be retested on a standardized susceptibility scale. They were promised a copy of the Morgan et al. (1974) article on the 10-year retest after concluding their participation.

Table 1
Adequacy of Mean Hypnotizability of Later Samples as Representative of Earlier Testing

Measure of hypnotizability	Potential subjects in 1985: Tested	Not tested
SHSS:A, 1970		
N	50	35
M	6.0	5.8
SD	3.6	3.8
SHSS:A or B, 1960		
N	50	35
M	5.9	6.1
SD	3.5	3.1
SHSS:A or B, Norms		
N	533	
M	5.62	
SD	3.27	

Note. SHSS:A or B = Stanford Hypnotic Susceptibility Scale, Form A or B (Weitzenhoffer & Hilgard, 1959). The norms (revised) are from E. R. Hilgard, 1965, p. 215. No significant mean differences between tested and not tested samples by t test are present; $p > .05$, two-tailed.

We used no other incentive to gain their participation, and they were not paid for participating.

A 98% return rate was obtained from the 31 men and 31 women sent an invitation; of those who replied, only 5 decided not to participate. Scheduling difficulties prevented 7 of the available respondents from being tested. Therefore, 50 individuals comprise the total sample with three complete protocols. Thirty-five subjects in the 10-year retest study were not tested in the 25-year retest. The resulting subject sample consisted of 81% of the 62 individuals who could possibly have been tested and 59% of the 85 available subjects from the 10-year retest.

To assess a subject selection bias, we compared the SHSS:A mean scores for the participating subjects with those respondents in the 10-year retest who were not tested in 1985 (N = 35). As can be seen in Table 1, there appears to be no systematic bias in the participating sample. There are only trivial, nonsignificant differences between the means of those tested in both Test 2 in 1970, $t(83) = .05$, and Test 1 in 1960, $t(83) = .06$, and those not tested a third time.

Furthermore, the means and standard deviations of the total scores for this sample of 50 subjects do not differ significantly by t test from the standardization sample of 533 subjects from which the respondents in the 1970 retest were drawn. Thus it appears that the current participants are representative in their hypnosis scores of the population of students tested during the same period of time.

Procedure

Each subject was individually tested following the standardized procedures for the administration of the SHSS:A (Weitzenhoffer & Hilgard, 1959). After the initial attempts to establish rapport, the experimenter read the standard instructions from the manual and scored the subject's responses in accordance with the behavioral criteria established by the scale. All testing was administered by the same researcher, who was unaware of the test scores on previous administrations until after the last respondent was tested. The interrogatory associated with the SHSS:A completed the formal testing.

Every attempt was made to test the respondent in a quiet room with comfortable seating arrangements. The location of the testing and the facilities were arranged for the subject's convenience. These facilities were university and hospital testing rooms, the offices of colleagues, mo-

Table 2
Test–Retest Correlation Coefficients of Measured Hypnotizability (Stanford Hypnotic Susceptibility Scale, Form A) for Total Sample and by Sex

Retest	Total (*N* = 50)	Male (*N* = 24)	Female (*N* = 26)
25 year (1960–1985)	.71	.69	.73
15 year (1970–1985)	.82	.82	.81
10 year (1960–1970)	.64	.62	.67

Note. All correlations are statistically significant, $p < .01$, but no one correlation differs significantly from another, $p > .05$, two-tailed.

tel rooms, or the home of a participating subject. Data from all of the subjects tested were used in the analysis of the results.

Results

Group Changes in Total Hypnotizability Scores

Stability and change were judged by criteria both of correlations and mean scores.

Test–retest correlations over time. The correlation between test scores over time is limited by the reliabilities of the tests. In this case, the internal consistencies were high enough to give an expectation of significant correlations over time if what was measured did in fact show some stability. The estimate of the internal consistency for the three testings is .86 for Test 1, .87 for Test 2, and .88 for Test 3, as determined by K–R 20 (all *N*s = 50).

The test-retest correlations over the 25-year period for the total SHSS:A scores are found in Table 2. For the 25-year, 15-year, and 10-year periods the retest correlations are .71, .82, and .64, respectively, all highly significant. A general chi-square test indicates that the three correlations for the total sample are drawn statistically from the same population, $\chi^2(2, N = 50) = 3.54$, $p > .05$ (Hays, 1973). None of the pairwise comparisons of the correlations was statistically significant by *z*-test, $p > .05$, two-tailed. The similarity between the test–retest correlation coefficients for the women and men in this study can also be seen in Table 2.

Mean score differences over time. Because this is a longitudinal study with repeated measures on the same subjects, it is appropriate to test the significance of mean score differences through analyses of variance (ANOVAS) based on this within-subjects variable.

A 2 × 3 (Sex × Test) repeated-measures ANOVA comparing the total SHSS:A scores of the men and women (sex) on each of the three tests (test) did not result in any statistically significant differences by test or sex. Table 3 presents the corresponding mean total SHSS:A scores for the group as a whole and separately for the women and men for the three tests at different ages. The mean total scores for the three tests over the 25-year period are not statistically different from each other, $F(2, 96) = 1.57$, *ns*. The absences of both a difference between the men's and women's total scores on the SHSS:A, $F(1, 48) = 0.00$, *ns*, and of an interaction effect, $F(2, 96) = 0.41$, *ns*, allow the data on sex to be collapsed.

Table 3
Retest Mean Hypnotizability Scores (Stanford Hypnotic Susceptibility Scale, Form A) for the Total Sample and by Sex

Test	Total (*N* = 50)	Male (*N* = 24)	Female (*N* = 26)
1985			
M	6.5	6.6	6.4
SD	3.6	3.7	3.6
1970			
M	6.0	5.8	6.2
SD	3.6	3.6	3.6
1960			
M	5.9	6.0	5.8
SD	3.5	3.8	3.4

Note. All differences between the means by sex and test are nonsignificant, $p > .05$.

Prediction of later test scores from earlier ones. The scores on Test 1 and Test 2 can be weighted through a regression analysis to account for the variance of scores in Test 3. The best fit was found to be the following linear equation: Test 3 score = .85 + .328 (Test 1 score) + .622 (Test 2 score). When applied, this combination of scores from Test 1 and Test 2 led to $R^2 = .724$. In other words, 72% of the variance in Test 3 scores is accounted for by the scores in Tests 1 and 2.

Individual Changes in Hypnotizability Scores

Despite the high group correlations, there is still room for substantial changes in scores by individuals. It is therefore important to analyze the flux in hypnotizability scores by individuals over time.

The absolute differences between each participant's total hypnotizability scores on the three protocols can be seen in Table 4. All score distributions had standard deviations of 3.4 or greater (Table 3). Hence, those individuals whose scores changed 3 points or less had changed less than 1 standard deviation. Eighty-four percent fell in this group over the 25-year retest, 88% in the 15-year retest, and 86% in the 10-year retest. The median change for the 50 subjects over each interval was very close to a single score point, with 52%, 48%, and 52% of

Table 4
Individual Change in Total Hypnotizability Scores (Stanford Hypnotic Susceptibility Scale, Form A)

	Absolute change scores					
					Total	
Retest	Δ0	Δ1	Δ2	Δ3	Δ3 or less	Δ4 or more
25 year (1960–1985)	8	18	10	6	42 (84%)	8 (16%)
15 year (1970–1985)	11	13	14	6	44 (88%)	6 (12%)
10 year (1960–1970)	13	13	10	7	43 (86%)	7 (14%)

Note. *N* = 50. For the three tests used in the comparisons, the standard deviations are between 3 and 4 scale points. A change score of 4 or more is greater than 1 standard deviation for any test.

Table 5
Corresponding General Level of Hypnotizability Scores (Stanford Hypnotic Susceptibility Scale, Form A) on the 10-Year Retest by Individuals

	Test 2 (1970)			
Test 1 (1960)	Low	Medium	High	Total
High	1	3	**10**	14
Medium	4	**12**	5	21
Low	**10**	4	1	15
Total	15	19	16	50

Note. Numbers in boldface indicate agreement in scoring level on both tests.

Table 7
Corresponding General Level of Hypnotizability Scores (Stanford Hypnotic Susceptibility Scale, Form A) on the 25-Year Retest by Individuals

	Test 3 (1985)			
Test 1 (1960)	Low	Medium	High	Total
High	1	2	**11**	14
Medium	3	**12**	6	21
Low	**8**	6	1	15
Total	12	20	18	50

Note. Numbers in boldface indicate agreement in scoring level on both tests.

the cases showing either no change or a 1-point change over the 10-year, 15-year, or 25-year retest, respectively.

Only 2 subjects had the same score on all three tests. The remaining 48 subjects in our sample changed their total hypnotizability score at least once during retest.

The overall stability of the test scores as revealed by these correlations is not informative about where the failures of stability lie. To ascertain which subjects moved up and which moved down over test periods, we recast the data in a scatterplot. A convenient adaptation of a scatterplot, yielding some information in addition to that provided more precisely by regression analysis, can be found by a correlation plot reduced to 9 cells by grouping subjects into three scoring levels on SHSS:A—high (scores 9–12), medium (scores 4–8), and low (scores 0–3)—on both of the correlated tests. This is shown for the three retest correlations in Tables 5, 6, and 7.

The correspondence of hypnotizability scores between Test 1 and Test 2 for individuals categorized as high, medium, and low on Test 1 is presented in Table 5. The retest correlation was .64, as previously shown in Table 2. The 32 individuals in the diagonal cells (in boldface) scored within the same level on both tests. Of the rest, 10 individuals scored in a higher level of hypnotizability on Test 2 from Test 1; the scores of 8 participants moved to lower levels in the 1970 retest.

A similar comparison between Tests 2 and 3, presented in Table 6, showed an increase in the number of individuals consistently scoring in the same level of hypnotizability. The stability coefficient was .82 between these two tests using the identical measure of hypnotizability, the SHSS:A. A total of 35 individuals (representing 70% of the sample of 50) were consistent on both tests. In 1985, no participant moved from the low level to the high or from the high level to the low.

Table 6
Corresponding General Level of Hypnotizability Scores (Stanford Hypnotic Susceptibility Scale, Form A) on the 15-Year Retest by Individuals

	Test 3 (1985)			
Test 2 (1970)	Low	Medium	High	Total
High	0	3	**13**	16
Medium	2	**12**	5	19
Low	**10**	5	0	15
Total	12	20	18	50

Note. Numbers in boldface indicate agreement in scoring level on both tests.

Over the 25-year period between Test 1 and Test 3 (with a correlation of .71), there were 31 individuals who scored at the same level of hypnotizability, as seen in Table 7. Unlike the 10-year retest, which had a similar number of individuals shifting their hypnotizability level upward or downward, from 1960 to 1985 there were more than twice as many individuals (13 to 6) with an upward shift in their levels of hypnotizability.

Retest Correlations and Means for Specific Items

As previously noted, a high coefficient of internal consistency is maintained subsequent to the repeated exposures to the SHSS:A. The retest correlations for the 12 specific items on the SHSS:A are also found to be positive and most of them significant, as shown in Table 8.

For a closer look at the results in Table 8, we have chosen to compare SHSS:A items in the 15-year retest, Test 2 versus Test 3. This is appropriate because SHSS:A was the only form used in both testings, whereas in Test 1 some of the subjects were given SHSS:B rather than SHSS:A.

Between Test 2 and Test 3, the tetrachoric correlation coefficients are above .45 and statistically significant for all of the 12 SHSS:A items; 9 of the items have a retest coefficient between .74–.95.

The changes or stability of the 12 items by percentage of subjects passing is also evidenced in their rank-order correlations (Table 8). The percentage of subjects passing each item resulted in some changes in rank order between Test 1 and Test 2 (10-year retest), yielding a positive but nonsignificant correlation between ranks (Spearman's $\rho = .49$), $t(10) = 1.78, p > .05$, two-tailed. The corresponding comparison between Test 2 and Test 3 (15-year retest) resulted in a statistically significant rank-order correlation (Spearman's $\rho = .95$), $t(10) = 9.50, p < .01$, two-tailed, possibly indicating a stabilization after the first retest. The third comparison, between Test 1 and Test 3 (25-year retest), yielded a significant rank-order correlation for item difficulty of .60 ($t = 2.37, p < .05$, two-tailed).

Table 8
Retest Measures on Specific Items of the Stanford Hypnotic Susceptibility Scale, Form A

Item	Percent passing					
	T1 (1960)	T2 (1970)	T3 (1985)	T1 vs. T2 (10-yr. retest)	T2 vs. T3 (15-yr. retest)	T1 vs. T3 (25-yr. retest)
Postural sway	64	68	70	.57	.60	.51
Eye closure	68[a]	74	82_a	.58	.91	.72
Hand lowering	84	74	84	.60	.75	.47*
Arm immobilization	28	34	36	.48	.74	.57
Finger lock	36_{ab}	44_b	50_a	.73	.85	.73
Arm rigidity	32	50	50	.54	.93	.77
Moving hands	66_b	84_b	74	.46	.60	.54
Verbal inhibition	24_{ab}	46_b	46_a	.54	.81	.81
Fly hallucination	52_b	32_b	44	.91	.75	.44
Eye catalepsy	34	36	46	.64	.87	.75
Posthypnotic suggestion	54_b	32_b	36	.19*	.45	.04*
Amnesia	44_b	24_b	30	.57	.95	.71

Note. T1 = Test 1. T2 = Test 2. T3 = Test 3. All r_t are significant at $p < .05$ except as indicated. The test items whose differences in percent passing proved significant by z test are marked by a same-letter subscript, in these cases, $p < .05$, two-tailed.
* $p > .05$.

The results in Table 8 supplement the more general findings in earlier tables by indicating the extent to which scores on individual test items contributed to the relative stability of the total hypnotizability scores.

Discussion

Hypnotizability, as measured by the SHSS:A proved relatively stable over 25 years. This stability occurred despite the changes in life experiences between the college years and mid-adult life. The flux in subjects' lives over a quarter of a century, through marriage and child-rearing, occupational shifts, traumas associated with illness, death of loved ones, and loss by divorce, cannot be assumed to be trivial.

Obtained Stability of Mean Hypnotizability

It would be possible for the retest correlations over time to be significant even though mean scores changed in some consistent manner with age. We found, however, that the means did not change significantly as a function of age.

Our finding of nonsignificant mean changes in hypnotic ability over 25 years conflicts with two major cross-sectional studies (Gordon, 1972; Morgan & Hilgard, 1973). In a study done with VA patients hospitalized for medical (nonpsychiatric) reasons, the decline between a group tested on the SHSS:A at ages 20–29 from one at ages 40–49 averaged 2.9 points (Gordon, 1972). Another study (Morgan & Hilgard, 1973) was based on 1,232 cases individually tested, including a large sample of students, and another sample of parents in the community. Morgan & Hilgard found a change of 2.1 scale points between the 265 subjects aged 17–20 and the 103 subjects aged 37 and older.

The advantage of a longitudinal study is that it deals with intraindividual modifications as a function of time rather than between individuals of different ages. Our findings suggest that, without special efforts at modification, hypnotizability may in fact be relatively stable between the college years and the early adult years. This result is tempered by the possibility that the retesting of the same individuals may accentuate stability. The absence of a decline in mean scores over the years has to be interpreted in line with these possibilities.

Stability of Hypnotizability Compared With Other Individual Difference Measures

It is pertinent to compare the stability of hypnotizability over longer time periods with the available evidence from other measures of individual differences.

Intelligence measurement. The stability of measured hypnotizability can be compared with the test–retest reliability of IQ scores. Over a retest period of similar length, the magnitude of the stability coefficients for the SHSS:A compares very well with those found for IQ. For a sample of similar size that was administered the Wechsler Adult Intelligence Scale at age 29 and again at age 42 (a 13-year interval) the test–retest correlations were .73 for the full scale IQ, .70 for Verbal IQ, and .57 for Performance IQ (Kangas & Bradway, 1971).

Personality tests. A comparison with a traditional personality assessment instrument is provided by the Study of Values (Allport & Vernon, 1931). The retest correlations ranged from .60 after a few years to an average of .50 after intervals spanning 10–25 years between testings (Huntley & Davis, 1983). The size of these correlations are representative of the more robust stability estimates of measures of personality (McCrae & Costa, 1984).

The stability of men's occupational interests as determined by scales on the Strong-Campbell Interest Inventory (SCII; Campbell & Hansen, 1981) provides yet another comparison. On the basis of data from an earlier version of the scale, the manual for the SCII reports a 20-year test–retest correlation of .72 for men 22–25 years old at first testing and .64 for those 19–21 years old at first testing.

The preceding comparisons indicate that the stability coefficients of the SHSS:A, despite its being only a 12-item test, compare favorably with the stability coefficients obtained with other measures of individual differences relevant to personality.

Issue of person versus situation. We are well aware of the attacks that have been made within personality theory against attributing relative stability of scores to persisting personality characteristics, such as aptitudes and traits, without recognition of the importance of the situation in which the behavior is observed. The significance of the interaction between person and situation is clearly recognized (Endler & Magnusson, 1976). If, therefore, we have called attention to the relatively high correlations over 25 years as an indication of a possibly persistent talent, a set of correlations and means cannot resolve the issue of why stability occurs.

There is, for example, the possibility of a hereditary component, as shown in studies of hypnotizability among twins and their parents. In this research all participants were hypnotized and tested separately but simultaneously, so that they had no opportunity to influence each other through discussion of their hypnotic performances (Morgan, 1973). However, as with the twin studies of intelligence, the data are subject to the same difficulties in estimating the effects of similarities in social and environmental influences.

Personality theorists would do well to attend to those aspects of human performance that override many situational influences. As far as our study is concerned, we can do little but point to the data that show a median change of but a single point over 25 years on a 12-item scale, despite the many situational changes that must have occurred over these years.

That hypnotizability scores remain resistant to modification with ordinary experiences normally encountered in daily life does not mean that scores are immutable through special interventions. The limits of score changes through special techniques directed at score modification are not, however, at issue in the present study. Most efforts to modify hypnotizability have resulted in very slight changes in test scores (Diamond, 1977; Perry, 1977). Large changes have been reported through the use of ingenious techniques to persuade and train the subject that everyone can learn to become highly hypnotizable (Gorassini & Spanos, 1986). Even with the generally successful manipulations of these efforts to raise scores of the initially low scorers, there are some limitations on success (Gfeller, Lynn, & Pribble, 1987). For example, in this study 14 of the 24 initially low scorers failed to score high on retest after training. Such large changes in test scores are subject to varying interpretations, just as enduring stabilities are.

Hypnotizability in Relation to Personality and Clinical Practice

With the introduction of the Stanford scales almost 30 years ago, numerous investigations have attempted to explain the individual differences found in hypnotic responsiveness, usually either by way of correlational studies or by changes in hypnotic procedures according to plausible hypotheses. Psychological processes that may be related include attention, imagery, daydreaming styles, psychophysiological changes, attitudes, expectancies, and many others investigated with limited success. (For a review, see Kihlstrom, 1985).

Measured hypnotizability and personality. Attempted correlations of hypnotizability scores with the Minnesota Multiphasic Personality Inventory (MMPI), the California Psychological Inventory (CPI), and projective tests such as the Rorschach have all resulted in trivial outcomes. Was this failure due to the limitations of the personality scales, or to the nature of hypnotic talent as perhaps something too unique to be captured by personality scales? Subsequently, the best evidence shows that the failure lay in the definition of personality implicit in these instruments and in their techniques of validation.

The study most relevant to a widely used personality inventory has proved illuminating (Tellegen & Atkinson, 1974). On the basis of efforts to predict hypnotizability from interviews, Josephine Hilgard (1970/1979) demonstrated the significance for hypnosis of what she called "imaginative involvement." Tellegen and Atkinson (1974) constructed a scale, based in part on what Hilgard had found in her interviews, that they called "absorption," which occurs in imagination in ordinary life with an altered sense of reality. Tellegen and Atkinson's hypnosis scale was a slight modification of the Harvard Group Scale of Hypnotic Susceptibility, Form A (HGSHS:A; Shor & Orne, 1962), a group form of SHSS:A. They conducted a careful study to select items representing absorption and the two prominent factors in the MMPI (stability–instability and introversion–extroversion). On cross-validation with a sample of $N = 171$, they found a modest but significant correlation between measured hypnotizability and absorption (.43, $p < .001$), but trivial negative correlations with the two MMPI factors (−.02 with stability–instability, −.18 with introversion–extroversion). They justifiably concluded that the MMPI, with its hundreds of items and validation on pathological populations, had failed to include items reflecting the personalities of the highly hypnotizable. Of course, the correlation of .43 is one of those significant but low correlations that plague personality measurement. However, the absence of even that much relation to hypnotic ability is more a weakness of the MMPI than it is of the hypnosis scale.

Some later support for the Tellegen and Atkinson (1974) findings, using other methods, has been reported (J. R. Hilgard, 1970/1979; O'Grady, 1980). O'Grady correlated the Tellegen–Atkinson absorption scale with a variety of personality measures and found, after a factor analysis, that one of the three factors (accounting for 17% of the total variance) was exclusively comprised of absorption. Although the correlation leaves much of the variance unaccounted for, a later study of exceptionally hypnotizable subjects confirmed that, independent of hypnosis, the highly hypnotic subjects were "fantasy prone" (Wilson & Barber, 1983).

Measured hypnotizability and clinical application. The results from this study support the findings on the functional utility of measured hypnotizability. For example, the predictability of the SHSS:A and similar tests has been established for the relation of hypnotic ability to the reduction of experimental and clinical pain (e.g., E. R. Hilgard, 1986; E. R. Hilgard & Hilgard, 1983; J. R. Hilgard & LeBaron, 1984). Because the effectiveness of psychological methods in clinical practice can depend on many aspects of the interpersonal relation between therapist and patient, it is desirable when that effectiveness is attributed to hypnosis to show that the modifications do indeed relate positively to measured hypnotizability. The heuristic of proposing and implementing the clinical treatment with the greatest probability of success depends on the use of reliable screening instruments. With these data supporting the stability of measured hypnotizability, the efficacy of clinical interventions using hypnosis can benefit from the predictive utility of hypnotic ability.

References

Allport, G. W., & Vernon, P. E. (1931). *Study of values.* Boston: Houghton Mifflin.

Campbell, D. P., & Hansen, J. C. (1981). *Manual for the Strong-Campbell Interest Inventory.* Palo Alto, CA: Consulting Psychologists Press.

Diamond, M. J. (1977). Hypnotizability is modifiable: An alternative approach. *International Journal of Clinical and Experimental Hypnosis, 25,* 147–166.

Endler, N. S., & Magnusson, D. (Eds.). (1976). *Interactional psychology and personality.* Washington, DC: Hemisphere.

Friedlander, J. W., & Sarbin, T. R. (1938). The depth of hypnosis. *Journal of Abnormal and Social Psychology, 33,* 453–475.

Gfeller, J. D., Lynn, S. J., & Pribble, W. E. (1987). Enhancing hypnotic susceptibility: Interpersonal and rapport factors. *Journal of Personality and Social Psychology, 52,* 586–595.

Gorassini, D. R., & Spanos, N. P. (1986). A social-cognitive skills approach to the successful modification of hypnotic susceptibility. *Journal of Personality and Social Psychology, 50,* 1004–1012.

Gordon, M. C. (1972). Age and performance differences of male patients on modified Stanford Hypnotic Susceptibility Scales. *International Journal of Clinical and Experimental Hypnosis, 20,* 152–155.

Hays, W. L. (1973). *Statistics for the social sciences* (2nd ed.). New York: Holt, Rinehart & Winston.

Hilgard, E. R. (1965). *Hypnotic susceptibility.* New York: Harcourt, Brace & World.

Hilgard, E. R. (1973). The domain of hypnosis, with some comments on alternative paradigms. *American Psychologist, 28,* 972–982.

Hilgard, E. R. (1978/1979). The Stanford Hypnotic Susceptibility Scales as related to other measures of hypnotic responsiveness. *The American Journal of Clinical Hypnosis, 21,* 68–83.

Hilgard, E. R. (1979, March). The measurement of hypnotic responsiveness: Purposes and available instruments. *Bulletin of the British Society of Experimental and Clinical Hypnosis* (No. 2), 6–10.

Hilgard, E. R. (1986). Hypnosis and pain. In R. A. Sternbach (Ed.), *The psychology of pain* (2nd ed., pp. 197–221). New York: Raven.

Hilgard, E. R., & Hilgard, J. R. (1983). *Hypnosis in the relief of pain* (2nd ed.). Los Altos, CA: William Kaufmann.

Hilgard, J. R. (1979). *Personality and hypnosis: A study of imaginative involvement* (2nd ed.). Chicago: University of Chicago Press. (Original work published 1970).

Hilgard, J. R., & LeBaron, S. (1984). *Hypnotherapy of pain in children with cancer.* Los Altos, CA: William Kaufmann.

Huntley, C. W., & Davis, F. (1983). Undergraduate Study of Values scores as predictors of occupation 25 years later. *Journal of Personality and Social Psychology, 45,* 1148–1155.

Kangas, J., & Bradway, K. (1971). Intelligence at middle age: A thirty-eight year follow-up. *Developmental Psychology, 5,* 333–337.

Kihlstrom, J. F. (1985). Hypnosis. *Annual Review of Psychology, 36,* 385–418.

McCrae, R. R., & Costa, P. T. (1984). *Emerging lives, enduring dispositions: Personality in adulthood.* Boston: Little, Brown.

Morgan, A. H. (1973). The heritability of hypnotic susceptibility in twins. *Journal of Abnormal Psychology, 82,* 55–61.

Morgan, A. H., & Hilgard, E. R. (1973). Age differences in susceptibility to hypnosis. *International Journal of Clinical and Experimental Hypnosis, 21,* 78–85.

Morgan, A. H., Johnson, D. L., & Hilgard, E. R. (1974). The stability of hypnotic susceptibility: A longitudinal study. *International Journal of Clinical and Experimental Hypnosis, 22,* 249–257.

O'Grady, K. E. (1980). The absorption scale: A factor-analytic assessment. *International Journal of Clinical and Experimental Hypnosis, 28,* 281–288.

Perry, C. (1977). Is hypnotizability modifiable? *International Journal of Clinical and Experimental Hypnosis, 25,* 125–146.

Shor, R. E., & Orne, E. C. (1962). *The Harvard Group Scale of Hypnotic Susceptibility, Form A.* Palo Alto, CA: Consulting Psychologists Press.

Tellegen, A., & Atkinson, G. (1974). Openness to absorbing and self-altering experiences ("absorption"), a trait related to hypnotic susceptibility. *Journal of Abnormal Psychology, 83,* 268–277.

Weitzenhoffer, A. M., & Hilgard, E. R. (1959). *Stanford Hypnotic Susceptibility Scale, Forms A and B.* Palo Alto, CA: Consulting Psychologists Press.

Wilson, S. C., & Barber, T. X. (1978). The Creative Imagination Scale as a measure of hypnotic responsiveness: Applications to experimental and clinical hypnosis. *The American Journal of Clinical Hypnosis, 20,* 235–249.

Wilson, S. C., & Barber, T. X. (1983). The fantasy-prone personality: Implications for understanding imagery, hypnosis, and parapsychological phenomena. In A. A. Sheikh (Ed.), *Imagery: Current theory, research, and application* (pp. 340–387). New York: Wiley.

Received November 10, 1987
Revision received June 27, 1988
Accepted June 28, 1988 ■

[16]

Imaginative Suggestibility and Hypnotizability

Irving Kirsch[1] and Wayne Braffman

Department of Psychology, University of Connecticut, Storrs, Connecticut

Abstract

More than a half-century of research aimed at identifying the predictors of hypnotic responding has been described as investigations of "hypnotizability." Most of that research, however, has disregarded the well-established findings that (a) people respond to suggestion without being hypnotized almost as much as they do following a hypnotic induction, and (b) nonhypnotic and hypnotic suggestibility are highly correlated. More recent studies have provided the first empirical data on predictors of individual differences in response to the induction of hypnosis. These studies indicate that individual differences in hypnotic suggestibility can be accounted for completely by nonhypnotic suggestibility, expectancy, motivation, and reaction time. Because the amount of variance accounted for is as great as the reliability of the hypnotic-suggestibility scale, and because nonhypnotic suggestibility has been controlled, no additional variables are necessary to account for hypnotic suggestibility.

Keywords

hypnosis; suggestibility; hypnotizability

Highly suggestible hypnotized subjects display and report automatic movements, partial paralyses, selective amnesia, insensitivity to painful stimulation, and hallucinations in all sensory modalities. These responses seem so astonishing that they have evoked two contrasting reactions. One is to doubt their veracity; the second is to assume that they must be due to a very unusual altered state, generally referred to as a hypnotic "trance." But research indicates that neither of these conclusions is justified.

Hypnotized subjects are not merely putting on an act to impress an observer. Unlike unsuggestible people who have been instructed to fake high levels of responding, highly suggestible people display hypnotic responses even when they think that they are alone (Perugini et al., 1998). The veracity of the experiential reports of hypnotized subjects has also been substantiated by brain-imaging studies. Rainville, Duncan, Price, Carrier, and Bushnell (1997), for example, reported that suggestions used to alter the unpleasantness of painful stimuli produced changes in brain activity that were consistent with those suggestions.

Although the experiences and behaviors reported and observed in hypnosis are real, data indicate that they are not due to a trance. Instead, hypnotic responses reveal an astounding capacity that some people have to alter their experience in profound ways. Hypnosis is only one of the ways in which this capacity is revealed. It can also be evoked—and almost to the same extent—without inducing hypnosis at all. These data and their implications are the subjects of this article.

HYPNOTIC AND NONHYPNOTIC SUGGESTIBILITY

One of the most salient aspects of hypnotic responding is its variability between people. Some people respond to almost all suggestions; others respond to none; most show moderate levels of response. Although responsiveness can be altered by changing people's expectations about how they will respond (e.g., Vickery & Kirsch, 1991) and by training (Gorassini & Spanos, 1999), in the absence of interventions of this sort, it is remarkably stable. This has led to the development of highly reliable standardized scales that measure individual differences in responding (e.g., Weitzenhoffer & Hilgard, 1962).

Because the behaviors measured by these scales were presumed to be due to the induction of an altered state of consciousness, the construct they measure was labeled "hypnotizability" or "hypnotic susceptibility." The presumption was that the observed behaviors were due to the induction of hypnosis, but the data tell a very different story. They reveal that hypnotizability is an inaccurate and misleading name for a very important trait, ability, or propensity that has little to do with the induction of hypnosis.

Hypnotic-suggestibility scales consist of two parts: a hypnotic-induction ritual and a series of test suggestions. A typical induction ritual consists of instructions for muscular and mental relaxation (similar to those given in relaxation training) with mention of the word "hypnosis." The test suggestions are of four types: motor productions (involuntary movements), motor inhibitions (paralyses), cognitive productions (hallucinations), and cognitive inhibitions (sensory inhibition, amnesia).

Because the induction rituals are separate from the test suggestions, it is possible to administer the suggestions with and without inducing hypnosis or following any other procedure aimed at increasing responsiveness to suggestion. This has been done in six studies (Barber & Glass, 1962; Braffman & Kirsch, 1999a, 1999b; Hilgard & Tart, 1966; Hull, 1933; Weitzenhoffer & Sjoberg, 1961), and the results reported in all of these studies are consistent. They reveal that the effect of hypnosis is relatively small—"probably far less than the classical hypnotists would have supposed had the question ever occurred to them," wrote Clark Hull in 1933 (p. 298)—and the correlation between hypnotic and nonhypnotic responding is very high. These data alone should lay to rest the altered-state hypothesis in its strongest form. Because responses to imaginative suggestions are almost as readily observed outside of hypnosis as in it, they cannot be ascribed to the presence of a hypnotic trance.[2]

Because of the small effect of hypnosis and the high correlation between hypnotic and nonhypnotic responding, the term hypnotizability is inaccurate and misleading as a label for the individual difference variable measured by so-called hypnosis scales. These scales do not measure differences in the effects of hypnosis. Instead, they measure differences in responses to a particular type of suggestion, more or less independent of the induction of hypnosis.

One might consider using the term "suggestibility" to denote the construct measured by these scales. But without further qualification, this term is too broad. There are diverse types of suggestibility that differ from each other in the nature of the suggestions given, and these different types of suggestibility are not highly correlated with each other. Most types of suggestion are deceptive. They are aimed at convincing the person that the world is (or was) different from the way it actually is (or was). For example, placebos are inert, but are presented as substances that contain active medications (Kirsch, 1997). Similarly, leading questions provide false information about past events (Mazzoni, in press). In contrast, the suggestions that are administered in hypnotic susceptibility scales are not deceptive. They are not aimed at convincing the person that the world outside his or her experience has changed or is different from the way it actually is. Instead, hypnotized subjects are asked to engage in fantasies, leading to subjective experiences that are at variance with what they know to be objectively true. Often, they are explicitly instructed to imagine the suggested state of affairs (e.g., "imagine a force acting on your hands to push them apart," Weitzenhoffer & Hilgard, 1962, p. 18). For this reason, we have termed this type of suggestibility *imaginative suggestibility*.

Imaginative suggestions are requests to experience an imaginary state of affairs as if it were real. These suggestions can be given in or out of hypnosis. Imaginative suggestibility is the degree to which the person succeeds in having the suggested experiences. It can be assessed in or out of hypnosis. Responsiveness to other types of suggestions can also be assessed with and without hypnosis, but the suggestions contained in the so-called hypnosis scales are imaginative suggestions, and it is the responsiveness to these suggestions that has been mislabeled hypnotizability. When we use the terms hypnotic suggestibility and nonhypnotic suggestibility, we are referring to imaginative suggestibility, assessed in and out of hypnosis, respectively.

THE IMPORTANCE OF LANGUAGE

Referring to hypnotic suggestibility as hypnotizability is not just inaccurate, it is also very misleading. Just how misleading it is can most clearly be appreciated by considering analogous situations. Imagine, for example, that a group of researchers wishes to determine the correlates of successful weight loss. In study after study, they put people on diets and then correlate their postdiet weight with potential predictor variables, without controlling for differences in prediet weight. They find that postdiet weight is correlated with height, waist size, gender, and weight of parents. They then conclude that short, thin women with thin parents have a natural ability to lose weight.

We suspect that the fallacy of this conclusion would be recognized immediately by virtually all members of the scientific community studying weight loss and that the manuscripts of these researchers would never find their way into print. A similar fate should await hypnosis researchers who commit the error of confusing hypnotic suggestibility with hypnotizability. Just as weight loss is the change in weight after a diet, hypnotizability is the change in suggestibility after hypnosis has been induced. Measuring suggestibility after a hypnotic induction and calling it hypnotizability is like assessing weight after a diet and calling it weight loss. Neither approach makes any sense unless the pretreatment data (i.e., nonhypnotic suggestibility and prediet weight, respectively) are taken into account. Because hypnotizability refers to the change in suggestibility that is produced by hypnosis, it can be measured as hypnotic suggestibility with nonhypnotic suggestibility statistically controlled.

THE CORRELATES OF HYPNOTIC SUGGESTIBILITY AND HYPNOTIZABILITY

Accounting for individual differences in hypnotic suggestibility (generally mislabeled hypnotizability or hypnotic susceptibility) has been an enigma that has eluded the best efforts of hypnosis researchers for the better part of a century. Excepting nonhypnotic suggestibility, only four variables have been shown to be reliably correlated with hypnotic suggestibility (e.g., Kirsch, Silva, Comey, & Reed, 1995). In descending order of the magnitude of association, these variables are response expectancy (i.e., the participant's prediction about the degree to which he or she will respond to suggestions), attitudes toward hypnosis, fantasy proneness, and absorption (i.e., the tendency to become absorbed in commonplace imaginative experiences). Until recently, however, studies of correlates of hypnotic suggestibility left out the most powerful one: nonhypnotic imaginative suggestibility.

We recently reported the first study in which nonhypnotic imaginative suggestibility was examined in conjunction with other correlates of hypnotic suggestibility (Braffman & Kirsch, 1999a). These data revealed significant correlations of hypnotic suggestibility with nonhypnotic imaginative suggestibility, response expectancy, the motivation to respond to suggestion, and fantasy proneness. The correlation between hypnotic suggestibility and absorption was not significant. This study also was the first attempt to find correlates of individual differences in hypnotizability, defined as the effect of hypnosis on response to suggestion. We did this via a series of regression analyses in which we analyzed the associations between hypnotic suggestibility and other variables after statistically controlling for individuals' nonhypnotic suggestibility. Thus, hypnotizability was defined operationally as hypnotic suggestibility with nonhypnotic suggestibility controlled. In these analyses, hypnotizability was significantly associated only with individual differences in expectancy and motivation to respond to suggestion.

A final analysis revealed that hypnotic suggestibility was predicted uniquely by nonhypnotic suggestibility, expectancy, and motivation. In other words, each of these variables was significantly associated with hypnotic suggestibility even with all other variables statistically controlled. It is conventionally assumed that the degree of variance that can be accounted for by predictor variables is limited to the reliability of the criterion variable (in this case, hypnotic suggestibility). All that is left after that is variance due to measurement error. However, the variance accounted for in this analysis exceeded the reliability of the suggestibility scale. This suggested to us that there was little left to learn about the immediate determinants of hypnotic suggestibility. They had been established. All that remained, we maintained, was to find more of the factors influencing individual differences in nonhypnotic imaginative suggestibility.

But we were wrong. In addition to replicating the results of our first study, our next study (Braffman & Kirsch, 1999b) revealed two more determinants of hypnotic suggestibility and hypnotizability (i.e., hypnotic suggestibility with nonhypnotic suggestibility statistically controlled). These were two of the first individual difference variables ever studied: simple and go/no-go reaction times (Donders, 1868).[3] With all other variables controlled, including nonhypnotic suggestibility, hypnotic suggestibility (and therefore hypnotizability) was associated positively with simple reaction time and negatively with go/no-go reaction time. With the addition of these two reaction time variables, the analysis accounted for even more of the individual differences in hypnotic suggestibility and hypnotizability than the analysis in our previous study did. Also, as before, the large proportion of individual differences accounted for indicated that there were no more predictors to find. At the risk of making the same mistake twice, we will climb out on the perilous limb of pertinacity and claim, once again, that the immediate determinants of hypnotic suggestibility have now been established. These are nonhypnotic suggestibility, expectancy, motivation for responding, and reaction time. Hypnotic suggestibility is simply nonhypnotic suggestibility augmented by a readiness to respond and modified by the changes in expectancy and motivation produced by the hypnotic context.

WHERE RESEARCH SHOULD GO FROM HERE

The immediate determinants of hypnotic suggestibility and hypnotizability have been empirically established, and there are apparently no additional determinants left to uncover. In contrast, there is much left to discover about their most powerful correlate, nonhypnotic imaginative suggestibility. We have established that nonhypnotic imaginative suggestibility is influenced by expectancy, motivation, absorption, and fantasy proneness (Braffman & Kirsch, 1999a). However, these variables account for only a small part of the variability in nonhypnotic suggestibility. Learning more about imaginative suggestibility will require additional studies in which it is assessed without the potentially confounding effects of a hypnotic induction. This should be done in correlational studies, brain-imaging studies, and studies using the wide variety of experimental paradigms that have been developed in hypnosis research.

Nonhypnotic imaginative suggestibility is an egregiously ignored construct, and understanding it is an exceptionally important task. Imaginative suggestibility is the ability or trait underlying the automatic movements, partial paralyses, selective amnesias, pain reduction, and hallucinations that are most commonly observed in the context of hypnosis. These behaviors mimic the symptoms of dissociative and conversion disorders, which until recent years were collectively known as "hysteria." One of the prominent symptoms of dissociative identity disorder (formerly termed multiple personality disorder), for example, is amnesia for behaviors supposedly carried out by an alternate personality. Similarly, conversion disorders are defined by psychologically produced physical symptoms, such as automatic movements and paralyses. Thus, it seems likely that the behaviors by which imaginative suggestibility is measured share some common underlying mechanisms with those disorders. But all of these responses and experiences can be elicited without hypnosis, and some of them can be produced easily by the vast majority of people. This indicates that the ability to respond to imaginative suggestions is a normal human characteristic, and its substantial effect in such important clinical areas as pain management indicates that it is a characteristic of great importance. Understanding this widely neglected phenomenon will require the combined efforts of cognitive, neuropsychological, social, and clinical psychologists.

Recommended Reading

Barber, T.X., Spanos, N.P., & Chaves, J.F. (1974). *Hypnosis, imagination, and human potentialities.* New York: Pergamon Press.

Hilgard, E.R. (1965). *Hypnotic susceptibility.* New York: Harcourt, Brace & World.

Kirsch, I., & Lynn, S.J. (1995). The altered state of hypnosis: Changes in the theoretical landscape. *American Psychologist, 50,* 846–858.

Kirsch, I., & Lynn, S.J. (1998). Dissociation theories of hypnosis. *Psychological Bulletin, 123,* 100–115.

Kirsch, I., & Lynn, S.J. (1999). Automaticity in clinical psychology. *American Psychologist, 54,* 504–515.

Notes

1. Address correspondence to Irving Kirsch, Department of Psychology, University of Connecticut, 406 Babbidge Rd., U-20, Storrs, CT 06269-1020.

2. In an attempt to save the altered-state hypothesis, some psychologists

have advanced the idea that people might slip into trance spontaneously, so that responses to suggestion can be taken as evidence that the person is in a hypnotic state. The circularity of this position has long been argued. People are hypothesized to be responding to suggestion because they have slipped into a trance, but the only reason for claiming they are in this trance is that they are responding to suggestion. Also, the ease and frequency with which people display responses to nonhypnotic suggestion render this hypothesis implausible. Almost 80% of the participants in our first study (Braffman & Kirsch, 1999a) responded to suggestions during the nonhypnotic trial. Thus, the altered-state hypothesis requires supposing that the vast majority of people spontaneously slip into a hypnotic trance in response to simple requests to imagine experiences like one's arms moving apart. If slipping into trance is that common a phenomenon, then perhaps we are all in a hypnotic state much of the time, and much psychological research has been unwittingly conducted on inadvertently hypnotized participants.

3. Simple reaction time measures the speed with which a person can respond (e.g., by pressing a key) to a stimulus. In go/no-go reaction time tasks, two different stimuli are presented in random order. The participant is instructed to respond to one of the two stimuli and not to respond to the other stimulus. Simple reaction time is facilitated when the person gets set to respond as soon as any stimulus is detected, thereby allowing the response to be activated automatically, much as are the routine behaviors associated with well-learned habits (e.g., typing or driving a car). However, the adoption of this response set is precluded by the instructions for go/no-go reaction time tasks.

References

Barber, T X , & Glass, L B (1962) Significant factors in hypnotic behavior. *Journal of Abnormal Psychology, 64,* 222–228

Braffman, W., & Kirsch, I (1999a) Imaginative suggestibility and hypnotizability: An empirical analysis. *Journal of Personality and Social Psychology, 77,* 578–587

Braffman, W , & Kirsch, I (1999b, November). *Reaction time as a predictor of imaginative suggestibility and hypnotizability.* Paper presented at the annual meeting of the Society for Clinical and Experimental Hypnosis, New Orleans, LA.

Donders, F C. (1868). On the speed of mental processes. *Acta Psychologica, 30,* 412–431.

Gorassini, D.R , & Spanos, N P. (1999). The Carleton Skill Training Program In I Kirsch, A. Capafons, E Cardeña, & S. Amigó (Eds), *Clinical hypnosis and self-regulation: Cognitive-behavioral perspectives* (pp. 141–177) Washington, DC: American Psychological Association.

Hilgard, E R , & Tart, C T (1966). Responsiveness to suggestions following waking and imagination instructions and following induction of hypnosis. *Journal of Abnormal Psychology, 71,* 196–208.

Hull, C L. (1933) *Hypnosis and suggestibility: An experimental approach.* New York: Appleton-Century-Crofts

Kirsch, I (1997) Specifying nonspecifics: Psychological mechanisms of placebo effects In A. Harrington (Ed), *The placebo effect: An interdisciplinary exploration* (pp 166–186). Cambridge, MA: Harvard University Press

Kirsch, I., Silva, C E., Comey, G., & Reed, S (1995). A spectral analysis of cognitive and personality variables in hypnosis: Empirical disconfirmation of the two-factor model of hypnotic responding *Journal of Personality and Social Psychology, 69,* 167–175

Mazzoni, G. (in press) False memories *European Psychologist.*

Perugini, E.M., Kirsch, I., Allen, S T , Coldwell, E., Meredith, J , Montgomery, G H , & Sheehan, J. (1998). Surreptitious observation of responses to hypnotically suggested hallucinations: A test of the compliance hypothesis. *International Journal of Clinical and Experimental Hypnosis, 46,* 191–203

Rainville, P.D., Duncan, G.H , Price, D.D , Carrier, B , & Bushnell, M C (1997). Pain affect encoded in human anterior cingulate but not somatosensory cortex. *Science, 277,* 968–971

Vickery, A.R., & Kirsch, I. (1991) The effects of brief expectancy manipulations on hypnotic responsiveness. *Contemporary Hypnosis, 8,* 167–171

Weitzenhoffer, A M., & Hilgard, E.R. (1962). *Stanford Hypnotic Susceptibility Scale: Form C.* Palo Alto, CA: Consulting Psychologists Press.

Weitzenhoffer, A.M., & Sjoberg, B.M , Jr. (1961). Suggestibility with and without "induction of hypnosis." *Journal of Nervous and Mental Disease, 132,* 204–220.

Part V
Investigating Hypnotic Phenomena

[17]

Pain and Dissociation in the Cold Pressor Test: A Study of Hypnotic Analgesia with "Hidden Reports" Through Automatic Key Pressing and Automatic Talking

Ernest R. Hilgard, Arlene H. Morgan, and Hugh Macdonald
Stanford University

To test whether pain blocked by hypnotic analgesia may still be perceived at some level, 20 highly hypnotizable subjects participated in an experiment involving cold pressor pain in the normal condition and in hypnotically suggested analgesia. Three reports were obtained reflecting felt pain within the hypnotic analgesia condition: the usual verbal report on a numerical scale, a manual report by "automatic key pressing," and a retrospective verbal report through "automatic talking." Nine subjects who were amnesic for both key pressing and automatic talking reported more pain in the automatic (hidden) reports than in their usual verbal reports. Eight of these nine, following release of amnesia, had a clear perception of two levels of awareness of the pain: the usual hypnotic experience of pain attenuated by analgesia suggestions, and a knowledge at another level of a more severe pain. In no case, however, did a subject give a retrospective report of normal suffering at this "hidden" level. The hypnotically analgesic subject may have reported no pain verbally because he was amnesic for it; when amnesia was removed he recalled the sensory pain, but without a suffering component, because suffering apparently did not occur.

Suggestions of analgesia following hypnotic induction have long been known to be effective in subjects responsive to hypnosis. The question of what happens to the perception of pain in hypnotic analgesia, however, has continued to challenge investigators. The bulk of experimental evidence suggests that whereas hypnotically analgesic subjects report much less pain than in normal waking (and occasionally none at all), the cardiovascular concomitants of the pain response continue as usual (Hilgard, Morgan, Lange, Lenox, Macdonald, Marshall, & Sachs, 1974).

It appears that some amnesialike process may conceal from the hypnotized person his or her own perception of the pain; the amnesia differs from ordinary posthypnotic amnesia in that the perception of pain is diverted from consciousness before it has ever become conscious. This concealed perception of pain can be brought to light if the amnesia is broken by the familiar technique of automatic writing, or by a related technique known by analogy as automatic talking. Preliminary evidence was presented by Hilgard (1973), and subsequent experimental evidence within ischemic pain by Knox, Morgan, and Hilgard (1974). The metaphor of a "hidden observer" was used to describe the reporting of the pain as concealed under the amnesic barrier, but of course no homunculus is implied. The point is that while the subject is honestly reporting no felt pain, some cognitive system within him is registering and processing the pain in a form that can be revealed by the adopted procedures for breaking the amnesic barrier. The existence of such a hidden report of pain has been known for many years, but systematic studies have been lacking (Estabrooks, 1957; James, 1889; Kaplan, 1960).

The study by Knox et al. (1974) relied on concurrent reports through the ordinary verbal reports of the hypnotically analgesic subject alternating with hidden reports through automatic talking. The automatic talking procedure temporarily broke the amnesic barrier, but the barrier was quickly restored. Such vacillations within hypnosis can be produced

This research was supported by Grant MH-03859 from the National Institute of Mental Health to Ernest R. Hilgard in the Laboratory of Hypnosis Research, Department of Psychology, Stanford University.

Requests for reprints should be sent to E. R. Hilgard, Department of Psychology, Stanford University, Stanford, California 94305.

readily, as Blum (1972) has frequently demonstrated. Knox and her colleagues found that during the period of suggested analgesia with eight highly susceptible subjects, there was no felt pain or suffering at all within ischemia, whereas the hidden reports revealed both pain and suffering of approximately the same level as found in normal waking ischemia. This was coherent with the preliminary data reported by Hilgard (1973), except that the expected reduction in suffering was not found. The intermittent reports may have caused a sampling of the pain and suffering, with the suffering following the intermittently sampled sensory pain before it was again concealed by amnesia, but further experimentation is required on the issue of pain versus suffering. Some subsequent pilot subjects in ischemia, in which the pain and suffering reports were obtained retrospectively (i.e., after the amnesia was broken when the painful stress had already been terminated), have reported essentially normal pain with an absence of suffering. The pain–suffering differentiation is therefore somewhat uncertain, and this report adds a few data relative to that distinction.

This study differs from that of Knox et al. (1974) by using the pain of circulating ice water (cold pressor test) as the source of laboratory pain, and by using automatic key pressing (the equivalent of automatic writing) as a means of regularly breaking the amnesia while the subject is also giving a verbal report, followed by retrospective reports when the amnesic barrier has been broken by automatic talking.

The total investigation involved other features, such as the suggestion of analgesia with and without a prior induction of hypnosis and two methods of suggesting analgesia, which will be made the basis of a separate report. We are here concerned primarily with the differences between the usual report and the hidden report within hypnotic analgesia, based on data from subjects larger in number and not quite as highly selected as those in the previous experiment. The selection criteria were relaxed slightly to determine, if possible, some of the limiting conditions bearing on the feasibility of the hidden report methods.

METHOD

Subjects

Subjects were 20 university students, half male and half female, who had been tested on hypnotic susceptibility scales and had scored at least 9 on a 10-point modification of the Harvard Group Scale of Hypnotic Susceptibility (HGSHS) (Shor & Orne, 1962) and a 10-point individual modified form of the Stanford Scale of Hypnotic Susceptibility, Form C (SHSS-C) (Weitzenhoffer & Hilgard, 1962). Each subject had successfully passed the criterion for amnesia within these scales ("passing" not requiring total amnesia) and an item of posthypnotic automatic writing (Form II, Item 9) adapted from the Stanford Profile Scales (Weitzenhoffer & Hilgard, 1967). They scored at approximately the upper 10% of the group of students tested. Apart from earning these high scores in the testing procedures, they had no previous experience of hypnosis and the scales included no prior testing of hypnotic analgesia.

Experimental Design

Subjects participated for 1 hour on each of 4 days, 2 practice days and 2 experimental days. The overall plan was as follows:

Day 1: Practice. Practice in pain reporting was conducted on a numerical scale, both verbally and manually on the keys. There were two keys in a box, the right key for digits and the left for tens. This period provided the waking control test of the ice water pain.

A second type of practice was in deepening hypnosis. Because the subjects were to participate in several sessions, the deepening procedures familiarized them with a numerical scale for reporting their own depth of hypnosis and provided practice both in self-deepening and in detecting whatever signs they used to assure themselves of their hypnotic involvement. The exact meaning of hypnotic depth is problematical, but it has subjective reality for highly responsive hypnotic subjects and serves to legitimize the demands made on them. It may be noted that demand characteristics are of the essence in hypnosis and suggestion: A hypnotic subject will find a rabbit in his lap only if he responds to the demand for a rabbit. The presence of demand characteristics as such does not invalidate hypnotic experiments; they serve special critical purposes in the quasi-control group design proposed by Orne (1972). In that design a difference between "instructed simulators" and "hypnotically reals" is used to show that hypnosis produces some behavior beyond that implied either overtly or covertly by the the hypnotist.

In this investigation, the usual demands of hypnosis (e.g., that an arm will become painless) are being offered quite openly, with the full consent of the subject. The evidence for the reality of the effects rests largely on the verbal reports of the subjects, with their honesty commonly shown by the extent to which they do not conform to the demands. The reality of hypnotic analgesia has, in fact, been earlier demonstrated in experiments from another laboratory using the simulator control. Subjects simulating hypnosis did indeed conceal the effects of painful shocks, but when questioned afterwards they admitted suffering the pain, whereas the hypnotized subjects reported that they felt no pain (Shor, 1959, 1962).

Practice also assumed the form of automatic talking, as a method of temporarily breaking and restoring the amnesic process. This method has been reported in the earlier papers. Essentially, it makes plausible the breaking of the amnesic process by using the metaphor that some "hidden part" of the person knows more of what is going on than the "hypnotized part" that has reported some distortion of reality. The practice session did not involve pain; instead, it involved breaking the hallucination that an arm, actually held high in the air, was in the subject's lap. Insensitivity of the upraised arm (an indication of dissociation without specific suggestion) was tested by touching it several times but without painful stimulation. The signal for breaking the amnesic barrier and getting into communication with the hidden part was for the hypnotist to place his hand on the subject's shoulder, and the amnesia was restored when he removed his hand. This procedure may not be essential in all its details, but it serves conveniently to reveal how genuine the component experiences are to the subject. When the amnesia was ultimately removed, the subject remembered everything that went on and what was said.

Day 2: Practice. The first practice procedure involved automatic keypressing while consciously naming colors. This portion of the practice was based on the availability of equipment and procedures used in a study of interfering tasks, one conscious, the other out of awareness (Knox, Crutchfield, & Hilgard, in press). The key-pressing task consisted of pressing the right and left keys in a standard pattern of three to the right and three to the left, repeating this pattern for a minute. Under hypnosis, the task can be performed by highly responsive subjects without their awareness that the fingers are pressing the keys. To provide a competing task, the subject named colors arranged on a chart before him. This task was fully conscious and served to occupy the time that he was also pressing the keys out of awareness.

Practice in automatic key pressing concurrently with a hypnotically induced dream was also conducted. Because we desired the subjects to acquire as varied an experience as possible of competing activities, with one out of awareness, we followed an earlier suggestion of Wiseman and Reyher (1962) that the hypnotic dream can be used to facilitate hypnotic amnesia. The usual suggestions were given for the key pressing to go on out of awareness. Following the suggested dream (produced while the key pressing continued), the subject was asked to describe "what happened in the last few minutes." Most subjects responded only with the content of their dreams, failing to mention the key pressing.

Days 3 and 4: Experimental days—waking and hypnotic analgesia. There were two ice water sessions on each day, both either in waking or in hypnosis; half of the subjects had waking on the first day, half on the second. Pain reduction suggestions were given on both days, via tape recordings, in two forms. One was based on the suggestion that the arm was numb and insensitive "as if just a piece of rubber," following as closely as possible the suggestions used by Spanos, Barber, and Lang (1974). The other was an "absent arm" suggestion, based on the frequent observation by early investigators that an arm out of awareness was also anesthetic. The details will be given at another time because the differences in objective results were not sufficiently great to require treating the two methods separately in this report. The data regarding waking analgesia will also be omitted now, except to indicate that there was no evidence, following waking suggestion of analgesia, that there had been any amnesic distortion of the pain experience. Thus, the hidden reports (obtained during a subsequent hypnosis) were just the same as the usual ones.

Day 4 was symmetrical with Day 3, except that those who had waking analgesia on Day 3 had hypnotic analgesia on Day 4, and vice versa. For the present account, only the data from the hypnotic analgesia day are to be presented. For half of the subjects the condition was on Day 3 and for half on Day 4; therefore, the appropriateness of combining the data must be justified. Statistical comparison of the pain reports of the two subgroups, one on each day, showed no difference in their pain reports, whether by the usual verbal reports within suggested analgesia, the reports obtained by key pressing, or the reports subsequently obtained by automatic talking. In all cases, significances of differences by t test yielded $p > .20$.

Each day was followed by an inquiry after amnesia was lifted regarding all aspects of the reported experiences. The inquiry was recorded on tape, transcribed, and made the basis for the discussion to be presented later.[1]

RESULTS

Pain Reduction Within Hypnotic Analgesia

It has previously been shown that pain reports, obtained in the waking state in the cold pressor test, are sufficiently stable for an initial test to serve as a baseline for normal responsiveness to pain. That is, there is little adaptation or learning, so that a second day's results correlate .79 with the initial results and there is no significant change in mean reports over the 2 days (Hilgard, Ruch, Lange, Lenox, Morgan, & Sachs, 1974). Hence, when a significant change from this baseline is reported within suggested analgesia, it can be taken as a satisfactory measure of the effectiveness of the analgesia suggestions. The amount of reduction is commonly found to correlate about .50 with measured hypnotic susceptibility (Evans & Paul, 1970; Hilgard,

[1] Verbatim instructions have been reproduced and will be supplied on request.

TABLE 1

PAIN REPORTED IN NORMAL WAKING CONDITION AND IN HYPNOTIC ANALGESIA

Subject	Maximum pain within 45 seconds in the ice water			
	Normal waking pain (Column 1)	Hypnotic analgesia		
		Usual verbal report (Column 2)	Report by concurrent automatic key pressing (Column 3)	Report by retrospective automatic talking (Column 4)
Less pain reported in analgesia				
1	13.0	0.0	6.5	14.0
2	12.0	.5	4.8	4.8
3	18.0	.5	.5	.5
4	8.0	1.0	9.0	9.0
5	25.0	1.0	8.5	8.5
6	25.0	1.0	1.0	1.0
7	9.0	3.0	6.2	10.0
8	11.0	3.0	2.5	3.0
9	13.0	3.0	15.5	18.0
10	15.0	3.8	3.0	3.0
Mean of subgroup (n = 10)	14.9	1.68	5.75	7.18
More pain reported in analgesia				
11	10.0	4.0	8.5	8.5
12	10.0	4.0	7.0	7.0
13	25.0	4.8	4.8	4.8
14	10.0	5.5	5.5	5.5
15	10.0	6.0	6.0	6.0
16	12.0	6.2	6.2	6.2
17	25.0	8.5	7.8	7.8
18	10.0	8.5	10.0	10.0
19	10.0	9.0	9.0	9.0
20	13.0	10.0	10.0	10.0
Mean of subgroup (n = 10)	13.5	6.65	7.48	7.48
Mean of total (n = 20)	14.2	4.16	6.62	7.33

1967; Shor, 1959). There is some uncertainty over the relative effectiveness of waking analgesic suggestions versus suggestions given in hypnosis, but this problem need not be considered here.

The results are given in Table 1, in which the first column shows the normal wakin paing and the second column shows the pain reported in the usual way in hypnotic analgesia. Attention is now directed to these two columns only.

The subjects have been placed in the order of their success in reducing felt pain through hypnotic analgesia (Column 2) and divided into two groups for purposes of studying later some of the correlates of this ability. The 20 subjects all experienced pain normally in the usual waking condition, with the maximum pain at 45 seconds in the ice water, exceeding the critical level of 10 for all but two of the subjects. Those who were better able to reduce pain did not differ significantly from those less able (Column 1). The subjects, although selected for high responsiveness to hypnosis, were not universally able to achieve drastic pain reduction, although all but one reported the maximum pain within hypnotic analgesia to be below the critical level of 10. The reduction of pain as a consequence of suggested analgesia was highly significant, $t(19) = 6.47$, $p < .001$, with every subject reporting some pain reduction. The data in the first two columns merely replicate what has been reported in a number of previous experiments

TABLE 2
Statistical Tests Based on Total Sample of Table 1

Hypnotic analgesia report	*t*	*r*
Verbal versus key pressing	−2.96*	.37
Verbal versus automatic talking	−2.94*	.15
Key pressing versus automatic talking	−1.70	.90

Note. $F(2, 38) = 8.18$, $p < .01$.
* $p < .01$.

from this laboratory (e.g., Hilgard, 1967, 1969, 1971).

Evidence for a Hidden Experience of Pain Within Analgesia

The evidence presented in Columns 3 and 4 distinguishes this study from earlier research by showing that subjects who have given the usual reports of little pain in analgesia (Column 2), at some other processing level report pain often approximating that of the normal waking pain. The reports of maximum pain in Columns 2, 3, and 4 are averages obtained from two trials within the day. The trials differed in the suggestion according to which analgesia was produced, but otherwise the procedures were identical. The type of suggestion did not yield significant differences between the means of analgesia obtained, and the scores on the two trials were significantly correlated, so there is ample justification for averaging them.

Primary interest centers in the interrelatedness of the data of Columns 2, 3, and 4, all being reports obtained within the same experimental period. Hence, the analysis of variance as reported in Table 2 is confined to these three columns; it proved satisfactorily significant, $p < .01$, so that t tests between the columns were justified. Both automatic key pressing and automatic talking yielded reports of significantly more pain than in the usual reports with hypnotic analgesia, but they did not differ significantly from each other.

Despite the significant mean results, it should be noted that not all subjects followed the typical trend. For example, whereas the pain reported in Column 4 is typically below that in Column 1 (normal pain), pain in Column 4 was not reduced over Column 1 for Subjects 1, 4, 7, and 9, all of whom had substantial pain reduction as reported in Column 2 (pain in analgesia). Similarly, pain in Column 4 was not reduced for Subjects 11, 18, 19, and 20, who were less successful in pain reduction as reported in Column 2. At the other end of the spectrum are those subjects who failed to report more pain in Column 4 than their reduced pains in Column 2, including Subjects 3, 6, 8, and 10 among the more successful pain reducers, and Subjects 13–17 among the less successful. These divergent responses will require further discussion.

Because both key pressing and automatic talking yielded pain reports above the usual reports in hypnotic analgesia, they gave evidence of some hidden experience of pain. The hidden pain was somewhat below the normally experienced pain, but that is not unreasonable in view of the quiescence of the hypnotized subject. The course of the hidden pain, as reported by automatic key pressing, compared with normal waking pain and hypnotically reduced pain, as usually reported, is shown in Figure 1. The curves are presented separately for the subjects, divided as in Table 1 between those more and less analgesic according to their usual verbal reports within hypnotic analgesia. The general relationships hold, apart from the attenuation of the results for the less analgesic.

Results of the Final Inquiry

Relevant information was obtained through the automatic talking reports after each hypnotic session and through subsequent questioning. Each subject was asked about his recollection of what he had said within hypnotic analgesia, and what he had reported by way of the keys and in the automatic talking account. He then elaborated on underlying experiences reflected in these reports. After his free report he was asked specifically about his awareness of the cold water and about the suffering associated with the recollected pain. He was also asked whether or not he had at any time been aware of the key pressing. Subjects did not universally conform to the obvious demands of the experiment. For example, a few were not completely oblivious to the fact that they were pressing the keys while giving their verbal reports; some heard the clicking of the keys while being unaware of the source of the sound. When the subject

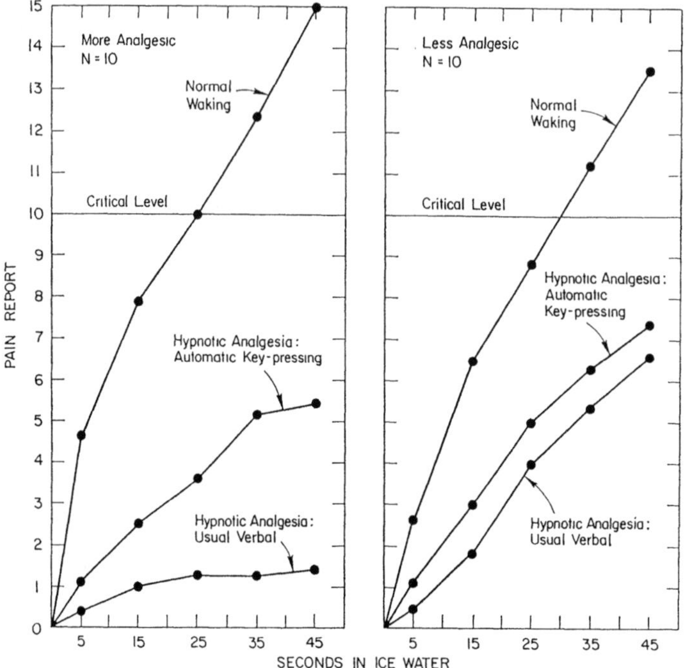

FIGURE 1. Pain reported verbally in the normal waking condition, and in the hypnotic analgesia condition, reported verbally and by automatic key pressing. (Subjects were divided according to the degree of pain reduction as reported verbally on hypnotic analgesia day.)

became fully aware of the keys, the difference between the usual verbal report and the key-pressing report tended to disappear. Another type of diasgreement with the implied demands of the experiment was shown by nine subjects, successful in hypnotic pain reduction, who failed to show any recovery of felt pain within the automatic reporting procedures. These were Subjects 3, 6, 8, 10, and 13–17 of Table 1, as previously noted.

The final inquiry, when the data had been collected, was conducted after all amnesia was removed and the subject was fully aware of what he had reported at all times. We were particularly interested in his phenomenal account of the nature of the cognitive system responsible for the hidden report that disagreed with his usual or open report within hypnotic analgesia, although other aspects of the experience were also noted.

The pain–suffering dichotomy. In the inquiry regarding the recollection of pain felt in hypnotic analgesia we asked the question whether the hidden pain was accompanied by suffering. In the case of eight subjects who most clearly sensed a distinction between the usual report of pain in analgesia and that revealed through the automatic methods, all reported that the recollected pain had been felt as a sensory or intellectual experience, and it caused *no distress or suffering*. This is coherent with the results mentioned above for some pilot subjects in an ischemia experiment, although it is at odds with aspects of the findings of Knox et al. (1974). It may very well prove to be the case that hypnotic analgesia relieves suffering more than it relieves sensory pain, but this cannot be considered proven. Were it to be the case, it would be congruent with aspects of the gate-control theory of pain as proposed by Melzack and Wall (1965).

Reactions to the exposure of the hidden experience of pain. We were interested in how the subjects reacted to their own discovery that, after having reported little or no pain in the usual way in analgesia, they reported more pain through the automatic techniques, thus exposing some felt pain that must either have been denied or in some manner hidden behind a cloak of amnesia. Because this experience was not a clear one for all of the subjects, the more illuminating answers depend on those who had the more vivid experience of change between usual and hidden report. These were 8 of the 20 subjects (Subjects 1, 2, 4, 5, 7, 9, 11, and 18 in Table 1). Of the rest, six (Subjects 3, 10, 12, 13, 14, and 17) reported some subjective differences in the roles of the two parts, that is, usual verbal reporting and the automatic reporting systems, but an incomplete separation of one from the other through amnesia. For them, some kind of interpretation in terms of divided attention may prove to be appropriate. The remaining six (Subjects 6, 8, 15, 16, 19, and 20) indicated no difference whatever between their usual reports and their automatic ones; either there was no amnesia, or the amnesia that existed was not relieved by the methods used. Obviously, more experimentation is required to produce a completely satisfactory explanation.

The eight who had a sense of separateness between the usual hypnotic analgesia experience and that uncovered by the automatic techniques described the differences in many ways, of which the following verbatim quotes are representative:

> I can separate my mind and my head from the rest of my body. The hidden part—reporting on the keys—was controlling my body. My mind was not counting key-pressing. My mind was reporting what it felt, verbally. I've always been aware of the difference between the mind and the body when I've been hypnotized.
>
> It's as though two things were happening simultaneously; I have two separate memories, as if the two things could have happened to different people. The memory of the hidden part is more intellectual, but I can't really comprehend or assimilate the two.
>
> Both parts were concentrating on what you said—not to feel pain. The water bothered the hidden part a little because it felt it a little, but the hypnotized part was not thinking of my arm at all.
>
> Part of me knew that my hand was in the water and it hurt as much as it did the other day [i.e., in the waking control]. The hypnotized part was vaguely aware of the presence of some pain, and that's why I had to concentrate really hard. [Subject reported zero pain.]
>
> When you're hypnotized, there are certain questions that just aren't answered, and you just don't probe them in your mind. I think you're aware that the pain exists, but it's not appropriate to deal with it just then.
>
> I don't think I'm totally unaware that there is some level at which I know exactly what was going on. But when you asked me what I had been doing [i.e., the inquiry within automatic talking], it was really hard to remember. I don't know if I could have. It was like a block.
>
> Today [to the hidden part] the pain was more general, and especially the second time [under the absent arm instruction]. I felt it in my shoulder. That part knew that my arm was there, but part of me knew it wasn't there. The pain was hidden from the hypnotized part.
>
> Part of me knows the pain is there, but I'm not sure I *feel* it. The hypnotized part *doesn't* feel it, but I'm not sure if the hypnotized part may have known it was there but didn't say it. The hypnotized part really makes an effort to not feel it.

Two aspects of the experience run through these comments. One is the activity of the hypnotized subject, a genuine cognitive effort involved in conforming to the demands of the experiment. It is by no means a completely passive experience controlled by the hypnotist. The other is the great difficulty in putting into words the fluctuations that occur within the experience—the fleeting glances at what is going on, even while the events are not fully cognized; separation and fusion; acceptance and denial. Much of this is familiar in subjective reports of posthypnotic amnesia.

The Amnesic Correlates of the Discrepancies Between Pain Reports

It has been repeatedly implied in the foregoing discussion that the concealment of pain that can be recovered through the automatic reporting methods must be amnesic in nature. If that is the case, some of the individual differences in the discrepant reports should correspond to differences in hypnotic amnesia measured in other ways. Two sets of such measures are available: responses within the items concerned with posthypnotic amnesia in the susceptibility tests that were given as part of the subject selection, and indications of amnesia within the training days preparatory to the experiment proper.

All subjects "passed" the amnesia tests according to criteria established in the test standardizations, but the criteria allow the recall of several items so that not all were equally amnesic. Despite the restricted range, it is possible to assign scores to the subjects according to their tested amnesia by making use of both the number of items recalled in the two amnesia tests they had taken and by weighting these scores according to the items recovered when told, "Now you can remember everything."[2] The true hypnotic amnesia is a recoverable one; if items are not recovered, the subject may simply have been inattentive to them or forgotten them for nonhypnotic reasons (Cooper, 1972; Kihlstrom & Evans, 1973). When subjects were scored for tested amnesia in this way, those who were more analgesic (Subjects 1–10 in Table 1) proved to have higher amnesia scores than those less analgesic (Subjects 11–20). The difference, as tested by the Mann–Whitney *U* test was significant at the .05 level. Of course, a correlation is expected among all tests of hypnotic susceptibility, so this relationship is not surprising, except that it holds within a very restricted range of hypnotic responsiveness and therefore points to a somewhat specific relation between amnesia and analgesia.

If the rise in pain between the usual report in analgesia and that in automatic talking were a consequence of lifting amnesia, this rise should also be related to amnesia. This did not prove to be the case. Among the more amnesic, 5 of 10 subjects reported substantial gains between the usual and the hidden reports in analgesia, whereas among the less amnesic, 4 of 10 reported corresponding gains. These differences are not significant, so the hypothesis that amnesia would predict the differential pain reports was not supported.

DISCUSSION

The phenomena of pain and suffering are puzzling in themselves and the phenomena of hypnosis are also puzzling, so it not surprising that their combination will yield data difficult to interpret. The data as reported are unequivocal in several respects, and indeterminate in others. It is again demonstrated that the subjective experience of pain and suffering can be reduced by hypnotic analgesia suggestions, especially among those whose hypnotic responsiveness, as measured by hypnotic susceptibility tests, is at a high level. Those who report complete absence of pain are in the minority, even among selected subjects; only 4 of the 20 subjects in this experiment reported complete absence of pain on one of their two test opportunities, although 14 of the 20 reduced their pain by half or more of that reported in the normal waking condition. This pain reduction through suggested analgesia is by now so firmly established that it is unequivocal. Those who are most successful feel neither pain nor suffering.

The second point now established is that for a substantial fraction of those who are able to reduce their pain through hypnotic analgesia, methods can be found to show that information about felt pain of greater magnitude has been processed and can be reported verbally. The methods used here (automatic writing and automatic talking) probably serve to break some sort of amnesic barrier, but the interpretation of how the methods work cannot be considered completely established. The general findings, until recently not confirmed by quantitative experiments, have been occasionally reported in the past, and can be accepted as firm.

A third point, less well established, is that at the hidden level there has been more reduction of suffering than of sensory pain. In the present experiment, all of those with the clearest account of a difference between their absent pain and their recovered pain through the automatic methods reported that there was strongly felt sensory pain but a minimum of suffering. This result might be taken as established, except for the previous findings from our laboratory that under some conditions, although neither pain nor suffering were reported in the usual conditions of hypnotic analgesia, both pain and suffering were reported by the automatic talking procedure (Knox et al., 1974). This uncertainty about the pain–suffering dimension does not reflect, however, on either the demonstration that both pain and suffering are relieved through hypnotic suggestion or that there is processing of the information at some concealed level.

---

[2] The short form of group test used did not provide data on the recovery of items following amnesia, so the correction could be made for only one of the two amnesia tests.

Because of the plausibility that some sort of amnesic process is responsible for the difference between the usual and the hidden analgesic reports, efforts were made to relate measured amnesia in these subjects to their success in the experiments. Unfortunately, the arrangements of the experiments make it difficult to conduct the investigation with subjects who are not capable of demonstrating hypnotic amnesia, so that, pending further experimentation, it was necessary to do the exploratory analyses with a very restricted range of amnesic abilities. Even so, there was a significant relationship between measured amnesia and the amount of hypnotic analgesia shown in the usual way, although there could not be demonstrated any relationship between measured amnesia and the recovery through the automatic techniques. There appears to be little doubt that an amnesic process of some sort is involved, but because it is an amnesia for something that has not been in awareness previously, it differs from usual posthypnotic amnesia.

If it should be substantiated that the recovery through automatic inquiry methods is of sensory pain, but not of suffering (a result found for a substantial group within this experiment), some interesting problems of interpretation would be involved. The two main problems, reminiscent of the James–Lange theory of emotion, are whether suffering is in reaction to sensory pain or is separately experienced. The separate pathways for pain and suffering that are stressed in the Melzack–Wall gate control theory allow for the second interpretation, although according to the theory there is an interaction between the two systems.

The hypnotic findings (were they to be confirmed) would be that the amnesic effect was only with respect to the sensory pain and there was no amnesic effect on suffering. Thus, recovery of pain but no recovery of suffering would occur. The deeper interpretation could take one of two forms: There might have been some psychophysiological blocking of the suffering mechanism through hypnotic suggestion that operated differently from the blocking of sensory pain, or felt suffering might be in fact only a response to felt pain so that when pain is not felt, no suffering occurs. It is evident in gross observation that the hypnotic subject does not show the usual signs of overt suffering when not experiencing pain; that is, he does not visibly squirm, or sigh, or tense his muscles. If suffering is felt as a reaction to these responses (in the James–Lange spirit), then he does not suffer if the reactions do not occur. There are, of course, some experimental approaches to the clarification of these issues; it is sufficient to point out that they are at present unresolved.

REFERENCES

Blum, G. S. Hypnotic programming techniques in psychological experiments. In E. Fromm & R. E. Shor (Eds.), *Hypnosis: Research developments and perspectives*. Chicago: Aldine-Atherton, 1972.

Cooper, L. M. Hypnotic amnesia. In E. Fromm & R. E. Shor (Eds.), *Hypnosis: Research developments and perspectives*. Chicago: Aldine-Atherton, 1972.

Estabrooks, G. H. *Hypnotism* (Rev. ed.). New York: Dutton, 1957.

Evans, M. B., & Paul, G. L. Effects of hypnotically suggested analgesia on physiological and subjective responses to cold stress. *Journal of Consulting and Clinical Psychology*, 1970, *35*, 362–371.

Hilgard, E. R. A quantitative study of pain and its reduction through hypnotic suggestion. *Proceedings of the National Academy of Sciences*, 1967, *57*, 1581–1586.

Hilgard, E. R. Pain as a puzzle for psychology and physiology. *American Psychologist*, 1969, *24*, 103–113.

Hilgard, E. R. Pain: Its reduction and production under hypnosis. *Proceedings of the American Philosophical Society*, 1971, *115*, 470–476.

Hilgard, E. R. A neodissociation interpretation of pain reduction in hypnosis. *Psychological Review*, 1973, *80*, 396–411.

Hilgard, E. R., Morgan, A. H., Lange, A. F., Lenox, J. R., Macdonald, H., Marshall, G. D., & Sachs, L. B. Heart rate changes in pain and hypnosis. *Psychophysiology*, 1974, *11*, 692–702.

Hilgard, E. R., Ruch, J. C., Lange, A. F., Lenox, J. R., Morgan, A. H., & Sachs, L. B. The psychophysics of cold pressor pain and its modification through hypnotic suggestion. *American Journal of Psychology*, 1974, *87*, 17–31.

James, W. Automatic writing. *Proceedings of the American Society for Psychical Research*, 1889, *1*, 584–564.

Kaplan, E. A. Hypnosis and pain. *Archives of General Psychiatry*, 1960, *2*, 657–658.

Kihlstrom, J. F., & Evans, F. J. Recovery of memory after posthypnotic amnesia. *Proceedings of the 81st Annual Convention of the American Psychological Association*, 1973, *8*, 1079–1080.

Knox, V. J., Morgan, A. H., & Hilgard, E. R. Pain and suffering in ischemia: The paradox of hypnotically suggested anesthesia as contradicted by reports from the "hidden observer." *Archives of General Psychiatry*, 1974, *30*, 840–847.

Knox, V. J., Crutchfield, L., & Hilgard, E. R. The nature of task interference in hypnotic dissociation. *International Journal of Clinical and Experimental Hypnosis*, in press.

Melzack, R., & Wall, P. D. Pain mechanisms: A new theory. *Science*, 1965, *150*, 971–979.

Orne, M. T. On the simulating subject as a quasi-control group in hypnosis research: What, why, and how. In E. Fromm & R. E. Shor (Eds.), *Hypnosis: Research developments and perspectives*. Chicago: Aldine-Atherton, 1972.

Shor, R. E. Hypnosis and the concept of the generalized reality-orientation. *American Journal of Psychotherapy*, 1959, *13*, 582–602.

Shor, R. E. Three dimensions of hypnotic depth. *International Journal of Clinical and Experimental Hypnosis*, 1962, *10*, 23–38.

Shor, R. E., & Orne, E. C. *The Harvard Group Scale of Hypnotic Susceptibility, Form A*. Palo Alto, Calif.: Consulting Psychologists Press, 1962.

Spanos, N. P., Barber, T. X., & Lang, G. Effects of hypnotic induction, suggestions of analgesia, and demands for honesty on subjective reports of pain. In H. London & R. E. Nisbett (Eds.), *Thought and feeling: Cognitive alteration of feeling states*. Chicago: Aldine, 1974.

Weitzenhoffer, A. M., & Hilgard, E. R. *The Stanford Scale of Hypnotic Susceptibility, Form C*. Palo Alto, Calif.: Consulting Psychologists Press, 1962.

Weitzenhoffer, A. M., & Hilgard, E. R. *Revised Stanford Profile Scales of Hypnotic Susceptibility, Forms I and II*. Palo Alto, Calif.: Consulting Psychologists Press, 1967.

Wiseman, R. J., & Reyher, J. A procedure utilizing dreams for deepening the hypnotic trance. *American Journal of Clinical Hypnosis*, 1962, *5*, 105–110.

(Received July 8, 1974; revision received January 10, 1975)

[18]

CONTEXTUAL DEMANDS, NEGATIVE HALLUCINATIONS, AND HIDDEN OBSERVER RESPONDING: THREE HIDDEN OBSERVERS OBSERVED

Nicholas P. Spanos, Deborah M. Flynn, and Maxwell I. Gwynn

Carleton University, Ottawa, Canada

Abstract

Highly susceptible hypnotic subjects were tested in an experimental paradigm which Zamansky and Bartis (1985) contended rigorously demonstrated the occurrence of hidden observer responding unconfounded by social expectancies and situational demands. Contrary to this assertion, the hidden observer responding of subjects was profoundly influenced by situational demands. In fact, following a negative visual hallucination suggestion subjects displayed "hidden observers" that (a) saw stimuli veridically, (b) saw stimuli in reverse, or (c) saw nothing at all, depending upon the pattern of situational demands administered. These findings run counter to dissociation accounts of hidden observer responding but provide strong evidence for social psychological accounts of such responding.

A number of studies from Hilgard's laboratory (reviewed by Hilard, 1979) were designed to assess cognitive dissociation during hypnotic responding. In these studies highly hypnotizable hypnotic subjects were administered a suggestion for pain reduction (or reduced hearing) and informed that their hypnotized "part" would feel reduced pain while a "hidden part" remained aware of everything that transpired in the experimental session. Subjects were further informed that their hypnotized and hidden "parts" could report on their respective levels of pain independently of one another. Many of the subjects administered these instructions reported relatively low levels of pain from their "hypnotized part" (i.e., overt pain) but relatively high levels of pain from their "hidden part." According to Hilgard (1979) hidden reports do not result from suggestion or from other contextual demands. Instead, hypnotically analgesic subjects supposedly experience high levels of hidden pain regardless of whether the experimenter gives them instructions for accessing hidden pain. However, hidden pain normally remains separated from hypnotic consciousness by an "amnesic barrier" unless and until the experimenter obtains hidden reports.

In contrast to Hilgard (1979), investigators who adopt a social psychological perspective toward hypnotic responding suggested that hidden reports reflect the instructional demands employed in hidden observer studies rather than the intrinsic operation of a dissociated cognitive subsystem (Coe & Sarbin, 1977; Spanos, 1983, 1986; Wagstaff, 1981). Three experiments (Spanos, Gwynn & Stam, 1983; Spanos & Hewitt, 1980; Spanos, Radtke & Bertrand, 1984) obtained support for the social psychological hypothesis by demonstrating that hidden reports could be varied in opposite directions by manipulating instructional demands. For example, Spanos, Gwynn and Stam (1983) found that the same highly hypnotizable subjects could be induced to sequentially report hidden pain that was the same as, higher than and lower than overt pain.

Recently, Zamansky and Bartis (1985) acknowledged the limitations of Hilgard's hidden observer studies. However, they also presented the results of a new study that they contended "help to place the notion of the hidden observer on a substantially more secure footing" (p. 246). To access the hidden observer notion Zamansky and Bartis (1985) made use of negative hallucination suggestions. For example, in one case hypnotic subjects were given a negative visual hallucination suggestion which informed them that they would see only a blank piece of paper. Subjects were then shown a piece of paper that had printed on it a highly visible number (e.g., the number 8). Subject passed this suggestion if they reported seeing nothing on the paper. The paper was then withdrawn and subjects were given explicit instructions informing them that hypnotized subjects have a special hidden part of their mind that remains aware of all that is really going on during hypnosis. Following these instructions subjects' "hidden part" was contacted and subjects were instructed to "be aware of things that you were not aware of or did not know before" (p. 245). Under these circumstances all of the subjects who initially indicated that the paper was blank now correctly reported the number that had actually been on the paper.

According to Zamansky and Bartis (1985) their procedures represent an improvement over those employed by Hilgard because (a) the verdicality of their subjects' reports could be determined (e.g., whether or not the number reported by subjects was the number on the paper could be verified), (b) hidden observer instructions were not introduced until after the stimuli had been withdrawn and (c) subjects were not given prior practice on dissociation tasks. Zamansky and Bartis (1985) argued that, because of these methodological "improvements," "the interpretation that the hidden observer report is simply a creation of experimental demands becomes much less tenable" (p. 244).

Despite statements of this kind Zamansky and Bartis (1985) provided no evidence whatsoever to support the contention that their procedural alterations reduced or controlled for the impact of contextual demands on hidden observer reports. On the contrary, the available data suggests that hidden reports are strongly influenced by instructional demands even when the procedural "improvements" employed by Zamansky and Bartis (1985) are in place. For example, Spanos et al. (1984) and Spanos et al. (1983) found that hidden reports could be easily manipulated in opposite directions even when subjects had no prior practice on dissociation tasks, and Spanos et al. (1984) obtained this "opposite direction" demand effect using responses whose verdicality could be easily determined (i.e., previously learned words). The hidden observer instructions employed by Zamansky and Bartis (1985) provided subjects with explicit information about the responses expected from them. Under these circumstances there is little reason to assume that the potency of those demands was appreciably reduced simply because subjects had not practised equally obvious tasks or because the stimulus number was not in view when subjects were instructed to give their hidden reports.

The social psychological hypothesis suggests that hidden reports reflect subjects' understandings of task demands. Contrary to the dissociation hypothesis, these reports need not veridically reflect the stimulus situation that was present when subjects were given a suggestion. Instead, these reports will be either verdical or nonverdical depending upon the specific demands conveyed by hidden observer instructions (Spanos, 1983, 1986). Such variation in hidden reports should occur even when the procedural "improvements" suggested by Zamansky and Bartis (1985) are in place.[1]

The present study tested these ideas by modifying the the negative hallucination-hidden observer sequence employed by Zamansky and Bartis (1985). Highly hypnotizable hypnotic subjects were given the suggestion that they would see a blank piece of paper. On the paper, however, was an easily visible number 18. Subjects who reported that the paper was blank were divided into two groups. Those in one group were informed that they possessed a hidden part of their mind that was aware of everything that they had seen (i.e., the Zamansky/Bartis sequence). Those in the other group were also told that they had a hidden part, but were further informed that their hidden part had the property of reversing everything that it saw. What had actually been on the left was seen by the hidden part as on the right, and so on. We predicted that subjects in the standard group would give hidden reports of having seen a number 18, while those in the alternate group would show a reversal and give hidden reports of having seen 81.

Because negative hallucination suggestions are very difficult, we anticipated that many of our subjects would fail the initial suggestion. These subjects, who despite the suggestion acknowleged seeing 18, were informed that a special part of their mind was so deeply hidden that it had not seen anything on the paper. We anticipated that at least some of these subjects would respond to these reinforced demands to "not see". In short, we anticipated that by manipulating hidden observer instructions in the context of Zamansky and Bartis' (1985) "rigorous" procedures we would obtain evidence for hidden observers who (a) saw accurately, (b) saw the reverse of what had been present, and (c) saw nothing at all. Such a pattern of findings would be inconsistent with the dissociation hypothesis but would provide strong evidence for the social psychological account of the hidden observer phenomenon.

Method

Subjects

Thirty six Carleton Univerity undergraduates (ages 18 to 30 years) who in previous testing obtained very high scores (6 or 7) on the objective dimension of the 7 item Carleton University Responsiveness to Suggestion Scale (CURSS:O; Spanos, Radtke, Hodgkins, Stam & Bertrand, 1983) agreed to participate in a single session study involving hypnosis. Subjects were either paid $5.00 or received course credit for participation. Although not employed as selection criteria, CURSS:S (subjective) and CURSS:OI (objective-involuntariness) scores were also available for these subjects.

Stimulus Material

During negative hallucination testing subjects were shown a rectangular white card 21.75 cm x 28 cm. In the centre of the card was printed a number 18 that was 5 cm in height.

Procedure

All subjects were tested individually by the same female experimenter. After being comfortably seated subjects were asked to close their eyes and were administered a 7 min hypnotic induction procedure modified from Barber (1969), followed by a 30s negative hallucination suggestion. The suggestion informed subjects repeatedly that they would be shown a blank card with nothing on it. Subjects were then instructed to open their eyes and to "look carefully at the blank piece of paper." While the stimulus card remained in view subjects were asked to "Please describe what you see." Those who reported that the card had nothing on it were further asked "Are you sure you see nothing?"

Following these procedures the card was removed from view and subjects were instructed to again close their eyes. Those who indicated to both probes that the card had nothing on it were assigned by prior randomization to either a standard or a reversal hidden observer testing sequence with the restriction of 5 subjects in each sequence. Subjects who reported seeing the number (or even part of the number) in response to either or both probes were assigned to a "less aware" hidden observer sequence.

Standard sequence. Subjects in this group were informed that they possessed a hidden mental part,

> ... that continues to perceive even when you are given a suggestion that you see nothing. Even though you, in hypnosis, are not aware of what you saw on the card, your hidden part knows. We can reach this hidden part of your mind and learn more about the things you were not able to see on the card even though they were present. In a moment I will count to three and the hidden information will no longer be hidden. You will be aware of what was on the card that you did not see before.

Following these instructions the experimenter counted to three and again asked subjects to describe the card. After making their response subjects were given "wake up" instructions, debriefed, and thanked for their participation.

Reversal sequence. The hidden observer instructions administered to these subjects were the same as those above with the following exception. These subjects were informed that,

> The hidden part of your mind has an interesting property. It reverses the information that was actually presented when you were told that you could see nothing ... suppose a hypnotized subject had been given the suggestion that they could see nothing on a piece of paper that contained an arrow pointing to the right. The hidden part of the person would see the arrow pointing to the left ...

Following their hidden observer instructions the sequence for these subjects was the same as described above.

Less aware sequence. Subjects who failed the negative hallucination suggestion by reporting that they saw the number (or some part of the number) on the card were informed that they possessed a hidden part that had not seen the number,

> [you have] a special part of your mind that was unable to perceive when you were given the suggestion ... Even though you, in hypnosis, were able to see what was on the card, the hidden part was so deeply hidden that it was completely unable to perceive what was on the card ...

Following these instructions the sequence for these subjects was the same as that in the other two groups.

Results

Ten subjects reported to both probes that they saw nothing at all on the card during the negative hallucination phase of testing. Five of these subjects were tested in the standard sequence and 5 in the reversal sequence. All of these subjects responded in terms of their hidden observer instructions. Thus, the five in the standard sequence all correctly reported that the number 18 had been on the card, while the five in the reversal sequence all reported incorrectly that the number 81 had been on the card. This difference in the number of correct hidden responses given by subjects in these two groups was, of course, highly significant, chi square (1) = 10.00, $p < .01$.

Twenty-six subjects failed the negative hallucination suggestion (i.e., reported all or part of the number on the card) and, therefore, were tested in the less aware hidden observer condition. Twelve of these 26 subjects (46%) reported that their less aware hidden part had not seen anything on the paper. The remaining 14 subjects reported the correct number despite their less aware instructions.

Subjects were grouped on the basis of whether they had responded in terms of their instructions (a) on both the suggestion trial and hidden observer trial (N = 10), (b) on the hidden observer trial but not on the suggestion trial (N = 12), or (c) on neither trial (N = 14). Separate one-way analyses of variance (ANOV As) indicated that these three groups failed to differ significantly on CURSS:0, CURSS:S or CURSS:OI dimensions.

Discussion

Zamansky and Bartis (1985) found that subjects who passed their negative visual hallucination suggestion always exhibited a hidden observer response. We obtained the same result. However, our findings make it very clear that hidden observer responding was determined by instructional demands rather than by intrinsic, nonsuggested dissociative processes. Without exception the hidden responses of subjects who passed our negative hallucination suggestion were in the direction specified by their instructions. Subjects instructed to give veridical hidden reports always did so while those informed that their "hidden part" reversed stimuli reported the number 81 instead of the number 18. Still a third type of hidden report occurred in almost half of the subjects who failed the negative hallucination suggestion. When informed that they possessed a less aware hidden part 46% of these subjects reported that they had not seen the very number 18 that they had correctly reported only a few moments earlier. It is worth emphasizing that all of these very clear demand effects occurred despite the fact that our study employed the specific "improvements" that, according to Zamansky and Bartis (1985) placed the notion of a nonsuggested hidden observer "on a substantially more secure footing" (p. 246).

The present findings are similar to the "opposite direction demand effects" obtained in our earlier hidden observer studies on pain and amnesia (Spanos et al., 1983; Spanos et al., 1984; Spanos & Hewitt, 1980). Together with the present results these findings provide very strong support for the prepotent role of contextual cueing in hidden observer responding. On the other hand, the nonsuggested dissociation hypothesis is simply unable to account for "hidden parts" that see things in reverse, are less (rather than more) aware of stimuli than "hypnotized parts", that have access to only concrete words in one case and only abstract words in another (Spanos et al., 1984), and so on.

In both the Zamansky and Bartis (1985) study and in the present study, subjects who passed the negative visual hallucination suggestion later gave hidden reports indicating that they had seen the "stimulus" number. What then should be made of the initial reports by these subjects that the stimulus card was blank? The theoretical account favoured by Zamansky and Bartis (1985) suggests that these subjects never consciously saw the number that was held before their eyes. Nevertheless, a hidden part of them saw the number unconsciously. This unconscious information remained hidden from subjects' phenomenal awareness until the administration of hidden observer instructions somehow released the unconsciously seen information into phenomenal awareness.

This theoretical account provides no explanation for how neurologically intact subjects can focus on but fail to see a meaningful, easily identifiable, sharply contoured, supraliminal, long duration stimulus placed in the centre of a homogeneous white background. This account also fails to explain why a nonsuggested "hidden part" that stores environmental information veridically, and is not "fooled" by suggestions, should respond in terms of demands to report stimuli as reversed.

A social psychological account of the reports proffered by our subjects escews the positing of esoteric psychological processes like the "unconscious seeing" of supraliminal stimuli. Our account suggests that subjects who passed the negative hallucination suggestion saw the stimulus number but, in response to the compliance pressures of the suggestion, denied having done so. Later, the hidden observer instructions altered instructional demands. In the standard sequence these instructions placed a premium on subjects reporting accurately that they had seen the number 18 on the card. Hidden reports were defined as providing information that had previously been out of awareness. Consequently, subjects could safely make such reports without fear of discrediting their earlier testimony of having seen a blank card (Spanos & McLean, 1986; Wagstaff, 1981).

The demands imposed on subjects in the reversal sequence called for them to report having seen the number 81. However, this response was possible only if subjects had, in fact, seen the 18 on the card and were aware that the reverse of 18 is 81. Subjects exposed to these demands always responded in just this way. These responses were clearly goal-directed. They indicate that these subjects were strategically gearing their behaviour to shifting contextual demands in order to present themselves as deeply hypnotized and highly responsive to suggestions.

10 *Spanos, Flynn and Gwynn*

Our account does not deny that subjects may have attempted to avoid seeing the stimulus number by not focussing their eyes on the card, trying to create a visual image that "blocked" the stimulus, and so on. However, any such attempts were less than completely successful and, for this reason, subjects were able to use accurate stimulus information when giving their hidden reports.

Footnotes

This research was supported by a grant to the first author from the Social Sciences and Humanities Research Council of Canada.

1 Perry and his associates (e.g., Nogrady, McConkey, Laurence & Perry, 1983) have attempted to cull evidence for a nonsuggested hidden observer effect by employing ambiguous hidden observer instructions and comparing the responses of highly susceptible hypnotic subjects with low susceptibles instructed to fake hypnosis. The results of these studies remain controversial and a social psychological reinterpretation of them was recently provided (Spanos, 1986).

References

Barber, T.X. (1969). *Hypnosis: A scientific approach.* New York: Van Nostrand Reinhold.

Coe, W.C. & Sarbin, T.X. (1977). Hypnosis from the standpoint of a contextualist. Annuals of the New York Academy of Sciences, *296,* 2-13.

Hilgard, E.R. (1979). Divided consciousness in hypnosis: The implications of the hidden observer. In E. Fromm & R.E. Shor (Eds.), *Hypnosis: Developments in research and new perspectives.* Chicago: Aldine, 45-79.

Nogrady, H., McConkey, K.M., Laurence, J-R. & Perry, C.W. (1983). Dissociation, duality and demand characteristics in hypnosis. *Journal of Abnormal Psychology, 92,* 223-235.

Spanos, N.P. (1983). The hidden observer as an experimental creation. *Journal of Personality and Social Psychology, 44,* 170-176.

Spanos, N.P. (1986). Hypnotic behaviour: A social psychological interpretation of amnesia, analgesia and "trance logic." *Behavioural and Brain Sciences, 9,* 449-502.

Spanos, N.P., Gwynn, M.I. & Stam, H.J. (1983). Instructional demands and ratings of overt and hidden pain during hypnotic analgesia. *Journal of Abnormal Psychology, 92,* 479-488.

Spanos, N.P. & Hewitt, E.C. (1980). The hidden observer in hypnotic analgesia: Discovery or experimental creation? *Journal of Personality and Social Psychology, 39,* 155-159.

Spanos, N.P. & McLean, J. (1986). Hypnotically created pseudomemories: Memory distortions or reporting biases? *British Journal of Experimental and Clinical Hypnosis, 3,* 155-159.

Spanos, N.P. Radtke, H.L. & Bertrand, L.D. (1984). Hypnotic anmesia as a strategic enactment: The successful breaching of hypnotic amnesia in high susceptible subjects. *Journal of Personality and Social Psychology, 47,* 1155-1169.

Spanos, N.P., Radtke, H.L., Hodgins, D.C., Stam, H.J. & Bertrand, L.D. (1983). The Carleton University Responsiveness to Suggestion Scale: Normative data and psychometric properties. *Psychological Reports, 53,* 523-535.

Wagstaff, G.F. (1981). *Hypnosis, compliance and belief.* Brighton: Harvester Press.

Zamansky, H.S. & Bartis, S.P. (1985). The dissociation of an experience: The hidden observer observed. *Journal of Abnormal Psychology, 94,*243-248.

Address for correspondence and reprints:

Nicholas P. Spanos, PhD.
Department of Psychology,
Carleton University,
Ottawa, Ontario,
Canada. K15 5B6

[19]

Increasing Contextual Pressures to Breach Posthypnotic Amnesia

William C. Coe
California State University, Fresno

Anne S. E. Sluis
Georgia State University

The study investigated conditions that produce strong social pressures on posthypnotically amnesic Ss to remember more before being given the cue to remove amnesia. Highly susceptible Ss who passed posthypnotic amnesia were classified as *voluntary* or *involuntary* (having high or low control over recall). Test Ss were serially subjected to 3 pressure situations before being given the cue to lift amnesia: (a) instructions to be honest, (b) lie detection, and (c) a replay of a video of the session. Control Ss sat for the same amount of time and were only asked if they could remember anything else while the experimental Ss received the pressure recalls. All but 1 S breached in the experimental condition. Only the voluntary Ss breached in the control condition. Results are discussed as they relate to breaching amnesia and the voluntary dimension.

In posthypnotic amnesia, as measured by standard scales of hypnotic susceptibility (e.g., Weitzenhoffer & Hilgard, 1962), subjects are told that they will not be able to remember anything that has happened during hypnosis until the hypnotist later gives a cue saying that they *can* remember. Subjects who report 3 or fewer items of the 11 possible are considered amnesic. However, when the hypnotist then gives the cue, many of these items are reported. The material, then, was not lost from memory, yet it seemed to have been temporarily unavailable for recall during the posthypnotic suggestion period. Breaching studies create pressure on subjects to recall more material before they are given the posthypnotic cue "lifting" amnesia.

The outcome of breaching studies hold relevance for contemporary theorizing. Contemporary explanations for posthypnotic amnesia differ in the way they view the subject's degree of control over remembering. One position views posthypnotic amnesia as similar to other memory phenomena. Subjects are seen as passive recipients of their memory processes; that is, their inability to recall "happens" to them. Hilgard's (1977a, 1977b) *neodissociation theory* and Kihlstrom and Evans's (1977, Kihlstrom, 1978) *disrupted retrieval hypothesis* are examples. According to these theorists, changes in subjects' cognitive abilities occur in ways that disrupt the usual communications among them. The cognitive region containing the previously learned material is presumably dissociated from the conscious region during amnesic recall, thereby rendering the material unavailable until the hypnotist's cue releases an amnesic barrier when the material once again becomes available.

The other position is represented by social psychological theories like *role theory* (Coe, 1978; Coe & Sarbin, 1977; Sarbin & Coe, 1972, 1979) and *cognitive, strategic enactment theory* (e.g., Barber, Spanos, & Chaves, 1974; Spanos, 1982, 1986). These theorists view good hypnotic subjects as actively engaged in cognitive skills in order to meet the demands of the hypnotic context. They are "doing" something that prevents them from remembering. For example, they focus their conscious awareness away from the not-to-be-remembered material, away from cues that would help them access it, or away from both.

If posthypnotic amnesia is a "happening," and subjects have little or no control over remembering, then adding social pressures to remember should have little or no effect on how much subjects recall. If, on the other hand, subjects are engaged in active strategies, or "doings," that prevent recall, then adding social pressures to remember should change their strategies in the direction of the demands of the situation, that is, to remember more, and to breach amnesia.

Breaching Paradigms

Breaching procedures have varied. Bowers (1966) designed a study that tricked subjects into believing that the experiment had ended before the cue releasing amnesia had been administered. The responses of highly susceptible subjects who were hypnotized and given the posthypnotic amnesia suggestion were compared to those of highly susceptible subjects who were simply read the suggestion while awake and told to pretend that they had been hypnotized. After both samples showed the usual amnesic response on testing, Bowers told them that the experiment had been completed and that another investigator wished to interview them to obtain pilot information. He also told them to be completely honest with that person, no matter what Bowers had said before.

Recognition testing has also been used in breaching amnesia. McConkey, Sheehan, and Cross (1980) and McConkey and Sheehan (1981) used a video replay of the hypnosis session to evaluate the extent to which subjects would breach. Their approach is called the Experiential Analysis Technique (EAT; Sheehan, McConkey, & Cross, 1978). In this approach, subjects are instructed to stop the tape at any time should they wish to comment on their experiences. The playback is believed to act as a variant of recognition testing for amnesic subjects. Showing the playback of the hypnosis session before amnesia is lifted should create the most stringent demands to breach.

This study was presented in modified form at the symposium Hypnosis and Memory, August 15, 1985, 10th International Congress of Hypnosis and Psychosomatic Medicine, Toronto, Canada. It met in part Anne S. E. Sluis' requirements for a master's degree at California State University, Fresno.

Correspondence concerning this article should be addressed to William C. Coe, Department of Psychology, California State University, Fresno, California 93740-0011.

In sum, these two paradigms had mixed results that could be interpreted as either breaching or not breaching amnesia (see Coe, 1989, for details).

Three studies have investigated breaching amnesia during hypnosis rather than posthypnotically. Spanos and Radtke (1982) hypothesized that good subjects do not breach amnesia because being unable to remember strengthens their self-presentation as someone who is deeply hypnotized. They tested the hypothesis on 8 very susceptible subjects who had consistently described their responses to suggestions as involuntary and who had repeatedly failed to breach amnesia despite exhortations to be honest (Spanos, Radtke, & Bertrand, 1984). These subjects were hypnotized and told that their minds possessed two "hidden parts." One part remained aware of everything in their left hemisphere while the other remained aware of everything in their right hemisphere. The parts could be contacted by a cue from the hypnotist. Half of the subjects had been told that their right hemisphere stored concrete words and their left hemisphere stored abstract words; the other half had been told the opposite. They were also told that the hidden parts would know these things even though they could not consciously remember them.

Subjects then learned a list of abstract and concrete words, and later demonstrated high levels of suggested amnesia for them. The experimenter then contacted the subjects' hidden parts and tested recall before cancelling amnesia. All subjects recalled all of the words for the suggested hemisphere but not the words for the other hemisphere. That is, all these deeply hypnotizable subjects breached amnesia completely in a context where breaching supported a self-presentation as being deeply hypnotized. Spanos (1986) concluded that describing even very hypnotizable, amnesic subjects as unable to remember was inaccurate.

Silva and Kirsch (1987) took a somewhat different approach. Their view is, however, similar to that of Spanos (1986) in that they view good subjects as striving to present themselves as deeply hypnotized. But they postulate that subjects' expectations for reinforcement largely determine the way that they will respond.

Preselected subjects for high susceptibility and posthypnotic amnesia were all told before being hypnotized that they would be given an amnesia suggestion for a list of words while they were hypnotized. They would be tested for remembering it, after which they would be put into a very deep hypnotic state. Half were told that they would then be able to remember even more while in the deep state (*enhanced*), and half were told that they would then be able to remember even less (*reduced*). A six-word list was learned to two perfect recalls, and then the subjects were hypnotized. They were (a) tested for continued knowledge of the list, (b) given an amnesia suggestion for the list, (c) tested for amnesia for the list, (d) given a procedure for deepening hypnosis, (e) again tested for memory of the list, (f) told to cancel the amnesia suggestion, and (g) tested for memory again before they were brought out of hypnosis.

The results were as predicted. Eight of the 10 enhanced subjects breached amnesia completely, and 8 of the 10 reduced subjects remained completely amnesic.

Radtke, Thompson, and Egger (1987) used retrieval cues to breach amnesia during hypnosis. They used a difficult learning task (48 items: 12 categories, 4 items per category, one presentation) and forced recall (guessing) of all 48 items. Subjects were hypnotized, asked to learn the list, then tested on free recall with instructions to draw a line under the last item they remembered. They then had to fill in any of the remaining 48 spaces with guesses. One sample then received an amnesia suggestion, whereas a comparison sample (control) received only relaxation suggestions. A second forced, free-recall trial was administered after which they were given different answer sheets. These sheets contained the 12 category names with four lines below each. Subjects were then told to fill in all of the lines, and to place an *X* by any word that was a guess. The amnesia suggestion was removed for the amnesia sample (more relaxation for the comparison sample) after the third recall. Finally, they were asked to recall again using the same procedure as the third recall. The results were interpreted as showing complete breaching in amnesic subjects.

Taken together, the aforementioned three studies of amnesia during hypnosis appear to support a doing interpretation of hypnotic amnesia. The first two studies demonstrated the strong effects that instructions can have on breaching amnesia, and the third showed the strong interfering effects that retrieval cues can have on maintaining amnesia.

Like the present study, other studies have raised the question of the relative strength of posthypnotic breaching conditions. Kihlstrom, Evans, Orne, and Orne (1980) evaluated four groups of subjects. Following the administration of the Harvard Group Scale of Hypnotic Susceptibility (HGSHS; Shor & Orne, 1962) all subjects were tested for posthypnotic amnesia (they were given 3 min to write down everything that they remembered). Different instructions were then given to each sample: (a) *retest* asked subjects to recall again, (b) *cue* asked subjects to list the items in chronological order, (c) *challenge* asked subjects to overcome amnesia by exerting more effort to recall, and (d) *honesty* cautioned subjects not to fail to report voluntarily what they actually remembered. Amnesia was tested a second time. Finally, the reversal cue was administered and followed by a final recall.

Subjects who were initially amnesic in all four samples did not differ from each other on Recalls 2 or 3. Because the three breaching groups (cue, challenge, and honesty) did not recall more than the retest group at Recall 2, the results were interpreted as evidence that posthypnotic amnesia was not breached. However, closer examination of the data made it clear that about 50% of the subjects in all four samples breached. That is, each of the instructions led about half of the initially amnesic subjects to recall significantly more. The results could therefore be as easily interpreted as demonstrating that all four instructions had a considerable effect on breaching amnesia. Kihlstrom (1978) did not agree. He offered the alternative hypothesis that posthypnotic amnesia, "at least in inexperienced subjects, remits with time regardless of demands" (p. 258). Kilstrom's hypothesis will be evaluated later.

Coe (1978) concluded that the potency of the situational demands for breaching was an important variable. Kihlstrom (1978) agreed, but also argued that until someone obtained positive evidence with stronger demands, posthypnotic amnesia remained robust in the face of demands for extra effort to recall and for honesty in reporting.

Coe and his colleagues (Coe & Yashinski, 1985; Howard & Coe, 1980; Schuyler & Coe, 1981, in press) have since been evaluating the effects of stronger breaching demands and also the interaction of breaching with subjects' ratings of their control over remembering. The present study is an extension of this approach.

In these studies, subjects are preselected for high hypnotic scores on a group hypnosis scale and for displaying amnesia. Half have rated themselves as in control of remembering, and half have rated themselves as not in control of remembering. In each of these studies, some initially amnesic subjects have breached and others have not.

Howard and Coe (1980), in a between-groups design, introduced three conditions before amnesia was tested: (a) *polygraph* told subjects that the physiological equipment they were connected to acted as a lie detector that could reveal whether or not information was being withheld, (b) *honesty* told subjects that it was absolutely crucial to the experiment that they answer questions honestly regarding their hypnotic experiences, and (c) *relax* allowed subjects to relax for the same duration of time needed to administer instructions to the other two groups. The polygraph and honesty conditions induced equally significant breaching compared to the relax condition. However, breaching occurred primarily in subjects who had rated their screening recall as in their control (*voluntary*). *Involuntary* subjects did not breach significantly under any condition, nor did they differ from voluntary subjects in the relax condition.

Schuyler and Coe (1981) again tested subjects under a polygraph and a relax condition, but tested for initial posthypnotic amnesia before introducing the breaching instructions. The interaction between the screening control ratings and breaching found in the Howard and Coe (1980) study was replicated; that is, subjects who had rated themselves as having control over remembering were more likely to breach.

Coe and Yashinski (1985) also used the polygraph versus relax conditions and classified subjects as voluntary or involuntary. Although the interaction was not significant, most of the breaching was accounted for by voluntary subjects in either condition, and involuntary subjects in the polygraph condition.

Other findings offered support for an attributional hypothesis for the control ratings. Subjects rated their control over remembering during the breaching session as well as during the selection session. It appeared that they rated their degree of control by observing their own level of recall. That is, (a) the more responsive subjects were to hypnosis in general, the more likely they were to rate their control during amnesia as lower, (b) the more items they recalled before amnesia was lifted, the more likely they were to rate themselves as having control, and (c) the relationships between control ratings and the number of items recalled were session-specific.

The second Schuyler and Coe (in press) study compared three breaching manipulations. One was the same as the polygraph (lie detector) condition used earlier. A second was *truth* where subjects were told that their physiological responses indicated they were telling all they knew. In the third they were told that their physiological responses indicated that they were not telling all they knew, a *lie* condition. Subjects were then asked if they remembered anything else.

The lie condition created more breaching than the truth or lie detector conditions, which were equal; and the interactions with the voluntary ratings were not significant, but voluntary subjects again accounted for most of the breaching.

Some support was also found for the attributional hypothesis for the control ratings. That is, the number of items recalled at breaching related positively to subjects ratings of control, and the number of items recalled at reversibility related negatively to subjects' ratings of control. Furthermore, although the correlation between the control ratings across the two sessions was significant ($r = .32$), its low level suggested that subjects' ratings may in large part be situation specific.

In this study, as in the Schuyler and Coe (1981) and the Coe and Yashinski (1985) studies, physiological measures and ratings of anxiousness were also observed. None of the measures related meaningfully to levels of recall in any study.

The findings of the four studies we have discussed can be summarized as follows:

1. The lie detector and honesty manipulation have resulted in more breaching as compared with the relax or truth conditions. However, none of the breaching manipulations have breached all of the initially amnesic subjects.

2. Ratings of control over remembering (premeasure) showed a significant interaction with breaching in the first two studies but not in the last two studies. However, voluntary subjects tended to breach more than involuntary subjects in all of the studies.

3. Findings from the last two studies supported an attributional accounting of the control ratings. That is, subjects seem to rate their degree of control over remembering after observing their degree of recall.

We have taken Bem's (1965, 1967) position that control ratings, as indicators of volition, are in part determined by subjects observing their own behavior. When a subject responds in the way a good subject is expected to, he or she concludes that the response was not volitional. Thus, we would expect a positive relationship between reports of voluntariness and the number of items recalled before amnesia is reversed. The relationship, of course, can be interpreted as supporting either a happening hypothesis or a doing hypothesis. The happening position would postulate that the control ratings are based on subjects' perceived change in their feelings of volition; therefore, subjects who have lost volition (do not have control) recall fewer items, and vice versa. The doing position would postulate that subjects observe their own responses (items recalled) and then rate their degree of control accordingly: The fewer items recalled the less control, and vice versa. Thus, a different analysis is required to evaluate the desirability of one theoretical position over the other.

A happening theory should reason that if subjects' ratings are based on their internal feelings of control, then their ratings should predict their future responsiveness. That is, ratings of control taken before the next recall should predict the level of the next recall, because the subject has lost (or gained) control. The reasoning is similar to that proposed by Tart (1970, 1979), concerning subjects' "state reports" (see, Wedemeyer & Coe, 1981, for an alternate view). On the other hand, doing theories should reason that if subjects are using their own level of recall to judge their level of control, then their ratings should more accurately reflect the previous level of recall rather than predict the level of future recall. We predict the latter results.

Although we have tried to understand volition by focusing on subjects' self-observations, voluntariness in hypnosis has also been investigated from other perspectives. Each suggests that attributions of involuntariness are a function of manipulatable variables. Kirsch (1985) summarized a number of studies that support a response expectancy construct in accounting for both behavior and experience. Because hypnotic inductions present involuntary responding as a characteristic of good hypnotic responsiveness, nonvolitional responses can be viewed at least in part as dependent on subject's positive expectancies about involuntary responding. Lynn and his colleagues (Lynn, Nash, Rhue, Frauman, & Scott, 1983; Lynn, Nash, Rhue, Frauman, & Sweeney, 1984; and Lynn et al., 1985) have also provided evidence that hypnotic contextual determinants encourage self-attributions of responsiveness to trance or involuntariness, and Spanos and his colleagues (e.g., Spanos & deGroh, 1983; Spanos & Gorassini, 1984; Spanos, Weekes, & deGroh, 1984) have focused on the content of preinstructions and hypnotic instructions as they determine subjects attributions of volition or nonvolition. Finally, Sarbin (1984) presented a semiotic analysis of nonvolition in hypnosis. He suggested that the good subject enters into a serious, sincere interaction with the hypnotist, as indicated by the setting and the hypnotist's demeanor. The subject then deceives both self and the hypnotist by using his or her skill of spelling out or not spelling out particular aspects of the ongoing scene. That is, the good subject is able to pick out and to report those parts of the interaction that will support the conclusion that he or she has actually lost control.

Spontaneous Recovery (Dissipation Hypothesis)

Several studies have shown that some amnesic subjects who are not pressured to recall more, but are given two successive attempts to recall before amnesia is removed, recall more on the second trial (Ham, Radtke, & Spanos, 1981; Kihlstrom, Easton & Shor, 1983; Kihlstrom et al., 1980). Kihlstrom et al. (1980) hypothesized that amnesia tends to "wear away" naturally with time. Presumably, the amnesic barriers wear down and the dissociated memories are allowed access to awareness.

Bertrand, Spanos, and Parkinson (1983) and Spanos, Tkachyk, Bertrand, and Weekes (1984) tested the dissipation hypothesis. They gave amnesic and partially amnesic subjects a second recall after the challenge trial, but varied the time interval between the initial recall and the second recall. In the first study, the second recall was administered either 60 or 120 seconds after the challenge (Recall 1). In the second study, the second recall was administered immediately or 15 min after the first recall. In both studies, recall increased at the second trial, but the time between the two recalls made no difference. Thus, simply asking subjects to recall again seemed to be the important variable in the dissipation of amnesia, not the passage of time alone.

Dubreil, Spanos, and Bertrand (1983) hypothesized that people expect to recall more on a second trial and that this expectation may be important with posthypnotic amnesia. Three groups of subjects were used to test the hypothesis. The first group was told that people usually remember *more* on a second trial, the second was told that people usually recall *less* on a second trial, and the third was told nothing. The results supported the hypothesis: All three groups recalled more on the second trial. The groups recalled in descending order: The *remember more* group recalled the most, the no instruction group recalled less, and the *recall* less group recalled the least. Thus, all groups recalled more, even the one told that less recall is expected, supporting the notion that people expect to recall more on a second trial even though they are given specific instructions that they will not.

The series of studies on breaching discussed earlier (Coe & Yashinski, 1985; Howard & Coe, 1980; Schuyler & Coe, 1981, in press) may shed some light on the issue of spontaneous recovery over time. In all of these studies, only one breaching recall was given after the challenge recall. Controls who were asked only to recall again (no breaching pressure) did not uniformly show increased recall at Recall 2. Generally, across the studies, subjects who had rated their first recall attempt as "mostly not in their control" (involuntaries) were not likely to recall more at the second trial. But, subjects who had rated their first recall as "mostly in their control" (voluntaries) were likely to recall more at Recall 2. Thus, these studies have so far suggested that, even with additional post-challenge recall requests, amnesia may be maintained in subjects who view their amnesia as mostly out of their control. The fact, however, that their involuntary counterparts who were under breaching pressures did not maintain amnesia, qualifies the observation. The involuntaries should not be viewed as having no control over remembering because of inner, cognitive workings, like amnesic barriers or dissociated subsystems. When pressures to recall are added, they may be able to recall. In any case, subject's reports of control over remembering may be an important variable to consider in researching the dissipation hypothesis.

The present study was designed to add to, and to clarify, the findings from these earlier studies. Past results may be interpreted as support for a happening theoretical position or for a doing theoretical position, depending on whether one places importance on the subjects who breached or on the subjects who did not breach. Therefore, our first goal was to create stronger breaching conditions. To this end, we combined three breaching manipulations in serial order attempting to increase considerably the pressures placed on subjects to breach. After the initial testing for posthypnotic amnesia, we presented the honesty condition from Howard and Coe (1980) followed by the lie condition of Schuyler and Coe (in press). These were then followed with a playback of the videotape of the hypnosis session and another recall (similar to that used in McConkey & Sheehan, 1981, and McConkey et al., 1980). The entire hypnosis and recall period lasted approximately 2 hr.

Our second goal was to investigate control ratings in more detail. The present design allowed us to examine the stability of control-over-recall ratings over a number of recalls. A premeasure rating followed the hypnotic screening session, a second rating was taken after the initial amnesia test of the individual session, then ratings were taken after each of the three breaching attempts. We hoped that the additional voluntary ratings would illuminate the processes by which subjects determine the voluntariness of their recall. We also wanted to evaluate further the possibility of an interaction between control ratings and breaching.

Our third goal was to evaluate further the dissipation hypothesis. The series of five recalls over a longer period of time than investigated before raises new questions. Specifically, how many recall requests over an extended period of time can involuntary subjects respond to with no added recall? Our control samples help to provide an answer.

Method

Subjects

First, 433 introductory psychology students were administered the HGSHS, Form A. Of these, we selected 40 subjects who scored 9 or above and who demonstrated posthypnotic amnesia. Subjects had rated their HGSHS posthypnotic amnesia experience on a 4-point scale (discussed shortly) to indicate the degree of control they believed they had over remembering (Rating #1). We selected 20 who had rated themselves on this scale as voluntary (a rating of 3 or 4) and 20 who had rated themselves as involuntary (a rating of 1 or 2). The following scale was printed on the self-scoring booklets. We did not read the instructions.

Control Rating Scale

Please say the number which best describes the amount of control you felt you had just now while you were trying to remember:

1. I felt like I had *no* control over remembering the things that happened.
2. I felt like I had *very little* control over remembering the things that happened.
3. I felt like I had *very much* control over remembering the things that happened.
4. I felt like I had *complete* control over remembering the things that happened.

Apparatus

Standard galvanic skin response (GSR) equipment was used to simulate the collection of electrodermal responses. Finger electrodes were placed on the index and middle fingers of the subject's nondominant hand. A portable Stoelting Executive Polygraph was used. A VHS (very high speed) recorder and camera were used for videotaping.

Procedure

Ten "voluntary" subjects and 10 "involuntary" subjects were randomly assigned to the experimental treatment groups. Ten voluntary and 10 involuntary subjects also served as time-only controls. The resulting HGSHS scores were not significantly different: Voluntary Control (M = 9.7, SD = 1.25), involuntary control, (M = 10.5, SD = 0.97), voluntary experimental (M = 9.4, SD = 0.84), and involuntary experimental, (M = 10.6, SD = 1.07), $F(3) = 3.14, p > .05$.

The Stanford Hypnotic Susceptibility Scale, Form C (SHSS:C; Weitzenhoffer & Hilgard, 1962) was administered to all subjects. Item 2 was deleted (subject holds hands in front and it is suggested they will move apart) because of the electrodes attached to subject's hands. The collection of electrodermal responses was simulated throughout the procedure. All subjects were secretly videotaped through a one-way mirror beginning just after the standard induction. The experimentals were only taped through testing amnesia. The controls continued to be taped during the entire session.

Subjects received the standard posthypnotic amnesia suggestion. They were told after "awakening" that they would be sitting for a while in order to explore their hypnotic experiences. All subjects were then asked to tell the experimenter, in their own words, everything that had happened since they began looking at the target (testing posthypnotic amnesia, Recall 1). All verbal responses were recorded, regardless of content, then subjects rated their control over remembering immediately (Rating 2). (Ratings of control were also taken after each of the next three experimental recalls: Ratings 3, 4, and 5.)

Subjects were then told that they had forgotten some of the things that had happened, and were asked to report what that experience felt like. After recording subjects' responses, the experimenter said that she was interested in seeing if there were changes in their memory over a period of time.

The following procedures were administered:

Breaching 1. Experimental subjects were pressured to be honest in reporting the events that had occurred during hypnosis (honesty instructions): "It is very important that you be honest about reporting what has happened since you began looking at the target." Subjects were reminded of their previous recollections, (i.e., "You've told me that you remembered such and such") and were then asked, "Now, is there anything else you can recall?"

After an equivalent amount of time had elapsed (30 s), control subjects were reminded of their previous comments and were then asked, "Can you recall anything else now?"

Breaching 2. Experimental subjects were next asked to relax for a few moments while the experimenter looked at the GSR printout and were then given the following false feedback: "The physiological recording device you were connected to works like a lie detector. It indicates that you haven't told me everything you know." Subjects were again reminded of their previous rememberings and then asked for additional recollections.

Control subjects were disconnected from the physiological recording device, but no comments were made about it. After 60 s, they were reminded of their previous rememberings, then asked for additional recollections.

Breaching 3. Experimental subjects were told that the experimenter would like them to watch a videotape of the things that had happened during the hypnosis session. They were told that they would be asked periodically to repeat what the last person had said on the videotape in order to ensure maximal attention during the viewing (tested three times). The videotape was shown in its entirety. Subjects were free to comment on their experience and performance as they wished.

After seeing the videotape, experimental subjects were reminded of what they had already recalled previously and then asked, "Now that you have seen the videotape, is there anything else you *really* remember having happened during hypnosis?" Comments were recorded and the final control rating was obtained.

Control subjects did not view their videotapes. Instead, they spent the viewing-time equivalent (approximately 20 min) sitting quietly with the experimenter, commenting at will about further recollections if they wished, but they were asked nothing. At the end of the time period, subjects were reminded of what they had recalled previously then asked for further recollections, after which a final control rating was requested. This period of time did not seem to be very comfortable for experimenter or subject. Just sitting quietly for 20 min seemed unusual. There were no specific guidelines for the experimenter to follow should subjects comment, but generally any response was noncommittal and the experimental procedures or purposes were not discussed.

Reversal. The previously suggested reversibility cue ("Now you can remember everything") was administered to all subjects and additional recollections were recorded. Subjects were told which items they had not recalled then thanked for their participation. Control subjects were fully debriefed regarding the time-elapse experience.

Results

Seven of the original subjects who recalled more than three items at Recall 1, testing amnesia, were eliminated from further analyses because they were considered not amnesic. On the basis of the HGSHS ratings, 4 subjects were from the voluntary control group, 1 was an involuntary control subject, and 2 were from the voluntary breaching sample. Out of a possible score of 11 on the SHSS:C, the four groups did not differ significantly, $F(3) = 1.23, p > .05$): Voluntary-Breaching (N = 8), M = 9.50, SD = 0.76; Voluntary-Control (N = 61), M = 9.83, SD = 1.47; Involuntary-Breaching (N = 10), M = 10.60, SD = 1.07; Involuntary-Control (N = 9), M = 10.56, SD = 1.01. The resulting

Table 1
Percentage of Subjects Breaching Posthypnotic Amnesia (Recalls 3 or More Items) After the Breaching Manipulation in Six Studies

Study	Honesty		Polygraph		Lie		Truth		Relax—no instruction		Three breaching recalls		Three recalls only		Two breaching recalls	
	V	I	V	I	V	I	V	I	V	I	V	I	V	I	V	I
Howard & Coe (1980)	55	20	78	20	—	—	—	—	11	10	—	—	—	—	—	—
Schuyler & Coe (1981)	—	—	44	9	—	—	—	—	0	0	—	—	—	—	—	—
Coe & Yashinski (1985)	—	—	30	0	—	—	—	—	0	0	—	—	—	—	—	—
Schuyler & Coe (in press)	—	—	0	10	44	11	11	0	—	—	—	—	—	—	—	—
Coe & Sluis (present study)	—	—	—	—	—	—	—	—	—	—	100	90	67	33	—	—
Coe & Tucibat (1989)	—	—	—	—	—	—	—	—	—	—	—	—	—	—	78	89
Average % each condition	55	20	38	9.8	44	11	11	0	3.7	3.3	100	90	67	33	78	89

Note. V = Voluntary Ratings of Control Over Remembering (3 or 4) and I = Involuntary Ratings of Control Over Remembering (1 or 2) on the basis of Harvard Group Scale of Posthypnotic Susceptibility. Dash signifies not applicable.

samples did not differ in their means on their SHSS:C. (Total Score = 11)—voluntaries: breaching (n = 8), M = 9.50, SD = 0.76; control (n = 6), M = 9.83, SD = 1.47; involuntaries: breaching (n = 10), M = 10.60, SD = 1.07; control (n = 9), M = 10.56, SD = 1.01).

Overall Analyses

We adopted our criterion for amnesia (recalling three or fewer items at testing) from the HGSHS and the SHSS:C. We defined breaching as recalling three additional items after Recall 1 but before amnesia was lifted (the same criterion used by Schuyler and Coe, in press) in order to compare percentages of subjects who had breached across various breaching conditions. Table 1 presents those comparisons, including the present study's findings and those of Coe & Tucibat (1989).[1]

We recognize that the breaching criterion may be challenged by other investigators. The most stringent criterion would require a high level of recall after the initial testing, with no additional recall after the reversal cue. Conversely, the weakest criterion would be any additional recall after initially testing amnesia but before reversal.

Table 2 shows the number of items recalled by each subject in each of the four experimental groups. It is presented in order to clarify individual differences and to allow other investigators to come to their own conclusions should they disagree with the criteria we have used for amnesia, for breaching, or for both.

By inspection, in the breaching samples, all of the voluntaries breached, and all but 1 of the Involuntaries breached. In the control samples, 4 of the 6 voluntaries breached, and 3 of the 9 involuntaries breached.

Using 4 (experimental conditions) × 5 (recalls) repeated measures mixed model analyses of variance (ANOVAS) we found that neither main effect was significant: conditions, $F(3, 29) < 1.0$; recalls, $F(4, 116) < 1.0$. In contrast, the Conditions × Recall interaction was significant, $F(4, 116) = 3.19, p < .01$.

We computed 1 × 4 ANOVAS at each recall in order to clarify the significant interaction. As expected, the samples did not differ at Recall 1 (testing amnesia), $F(3, 29) = 1.50, p > .05$; Recall 2 (honesty), $F(3, 29) = 1.59, p > .05$; Recall 3 (lie), $F(3, 29) = < 1.00, p > .05$; or Recall 4 (video), $F(3, 29) = 1.88, p > .05$. The samples did, however, differ significantly at Recall 5 (reversability), $F(3, 29) = 7.59, p < .01$, when the involuntary control group recalled significantly more items (Tukey's $p < .01$) than any of the other three samples, which did not differ from each other (Tukey's $p > .05$ for each comparison).

Repeated measures ANOVAS were computed across recalls. None of the groups showed significant differences in items recalled at each trial. The involuntary control sample approached significance, $F(4, 116) = 2.63, p < .10 > .05$, with Recall 5 being higher than Recalls 1, 2, 3, and 4, which did not differ from each other. However, the small sample sizes give little confidence in the power of the test. All of the other Fs were < 1.0.

Thus, the significant interaction is accounted for by the involuntary control group producing more items at Recall 5 (revers-

[1] We recently tested subjects following the individual SHSS:C under the first two breaching conditions of the present study (*honesty* and *lie*). Sixteen of the 21 breached almost completely. Three of the 5 remaining subjects were "pseudoamnesics," recalling only one or two items over all four recalls. Only 2 subjects remained amnesic until the reversal cue. The HGSHS voluntary–involuntary designation was not related to breaching. In fact, all but three subjects rated their first recall on the SHSS:C as involuntary. As they recalled more items at breaching trials, their ratings changed in the voluntary direction (Coe & Tucibat, 1989). Criticisms and discussions of other breaching studies can be found in Coe (1978) and Kihlstrom (1978). A recent review of research on posthypnotic amnesia may be found in Coe (1989).

ibility) than the other three samples, which did not differ from each other.[2]

Breaching

These analyses suggest that the involuntary control subjects maintained amnesia until the reversal cue, in contrast to the other three samples, which gradually recalled more at each recall, having fewer items left to recall at reversibility. Because samples were equal at Recall 1 and for total recall, planned comparisons across the three breaching recalls were computed in order to test the breaching hypothesis more clearly.

A 4 × 3 mixed model ANOVA was computed over the three breaching recalls for samples on the basis of their HGSHS control ratings. The main effect for conditions (treatment) was significant, $F(3, 29) = 3.94, p < .05$. The repeated main effect for time (recalls) was not significant, $F(2, 58) = 1.41, p > .05$, nor was the interaction, $F(2, 58) < 1.0$. Tukey's comparisons showed that (a) the involuntary control group recalled significantly less ($M = 2.11$) than the other three groups (voluntary control = 4.17; voluntary breaching = 5.63; involuntary breaching = 4.60) (all $ps < .01$); (b) the voluntary breaching sample recalled significantly more than the other three samples ($ps < .05$), and (c) the voluntary control sample and the involuntary breaching sample did not differ ($p > .05$).[3]

Table 1 shows the percentage of subjects classified as voluntary or involuntary on the HGSHS rating who breached (three or more items) across all conditions of six studies on breaching. The percentages are not distributed normally, making statistical comparisons inappropriate. However, in the present study the three breaching recalls, one after the other, resulted in a high level of breaching (all of the voluntary subjects and about 90% of the involuntary subjects).

Criteria for Self-Ratings of Control (Volition)

Correlational analyses were computed for the 40 original subjects between their self-ratings of control over remembering (volition) and the number of items they recalled.[4] The correlation between the sum of subjects' four control ratings on the SHSS:C before amnesia was lifted and the total number of items they recalled was significant ($r = .56, p < .01$). That is, the more subjects rated themselves in control of remembering, the more items they were likely to have recalled, and vice versa.

Table 3 shows the correlations of control ratings taken before and after each recall (Recall 1 had no preceding rating). All four of the correlations taken after a recall significantly reflected the level of the previous recall. None of the three control ratings taken before the next recall was significant in predicting the next level of recall.

Spontaneous Recovery

Although we did not have subjects who only sat for the same amount of time, the results are of interest for the dissipation of posthypnotic amnesia overtime. The involuntary control subjects recovered significantly fewer items than any of the other samples (see the 4 × 3 mixed model ANOVA discussed earlier). Thus, subjects who rate their recall on the HGSHS (or the SHSS: C) as involuntary and have no pressure to recall more (other than being asked again if they remember) show little spontaneous recovery. On the other hand, most of their counterparts under strong pressures to recall, recall significantly more.

Discussion

In this section, we will discuss breaching, volitional ratings, and the dissipation of posthypnotic amnesia.

Breaching

The combination of procedures used in the present study came very close, by our criterion, to causing breaching in all subjects. All but one of the 20 subjects under breaching conditions recalled three or more items during the breaching period. The one breaching subject who did not breach recalled two items after being told that she was lying (Recall 2) then recalled nothing else until she recalled seven more items at reversibility (Table 1, Subject 2, involuntary breaching). This subject rated herself as not being in control of remembering at all recalls. On the basis of her performance, one could argue that at least some amnesic subjects have no control over remembering. However, there are other, more obvious ways to account for her behavior. For example, she may have purposely withheld information for some reason. The present results cannot provide a satisfactory answer. However, Table 1 shows that just the three recalls by themselves over time, without manipulated pressures, have resulted in more breaching in both voluntaries and involuntaries than any of the other studies reviewed herein, except perhaps for the voluntary subjects in the Howard and Coe (1980) honesty and polygraph conditions and the Coe and Tucibat (1989) study (see Footnote 1).

However, because breaching is a matter of degree, interpreting the results in regards to breaching becomes subjective. As mentioned earlier, we used a criterion of recalling three more items during breaching. However, if the most stringent criterion for breaching was used (i.e., no items recalled after the reversibility cue) only 38.9% of our sample (7 of 18) would be considered to have breached completely.

The present design does not allow us to evaluate the comparative strengths of the individual breaching manipulations. They were always given in the same order and were not compared to each other independently. Our goal was to create strong pressures to breach, not to compare breaching conditions.

Volitional Ratings

Breaching occurred equally across the three experimental manipulations for both voluntary and involuntary subjects.

---

[2] Subjects were reclassified as voluntary or involuntary on the basis of the mean of their four ratings of control during SHSS:C. The results based on those ratings of a 4 × 5 mixed model ANOVA were essentially the same as the voluntary classifications based on the HGSHS screening.

[3] The same analysis for samples based on their average control reports during the experimental recalls results in virtually identical findings and is therefore not reported.

[4] The data for the 7 subjects who recalled more than three items at Recall 1 are included in the remaining analyses because they continued making ratings and recalling even though by our criterion we did not consider them to demonstrate posthypnotic amnesia. Their results are useful and relevant in these computations.

Table 2
Number of New Items Recalled at Each Trial by Experimental Condition (HGS Voluntary Classification)

Subject no.	Recall 1 (test amnesia)	Recall 2 (honesty)	Recall 3 (lie)	Recall 4 (video)	Sum over recalls 2, 3, & 4	Recall 5 (lifting)	Total[a] of all recalls
			Breaching samples: Voluntary				
1	3	0	1	3	4	1	8
2	2	1	1	4	6	0	8
3	1	4	1	1	6	0	7
4	3	1	0	3	4	1	8
5	0	1	2	4	7	2	9
6	0	0	1	4	5	3	8
7	1	1	3	0	4	1	6
8	0	6	1	2	9	0	9
M	1.25	1.75	1.25	2.63	5.63	1.00	7.88
SD	1.28	2.12	0.89	1.51	1.77	1.09	0.99
			Breaching samples: Involuntary				
1	2	5	1	2	8	0	10
2	0	0	2	0	2	7	9
3	0	2	2	0	4	1	5
4	3	1	1	1	3	1	7
5	3	2	1	3	6	0	9
6	3	2	3	0	5	0	9
7	0	1	1	2	4	3	7
8	1	0	0	6	6	0	7
9	3	0	1	2	3	1	7
10	2	4	0	1	5	1	8
M	1.70	1.70	1.20	1.70	4.60	1.40	7.80
SD	1.34	1.70	0.92	1.83	1.78	2.17	1.48
			Control samples: Voluntary				
1	2	4	2	1	7	1	10
2	3	2	0	3	5	0	8
3	0	0	0	0	0	5	5
4	3	1	1	2	4	0	7
5	0	3	4	1	8	0	8
6	3	1	0	0	1	1	5
M	1.83	1.83	1.17	1.17	4.17	1.17	7.17
SD	1.47	1.47	1.60	1.17	3.19	1.94	1.94
			Control samples: Involuntary				
1	2	0	0	0	0	2	4
2	0	1	0	1	2	7	9
3	0	1	0	2	3	3	6
4	1	0	1	0	1	5	7
5	0	0	1	1	2	7	9
6	0	0	1	1	2	6	8
7	0	0	0	0	0	4	4
8	2	1	2	3	6	0	8
9	1	1	0	2	3	5	9
M	0.67	0.44	0.56	1.11	2.11	4.22	7.11
SD	0.87	0.53	0.73	1.05	1.83	2.28	2.03

[a] Total possible = 10.

The voluntary control subjects, who were only asked three times if they recalled anything else, breached as much as the involuntary experimental subjects. The involuntary control sample remained convincingly more amnesic than the other three samples before reversibility.

With one exception, the initially voluntary subjects, whether under breaching pressures or not, breached amnesia. The one who did not was in the control condition (see Table 2, subject 3, voluntary control). He recalled nothing until the reversal cue, then recalled five items. He also rated his control in the direction of involuntary after each of the SHSS:C recalls. Unfortunately, the present results cannot help us to understand this subject's behavior. However, the involuntary control subjects, based on either the HGSHS rating or the ratings during breach-

Table 3
Correlation Coefficients of Control Ratings Taken Before or After Recall With the Number of Items Recalled

Timing of ratings	Recall 1	Recall 2	Recall 3	Recall 4
After recall	.534**	.528**	.343*	.345*
Before recall[a]	—	.183	.134	.154

Note. $N = 40$.
[a] None of the correlations of ratings taken before recall were significant.
* $p < .05$. ** $p < .01$.

ing, tended to remain amnesic. The correlation between subjects' overall ratings of control and the number of items they remembered ($r = .56$, $p < .01$) also indicates that ratings of increasing control are predictive of increasing breaching.

The results also help to clarify what the volitional ratings appear to be measuring. The correlations between subjects' volitional ratings and their responses to the recall immediately preceding the ratings were all positive and significant. On the other hand, correlations between subjects' volitional ratings and their responses to the recall immediately after the ratings were all small and insignificant. Thus, the ratings appear to be based on subjects' observations of their own level of recall rather than some change in themselves that reduces volition and creates a happening. It would seem that happening theorists would have to modify their position to account for the findings. The present results suggest support for a doing interpretation.

We recognize that because our rating instructions specifically asked subjects to rate the control they believed they had over their previous recall, it can be argued that the correlations between ratings and recalls could simply reflect the instructional bias. Nevertheless, theorists who postulate that posthypnotic amnesia is a happening, and that subjects have lost control in the same way as subjects do with other defects of memory (like misplacing one's keys), will have a difficult time explaining subjects who rate themselves as not in control, yet who still breach amnesia; for example, the involuntary subjects on the SHSS:C ratings in the breaching condition.

Dissipation of Amnesia

Although no "time-alone" control condition was examined (subjects who are only asked to recall again at the end of the session), the results appear to provide some evidence on the natural dissipation of posthypnotic amnesia over time. Spontaneous recovery occurred in 46.67% of our control subjects who had no more pressure to recall than being asked to try again. Of these subjects, however, 67% who initially judged themselves as *having control* over remembering showed dissipation of amnesia, whereas only 33% (HGSH-A) to 42% (SHSS-C) of those who initially judged themselves as *not in control* showed it. Thus, one can probably expect that around 50% of subjects over an extended period (45–60 min) will breach amnesia if they are simply asked to try to recall again.

In conclusion, the high degree of breaching demonstrated appears to support a social psychological analysis, a doing analysis, of posthypnotic amnesia. Given strong enough pressures, probably all subjects will breach amnesia to a large extent before the posthypnotic cue for removing it is administered. If a happening analysis is postulated, it must be qualified with post-hoc explanations that attribute varying and unpredictable internal changes to account for changes in recall, volition, or both.

A doing analysis was also supported by the finding that subjects appear to use their own responses as primary criteria for judging their degree of control over remembering. Their judgments of control do not predict their future responsiveness as they should if their ratings were based on internal changes causing them to lose control. However, like breaching, the doing–happening dimension is not all or none. A subject may, for example, be focusing attention away from the material to be forgotten (a doing), and then attribute "forgetting" to a loss of control (a happening). When attention is forced back to the material by pressures to recall, the subject may "discover" the material, report it, and then attribute recall to a loss of control, or to gaining control. On the other hand, it may be more accurate to view the subjects' attributions as the result of a strategic action in presenting themselves as good subjects (e.g., Silva & Kirsch, 1987; Spanos & Radtke, 1982). In either event, subjects are doing something to arrive at their decisions. Our perception of the circumstances are the most important factor in deciding which interpretation, doing or happening, has the most heuristic value. We support the doing interpretation because it seems to open more variables for investigation. A happening interpretation tends to limit the focus to internal subject variables. More work is certainly needed to clarify the interactional processes leading to interpretations of doings and happenings.

References

Barber, T. X., Spanos, N. P., & Chaves, J. F. (1974). *Hypnotism, imagination and human potentialities.* Elmsford, NY: Pergamon Press.

Bem, D. J. (1965). An experimental analysis of self-persuasion. *Journal of Experimental and Social Psychology, 1,* 199–218.

Bem, D. J. (1967). Self-perception: An alternative interpretation of cognitive dissonance phenomena. *Psychological Review, 74,* 183–200.

Bertrand, L. D., Spanos, N. P., Parkinson, B. (1983). Test of the dissipation hypothesis of hypnotic amnesia. *Psychological Reports, 52,* 667–671.

Bowers, K. S. (1966). Hypnotic behavior: The differentiation of trance and demand characteristic variables. *Journal of Abnormal Psychology, 71,* 42–51.

Coe, W. C. (1978). The credibility of posthypnotic amnesia: A contextualist's view. *International Journal of Clinical and Experimental Hypnosis, 26,* 218–245.

Coe, W. C. (1989). Posthypnotic amnesia: Theory and research. In N. P. Spanos & J. F. Chaves (Eds.), *Hypnosis: A social psychological view* (pp. 110–148). New York: Praeger.

Coe, W. C., & Sarbin, T. R. (1977). Hypnosis from the standpoint of a contextualist. *Annals of New York Academy of Sciences, 296,* 2–13.

Coe, W. C., & Tucibat, M. (1989). *More on breaching posthypnotic amnesia and its correlates.* Manuscript submitted for publication.

Coe, W. C., & Yashinski, E. (1985). Volitional experiences associated with breaching posthypnotic amnesia. *Journal of Personality and Social Psychology, 48,* 716–722.

Dubreil, D. L., Spanos, N. P., & Bertrand, L. D. (1983). Does hypnotic amnesia dissipate with time? *Imagination, Cognition and Personality, 2,* 103–113.

Ham, M. L., Radtke, L. H., & Spanos, N. P. (1981). *The effects of suggestion type and the experience of involuntariness on the breaching of posthypnotic amnesia.* Unpublished manuscript, Carelton University, Ottawa, Ontario, Canada.

Hilgard, E. R. (1977a). *Divided consciousness.* New York: Wiley.

Hilgard, E. R. (1977b). The problem of divided consciousness: A neodissociation interpretation. *Annals of New York Academy of Sciences, 296,* 48–59.

Howard, M. L., & Coe, W. C. (1980). The effects of context and subjects' perceived control in breaching posthypnotic amnesia. *Journal of Personality and Social Psychology, 46,* 342–359.

Kihlstrom, J. F. (1978). Context and cognition in posthypnotic amnesia. *International Journal of Clinical and Experimental Hypnosis, 26,* 246–267.

Kihlstrom, J. F., Easton, R. D., & Shor, R. E. (1983). Spontaneous recovery of memory during posthypnotic amnesia. *International Journal of Clinical and Experimental Hypnosis, 31,* 309–323.

Kihlstrom. J. F., & Evans, F. J. (1977). Residual effects of suggestions for posthypnotic amnesia: A reexamination. *Journal of Abnormal Psychology, 86,* 327–333.

Kihlstrom, J. F., Evans, F. J., Orne, M. T., & Orne, E. C. (1980). Attempting to breach posthypnotic amnesia. *Journal of Abnormal Psychology, 89,* 603–616.

Kirsch, K. (1985). Response expectancy as a determinant of experience and behavior. *American Psychologist, 40,* 1189–1202.

Lynn, S. J., Nash, M. R., Rhue, J. W., Carlson, V., Sweeney, C., Frauman, D., & Givens, D. (1985). Nonvolition and hypnosis, reals vs. simulators: Experiential and behavioral differences in response to conflicting suggestions during hypnosis. In D. Waxman, P. C. Misra, M. Gibson, & A. Basker (Eds.), *Modern trends in hypnosis* (pp. 100–127). New York: Plenum Press.

Lynn, S. J., Nash, M. R., Rhue, J. W., Frauman, D., & Scott, S. (1983). Hypnosis and the experience of nonvolition. *International Journal of Clinical and Experimental Hypnosis, 21,* 293–308.

Lynn, S. J., Nash, M. R., Rhue, J. W., Frauman, D. C., & Sweeney, C. A. (1984). Nonvolition, expectancies, and hypnotic rapport. *Journal of Abnormal Psychology, 93,* 295–303.

McConkey, K. M., & Sheehan, P. W. (1981). The impact of videotape playback of hypnotic events on posthypnotic amnesia. *Journal of Abnormal Psychology, 90,* 46–54.

McConkey, K. M., Sheehan, P. W., & Cross, D. G. (1980). Posthypnotic amnesia: Seeing is not remembering. *British Journal of Social and Clinical Psychology, 19,* 99–107.

Radtke, H. L., Thompson, V. A., & Egger, L. A. (1987). Use of retrieval cues in breaching hypnotic amnesia. *Journal of Abnormal Psychology, 96,* 335–340.

Sarbin, T. R. (1984). Nonvolition in hypnosis: A semiotic analysis. *Psychological Record, 34,* 537–549.

Sarbin, T. R., & Coe, W. C. (1972). *Hypnosis: A social psychological analysis of influence communication.* New York: Holt, Rinehart & Winston.

Sarbin, T. R., & Coe, W. C. (1979). Hypnosis and psychopathology: Replacing old myths with fresh metaphors. *Journal of Abnormal Psychology, 88,* 506–526.

Schuyler, B. A., & Coe, W. C. (1981). A physiological investigation of volitional and nonvolitional experience during posthypnotic amnesia. *Journal of Personality and Social Psychology, 40,* 1160–1169.

Schuyler, B. A., & Coe, W. C. (in press). Volitional and nonvolitional experiences during posthypnotic amnesia. *International Journal of Clinical and Experimental Hypnosis.*

Sheehan, P. W., McConkey, K. M., & Cross, D. (1978). Experiental analysis of hypnosis: Some new observations on hypnotic phenomena. *Journal of Abnormal Psychology, 87,* 570–573.

Shor, R. E., & Orne, E. C. (1962). *The Harvard Group Scale of Hypnotic Susceptibility, Form A.* Palo Alto, CA: Consulting Psychologists Press.

Silva, C. E., & Kirsch, I. (1987). Breaching hypnotic amnesia by manipulating expectancy. *Journal of Abnormal Psychology, 96,* 325–329.

Spanos, N. P. (1982). A social psychological approach to hypnotic behavior. In G. Weary & H. L. Mirlls (Eds.), *Integrations of clinical and social psychology* (pp. 231–271). New York: Oxford University Press.

Spanos, N. P. (1986). Hypnotic behavior: A social psychological interpretation of amnesia, analgesia and "trance logic." *Behavioral and Brain Sciences, 9,* 449–502.

Spanos, N. P., & deGroh, M. (1983). Communication structure and involuntariness reports in hypnotic and nonhypnotic subjects. *Perceptual and Motor Skills, 57,* 1179–1186.

Spanos, N. P., & Gorassini, D. R. (1984). The structure of hypnotic test suggestions and attributions of responding involuntarily. *Journal of Personality and Social Psychology, 46,* 688–696.

Spanos, N. P., & Radtke, H. L. (1982). Hypnotic amnesia as a strategic enactment: A cognitive, socialpsychological perspective. *Research Communications in Psychology, 7,* 215–231.

Spanos, N. P., Radtke, H. L., & Bertrand, L. D. (1984). Hypnotic amnesia as a strategic enactment: The successful breaching of hypnotic amnesia in high susceptible subjects. *Journal of Personality and Social Psychology, 47,* 1155–1169.

Spanos, N. P., Tkachyk, M., Bertrand, L. D., & Weekes, J. R. (1984). The dissipation hypothesis of hypnotic amnesia: More disconfirming evidence. *Psychological Reports, 55,* 191–196.

Spanos, N. P., Weekes, J. R., & deGroh, M. (1984). The "involuntary" countering of suggested requests: A test of the ideomotor hypothesis of hypnotic responsiveness. *British Journal of Experimental and Clinical Hypnosis, 1,* 3–11.

Tart, C. T. (1970). Self-report scales of hypnotic depth. *International Journal of Clinical and Experimental Hypnosis, 18,* 105–125.

Tart, C. T. (1979). Measuring the depth of an altered state of consciousness, with particular reference to self-report scales of hypnotic depth. In E. Fromm & R. E. Shor (Eds.), *Hypnosis: Developments in research and new perspectives* (pp. 567–601). Hawthorne, NY: Aldine.

Wedemeyer, C., & Coe, W. C. (1981). Hypnotic state reports: Contextual variation and phenomenological criteria. *Journal of Mental Imagery, 5,* 107–118.

Weitzenhoffer, A. M., & Hilgard, E. R. (1962). *The Stanford Scale of Hypnotic Susceptibility, Form C.* Palo Alto, CA: Consulting Psychologists Press.

Received August 31, 1988
Revision received March 23, 1989
Accepted May 9, 1989

[20]

HYPNOTIC AND POSTHYPNOTIC SUGGESTION: *Finding Meaning in the Message of the Hypnotist*[1]

AMANDA J. BARNIER AND KEVIN M. McCONKEY[2]

University of New South Wales, Sydney, Australia

Abstract: High hypnotizable subjects were asked a question before, during, and after hypnosis and were given a suggestion before, during, or after hypnosis to rub their earlobe when they were asked this question. In this way, the experiment placed a question that required a verbal response in contrast with a suggestion that only sometimes required a behavioral response. Subjects were more likely to respond behaviorally when the question was associated with the suggestion but more likely to respond verbally when the question was a social interaction; furthermore, the likelihood of subjects responding behaviorally and/or verbally shifted across the tests with the changing message of the hypnotist. The findings highlight hypnotized subjects' attempts to interpret the hypnotist's communications and their ability to resolve ambiguity in the nexus of those messages in a way that promotes their hypnotic behavior and experience.

The complexity of the interaction between hypnotist and subject derives in large part from the formal and informal messages that are conveyed by the communications of the hypnotist and the nature of the hypnotic setting. Weitzenhoffer (1974), for instance, demonstrated that intended instructions aimed at producing "merely cooperative social behavior" could act as hypnotic suggestions to elicit experientially involuntary (as well as voluntary) behavior, whereas intended suggestions aimed at producing a hypnotic response could act as an instruction to elicit voluntary (as well as experientially involuntary) behavior. He argued that when a hypnotist gives a verbal communication to a subject, there is no way to tell a priori (i.e., before the communication is given) how it will be interpreted and responded to by a subject (Weitzenhoffer, 1974; see also Sheehan & McConkey, 1982).

Manuscript submitted August 12, 1997; final revision received July 21, 1998.

[1]This research was supported in part by a grant from the Australian Research Council to Kevin M. McConkey and an Australian Postgraduate Award to Amanda J. Barnier. We are grateful to Heather Wilton for research assistance.

[2]Address correspondence to Kevin M. McConkey, School of Psychology, University of New South Wales, Sydney NSW 2052, Australia or K.McConkey@unsw.edu.au.

When faced with communications that can be interpreted in various ways, hypnotized subjects must work to understand the intentions behind the hypnotist's message and to respond in a way that is appropriate to those intentions and that is compatible with their abilities and motivations. This view is consistent with Kihlstrom's (1995; see also Grice, 1975; McConkey, Glisky, & Kihlstrom, 1989; Orne, 1959) characterization of the hypnotic experiment (and indeed all psychological experiments) as involving a conversation and a collaboration between experimenters and subjects. Kihlstrom (1995) argued that subjects are continually trying to determine how to respond to both the formal and the informal messages that are emanating from the hypnotist and the setting. Moreover, this interpretation occurs in the context of a particular type of social encounter (labeled the "experiment") that has particular rules and that guides and constrains all participants' understandings of their interaction. From this perspective, subjects engage in "effort after meaning" within the context of a general understanding about what they can expect to happen during a hypnosis session in an experimental laboratory.

Experiments on conflicting hypnotic communications, countering preconceptions, the hidden observer effect, and trance logic (e.g., McConkey, 1983; McConkey, Bryant, Bibb, & Kihlstrom, 1991; Nogrady, McConkey, Laurence, & Perry, 1983; Sheehan, 1971) have all pointed to ambiguities in the communications of the hypnotist and to the ways in which hypnotized subjects may resolve those ambiguities and respond. Recent experiments on posthypnotic suggestion have demonstrated that ambiguities can arise not only from multiple, conflicting verbal communications but also from the way in which those messages are embedded within the context of the overall hypnotic interaction (Barnier & McConkey, 1996, 1998, in press). For instance, Barnier and McConkey (in press) gave real and simulating subjects either a general suggestion to respond when they heard a cue or a posthypnotic suggestion to respond when they heard a cue after hypnosis; half of the subjects were given the cue before hypnosis and half were given it after hypnosis. We found that subjects' behaviors and experiences were influenced by the level of congruence between information conveyed by the suggestion about when they should respond and the timing of the test. Our findings indicated that hypnotized subjects work actively to interpret the message of the hypnotist within the context of their interaction with him or her. Given these findings, we believed it would be valuable to examine further subjects' search for meaning in the hypnotic context, particularly when the conditions or circumstances of that setting were changing.

Accordingly, we explored shifts in subjects' interpretations of and responses to the hypnotist's communications as the context of testing changed. In the present experiment, high hypnotizable subjects were asked a question ("Do you think it will rain tonight?") three times during an experimental session: before hypnosis, during hypnosis, and after hypnosis. In addition, subjects were given a suggestion that they would rub their right earlobe when they were asked this question. In one condition, subjects were given the suggestion before hypnosis; in the second condition, they were given the suggestion during hypnosis; and in the third condition, they were given the suggestion after hypnosis.

The design of our experiment placed a message from the hypnotist that always required a verbal response (viz., the question "Do you think it will rain tonight?") against a hypnotic-like message that sometimes required a behavioral response (viz., the suggestion for subjects to rub their earlobe when they hear the phrase "Do you think it will rain tonight?"). The verbal response could be said to reflect routine social interaction; in other words, the hypnotist asked a benign question and subjects were expected to give a simple answer. The behavioral response, however, reflected a hypnotic interaction. That is, the hypnotist suggested that when she asked a question, subjects would give an unusual (hypnotic) response.

We expected that when the message of the hypnotist was interpreted as a formal hypnotic communication (viz., a suggestion to rub the earlobe) and the context was explicitly hypnotic, then subjects would rub their earlobe more so than answer the question. We expected that when the message was interpreted as a social interaction (viz., a question to answer) and the context was not explicitly hypnotic, then subjects would answer the question more so than rub their earlobe. However, we expected that the likelihood of subjects responding behaviorally and/or responding verbally would fluctuate across the tests in line with the changing message of the hypnotist (note that for each test, subjects could respond either behaviorally or verbally, or they could do both). In this way, we examined how subjects dealt with the ambiguity and conflict generated by the meaning of the hypnotist's message across different circumstances within the context of a hypnotic interaction.

To better appreciate the experience of hypnotized subjects, we used the Experiential Analysis Technique (EAT; Sheehan & McConkey, 1982). The EAT involves subjects commenting on a videotape record of their hypnotic session in the presence of an independent experimenter (the inquirer). We used this technique to explore experiential and interpretive processes that would not be captured by behavioral data. In this respect, we used it to better understand the participant's point of view as a central process in the hypnotic interaction (see also Kihlstrom, 1995; McConkey et al., 1989). More specifically, the EAT allowed an examination of the extent to which subjects' commitment to the communications of the hypnotist was related to behavioral responding. Sheehan (1991) argued that the deeply hypnotized subject is characterized by a motivated cognitive commitment, which reflects the ability and motivation of the individual to process the hypnotist's communications in a cognitively active way and thus to respond in an appropriate fashion. Accordingly, we considered that subjects' comments about their responses to the various tests would provide insight into the processes and influences that were associated with hypnotic and posthypnotic responding. We believed that those who demonstrated a cognitive commitment to the message of the hypnotist would be more likely to process the ambiguous, conflicting, and confusing information across the tests in a way that led to hypnotic responding.

Method

Participants

Twenty-one (7 male and 14 female) high hypnotizable participants of mean age 22.05 years (*SD* = 8.45) who were undergraduate psychology students at the University of New South Wales, Sydney, Australia, voluntarily participated in return for research credit of 1 hour. Subjects were preselected on the basis of their scores in the range of 10 to 12 on the 12-item Harvard Group Scale of Hypnotic Susceptibility, Form A (HGSHS:A; Shor & Orne, 1962; *M* = 10.88, *SD* = 0.66); their high hypnotizability was confirmed by their scores in the range of 8 to 10 on a 10-item tailored version of the Stanford Hypnotic Susceptibility Scale, Form C (Hilgard, Crawford, Bowers, & Kihlstrom, 1979; SHSS:C; Weitzenhoffer & Hilgard, 1962; *M* = 9.33, *SD* = 0.58).

Apparatus

A video camera and a videocassette recorder were used to record both the hypnosis and the inquiry session onto videocassettes; the video camera was focused on the participant throughout. A videocassette recorder and a color monitor were used to play back the recording of the hypnosis session.

Procedure

The experiment involved a hypnosis session and an EAT inquiry session. The hypnosis session was conducted by the first experimenter (the hypnotist), and the EAT inquiry session was conducted by a second, independent experimenter (the inquirer). The suggestion to rub the right earlobe in response to the cue was given either before hypnosis (prehypnotic condition), during hypnosis (hypnotic condition), or after hypnosis (posthypnotic condition); subjects were allocated to one of these three conditions. Response to the question/cue (viz., "Do you think it will rain tonight?") was tested on three occasions: before hypnosis (Test 1), during hypnosis (Test 2), and after hypnosis (Test 3); all subjects were given each test. Table 1 sets out the experimental design. For both the administration of the suggestion and the test(s), "before hypnosis" refers to the period of time before the hypnotic induction procedure was administered, "during hypnosis" refers to the period of time between the administration of the induction and the deinduction procedures, and "after hypnosis" refers to the period of time after the hypnotic deinduction was administered.

Hypnosis session. The hypnotist welcomed subjects, gave them an informed consent form to read and sign, and told them to make themselves comfortable. Following this, she gave the suggestion to those in the prehypnotic condition. Subjects in this condition were told that they would rub their right earlobe with the thumb and forefinger of their right hand when the hypnotist said, "Do you think it will rain tonight?"[3] The hypnotist then allowed 10 seconds to elapse before she administered Test 1, the prehypnotic test of the question/cue. Subjects in the hypnotic and posthypnotic conditions were not given the suggestion at this point; for these individuals, the hypnotist allowed 10 seconds to elapse from her initial instruction to allow the subjects to make themselves comfortable before administering Test 1. That is, following either the suggestion (prehypnotic condition) or the initial instruction (hypnotic and posthypnotic conditions), the hypnotist asked subjects, "Do you think it will rain tonight?" She avoided eye contact, allowed 30 seconds to elapse from the end of the cue, and noted their behavioral and verbal responses; if subjects asked for clarification, the hypnotist did not respond until the 30 seconds had elapsed.

The hypnotist then administered a standard induction procedure and tested all subjects on the four hypnotic items of moving hands apart, finger lock, verbal inhibition, and heat hallucination. She then gave the suggestion to those in the hypnotic condition. That is, subjects in this condition were told that they would rub their right earlobe with the thumb and forefinger of their right hand when the hypnotist said, "Do you think it will rain tonight?" The hypnotist allowed 10 seconds to elapse before she administered Test 2, the hypnotic test of the question/cue. Subjects in the prehypnotic condition previously had been given the suggestion, and those in the posthypnotic condition were not given the suggestion at this point; for these individuals, the hypnotist allowed 10 seconds to elapse from the end of the heat hallucination item before administering Test 2. Thus, following either the suggestion (hypnotic condition) or the conclusion of the heat hallucination item (prehypnotic and posthypnotic conditions), the hypnotist asked participants, "Do you think it will rain tonight?" Again, she allowed 30 seconds to elapse from

[3]The verbatim suggestion was as follows: "Now I'd just like you to listen closely to what I tell you next. When I say to you, 'Do you think it will rain tonight?' you will rub your right earlobe with the thumb and forefinger of your right hand. You will rub your right earlobe. No matter what you are doing, when you hear me say, 'Do you think it will rain tonight?' you will rub your right earlobe with the thumb and forefinger of your right hand. You will rub your right earlobe. This will happen by itself and you will not remember that I asked you to do this when I say these words. When I say to you, 'Do you think it will rain tonight?' you will rub your right earlobe with the thumb and forefinger of your right hand."

Table 1
Summary of Experimental Design

Suggestion Condition	Experimental Periods: Before Hypnosis	During Hypnosis	After Hypnosis
Prehypnotic	**Suggestion** Test 1 (question/cue)	Test 2 (question/cue)	Test 3 (question/cue)
Hypnotic	Test 1 (question)	**Suggestion** Test 2 (question/cue)	Test 3 (question/cue)
Posthypnotic	Test 1 (question)	Test 2 (question)	**Suggestion** Test 3 (question/cue)

Note. The possible interpretations of each test (viz., question to answer and/or cue to respond) are presented in parentheses.

the end of the cue and noted their behavioral and verbal responses; if subjects asked for clarification, the hypnotist did not respond until the 30 seconds had elapsed. After the hypnotic test of responding, the hypnotist allowed 10 seconds to elapse before she administered a standard deinduction procedure to all subjects.

Posthypnotic inquiry session. Immediately following the deinduction procedure, the hypnotist gave the suggestion to those in the posthypnotic condition. That is, subjects in this condition were told that they would rub their right earlobe with the thumb and forefinger of their right hand when the hypnotist said, "Do you think it will rain tonight?" The hypnotist then allowed 10 seconds to elapse before she administered Test 3, the posthypnotic test of the question/cue. Subjects in the prehypnotic and hypnotic conditions had been given the suggestion before and during hypnosis, respectively; for these individuals, the hypnotist allowed 10 seconds to elapse from the end of the deinduction procedure before administering Test 3. Thus, following either the suggestion (posthypnotic condition) or the deinduction procedure (prehypnotic and hypnotic conditions), the hypnotist asked subjects, "Do you think it will rain tonight?" She avoided eye contact, allowed 30 seconds to elapse from the end of the cue, and noted their behavioral and verbal responses; if subjects asked for clarification, the hypnotist did not respond until the 30 seconds had elapsed. Following this, the hypnotist cancelled the suggestion and conducted a brief inquiry into subjects' reactions to the hypnosis session.

EAT inquiry session. The inquirer told subjects that they would be shown a videotape of the hypnosis session that they had just completed and that they should ask her to stop the videotape at any point and describe their experiences. The decision to stop the videotape was left primarily to participants, but if they did not comment spontaneously on their responses to the suggestion and the question/cue across the three tests, the inquirer stopped the videotape and asked them to comment on their experiences. For instance, during the playback of the suggestion (whether prehypnotic, hypnotic, or posthypnotic), the inquirer asked questions such as, "What sorts of things were you thinking as you were listening to the hypnotist?" and "How were you feeling about this instruction?" During the playback of the question/cue for each of the tests, she asked questions such as, "Did that phrase have any meaning for you?" and "Tell me about the feelings you were experiencing at this point." During the playback of participants' responses to the tests, she asked subjects to: "Tell me about the thoughts that were going through your mind at this time" and "Is there anything you might have liked to say to the hypnotist?" In addition to these questions, the inquirer asked subjects who responded on the tests to rate how much of an urge they felt to rub their earlobe on each occasion (where 0 = *none at all* and 6 = *an extremely strong urge*). Finally, the inquirer answered any questions, thanked subjects, and ended the session.

RESULTS

Behavioral and verbal responses on the three tests and EAT comments were categorized from the video record by the hypnotist or the inquirer and an independent rater who was unaware of the aims of the experiment. Behavioral responses were categorized as either positive (a behavioral reaction consistent with the suggestion within 30 seconds of the question/cue) or negative (no behavioral reaction within 30 seconds of the question/cue); verbal responses were categorized as either a response (any verbal response to the question) or as no response. EAT comments about the suggestion were categorized in terms of whether it was confusing, considered to be unusual, and whether subjects expected to respond; comments about the question/cue were categorized in terms of the meaning it held for subjects and whether they felt confused by its presentation across the three tests; and comments about responding were categorized in terms of the nature of their response and the similarities and differences in their reactions to the repeated tests.[4]

[4]Overall interrater reliability for behavioral responses was $k = 0.91$ (Kappa statistic; see Cohen, 1960; Test 1: $k = 0.72$, Test 2: $k = 1.00$, Test 3: $k = 0.92$); overall interrater reliability for verbal responses was $k = 0.90$ (Test 1: $k = 1.00$, Test 2: $k = 0.90$, Test 3: $k = 0.79$). Interrater reliability for the categorization of Experiential Analysis Technique (EAT) comments ranged from $k = 0.76$ to $k = 1.00$. Behavioral and verbal data are those provided by the hypnotist; EAT data are those provided by the inquirer; analyses of the independent rater's data showed the same pattern of findings.

Figure 1 presents the percentage of behavioral and verbal responding for subjects in the prehypnotic, hypnotic, and posthypnotic conditions across the three tests. During Test 1, 4 (57.1%) subjects in the prehypnotic condition responded behaviorally, whereas only 1 (14.3%) responded verbally. No subject in the hypnotic and posthypnotic conditions responded behaviorally, but 6 (85.7%) and 7 (100%) subjects in these conditions, respectively, responded verbally. Chi-square analysis[5] confirmed that whereas more subjects in the prehypnotic condition than in the hypnotic and posthypnotic conditions responded behaviorally, $\chi^2(2, N = 21) = 9.88, p < .01$, fewer responded verbally, $\chi^2 (2, N = 21) = 13.29, p < .01$. Thus, during Test 1, and consistent with our expectations, subjects were more likely to respond behaviorally when the question/cue was associated with a hypnotic suggestion, but they were more likely to respond verbally when it was associated with a social interaction.

During Test 2, 7 (100%) subjects in the prehypnotic condition and 4 (57.1%) in the hypnotic condition responded behaviorally, whereas only 2 (28.6%) and 1 (14.3%) subject in these conditions, respectively, responded verbally. In contrast, no subject in the posthypnotic condition responded behaviorally, but all (100%) responded verbally. Chi-square analysis indicated that more subjects in the prehypnotic than in the hypnotic condition responded behaviorally, $\chi^2(1, N = 14) = 3.82, p < .05$, and more subjects in the posthypnotic condition than in the prehypnotic and hypnotic conditions responded verbally, $\chi^2(2, N = 21) = 11.84, p < .01$. Thus, as in Test 1, subjects were more likely to respond behaviorally when the question/cue was associated with a hypnotic suggestion, but they were more likely to respond verbally when it was associated with a social interaction.

During Test 3, 5 (71.4%), 3 (42.9%), and 5 (71.4%) subjects in the prehypnotic, hypnotic, and posthypnotic conditions, respectively, responded behaviorally, and 3 (42.9%), 4 (57.1%), and 6 (85.7%) subjects in these conditions, respectively, responded verbally. Analysis indicated that there was no difference in the pattern of responding between conditions. Subjects were equally likely to respond behaviorally and verbally when the question/cue was associated with the suggestion.

These data suggest that within each test period, subjects' responses depended on whether they interpreted the hypnotist's message as a question to answer or as a cue to respond. Looking across the three tests, the responses of some subjects fluctuated depending on the context of the test. For instance, analysis (Cochran's Q tests, $p < .05$) indicated that both the behavioral and verbal responding of subjects in the hypnotic

[5]For some of the chi-square analyses reported in this section, cell sizes were less than five. It is often assumed that when $df = 1$ and expected frequencies are less than 5, the chi-square test is not reliable (e.g., Siegel, 1956). However, recent research has suggested that this test does, in fact, generate accurate probabilities under these circumstances and that no correction procedure is required (Bradley, Bradley, McGrath, & Cutcomb, 1979; Camilli & Hopkins, 1978).

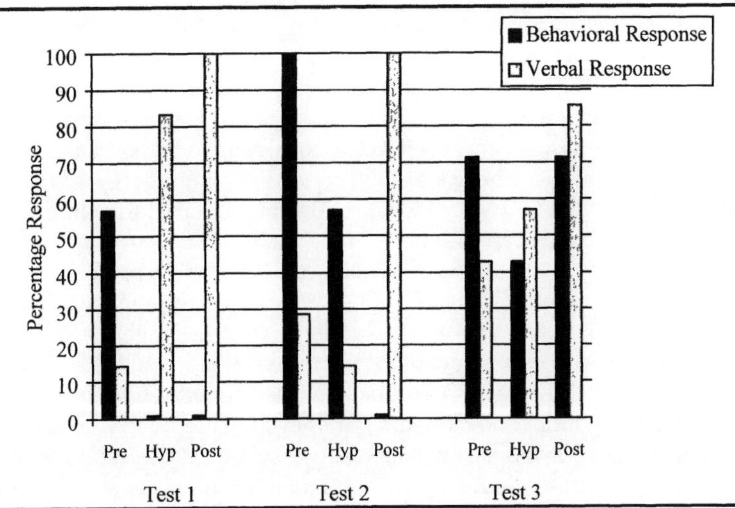

Figure 1. **Percentage behavioral and verbal response across the tests.**
Note. Pre = prehypnotic condition, Hyp = hypnotic condition, Post = posthypnotic condition.

condition changed significantly across the tests. Specifically, 0 (0%), 4 (57.1%), and 3 (42.9%) subjects in this condition responded behaviorally on Tests 1, 2, and 3, respectively; 6 (85.7%), 1 (14.3%), and 4 (57.1%) responded verbally. Thus, more subjects responded behaviorally to Tests 2 and 3 than on Test 1, and fewer subjects responded verbally on Test 2 than on Tests 1 and 3. Similarly, analysis indicated that whereas the verbal responding of subjects in the posthypnotic condition did not change significantly across the tests, their behavioral responding increased. Specifically, 0 (0%), 0 (0%), and 5 (71.4%) subjects responded behaviorally on Tests 1, 2, and 3, respectively; 7 (100%), 7 (100%), and 6 (85.7%) responded verbally. Thus, for these subjects, the question/cue remained a social interaction across the tests but became associated with the hypnotic suggestion during the final test, and this led to both behavioral and verbal responses. In contrast to subjects in these conditions, the behavioral and verbal responding of subjects in the prehypnotic condition remained relatively stable across the tests. Specifically, 4 (57.1%), 7 (100%), and 5 (71.4%) subjects responded behaviorally on Tests 1, 2, and 3, respectively; 1 (14.3%), 2 (28.6%), and 4 (57.1%) responded verbally. Most subjects responded behaviorally to the question/cue, whereas few responded verbally. These findings suggest that subjects' responding was influenced by both the hypnotist's message as well as by the context in which it was given.

During the EAT, subjects were asked to describe what they were thinking as they were administered the suggestion and the question/cue during each of the tests. These comments help to elucidate subjects' behavioral and verbal responding by highlighting the interpretations that they placed on the question/cue across the three tests. During Test 1, 6 (85.7%) subjects in the prehypnotic condition commented that they interpreted the question as a signal to respond behaviorally; only 1 (14.3%) subject interpreted it as both a cue to respond and a question to answer. The majority of subjects in the hypnotic ($N = 6/7$; 85.7%) and posthypnotic ($N = 7/7$; 100%) conditions said that they interpreted the cue as a question to answer, $\chi^2(4, N = 20) = 20.00, p < .01$.

During Test 2, the majority of subjects in the prehypnotic ($N = 6/7$; 85.7%) and hypnotic ($N = 4/7$; 57.1%) conditions commented that they interpreted the question as a signal to respond behaviorally. For instance, one said, "I just meant to rub my earlobe. I didn't think about it as a question to answer." One subject in the prehypnotic condition and two in the hypnotic condition said that they interpreted it as both a cue to respond and a question to answer, and one subject in the hypnotic condition said that it was just a question to answer. In contrast, all subjects (100%) in the posthypnotic condition said that they interpreted the cue as a question to answer, $\chi^2(4, N = 21) = 18.35, p < .01$.

During Test 3, 6 (85.7%) subjects in the prehypnotic condition, 4 (57.1%) in the hypnotic condition, and 5 (71.4%) in the posthypnotic condition interpreted the question as a signal to respond; 2 (28.6%) subjects in the hypnotic and 2 (28.6%) in the posthypnotic conditions interpreted the cue as both a signal to respond and as a question to answer; the remaining subjects interpreted the cue as a question to answer or said that it had no meaning for them. There was no difference in these comments across conditions. Overall, subjects' EAT comments indicate that their interpretation of the question/cue as a signal to respond behaviorally or as a social interaction differed across the tests.

During the EAT, subjects who responded were asked to rate how much of an urge they felt to rub their earlobe on each test (where 0 = *none at all* and 6 = *an extremely strong urge*). These data help to address the question of whether those subjects who responded to the hypnotic-like suggestion even when it was administered either prior to the induction of hypnosis (prehypnotic condition) or after formal hypnosis had been terminated (posthypnotic condition) did so due to behavioral compliance or whether they reported an accompanying experience of compulsion. Of those who responded to one or more of the tests, the mean compulsion rating was 3.67 ($SD = 2.24$) and the median rating was 4.00. On Test 1, 4 (all prehypnotic) subjects responded. Two (50%) gave ratings above the median (1 gave the highest rating) and 2 (50%) gave ratings below the median; the mean rating was 3.00 ($SD = 2.58$). On Test 2, 11 (7 prehypnotic, 4 hypnotic) subjects responded. Nine (81.8%) gave ratings above the median (5 gave the highest rating) and 2 (18.2%) gave ratings below the median; the mean rating was 4.64 ($SD = 1.86$). On Test 3, 13 (5 prehypnotic, 3 hypnotic, and 5 posthypnotic) subjects responded. Five

(38.5%) gave ratings above the median (4 gave the highest rating) and 8 (61.5%) gave ratings below the median; the mean rating was 3.23 (*SD* = 2.35). Notably, there was no difference in the ratings of subjects across the suggestion conditions on any test. Thus, although behavioral responding during hypnosis (Test 2) was more often associated with a strong compulsive experience (defined as a compulsion rating above the median), a number of subjects who responded either before (Test 1) or after (Test 3) hypnosis also experienced a strong sense of compulsion. Thus, responding at these times was not necessarily motivated by behavioral compliance.

Discussion

We expected that subjects would rub their earlobe more so than answer the question when the question/cue was interpreted as a formal hypnotic communication but that they would answer the question more so than rub their earlobe when the question/cue was interpreted as a social interaction. Consistent with this, for Tests 1 and 2, subjects were more likely to respond behaviorally when the question, "Do you think it will rain tonight?" was associated with a hypnotic suggestion but were more likely to respond verbally when it was associated with a social interaction. For Test 3, subjects were equally likely to respond behaviorally and verbally when the question was associated with the suggestion. We expected also that the likelihood of some subjects responding behaviorally and/or verbally would shift across the tests in line with the changing message of the hypnotist. Consistent with this, we found that both the behavioral and verbal responding of subjects in the hypnotic condition changed across the tests; also, whereas the verbal responding of subjects in the posthypnotic condition did not change across the tests, their behavioral responding increased. Subjects' EAT comments indicated that their interpretation of the message of the hypnotist as either a signal to respond behaviorally or as a question to answer depended on both the hypnotist's message and the context in which it was given. Moreover, the interpretation of many subjects shifted across the tests to follow the context of the interaction and the implied intent of the hypnotist's message.

These findings indicate that subjects strive to interpret the hypnotist's communications and attempt to match their behavior to this understanding (Kihlstrom, 1995; Orne, 1959; Weitzenhoffer, 1974). In some cases, this process of interpretation may be relatively straightforward. For instance, subjects were less likely to report feeling confused about what they should do when the suggestion and/or the question/cue were presented during hypnosis than when these messages were presented either before or after hypnosis. Also, subjects in the prehypnotic condition were more likely to respond behaviorally when presented with the question/cue during rather than before hypnosis. In other words, certain configurations of the hypnotist's communications and of the context were less likely to create ambiguity or confusion; typically, this was when the communications of the hypnotist were compatible with the context in which they were administered. Notably, subjects' ratings of compulsion, given during the EAT, indicated that behavioral responses made during hypnosis were more likely to be accompanied by an experience of compulsion than responses made either before or after hypnosis. These findings are consistent with other work on posthypnotic suggestion that has found that subjects show a high level of response on formal posthypnotic tests for which they are prepared (e.g., Barnier & McConkey, 1996, in press; Orne, Sheehan, & Evans, 1968; Spanos, Menary, Brett, Cross, & Ahmed, 1987). This high level of response can be said to reflect the relatively unambiguous message conveyed by both the hypnotist's suggestion and the formal tests used in those experiments. In some situations, the process of interpretation may not be as straightforward.

In the present experiment, subjects' interpretation of the hypnotist's suggestion was complicated by its administration in an unexpected, nonhypnotic context (i.e., prehypnotic and posthypnotic conditions) and by the unusual nature of the question/cue. For instance, most of the subjects in the prehypnotic condition and almost half of those in the posthypnotic condition thought that the suggestion was confusing and out of the ordinary. One subject in the prehypnotic condition said, "Actually, I was a bit confused about this bit because I wasn't sure whether I was expected to do it, because she said it before I was under. So I wasn't really sure if that had any relevance." Notably, only one subject in the hypnotic condition thought that the suggestion was confusing or unusual. When asked about her reactions to the suggestion, she said, "I was thinking that [the hypnotist] has already asked me that before and it's not a real question." For others, the question, "Do you think it will rain tonight?" which was intended to reflect a benign, social interaction, led to confusion even when it was not associated with the suggestion. For instance, one subject in the posthypnotic condition commented about the first test, "Why, why ask that? What a silly thing to ask. It didn't fit." For some subjects, the confusion created by the ambiguity in the hypnotist's communications and the time at which responding was indexed influenced both their interpretation of the question/cue and their responding. This is reflected not only in subjects' behavioral responses but in their ratings of compulsion as well, which were generally lower before and after, rather than during, hypnosis.

Despite experiencing some confusion during some tests, other individuals resolved this ambiguity in a way that allowed a behavioral and phenomenal experience of hypnotic responding. Often this resolution was personal and idiosyncratic. For example, one subject in the prehypnotic condition believed that she had been fully hypnotized during the suggestion and test, which were administered prior to the formal induction procedure. Although it could be argued that this subject was "hypnotized" from the moment the experiment began, her belief allowed her to respond to the suggestion at a time when others found it strange and confusing. Similarly, a posthypnotic subject believed that the purpose of the cue was to elicit or test his "true response" to the question; for him, the suggestion to rub his earlobe was secondary (although he responded behaviorally) to the nature of his verbal response. Of importance, such responding in a seemingly "nonhypnotic" context cannot be said to necessarily reflect behavioral compliance because some subjects gave extremely high ratings of compulsion for responses made during these times. In other words, some subjects experienced their responding either before or after hypnosis as compelling and genuine.

We considered that the individuals most likely to process the ambiguous and conflicting information presented by the suggestion and the tests would be those who demonstrated a motivated cognitive commitment to the hypnotist. Our results confirmed this prediction and indicated that many subjects who responded successfully, particularly those who were given the suggestion either before or after hypnosis, placed a great deal of meaning and emphasis on the hypnotist's communications and ignored information that was inconsistent with the essence of their hypnotic interaction. For example, one subject in the posthypnotic condition described her reaction to the administration of the suggestion (after hypnosis) in the following way:

> You see, I think that's kind of unusual because we'd counted down and here we are and I'm wide awake, presumably in my waking state. I'm looking at her [the hypnotist] and going along exactly with what she's going to say and asking me to do. So that when she says about the weather, "Do you think it will rain tonight?" I'm going to rub my earlobe. I can see the look on my face. I'm seriously listening; it doesn't seem bizarre at all. It doesn't seem outrageous that she's going to ask me to do an action in relation to something that she's said twice before. So, I think that is interesting.

Overall, our findings point to two important theoretical issues. First, they suggest that to respond to a hypnotic or posthypnotic suggestion, subjects must develop an appropriate motivated set or preparedness to respond in a hypnotic fashion. It is not sufficient for subjects to have received the suggestion and for the test simply to be presented; rather, they must actively process the information in a way that helps them to prepare to display hypnotic behavior. This information processing will be influenced by the extent to which the suggestion meets subjects' expectations, the availability of cues in the setting that reinforces appropriate responding, and the degree to which subjects are able to tolerate and manage ambiguity in the totality of messages and cues available to them (see also Orne, 1959). Second, the finding that some subjects gave priority to the hypnotic features of the message underscores the potency of the hypnotist's message, the relevance of the relationship between the subject and the hypnotist, and the hypnotized individual's cognitive predisposition and ability to assimilate conflicting and ambiguous information in a way that defines and promotes their experience as hypnotic rather than routine (McConkey, 1991; Sheehan, 1991).

The findings of our experiment also suggest that insight into the processes underlying hypnotic and posthypnotic behavior may be gained by focusing on talented hypnotic subjects faced with difficult or challenging experiences (see also McConkey et al., 1989). In particular, processes such as tolerance and management of ambiguity, preparedness to respond, and commitment to the hypnotist's communications were more often highlighted by subjects' attempts to find meaning when faced with conflicting rather than straightforward messages and influences in the present experiment. Furthermore, this ability to manage ambiguity is almost certainly related to hypnotizability; in this sense, our findings highlight the value of considering the personal and motivational characteristics of those who are able to respond in this way. Despite a relatively small subject number in the present experiment, we observed informally that virtuoso hypnotic subjects seemed less concerned by the confusion that limited the responding of the other high hypnotizable subjects and also seemed more likely to describe their experience as compelling and effortless. It would be worth following up these observations in a systematic way with a larger sample.

At a more general level, many subjects indicated a concern with the level of consistency between the hypnotist's communications and their expectations about the conduct of the hypnosis experiment. For instance, one subject in the posthypnotic condition responded to the administration of the question/cue before hypnosis (Test 1) in the following way: "I was assuming that the thing had started, and it seemed a strange question . . . it was just nonsensical . . . it was a statement that didn't belong to the context that I was expecting." Comments such as these suggested that subjects had a set of tacit rules about what was appropriate during an experimental, hypnotic interaction; in other words, they held clear expectations for the conduct and content of the hypnotic interaction. Although those expectations were broader for some rather than for others, the administration of the suggestion either before or after hypnosis and the question "Do you think it will rain tonight?" often represented a transgression of subjects' expectations. Furthermore, although we labeled only the period of time between the administration of the hypnotic induction and deinduction procedures as "during hypnosis," such an operationalization of "hypnosis" may underestimate the degree to which subjects perceived the entire experimental interaction, from the time they entered the room until they left, as hypnotic in nature.

Overall, and consistent with the comments of Orne (1959) and Kihlstrom (1995), these findings underscore that the hypnosis experiment is a rule-bound, social interaction. Most broadly, this is important to keep in mind when we are investigating hypnosis in the experimental setting, in which there are three experiments actually going on: the one the subject thinks they are in, the one the hypnotist thinks they are doing, and the one that is actually occurring (Kihlstrom, 1995; Orne, 1959). Just as subjects strive to bring meaning to the communications of the hypnotist, investigators must strive to interpret the subjects' actions and words. To do that effectively, we need to understand how hypnotized individuals find meaning in the message of the hypnotist.

References

Barnier, A. J., & McConkey, K. M. (1996). Action and desire in posthypnotic responding. *International Journal of Clinical and Experimental Hypnosis, 44*, 120-139.

Barnier, A. J., & McConkey, K. M. (1998). Posthypnotic responding: Knowing when to stop helps to keep it going. *International Journal of Clinical and Experimental Hypnosis, 46*, 204-219.

Barnier, A. J., & McConkey, K. M. (in press). Posthypnotic responding: The relevance of suggestion and test congruence. *International Journal of Clinical and Experimental Hypnosis.*

Bradley, D. R., Bradley, T. D., McGrath, S. G., & Cutcomb, S. D. (1979). Type I error rate of the chi-square test of independence in R × C tables that have small expected frequencies. *Psychological Bulletin, 86*, 1290-1297.

Camilli, G., & Hopkins, K. D. (1978). Applicability of chi-square to 2 × 2 contingency tables with small expected cell frequencies. *Psychological Bulletin, 85*, 163-167.

Cohen, J. A. (1960). A coefficient of agreement for nominal scales. *Educational and Psychological Measurement, 20*, 37-46.

Grice, H. P. (1975). Logic and conversation. In P. Cole & J. L. Morgan (Eds.), *Syntax and semantics 3: Speech acts* (pp. 41-58). New York: Academic Press.

Hilgard, E. R., Crawford, H. J., Bowers, P., & Kihlstrom, J. F. (1979). A tailored SHSS:C, permitting user modification for special purposes. *International Journal of Clinical and Experimental Hypnosis, 27*, 125-133.

Kihlstrom, J. F. (1995, June). *From the subject's point of view: The experiment as conversation and collaboration.* Keynote address presented at the Seventh Annual Convention of the American Psychological Society, New York.

McConkey, K. M. (1983). The impact of conflicting communications on response to hypnotic suggestion. *Journal of Abnormal Psychology, 92*, 351-358.

McConkey, K. M. (1991). The construction and resolution of experience and behavior in hypnosis. In S. J. Lynn & J. W. Rhue (Eds.), *Theories of hypnosis: Current models and perspectives* (pp. 542-563). New York: Guilford.

McConkey, K. M., Bryant, R. A., Bibb, B. C., & Kihlstrom, J. F. (1991). Trance logic in hypnosis and imagination. *Journal of Abnormal Psychology, 100*, 464-472.

McConkey, K. M., Glisky, M. L., & Kihlstrom, J. F. (1989). Individual differences among hypnotic virtuosos: A case comparison. *Australian Journal of Clinical and Experimental Hypnosis, 17*, 131-140.

Nogrady, H., McConkey, K. M., Laurence, J.-R., & Perry, C. (1983). Dissociation, duality, and demand characteristics in hypnosis. *Journal of Abnormal Psychology, 92*, 223-235.

Orne, M. T. (1959). The nature of hypnosis: Artifact and essence. *Journal of Abnormal and Social Psychology, 58,* 277-299.
Orne, M. T., Sheehan, P. W., & Evans, F. J. (1968). Occurrence of posthypnotic behavior outside the experimental setting. *Journal of Personality and Social Psychology, 9,* 189-196.
Sheehan, P. W. (1971). Countering preconceptions about hypnosis: An objective index of involvement with the hypnotist. *Journal of Abnormal Psychology, 78,* 299-322.
Sheehan, P. W. (1991). Hypnosis, context, and commitment. In S. J. Lynn & J. W. Rhue (Eds.), *Theories of hypnosis: Current models and perspectives* (pp. 520-541). New York: Guilford.
Sheehan, P. W., & McConkey, K. M. (1982). *Hypnosis and experience: The exploration of phenomena and process.* Hillsdale, NJ: Lawrence Erlbaum.
Shor, R. E., & Orne, E. C. (1962). *Harvard Group Scale of Hypnotic Susceptibility, Form A.* Palo Alto, CA: Consulting Psychologists Press.
Siegel, S. (1956). *Nonparametric statistics for the behavioral sciences.* New York: McGraw-Hill.
Spanos, N. P., Menary, E., Brett, P. J., Cross, W., & Ahmed, Q. (1987). Failure of posthypnotic responding to occur outside the experimental setting. *Journal of Abnormal Psychology, 96,* 52-57.
Weitzenhoffer, A. M. (1974). When is an "instruction" an "instruction"? *International Journal of Clinical and Experimental Hypnosis, 22,* 258-269.
Weitzenhoffer, A. M., & Hilgard, E. R. (1962). *The Stanford Hypnotic Susceptibility Scale, Form C.* Palo Alto, CA: Consulting Psychologists Press.

Hypnotische und posthypnotische Suggestion: Suche nach einer Bedeutung in den Kommunikationen des Hypnotherapeuten

Amanda J. Barnier und Kevin M. McConkey

Zusammenfassung: Hoch-hypnotisierbaren VPn. wurde vor, während und nach Hypnose eine Frage gestellt, und vor, während und nach der Hypnose wurden sie angewiesen, bei dieser Frage ihr Ohrläppchen zu reiben. Das Experiment kontrastierte also eine Frage, die eine verbale Reaktion erforderte, mit einer Suggestion, die nur manchmal eine verhaltensmäßige Reaktion erforderte. Die Vpn. tendierten mit größerer Wahrscheinlichkeit zu einer verhaltensmäßigen Reaktion, wenn die Frage mit der Suggestion assoziiert war, aber mit größerer Wahrscheinlichkeit zu einer verbalen Reaktion, wenn es sich bei der Frage um eine soziale Interaktion handelte; außerdem verschob sich die Wahrscheinlichkeit einer verhaltensmäßigen und/oder verbalen Reaktion der Vpn. bei den Tests, wenn sich die Botschaft des Hypnotherapeuten veränderte. Die Resultate heben das Bestreben der Vpn. hervor, die Kommunikationen des Hypnotherapeuten zu interpretieren, und im Kontext dieser Kommunikationen Ambiguität auf solche Weise zu lösen, daß es ihr hypnotisches Verhalten und ihre hypnotische Erfahrung unterstützt.

ROSEMARIE GREENMAN
University of Tennessee, Knoxville, USA

La suggestion hypnotique et post-hypnoptique: à la recheche d'un sens dans le message de l'hypnotiseur

Amanda J. Barnier et Kevin M. McConkey

Résumé: Il a été posé à des sujets hautements hypnotisables, une question avant, pendant et après hypnose et il leur fut donné une suggestion avant,

pendant ou après hypnose, d'effacer leur oreille quand on leur posait la question. De cette manière, l'expérience plaçait une question qui nécessitait une réponse verbale en contraste avec une suggestion que nécessitait seulement une réponse comportementale. Les sujets ont davantage répondu sur le plan comportemental quand la question était associée à la suggestion., mais davantage sur le mode verbal quand la question était une interaction sociale; en outre, la probabilité de la réponse comportementale et/ou verbale a changé pendant les tests par le changement de message de l'hypnotiseur. Les résultats sont les plus importants quand les sujets hypnotisés ont tenté d'interpréter la communication de l'hypnotiseur ainsi que leur capacité à résoudre l'ambiguité de ces messages de façon qu'elle puisse promouvoir leur expérience et comportement hypnotique.

VICTOR SIMON
Psychosomatic Medicine & Clinical Hypnosis Institute, Lille, France

Sugestión hipnótica y posthipnótica:
El significado del mensaje del hipnotista

Amanda J. Barnier y Kevin M. McConkey

Resumen: Se formuló una pregunta a sujetos muy hipnotizables antes de, durante y después de la hipnosis, y se les dio una sugestión antes de, durante o después de la hipnosis de que se frotarían el lóbulo de la oreja cuando escucharan esta pregunta. Así pues, el experimento consistía en una pregunta que requería una respuesta verbal, en contraste con una sugestión que sólo en ocasiones requería una respuesta conductual. Resultó más probable que los sujetos respondieran conductualmente cuando la sugestión estaba asociada con la pregunta, y más probable que respondieran verbalmente cuando la pregunta se relacionaba con una interacción social. Otro resultado es que la probabilidad de que los participantes respondieran conductual y/o verbalmente varió según las pruebas y los cambios en el mensaje del hipnotista. Estos resultados subrayan los intentos de los sujetos hipnotizados por interpretar las comunicaciones del hipnotista y la habilidad de los sujetos para resolver ambigüedades en el nexo de esos mensajes con el objeto de fomentar la conducta y experiencia hipnóticas.

ETZEL CARDEÑA
Uniformed Services University of the Health Sciences, Bethesda, Maryland, USA

Part VI
Neuropsychological and Neurophysiological Research and Theories

[21]

BRAIN DYNAMICS AND HYPNOSIS:
Attentional and Disattentional Processes[1, 2]

HELEN J. CRAWFORD[3, 4]

Virginia Polytechnic Institute and State University, Blacksburg

Abstract: This article reviews recent research findings, expanding an evolving neuropsychophysiological model of hypnosis (Crawford, 1989; Crawford & Gruzelier, 1992), that support the view that highly hypnotizable persons (highs) possess stronger attentional filtering abilities than do low hypnotizable persons, and that these differences are reflected in underlying brain dynamics. Behavioral, cognitive, and neurophysiological evidence is reviewed that suggests that highs can both better focus and sustain their attention as well as better ignore irrelevant stimuli in the environment. It is proposed that hypnosis is a state of enhanced attention that activates an interplay between cortical and subcortical brain dynamics during hypnotic phenomena, such as hypnotic analgesia. A body of research is reviewed that suggests that both attentional and disattentional processes, among others, are important in the experiencing of hypnosis and hypnotic phenomena. Findings from studies of electrocortical activity, event-related potentials, and regional cerebral blood flow during waking and hypnosis are presented to suggest that these attentional differences are reflected in underlying neurophysiological differences in the far fronto-limbic attentional system.

There is a resurgence of interest in brain dynamics associated with hypnosis due to the increased availability of physiological neuroimaging methods such as computerized electroencephalographic (EEG) fre-

Manuscript submitted October 26, 1992; final revision received January 12, 1994.

[1]This article is based on the author's Presidential Address presented at the 42nd Annual Scientific Meeting of The Society for Clinical and Experimental Hypnosis, New Orleans, LA, October 12, 1991.

[2]The research presented in this article was supported by The Spencer Foundation, the National Institutes of Health, NIH Biomedical Research Support Grant, Virginia Tech College of Arts and Sciences' small grant program, Virginia Tech Creative Match Program, and the University of Wyoming College of Arts and Sciences' small grant program. Additional support came from a fellowship from the U.S. National Academy of Sciences and Hungarian Academy of Sciences Cooperative Scientific Exchange Program and a visiting fellowship (research scholar) from the University of Rome. The author gratefully acknowledges this support.

[3]The author is particularly appreciative of Karl Pribram's thoughtful evaluation and determination of the correctness of the neurophysiological discussion.

[4]Requests for reprints should be addressed to Helen J. Crawford, Ph.D., Department of Psychology, Virginia Polytechnic Institute and State University, Blacksburg, VA 24061-0436. (Electronic mail may be sent to CRAWFORD @ VTVM1.CC.VT.EDU.)

quency analysis, EEG topographic brain mapping, event-related potential (ERP) analysis, regional cerebral blood flow (CBF), positron emission tomography (PET), and single photon emission computer tomography (SPECT). This article reviews converging evidence from recent studies that suggests that hypnosis activates an interplay between cortical and subcortical brain dynamics. Both sustained attention and disattention are two major higher level, cognitive control processes associated with the "executive control system" (E. R. Hilgard, 1986; Pribram, 1991) or the "supervisory attentional system" (Shallice, 1988) that are of importance in our understanding of hypnosis and individual differences in hypnotic susceptibility. Research is presented that suggests that highly hypnotizable persons possess greater sustained attentional and disattention abilities that are reflected in underlying neurophysiological differences in the fronto-limbic attentional system. Finally, evidence suggesting shifts in brain dynamics during hypnosis, as moderated by hypnotic level, is provided in support of a recently developed, but still evolving, neuropsychophysiological model of hypnosis (Crawford, 1989, 1991; Crawford & Gruzelier, 1992).

Attentional Correlates of Hypnotizability

What is attention? In his *Principles of Psychology*, William James (1890/1983) described attention eloquently:

> Everyone knows what attention is. It is the taking possession by the mind, in clear and vivid form, of one out of what seem several simultaneously possible objects or trains of thought. Focalization, concentration, of consciousness are of its essence. It implies withdrawal from some things in order to deal effectively with others, and is a condition which has a real opposite in the confused, dazed, scatter-brained state which in French is called distraction, and Zerstreutheit in German. (pp. 403-404)

Attention is a multidimensional phenomenon. While knowledge of its structure is incomplete, there is evidence for different neurophysiological systems of attention (e.g., for reviews, see Posner & Petersen, 1990; Pribram & McGuinness, 1975, 1992).

We all know of individuals who often cannot focus their attention and are quickly inattentive and drawn to distracting, irrelevant stimuli. We know, as well, of individuals who can become so focused on their projects or inner thoughts and fantasies that they appear oblivious to the world around them. Individual differences in attentional processing are observed in the cognitive literature (e.g., Berch & Kanter, 1984; Crawford, Brown, & Moon, 1993; Davies, Jones, & Taylor, 1984; Sack & Rice, 1974) for four major attentional dimensions: (a) focused and sustained attention: the ability to focus and sustain attention over time without distraction; (b) selective attention: the ability to select and discriminate between stimuli; (c) divided or dual attention: the ability to divide attention between two tasks, often one primary and the other secondary; and (d) ambient attention: the ability to attend to one task but also to have diffuse attention in preparation to respond to other stimuli.

Behavioral and Evoked Potential Attentional Correlates of Hypnotizability

Numerous studies have demonstrated that hypnotizability, as measured by standardized hypnotic susceptibility scales, is related to the abilities of extremely focused and sustained attention. [Other contributing factors (e.g., role-playing, imagery) are acknowledged as being important mediators of hypnotic behavior, but are not addressed in this article.] Concentration and suppression may be two sides of the same cognitive process—the willful movement of attention towards some things and away from others.[5] It is for this reason that we have argued that both sustained attentional and disattentional abilities are correlates of hypnotizability (Crawford, 1989, 1991; Crawford, Brown, & Moon, 1993; Crawford, Corby, & Kopell, 1994).

Correlational studies of hypnotizability have often used the Tellegen Absorption Scale (TAS; Tellegen, 1982), a measure of involvement in various imaginative activities suggestive of passive, effortless rather than active attention. The correlations between absorption and hypnotizability are usually in the .40s (e.g., Crawford, 1982b; Crawford, Brown, & Moon, 1993; Finke & Macdonald, 1978; Kilhstrom et al., 1980; Nadon, Laurence & Perry, 1987; Tellegen & Atkinson, 1974; for a review, see Roche & McConkey, 1990). An analysis of this literature and interview studies (e.g., J. R. Hilgard, 1970) led us to conclude that we are often intermingling two separate focused attentional abilities: (a) moderately focused attention: the ability to attend moderately so that noise in the environment is no longer disruptive, but may still be attended to some; and (b) extremely focused attention and disattention: the ability to attend so fully to a task that noise and irrelevant stimuli in the environment are apparently not even noticed and provide no distraction. The first is more closely related to ambient attention. The second, extremely focused and sustained attention, has been found to be more closely related to hypnotizability and to load with the TAS in factor analyses (Crawford, Brown, & Moon, 1993; Lyons & Crawford, 1991; Yanchar, 1983, 1984). This latter research used a questionnaire, the Differential Attentional Processes Inventory (DAPI; Crawford, 1981a; Grumbles & Crawford, 1981), that has separate scales for these two attentional dimensions along with two dual attention scales. Further, Lyons and Crawford (1991) found hypnotic susceptibility did not load on measures of arousability (e.g., extraversion as measured by the Eysenck Personality Inventory), another

[5]Treisman (1964) was one of the first to propose that inhibition of information plays a role in attention. The degree to which irrelevant information is processed, and how closely inhibitory processes are related to selective attentional processes, has been the center of considerable debate in the cognitive and neuropsychological literatures. A coverage of such issues is beyond the scope of this article.

attentional system wherein a person modulates and maintains one's homeostasis by either seeking out or retreating from highly arousing stimuli in the environment.

Relationships between hypnotic susceptibility and cognitive task performance, interpreted as a measure of attentional processing, have been reported. Hypnotic susceptibility was found to be associated with superior performance on visual search tasks (Wallace & Patterson, 1984), perception of fragmented stimuli (e.g., gestalt closure) tasks (Crawford, 1981b; Wallace, 1990), and searches for an object embedded within a pictorial scene (Priebe & Wallace, 1986; Wallace, 1988). In addition, Wallace (1990) has shown that highs who self-reported high vivid imagery perceived fragmented stimuli better than highs who reported less vivid imagery. In these studies by Wallace and his students, highs were more likely to report holistic, rather than detail, search strategies, similar to what Crawford (1981b) and Crawford and Allen (1983) have described. An intensification of such holistic strategies was found in hypnosis among highs who reported increased holistic processing accompanying increased successive visual discrimination memory (Crawford & Allen, 1983) and eidetic-like memory (Crawford, Wallace, Nomura, & Slater, 1986) performance.

Highs are more responsive to reversible figures and visual illusions, as evidenced in studies of the Necker Cube and Schroeder staircase (Crawford, Brown, & Moon, 1993; Wallace, 1986, 1988; Wallace, Knight, & Garrett, 1976) and the Ponzo illusion (R. J. Miller, 1975). Highs report significantly more autokinetic movement in a dark environment (Atkinson & Crawford, 1992; Wallace & Garrett, 1973; Wallace, Garrett, & Anstadt, 1974) and even greater movements during hypnosis (Atkinson, 1991). We propose that these findings are due to highs possessing greater sustained attentional and disattentional abilities.

Recent ERP research by Crawford, Corby, and Kopell (1994) provides neurophysiological evidence in support of the hypothesized attentional differences between low and high hypnotizables during waking. They recorded auditory ERPs at central sites (Cz, C3, C4) to 50 msec 1961 Hz tone pips of 50, 60, 70, and 80 dB intensities, in counterbalanced conditions where subjects were instructed to ignore the tones while reading a novel or counting their pulses. Highs showed significantly smaller N1 and P2 amplitudes than did lows. Typically, as seen in previous work using the augmenting-reducing paradigm (for a review, see Hillyard & Picton, 1979), as stimuli intensities increase, N1 latencies decrease. Such latency decreases are interpreted as an index of increased attentional processing allocated to the distracting or novel stimuli. The lows showed the expected decrease in N1 latencies as the stimuli intensities increased, but the highs did the opposite and showed a slowing down of the processing of distracting stimuli (longer N1 latencies) with increased intensities. This differential latency change was positively associated with both hypnotic susceptibility ($r = .44$, $p < .05$) and absorption as measured by the TAS ($r = .58$, $p < .01$). Kunzendorf and Boisvert (in press) provided preliminary evidence that inhibitory processing may even be seen in brain stem auditory ERPs of some highly hypnotizable persons.

It is well-known that there are descending inhibitory pathways that parallel the ascending sensory systems and can modulate quite early responses to sensory information. Thus this research suggests that high hypnotizables can better inhibit incoming sensory stimuli. Based upon Skinner and Yingling's (1977) and Pribram and McGuinness's (1975, 1992) models of attention that propose that the far frontal cortex regulates the limbic system in the active gating of incoming sensory stimuli, Crawford, Pribram, Kugler, Xie, Zhang, and Knebel (1992, 1993) have reported somatosensory ERP evidence (discussed further in a subsequent section) for a hypothesized far frontal (Fp1, Fp2) regional involvement in the inhibition of the conscious perception of pain in highly hypnotizable individuals. Thus there is some neurophysiological evidence to support the hypothesis that high hypnotizables have a more efficient far fronto-limbic attention system (e.g., Crawford, 1991; Crawford, Brown, & Moon, 1993; Crawford, Pribram, et al., 1992, 1993).

Far-Frontal Attentional System and Hypnosis

The disattending to extraneous stimuli in the environment so that one can sustain attention, also referred to as cognitive inhibition, may involve higher order neurophysiological control systems. Injury to the anterior region of the brain, more precisely the far frontal (prefrontal) cortex, often leads to major problems in controlled attentional focusing over time and sensitivity to interference (e.g., for reviews, see Graf, 1989; Stuss & Benson, 1986). By contrast, damage to the posterior region of the brain does not lead to such attentional deficits, but rather deficits in selective attention such as the ability to disengage and engage attention (Posner, Petersen, Fox, & Raichle, 1988; Stuss & Benson, 1986).

Human and animal studies of the localization of attention have led various neuropsychological researchers, including Posner (e.g., Posner et al., 1988) and Pribram (Pribram, 1991; Pribram & McGuinness, 1992), to propose at least two major attentional systems: (a) a posterior attention system that involves processing and encoding of incoming information, and is where selective attentional processes of engaging and disengaging occur; and (b) an anterior attention system that involves "attention for action" (Posner et al., 1988, p. 1628) and effortful attention over time (Pribram, 1991; Pribram & McGuinness, 1992). These higher attentional control processes involve both the frontal lobes and the limbic system to which there are major connecting fibers.

Thus neurophysiological evidence has shown that resistance to distraction, accompanied by sustained attention, is a function of the fronto-limbic attentional system, while selective attention is a function of the posterior cerebral cortex (e.g., Posner & Petersen, 1990; Pribram, 1991; Pribram & McGuinness, 1975). In addition, the fronto-limbic attentional system is involved in the modulation of emotionality and comfort-discomfort (e.g., Pribram, 1991; Stuss & Benson, 1986).

In light of these neurophysiological findings, a reanalysis of the hypnosis literature suggests that highs may also show greater performance on tasks that involve sustained attention without distraction and are associated with far-frontal lobe functioning. The perception of reversals in figures, such as the Necker Cube, is greatly reduced by frontal lobe pathology (Cohen, 1959; for a review, see Stuss & Benson, 1986). It is thought that perceptual judgments of figural reversals require sustained concentration without distraction. As discussed above, studies (Crawford, Brown, & Moon, 1993; R. J. Miller, 1975; Wallace, 1986; Wallace et al., 1976) have shown that hypnotizability correlated with frequency of reversals of the Necker Cube as well as other visual illusions. We (Crawford, Brown, & Moon, 1993) found approximately 70% of low and high hypnotizables were correctly discriminated between by tasks that represented two sustained attentional processing factors. Both involved focused attention without interference from distraction: (a) extremely focused and sustained attention, as reflected by the TAS and the extreme, focused attention scale of the DAPI, and (b) sustained attention in an impoverished environment, as shown by the Necker Cube and the autokinetic illusion tasks.

Stroop effects, a hallmark of focused attentional processing affected by distraction (MacLeod, 1991; Shiffrin & Schneider, 1977) that may involve the frontal cortex (Martinot et al., 1990; Perret, 1974), can also differentiate lows from highs. Dixon and his associates (Dixon, Brunet, & Laurence, 1990; Dixon & Laurence, 1992) have demonstrated that highly hypnotizable subjects process words more automatically than do low hypnotizables in a paradigm that separated strategic from automatic processes in the Stroop color-naming test. Reduced Stroop effects were obtained only among highs when they were given attentional focusing instructions during hypnosis (Sheehan, Donovan, & MacLeod, 1988), or outside of the hypnotic context (Dixon & Laurence, 1992). Highs may be able to better respond to directed attention instructions due to their greater cognitive flexibility (Crawford, 1989; Crawford & Allen, 1983) and ability to suppress irrelevant information.

Gruzelier and his colleagues (for reviews, see Crawford & Gruzelier, 1992; Gruzelier, 1990) have investigated hemispheric frontal lobe dynamics of lows and highs during waking and hypnosis by employing neuropsychological tests. In waking control conditions, highs (in comparison to lows) showed evidence of greater left hemisphere dominance in studies of tactile processing (Gruzelier, Brow, Perry, Rhonder, & Thomas, 1984) and bilateral electrodermal orienting (Gruzelier & Brow, 1985). Most recently, Gruzelier and Warren (1993) reported that highs showed greater word fluency to letter categories, implicated to involve frontal lobe functions primarily of the left hemisphere (Benton, 1968), during waking than did lows. Each of these studies demonstrated shifts in hemispheric dominance during hypnosis: only highs demonstrated inhibitory left hemispheric functioning on these tasks. Such research supports our argument (Crawford, 1989, 1990a; Crawford & Allen, 1983; Crawford & Gruzelier, 1992) that highs are characterized by greater cognitive flexibility, a greater adroitness to shift cognitive strategies in accordance with task demands that may be accompanied by greater neurophysiological hemispheric specificity.

EEG Correlates of Hypnotic Susceptibility and Hypnosis

Of particular interest to my thesis is the theta band (3 - 7 or 8 Hz) of the EEG. Theta power increments have been associated with problem solving as shown in studies of perceptual processing, cognitive processing, and during the production of imagery (for a review, see Schacter, 1977). Vogel, Broverman, and Klaiber (1968) differentiated between two classes of theta: (a) "Class I inhibition" which is associated with general inactivity or drowsiness, and sleep; and (b) "Class II inhibition" which is associated with efficient and attentive performance. According to them, this second class of theta represents "a selective inactivation of particular responses so that a continuing excitatory state becomes directed or patterned" (p. 172). It is apparent that this second class of theta may be associated with what I refer to as focused attention and disattention. Theta that is associated with Class I drowsiness is irregular and low voltage, whereas theta associated with Class II attention is more regular and higher in amplitude (Schacter, 1977).

Diverse studies have consistently found that theta power increases during performances that involve "narrowly focused processing, and intensive 'mental effort' " (Schacter, 1977, p. 59). Enhanced theta density and power are reported in studies of mental arithmetic (Nakagawa, 1988), concept formation (Lang, Lang, Kornhuber, Diekmann, & Kornhuber, 1988), and verbal and spatial tasks (Gutierrez & Corsi-Cabrera, 1988). A particularly distinct theta activity in the 6-7 Hz range, as measured by density and power, has been found anterior to the Fz derivation, an area in the midline of the forehead, and is associated with improved performance (e.g., Nakagawa, 1988; Yamamoto & Matsuoka, 1990). While subjects were observing the Necker Cube, Knebel (1993) found greater right (F4) than left (F3) frontal theta power, more so in active than passive conditions, while posteriorly there was greater left (P3) than right (P4) theta power. Interestingly, some subjects do not generate theta during task performance, while others generate high amplitude theta that is present in long, regular bursts and associated with better performance (Nakagawa, 1988). Not yet integrated into this body of literature are findings (e.g., Evans, 1992; Galin et al., 1992; Lubar, 1991) that individuals with brain-damage or attention-deficit disorders with hypothesized cortical-subcortical disruptions of attentional mechanisms may also exhibit enhanced theta (only 3 - 8 Hz range reported). We (Barabasz, Crawford, & Barabasz, 1993) found substantially more low theta, but not high theta, power present in attention-deficit children than in normal children.

One robust finding has related hypnotic susceptibility to enhanced theta power. Several early studies (e.g., Galbraith, London, Leibovitz, Cooper, & Hart, 1970; Tebecis, Provins, Farnbach, & Pentony, 1975; Ulett, Akpinar, & Itil, 1972; for reviews, see Crawford & Gruzelier, 1992; Schacter, 1977) reported that enhanced theta recorded in posterior regions (often occipital) was an important predictor of hypnotizability. More recent studies have evaluated various regions of the brain with multiple electrode placements. Sabourin, Cutcomb, Crawford, and Pribram (1990) reported substantial differences in mean theta power between extreme lows and highs who had been screened on three different measures of hypnotizability. Subjects had their EEG recorded while in waking rest, with eyes open and closed; in hypnotic rest, with eyes closed; and during certain hypnotic suggestions from the Stanford Hypnotic Susceptibility Scale, Form C (SHSS:C; Weitzenhoffer & Hilgard, 1962) test items. As seen in Figure 1, the major finding was that highs had substantially greater mean theta power than lows in both the left and right regions of the frontal (F3, F4), central (C3, C4), and occipital (01, 02) regions across conditions of waking rest, hypnotic rest, SHSS:C hypnotic suggestion items, and waking rest. Interestingly, during hypnosis there was a substantial increase of theta power in both lows and highs, but the difference between the two groups remained. Lows and highs did not differ in total alpha and beta power, although highs showed greater hemispheric asymmetry than lows in the beta power band.

In research carried out in Hungary, we (Crawford, 1989; Crawford, Mészáros, & Szabó, 1989; Mészáros, Crawford, Szabó, Nagy-Kovács, & Révész, 1989) found enhanced theta power in the right hemisphere among highs while engaged in eyes-closed arithmetic, visual discrimination, and imaginal tasks. In addition, we found hemispheric asymmetry differences for lows and highs in the anterior and posterior regions of the brain. Generalized functional changes were not evident throughout the entire hemisphere; rather, differential influences within hemispheres along an anterior-posterior axis were found (e.g., Gruzelier, 1987, 1990).

In a study of induced positive and negative emotional states during waking and hypnosis, we (Crawford, Clarke, & Kitner-Triolo, 1989; Crawford, Kitner-Triolo, Clarke, & Brown, 1988) found highs showed significantly more mean theta power than did lows. Highs showed significantly more theta power in the right than left hemisphere, while

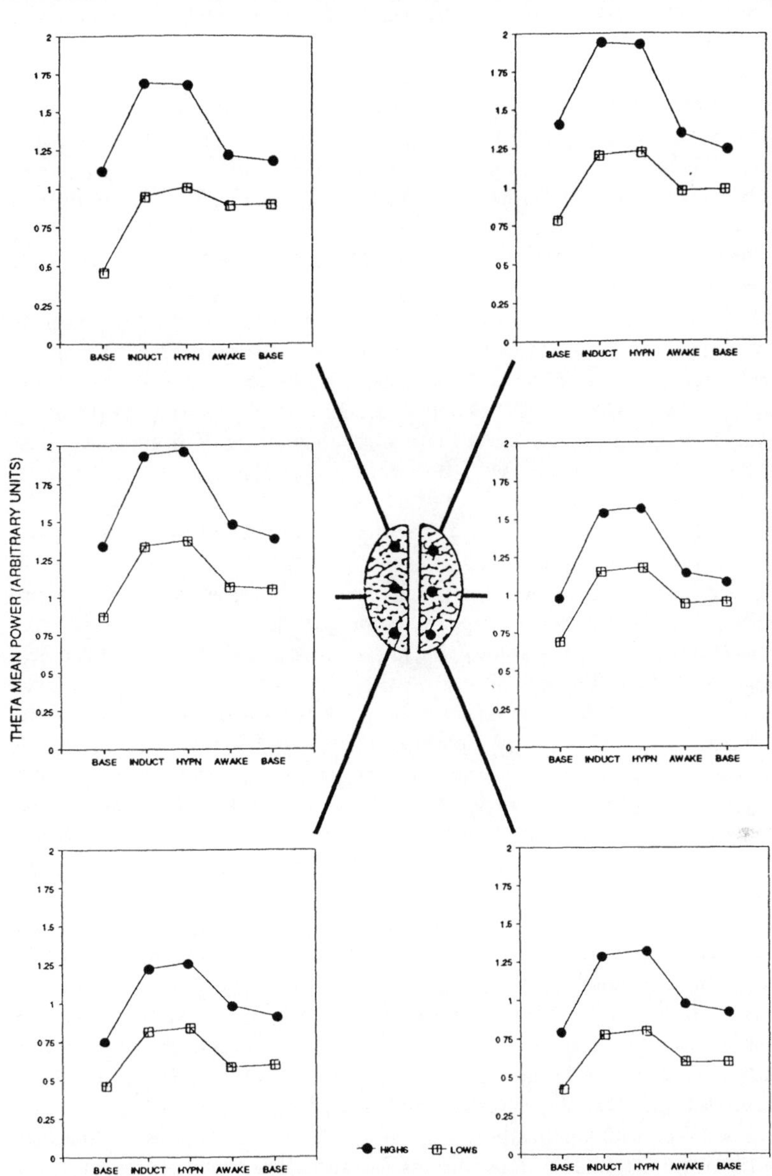

Figure 1. **Mean theta power differences across waking and hypnosis conditions at frontal (F3, F4), central (C3, C4), and occipital (01, 02) regions in low and high hypnotizables.**
Note. From "EEG Correlates of Hypnotic Susceptibility and Hypnotic Trance: Spectral Analysis and Coherence," by M. E. Sabourin, S. D. Cutcomb, H. J. Crawford, and K. Pribram, 1990, *International Journal of Psychophysiology, 10,* p. 132. Copyright 1990 by Elsevier. Reprinted by permission.

lows showed no significant hemispheric differences for either happy or sad emotional states.

During hypnosis when experiencing cold pressor pain and following suggested analgesia, highs were found to generate more high theta power (5.5 - 7.5) Hz in both hemispheres of the frontal (F3, F4), temporal (T3, T4), parietal (P3, P4), and occipital (01, 02) regions (Crawford, 1990a, 1990b) (see Figure 2). This study will be discussed in greater detail later in this article.

Increased theta power similar to that observed in hypnosis has been reported following restricted environmental stimulation (Barabasz, 1990), and during quiescent meditative states among experienced meditators (Banquet, 1973; Corby, Roth, Zarcone, & Kopell, 1978; Delmonte, 1984; Elson, Hauri, & Cunis, 1977; Hebert & Lehmann, 1979; Kasamatsu & Hirai, 1969; Saletu, 1987; Taneli & Krahne, 1987), autogenic training (Jacobs & Lubar, 1989), and a "self-regulation method" that is similar to self-hypnosis (Ikema, 1988; Ikema, Tomita, Kuroda, Hayashida, & Ikema, 1986). These related alternate states of awareness all involve the redistribution of attention, and are often accompanied by self-reports of enhanced focused attention.

Can theta recorded at the surface of the scalp reflect theta generators indigenous to the hippocampal system, a phylogenetically ancient cortex? Michel, Lehmann, Henggeler, and Brandeis (1992) reported the first dipole study evidence indicating that theta recorded at the cortical surface is of a bihemispheric origin from the hippocampal region of the human brain. A study (Arnolds, Lopes Da Silva, Aitink, Kamp, & Boeijinga, 1980) of an epileptic patient with electrodes implanted in the hippocampal area reinforced the relationships between theta in the hippocampus and focused attention. When the patient was concentrating on a task, there were enhanced theta bursts being generated in the hippocampal area.

There is strong evidence from animal studies (e.g, Isaacson, 1982; Isaacson & Pribram, 1986; R. Miller, 1991) that increased firing of theta generators (increased theta bursts) in the hippocampal region occurs when animals (e.g., cats, rats, rabbits, primates) are actively engaged in exploratory and other attentional behaviors. Pribram and his associates (Crowne, Konow, Drake, & Pribram, 1972; see also, Pribram, 1991) demonstrated that the hippocampus is "ordinarily involved in processing the nonreinforced rather than the reinforced aspects of a situation" (Pribram, 1991, p. 224). This implies that the hippocampus is assisting in processing the nonimportant stimuli in the environment that are to be subsequently ignored. R. Miller (1989, 1991) suggested that the hippocampus through a cortico-hippocampal relay transmits information by theta wave modulation and Hebbian synaptic modification so that there is selective disattention. Crowne et al. (1972) found theta electrical activity from the hippocampus while monkeys were performing discrimina-

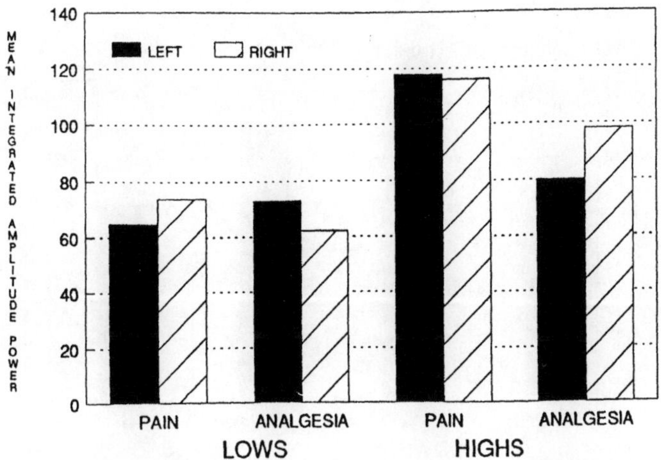
FRONTAL: HIGH THETA
MEAN INTEGRATED AMPLITUDE POWER
LEFT
RIGHT
0
20
40
60
80
100
120
140
PAIN
ANALGESIA
PAIN
ANALGESIA
LOWS
HIGHS

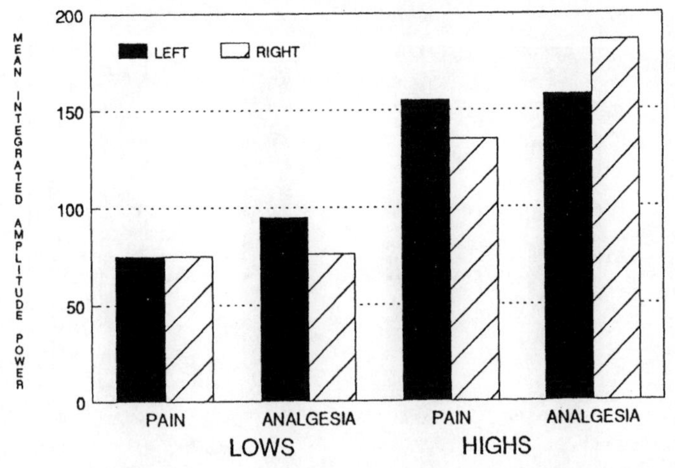
PARIETAL: HIGH THETA
MEAN INTEGRATED AMPLITUDE POWER
LEFT
RIGHT
0
50
100
150
200
PAIN
ANALGESIA
PAIN
ANALGESIA
LOWS
HIGHS

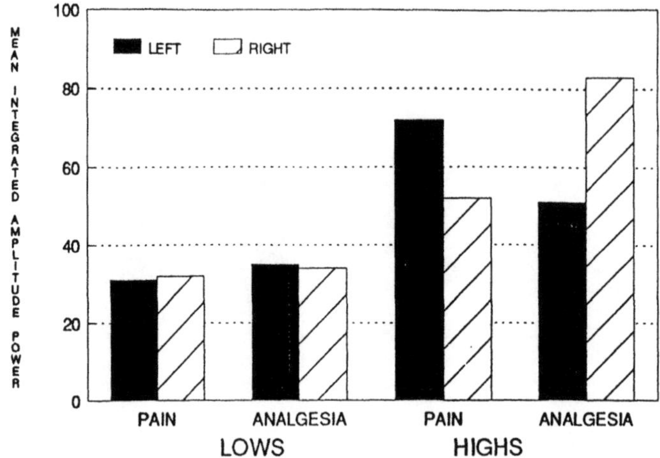

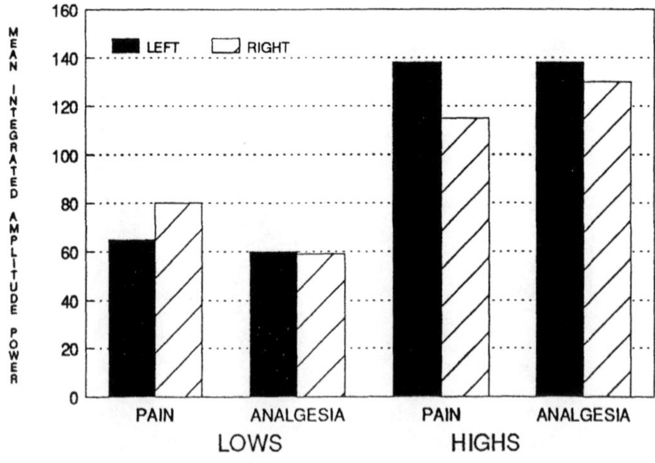

Figure 2. **Mean integrated theta power in the left and right hemispheres during hypnosis with and without suggested analgesia in low and high hypnotizables.**

Note. From "Cognitive and Psychophysiological Correlates of Hypnotic Responsiveness and Hypnosis," by H. J. Crawford, in M. L. Fass and D. Brown (Eds.), 1990, *Creative Mastery in Hypnosis and Hypnoanalysis: A Festschrift for Erika Fromm* (p. 53); Hillsdale, NJ: Lawrence Erlbaum. Copyright 1990 by Lawrence Erlbaum Associates. Reprinted by permission of the author.

tion tasks. When monkeys learned not to respond in no-go conditions, hippocampal theta was generated. As Pribram (1991) stated, "It is as if these systems were processing 'don't look there' rather than 'look-here' " (p. 224). This suggests that the willing of both attention and disattention may be correlated with theta activity.

De Benedittis and Sironi (1986, 1988) have directly examined hippocampal and amygdala electrical activity in epileptic patients with deeply implanted intracranial electrodes. During hypnosis, repeated stimulations of the left and right amygdala aroused a moderately hypnotizable patient from hypnosis, whereas stimulation of the temporal neocortices and the right Ammon's horn of the hippocampus did not. Unknown is whether any segment of the arousal system that includes the amygdala, when stimulated may bring an individual out of hypnosis. They postulated "that hypnotic behavior is mediated, at least in part, by a dynamic balance of antagonizing effects of discrete limbic structures—the amygdala and the hippocampus. In fact, the trance state is associated with the hippocampal activity, concomitant with a partial angdaloid [*sic*] complex functional inhibition" (p. 104).

What might this related physiological research say about the robust finding of greater theta power in high than low hypnotizable persons during task performance that requires focused and sustained attention? I would like to suggest that highly hypnotizable persons demonstrate greater efficiency in processing relevant and irrelevant environmental stimuli—the process of cognitive inhibition and ignoring stimuli requires first the recognition of it and then the decision to not look there. It is hypothesized that this disattending ability is related to greater theta power, a reflection of the fronto-limbic system of attention. If this is true, then to eliminate the perception of pain or to experience other positive or negative hallucinations, the highly hypnotizable person must have the ability to disattend and may generate substantial theta power during such attentive/disattentive states. Several hypnotic analgesia studies, reviewed in the next section, provide support for this hypothesis.

Finally, related neurophysiological work from Gruzelier's laboratory provides further support for our argument of greater fronto-limbic inhibitory processing found among highs. Gruzelier and Brow (1985) found that there were fewer orienting responses and increased habituation to relevant auditory clicks during hypnosis for highs, but not lows. Such changes reflect increased activity in fronto-limbic attentional systems having an inhibitory action (Gruzelier, 1990; Gruzelier & Venables, 1972).

Hypnotic Analgesia: Shifts in Attentional Processing

Pain and hypnotic analgesia is a particularly fertile ground to explore attentional and disattentional processes and their relationships to hypnotic susceptibility. The effectiveness of hypnosis in the relief of pain is a topic not in need of review here (for a review, see E. R. Hilgard & J. R. Hilgard, 1983). Typically, standardized measures of hypnotic susceptibility correlate about .50 with pain reduction during hypnotically suggested analgesia.

Neurophysiology of Pain

Pain is "an unpleasant sensory and emotional experience associated with actual or potential tissue damage, or described in terms of such pain" (Mersky, 1986, p. 215). First, there is the nociception or sensory aspect of pain. Second, there are the emotional-motivation and cognitive aspects of pain, often referred to as psychological distress. Much work (for a review, see Price, 1988) has been done to elucidate the complex interactions between primary sensory afferents and neuronal responses within the dorsal horn of the spinal cord and the subcortical structures, but much less is known about the cortical-subcortical involvement during pain.

Two processes present in pain and temperature are associated with different regions of the brain. The epicritic, sensory aspects of pain are more associated with the central and posterior regions of the brain, while the protocritic, distress, comfort-discomfort aspects of pain are associated with the fronto-limbic region (e.g., Pribram, 1991). The sensory experience that is critically located in space and time is sent to the posterior region of the brain, particularly the parietal cortex. Anatomical studies have linked the multisynaptic pain pathways from the thalamus not only to the posterior cortex but also to the amygdala and related limbic-cortical structures, as well as to the orbito-frontal cortex (e.g., Morin, Schwartz, & O'Leary, 1951; Pribram, 1991; Price, 1988; Roland, 1992). Electrical activity from the frontal cortex shows arousal when pain is experienced. As attention is directed away from pain, it is hypothesized that one should see changes in the activation of this anterior protocritic sensory process that may differ from changes observed in the posterior epicritic process.

Using magnetic resonance imaging and PET in humans, Talbot and her colleagues (Talbot et al., 1991) have demonstrated that the parietal and frontal cortical areas are involved in different aspects of heat perception (41-42° C; 48-49° C). Mild heat and pain are evaluated in terms of their temporal and spatial features in the posterior primary and secondary somatosensory cortex and in terms of emotional reactions of distress in the limbic regions of the frontal cortex, particularly the anterior cingulate cortex. The heterogeneous anterior cingulate cortex is activated during word association, recognition of visual material, and lactate-induced panic (for a review, see Raichle, 1990). Jones, Brown, Friston, Qi, and Frackowiak (1991) administered painful thermal stimuli (46-47° C) to the forearm. With PET subtractive techniques they found that the contralateral thalamus, anterior cingulate cortex, and lenticular nucleus are activated when strong pain is experienced. Removal of the frontal or cingulate cortex in patients with intractable pain leads to the amelioration of distress while not eliminating sensory pain (for a review, see Bouckoms, 1989). These diverse physiological studies suggest that the frontal cortex and the cingulate mediate thalamic pain input from the spinothalamic tract.

Neurophysiological Changes During Hypnotic Analgesia

Highly hypnotizable pain patients or laboratory subjects are more likely to learn to decrease or eliminate the perception of pain during suggested analgesia (for review, see E. R. Hilgard & J. R. Hilgard, 1983). Those who can eliminate the distress or emotional involvement but still experience some sensory pain give reports similar to frontal lobotomized patients (Bouckoms, 1989). The virtuoso hypnotic individual, whom we study after extensive screening and training, can eliminate absolutely all perception of sensory pain and distress. Brain dynamic changes accompanying hypnotic analgesia in such virtuoso highs have been observed in recent EEG, ERP, and CBF studies.

Electroencephalographic activity. In an earlier section was a discussion of enhanced theta being associated with focused attention. Recently I (Crawford, 1990a, 1990b) have initiated research to investigate EEG correlates of cold pressor pain during counterbalanced conditions of attend to and suggested analgesia in conditions of waking and hypnosis. Subjects were highs who had been able to reduce the perception of pain to absolutely no experience during cold pressor training sessions and lows who could not eliminate such pain perceptions, although their pain and distress perceptions were sometimes reduced during suggested hypnotic analgesia. Using the same recording technique as Sabourin et al. (1990), EEG was recorded monopolarly at frontal (F3, F4), temporal (T3, T4), parietal (P3, P4), and occipital (01, 02) regions while subjects had their left hand dipped into cold water for 60 seconds.

In all measured brain regions, highs showed significantly more high theta (5.5 - 7.5 Hz) power than did lows during pain and analgesia during hypnosis. Of the four regions of the brain (Figure 2), the anterior temporal region (T3, T4) showed the greatest differences between pain and analgesia conditions. In the anterior temporal region, during pain and analgesia, low hypnotizables showed no significant asymmetries between the left and right hemispheres. By contrast, the highs were significantly more left hemisphere dominant in the pain dip and showed a dramatic reversal in hemispheric dominance during analgesia. Left hemisphere theta power decreased significantly while right hemisphere theta power increased in the anterior temporal region (T3, T4).

Complementary support is provided by Larbig and his colleagues (Larbig et al., 1982) in a study of the EEG and evoked potentials in fakirs trained to hang from hooks or put needles through their skin or tongue without perception of pain. Substantially higher theta power was shown in the parietal, but not central, midline derivations in fakirs who demonstrated pain control, in comparison to controls who showed no change when asked to reduce pain perception but were unsuccessful. Chen, Dworkin, and Bloomquist (1981) reported shifts in EEG theta and alpha power during hypnotic analgesia in one dental patient undergoing surgery.

If cortically recorded theta is reflective of underlying theta generators in the hippocampal region as found by Michel et al. (1992), these data suggest the fronto-hippocampal attentional system may be involved during suggested analgesia. Shifts in theta power dominance, as seen in Crawford (1990a, 1990b), suggest possible shifts in hippocampal dominance during conditions of pain and analgesia. When pain is experienced, the subject—particularly the highly hypnotizable subject—is immersed in and focused on the external pain. This focusing of attention on the environment is suggestive of left hemisphere involvement. When hypnotic analgesia occurs, the subject may turn away from the pain and be immersed in and focused on ongoing self-generated imagery. While this imagery activity may be associated with right hemisphere functioning (e.g., Kosslyn, 1988), we must also consider more complex brain dynamics as the left hemisphere has also been implicated in self-generated visual imagery (e.g., Farah, 1988; for a review, see Crawford, in press). Research with topographical EEG is under way in my laboratory to explore further brain dynamics, both anterior-posterior and left-right, during cold pressor pain.

Somatosensory evoked potentials. The later components of pain-associated ERP amplitudes correlate positively with perceived pain level (e.g., Chen, Chapman, & Harkins, 1979; Stowell, 1984). When given successful suggestions of hypnotic analgesia or reduced feeling, the amplitudes of the early, sensory components of evoked potentials (less than 100 msec) to somatosensory electrical (e.g., Mészáros, Bányai, & Greguss, 1981; Spiegel, Bierre, & Rootenberg, 1989) and heat (e.g., Sharev & Tal, 1989) stimuli are apparently unaffected. But the latter components of the evoked potential are often, but not always (e.g., Barabasz & Lonsdale, 1983), reduced in amplitude. Mészáros et al. (1980) reported decreases in P200 somatosensory (SERP) amplitudes to short electrical impulses to the median nerve during hypnotic analgesia. Spiegel et al. (1989) demonstrated that there were greater reductions in the SERP components to mildly uncomfortable stimuli in the right hemisphere than in the left hemisphere, as early as P100. We (De Pascalis, Crawford, & Marucci, 1992a, 1992b) found reductions of the amplitude of the N150-P260, more so in the left hemisphere, to quite painful somatosensory stimuli administered to the median nerve during suggested hypnotic analgesia. Like

I. Mészáros (personal communication, July 1990), we found the P200 (which correlates with perceived pain level in other studies) contributed to this reduced amplitude.

In ongoing research, we (e.g., Crawford, Pribram et al., 1992, 1993; Crawford, Pribram, Xie, & Zhang, 1993a, 1993b) are evaluating topographical SERP brain maps of highs who can completely eliminate the perception of pain with lows during conditions of attend to and ignore noxious electrical stimulations. During hypnotic analgesia, in the far frontal region there is often a complete amelioration of the SERP at least as early as N100, while in the primary sensory central region, we observe dramatic decreases of the N100 and P200 often with no later components evident. At times we have seen contingent negative variations in the pre-500-msec period, associated with preparation to respond or inhibit responses (Birbaumer, Elbert, Canavan, & Rockstroh, 1990), occur during hypnotic analgesia mainly in the far frontal region. This ongoing research supports prior research (e.g., Jones et al., 1991; Talbot et al., 1991) suggesting two attentional systems associated with pain. During hypnotic analgesia, the far frontal cortex appears to be involved in a topographically specific inhibitory feedback circuit that cooperates in the regulation of thalamocortical activities (for a review, see Birbaumer et al., 1990). Thus we propose that during hypnotic analgesia the far frontal cortex "determines" that the incoming painful events are irrelevant and is involved in the inhibition of somatosensory information coming from the thalamic region.

Cerebral blood flow. Regional cerebral blood flow (CBF) provides a window on regional brain metabolism activity that is sensitive to the effects of cognitive tasks (e.g., Gur & Reivich, 1980; Risberg, 1986). In the first study to address CBF activation patterns by the 133-xenon inhalation method during hypnotic analgesia, Crawford, Gur, Skolnick, Gur, and Benson (1993) studied virtuoso highs who could completely eliminate the perception of pain with lows. Following an eyes-closed rest condition, they were administered ischemic pain to both arms under counterbalanced conditions of attend to pain and suggested analgesia in waking and hypnosis. Previously, they had been administered three standardized hypnotizability scales as well as training in both the typical cold pressor pain and ischemic pain experimental regimes.

Both low and highly hypnotizable men had essentially the same initial slope of regional blood flow metabolism during the waking condition, regardless of the presence or absence of pain. During hypnosis, the lows continued to show similar cerebral metabolism, while the highs showed a significant increase in overall CBF during hypnosis (see Figure 3). This finding of enhanced CBF during hypnosis has been substantiated elsewhere (De Benedittis & Longostreui, 1988; Halama, 1989; Meyer, Diehl, Ulrich, & Meinig, 1989; Walter, 1992). We believe this process may reflect increased cortical involvement in the focusing of attention and disatten-

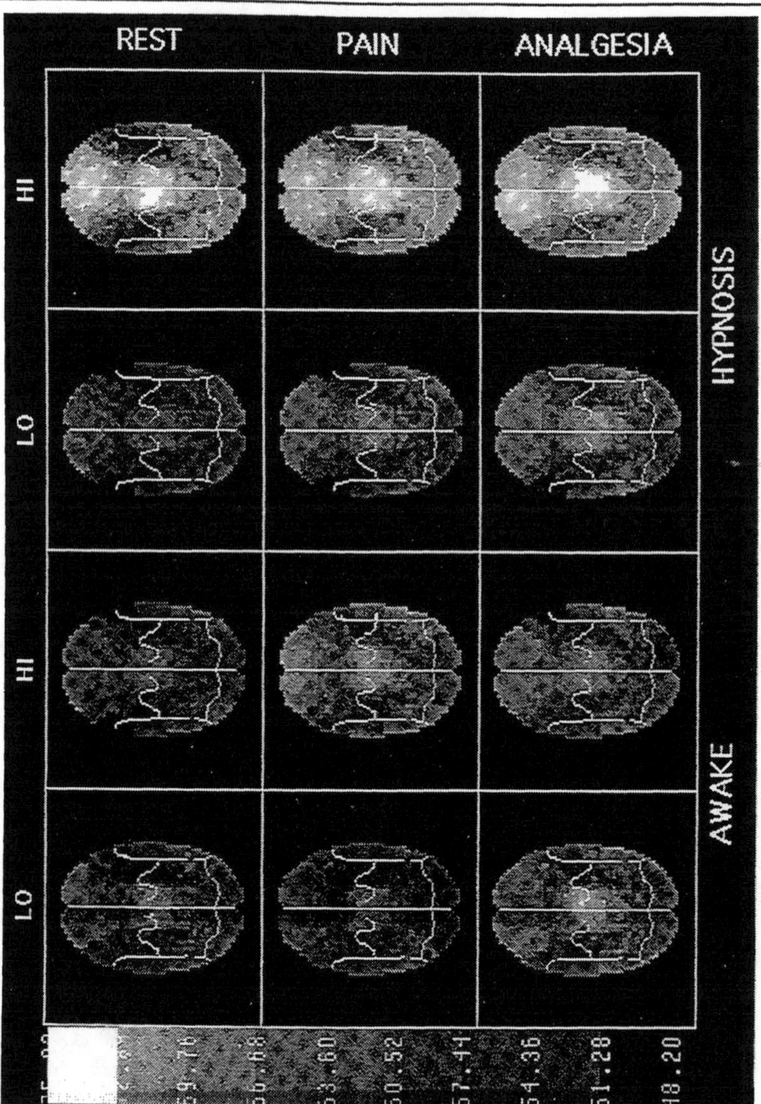

Figure 3. **A topographical display of CBF grey-matter values in three conditions: Rest (Column 1), Pain (Column 2), Pain with Suggested Analgesia (Column 3). The waking, nonhypnosis state is the first two rows: low (bottom row) and highly (second row) hypnotizable subjects. The hypnosis state is the top two rows: Low (third row) and highly (fourth row) hypnotizable subjects. The lighter the color, the greater the CBF.**

Note. From "Effects of Hypnosis on Regional Cerebral Blood Flow During Ischemic Pain With and Without Suggested Hypnotic Analgesia," by H. J. Crawford, R. C. Gur, B. Skolnick, R. E. Gur, and D. Benson, 1993, *International Journal of Psychophysiology, 15,* p. 189.

tion during hypnosis (e.g., E. R. Hilgard, 1965, 1986; Krippner & Bindler, 1974). While hypnosis may be experienced as being involuntary and effortless, at another level the cerebral metabolism increases suggest that hypnosis may be a state in which there is increased cognitive effort and activity occurring. Thus, in view of the consistent demonstrations of increased CBF during mental effort (for a review, see Frith, 1991), this research supports a growing belief (e.g., Crawford & Gruzelier, 1992; E. R. Hilgard, 1986) that hypnosis takes effort and is a cognitive task that demands attentional and disattentional allocations.

During ischemic pain there was the anticipated increased CBF in the somatosensory cortex, consistent with other neuroimaging studies. During hypnotic analgesia, there were significant CBF increases only among the highs, beyond that noted in the attend to pain condition, in the orbito-frontal cortex and the sensorimotor cortex. Crawford, Gur, et al. (1993) suggest "that the increased orbito-frontal CBF activation in highs is reflective of increased attentional effort during hypnotic analgesia by the 'executive control system' (E. R. Hilgard, 1986; Pribram, 1991) or 'supervisory attentional system' (Shallice, 1988). PET studies (for a review, see Frith, 1991) show an increase of activity in the frontal cortex during the performance of willed actions" (p. 192). They concluded that their data provide further support to the hypothesis that hypnotic analgesia activates a topographically specific inhibitory feedback circuit that cooperates in the regulation of thalamocortical activities (e.g., Birbaumer et al., 1990).

Such CBF data, in conjunction with previously reviewed SERP (Crawford, Pribram, et al., 1992, 1993; 1993a, 1993b) and habituation (Gruzelier & Brow, 1985) findings suggestive of enhanced frontal lobe inhibitory processing during hypnosis, fail to support Bowers' (1990; see also, Miller & Bowers, 1986, 1993) conclusion that "hypnotic analgesia does not seem to require executive initiative and/or the sustained effort of higher, conscious processes" (Bowers, 1990, p. 171) but rather unspecified "lower levels" (p. 171) of cognitive control. Rather, I would argue that "dissociated control" still requires higher order cognitive and attentional effort (even though experienced as effortless or out of awareness). Morton Prince (1910) argued that dissociated hypnotic phenomena were due to "consciousness occur(ing) without self-consciousness" (p. 29). While there may be a lack of self-concept (see Kihlstrom, 1987; Kunzendorf, 1989-90) and thus a dissociation during hypnosis, this does not negate processes still occurring during dissociated hypnotic phenomena that may involve higher cognitive processing and the executive control system. My laboratory is presently pursuing research that investigates the interplay between cortical-subcortical processes during hypnotic phenomena out of awareness to self-consciousness.

Conclusions

Experimental evidence has been provided that highly hypnotizable persons demonstrate greater cognitive flexibility, the ability to shift cognitive strategies and states of awareness, than do lows (e.g., Crawford, 1982a; 1989; Crawford & Allen, 1983; Crawford & Gruzelier, 1992; Crawford et al., 1986). Highs can shift from detail to holistic strategies with greater ease than lows (e.g., Crawford & Allen, 1983). Highs can also shift from left to right anterior functioning as demonstrated by neuropsychological tests (e.g., Gruzelier, 1990; Gruzelier & Warren, 1993). These cognitive strategy shifts appear to be accompanied by greater neurophysiological hemispheric specificity or dominance across tasks (e.g., Crawford, 1989, 1990a, 1990b, 1991; Crawford, Mészáros, & Szabó, 1989; for reviews, see Crawford & Gruzelier, 1992; Gruzelier, 1987, 1990).

In the present article, evidence was presented to suggest that highly hypnotizable persons possess stronger attentional filtering abilities that may be associated with the fronto-limbic attentional system. As shown in behavioral and cognitive studies, highly hypnotizable individuals have a greater ability to sustain focused attention on relevant activities and to disattend nonimportant stimuli in the environment than do low hypnotizable persons. The importance of the anterior fronto-limbic system in the control processes of attention is supported by independent studies of EEG, evoked potentials, cerebral blood flow, electrodermal, and neuropsychological functioning. These studies demonstrate individual differences in the brain dynamics of lows and highs in waking or hypnosis. Despite these propositions, much has still to be empirically demonstrated and explained. While an emphasis has been placed upon neurophysiological mechanisms associated with focused attention and disattention, we must also still consider other additionally important information processing abilities of highs and what neurophysiological correlates may be associated with them (e.g., Crawford, in press). These include the abilities to give up reality testing and become deeply involved in imaginative activities, to produce imagery (even of an hallucinatory nature) vividly and effortlessly, and the ability to shift to greater holistic information processing styles.

Most exciting then is that our field of hypnosis research can provide a unique window on individual differences in cognitive and attentional processing and their accompanying brain dynamics. As B. F. Skinner (1989) wrote just prior to his death:

> There are two unavoidable gaps in any behavioral account: one between the stimulating action of the environment and the response of the organism and one between consequences and the resulting change in behavior. Only brain science can fill those gaps. In doing so it completes the account; it does not give a different account of the same thing. (p. 18)

Thus brain research is validating and extending our behavioral observations—it is completing our account of how and why individuals differ in their abilities to attend and to disattend and helping us understand why there are individual differences in hypnotic susceptibility.

REFERENCES

Arnolds, D., Lopes Da Silva, F. H., Aitink, J. W., Kamp, A., & Boeijinga, P. (1980). The spectral properties of hippocampal EEG related to behavior in man. *Electroencephalography and Clinical Neurophysiology, 50*, 324-328.

Atkinson, R. P. (1991, October). *Individual differences in afterimage persistence during waking and hypnosis: Effects of hypnotizability and visuospatial skills*. Paper presented at the 42nd Annual Scientific Meeting of the Society for Clinical and Experimental Hypnosis, New Orleans, LA.

Atkinson, R. P., & Crawford, H. J. (1992). Individual differences in afterimage persistence: Relationships to hypnotic responsiveness and visuospatial skills. *American Journal of Psychology, 105*, 527-539.

Banquet, J. P. (1973). Spectral analysis of the EEG in meditation. *Electroencephalography and Clinical Neurophysiology, 35*, 143-151.

Barabasz, A. F. (1990, July). *Effects of sensory deprivation on EEG theta and skin conductance*. Paper presented at the Fifth International Congress of Psychophysiology, Budapest, Hungary.

Barabasz, A. F., Crawford, H. J., & Barabasz, M. (1993, October). *EEG topographical map differences in attention deficit disordered and normal children: Moderating effects from focused active alert instructions during reading, math and listening tasks*. Paper presented at the annual meeting of the Society for Psychophysiological Research, Rottach-Egern, Germany.

Barabasz, A. F., & Lonsdale, C. (1983). Effects of hypnosis on P300 olfactory evoked potential amplitudes. *Journal of Abnormal Psychology, 92*, 520-523.

Benton, A. L. (1968). Differential behavioral effects in frontal lobe disease. *Neuropsychologia, 6*, 53-60.

Berch, D. B., & Kanter, D. R. (1984). Individual differences. In J. S. Warm (Ed.), *Sustained attention in human performance* (pp. 143-178). New York: Wiley.

Birbaumer, N., Elbert, T., Canavan, A.G.M., & Rockstroh, B. (1990). Slow potentials of the cerebral cortex and behavior. *Physiological Reviews, 70*, 1-41.

Bouckoms, A. J. (1989). Psychosurgery for pain. In P. D. Wall & R. Melzack (Eds.), *Textbook of pain* (2nd ed., pp. 868-881). Edinburgh, Scotland: Churchill Livingstone.

Bowers, K. S. (1990). Unconscious influences and hypnosis. In J. L. Singer (Ed.), *Repression and dissociation: Implications for personality, theory, psychopathology, and health* (pp. 143-178). Chicago: University of Chicago Press.

Chen, A.C.N., Chapman, C. R., & Harkins, S. W. (1979). Brain evoked potentials are functional correlates of induced pain in man. *Pain, 6*, 305-314.

Chen, A.C.N., Dworkin, S. F., & Bloomquist, D. S. (1981). Cortical power spectrum analysis of hypnotic pain control in surgery. *International Journal of Neuroscience, 13*, 127-136.

Cohen, L. (1959). Perception of reversible figures after brain injury. *Archives of Neurology and Psychiatry, 81*, 765-775.

Corby, J. C., Roth, W. T., Zarcone, V. P., & Kopell, B. S. (1978). Psychophysiological correlates of the practice of Tantric Yoga meditation. *Archives of General Psychiatry, 35*, 571-577.

Crawford, H. J. (1981a). *Differential Attentional Processes Inventory*. Unpublished questionnaire.

Crawford, H. J. (1981b). Hypnotic susceptibility as related to gestalt closure. *Journal of Personality and Social Psychology, 40*, 376-383.

Crawford, H. J. (1982a). Cognitive processing during hypnosis: Much unfinished business. *Research Communications in Psychology, Psychiatry, and Behavior, 7*, 169-179.

Crawford, H. J. (1982b). Hypnotizability, daydreaming styles, imagery vividness, and absorption: A multidimensional study. *Journal of Personality and Social Psychology*, 42, 915-926.

Crawford, H. J. (1989). Cognitive and physiological flexibility: Multiple pathways to hypnotic responsiveness. In V. Ghorghui, P. Netter, H. Eysenck, & R. Rosenthal (Eds.), *Suggestion and suggestibility: Theory and research* (pp. 155-168). New York: Springer-Verlag.

Crawford, H. J. (1990a). Cognitive and psychophysiological correlates of hypnotic responsiveness and hypnosis. In M. L. Fass & D. Brown (Eds.), *Creative mastery in hypnosis and hypnoanalysis: A Festschrift for Erika Fromm* (pp. 47-54). Hillsdale, NJ: Lawrence Erlbaum.

Crawford, H. J. (1990b). *Cold pressor pain with and without suggested analgesia: EEG correlates as moderated by hypnotic susceptibility level*. Paper presented at the Fifth International Congress of Psychophysiology, Budapest, Hungary.

Crawford, H. J. (1991, October). *The hypnotizable brain: Attentional and disattentional processes*. Presidential address delivered at the 42nd Annual Scientific Meeting of The Society for Clinical and Experimental Hypnosis, New Orleans, LA.

Crawford, H. J. (in press). Cerebral brain dynamics of mental imagery: Evidence and issues for hypnosis. In R. G. Kunzendorf, N. Spanos, & B. Wallace (Eds.), *Imagination and hypnosis*. Amityville, NY: Baywood.

Crawford, H. J., & Allen, S. N. (1983). Enhanced visual memory during hypnosis as mediated by hypnotic responsiveness and cognitive strategies. *Journal of Experimental Psychology: General*, 112, 662-685.

Crawford, H. J., Brown, A., & Moon, C. (1993). Sustained attentional and disattentional abilities: Differences between low and high hypnotizable individuals. *Journal of Abnormal Psychology*, 102, 534-543.

Crawford, H. J., Clarke, S. N., & Kitner-Triolo, M. (1989). EEG activity pattern differences in low and high hypnotizables: Reflections of cognitive strategy differences? *International Journal of Psychophysiology*, 7, 165-166.

Crawford, H. J., Corby, J. C., & Kopell, B. S. (1994). *Auditory event-related potentials while ignoring tone stimuli: Attentional differences in stimulus intensity responses in low and highly hypnotizable individuals*. Manuscript submitted for publication.

Crawford, H. J., & Gruzelier, J. (1992). A midstream view of the psychoneurophysiology of hypnosis: Recent research and future directions. In E. Fromm & M. Nash (Eds.), *Hypnosis: Research developments and perspectives* (pp. 227-266). New York: Guilford.

Crawford, H. J., Gur, R. C., Skolnick, B., Gur, R. E., & Benson, D. (1993). Effects of hypnosis on regional cerebral blood flow during ischemic pain with and without suggested hypnotic analgesia. *International Journal of Psychophysiology*, 15, 181-195.

Crawford, H. J., Kitner-Triolo, M., Clarke, S. W., & Brown, A. M. (1988). EEG activation patterns accompanying induced happy and sad moods: Moderating effects of hypnosis and hypnotic responsiveness level. *International Journal of Clinical and Experimental Hypnosis*, 36, 229. (Abstract)

Crawford, H. J., Mészáros, I., & Szabó, Cs. (1989). EEG differences in low and high hypnotizables during waking and hypnosis: Rest, math and imaginal tasks. In D. Waxman, D. Pedersen, I. Wilkie, & P. Mellett (Eds.), *Hypnosis* (pp. 76-85). London: Whurr.

Crawford, H. J., Pribram, K., Kugler, P., Xie, M., Zhang, B., & Knebel, T. (1992, September). *EEG and somatosensory evoked potential brain topographical changes during suggested hypnotic anesthesia*. Invited paper presented at the Sixth International Congress of Psychophysiology, Berlin, Germany.

Crawford, H. J., Pribram, K., Kugler, P., Xie, M., Zhang, B., & Knebel, T. (1993). EEG and somatosensory evoked potential brain topographical changes during suggested hypnotic anesthesia. *International Journal of Psychophysiology*, 14, 118. (Abstract)

Crawford, H. J., Pribram, K., Xie, M., & Zhang, B. (1993a, October). *Far frontal "Executive" control over disattention to pain during hypnotic analgesia: Evidence from somatosensory event-related potential research*. Paper presented at the 43rd Annual Scientific Meeting of The Society for Clinical and Experimental Hypnosis, Chicago, IL.

Crawford, H. J., Pribram, K., Xie, M., & Zhang, B. (1993b). *Somatosensory event-related potentials and preparatory processing to painful stimuli: Effects of hypnotically suggested analgesia as moderated by hypnotic level.* Paper presented at the annual meeting of the Society for Psychophysiological Research, Rottach-Egern, Germany.

Crawford, H. J., Wallace, B., Nomura, K., & Slater, H. (1986). Eidetic-like imagery in hypnosis: Rare but there. *American Journal of Psychology, 99*, 527-546.

Crowne, D. P., Konow, A., Drake, K. J., & Pribram, K. H. (1972). Hippocampal electrical activity in the monkey during delayed alternation problems. *Journal of EEG and Clinical Neurophysiology, 33*, 567-577.

Davies, D. R., Jones, D. M., & Taylor, A. (1984). Selective- and sustained-attention tasks: Individual and group differences. In R. Parasuraman & D. R. Davies (Eds.), *Varieties of attention* (pp. 395-447). San Diego, CA: Academic Press.

De Benedittis, G., & Longostreui, G. P. (1988, July). *Cerebral blood flow changes in hypnosis: A single photon emission computerized tomography (SPECT) study.* Paper presented at the Fourth International Congress of Psychophysiology, Prague, Czechoslovakia.

De Benedittis, G., & Sironi, V. A. (1986). Deep cerebral electrical activity in man during hypnosis. *International Journal of Clinical and Experimental Hypnosis, 34*, 63-70.

De Benedittis, G., & Sironi, V. A. (1988). Arousal effects of electrical deep brain stimulation in hypnosis. *International Journal of Clinical and Experimental Hypnosis, 36*, 96-101.

Delmonte, M. M. (1984). Meditation: Similarities with hypnoidal states and hypnosis. *International Journal of Psychosomatics, 31*, 24-34.

De Pascalis, V., Crawford, H. J., & Marucci, F. S. (1992a). Analgesia ipnotica nella modulazione del dolore: Effeti sui potenziali somatosensoriali [Hypnotic analgesia moderates pain: Effects on somatosensory potentials]. *Comunicazioni Scientifice di Psicologie Generale*, 71-89.

De Pascalis, V., Crawford, H. J., & Marucci, F. S. (1992b, September). *Effects of hypnosis and hypnotic analgesia on somatosensory evoked potentials during painful stimulations.* Paper presented at the Sixth International Congress of Psychophysiology. Berlin, Germany.

Dixon, M., Brunet, A., & Laurence, J-R. (1990). Hypnotizability and automaticity: Toward a parallel distributed processing model of hypnotic responding. *Journal of Abnormal Psychology, 99*, 336-343.

Dixon, M., & Laurence, J-R. (1992). Hypnotic susceptibility and verbal automaticity: Automatic and strategic processing differences in the Stroop color-naming task. *Journal of Abnormal Psychology, 101*, 344-347.

Elson, B. D, Hauri, P., & Cunis, D. (1977). Physiological changes in Yoga meditation. *Psychophysiology, 14*, 52-57.

Evans, B. M. (1992). Periodic activity in cerebral arousal mechanisms—the relationship to sleep and brain damage. *Electroencephalography and Clinical Neurophysiology, 83*, 130-137.

Farah, M. J. (1988). The neuropsychology of mental imagery: Converging evidence from brain-damaged and normal subjects. In J. Stiles-Davis, M. Kritchevsky, & U. Bellugi (Eds.), *Spatial cognition: Brain bases and development*. Hillsdale, NJ: Lawrence Erlbaum.

Finke, R. A., & Macdonald, H. (1978). Two personality measures relating hypnotic susceptibility to absorption. *International Journal of Clinical and Experimental Hypnosis, 26*, 178-183.

Frith, C. D. (1991). Positron emission tomography studies of frontal lobe function: Relevance to psychiatric disease. In D. H. Chadwick & J. Whelan (Eds), *Exploring brain functional anatomy with positron tomography* (pp. 181-197). New York: Wiley. (Ciba Foundation Symposium 163)

Galbraith, G. C., London, P., Leibovitz, M. P., Cooper, L. M., & Hart, J. T. (1970). EEG and hypnotic susceptibility. *Journal of Comparative and Physiological Psychology, 72*, 125-131.

Galin, D., Raz, J., Fein, G., Johnston, J., Herron, J., & Yingling, C. (1992). EEG spectra in dyslexic and normal readers during oral and silent reading. *Electroencephalography and Clinical Neurophysiology, 82*, 87-101.

Graf, J. (1989). Plans, actions, and mental sets: Managerial knowledge units in the frontal lobes. In E. Perecman (Ed.), *Integrating theory and practice in clinical neuropsychology* (pp. 93-138). Hillsdale, NJ: Lawrence Erlbaum.

Grumbles, D., & Crawford, H. J. (1981, October). *Differential attentional skills and hypnotizability.* Paper presented at the 33rd Annual Scientific Meeting of The Society for Clinical and Experimental Hypnosis, Portland, OR.

Gruzelier, J. H. (1987). The neuropsychology of hypnosis. In M. Heap (Ed.), *Hypnosis: Current clinical, experimental and forensic practices* (pp. 68-76). London: Croom Helm.

Gruzelier, J. H. (1990). Neuropsychophysiological investigations of hypnosis: Cerebral laterality and beyond. In R. Van Dyck, P. H. Spinhoven, & A.L.W. Van Der Does (Eds.), *Hypnosis: Theory, research and clinical practice* (pp. 38-51). Amsterdam: Free University Press.

Gruzelier, J. H., & Brow, T. D. (1985). Psychophysiological evidence for a state theory of hypnosis and susceptibility. *Journal of Psychosomatic Research, 29,* 287-382.

Gruzelier, J. H., Brow, T. D., Perry, A., Rhonder, J., & Thomas, M. (1984). Hypnotic susceptibility: A lateral predisposition and altered cerebral asymmetry under hypnosis. *International Journal of Psychophysiology, 2,* 131-139.

Gruzelier, J. H., & Venables, P. H. (1972). Skin conductance orienting activity in a heterogeneous sample of schizophrenics: Possible evidence of limbic dysfunction. *Journal of Nervous and Mental Diseases, 155,* 277-287.

Gruzelier, J., & Warren, K. (1993). Neuropsychological evidence of reductions on left frontal tests with hypnosis. *Psychological Medicine, 23,* 93-101.

Gur, R. C., & Reivich, M. (1980). Cognitive task effects on hemispheric blood flow in humans: Evidence for individual differences in hemispheric activation. *Brain and Language, 9,* 78-92.

Gutierrez, S., & Corsi-Cabrera, M. (1988). EEG activity during performance of cognitive tasks demanding verbal and/or spatial processing. *International Journal of Neuroscience, 42,* 149-155.

Halama, P. (1989). Die Veranderung der corticalen Durchblutung vor under in Hypnose [The change of the cortical blood circulation before and during hypnosis]. *Experimentelle und Klikische Hypnose, 5,* 19-26.

Herbert, R., & Lehmann, D. (1979). Theta bursts: An EEG pattern in normal subjects practicing the transmeditational technique. *Electroencephalography and Clinical Neurophysiology, 42,* 397-405.

Hilgard, E. R. (1965). *Hypnotic susceptibility.* New York: Harcourt, Brace & World.

Hilgard, E. R. (1986). *Divided consciousness: Multiple controls in human thought and action* (rev. ed.). New York: Wiley.

Hilgard, E. R., & Hilgard, J. R. (1983). *Hypnosis in the relief of pain.* Palo Alto, CA: Kaufmann.

Hilgard, J. R. (1970). *Personality and hypnosis: A study of imaginative involvement.* Chicago: University of Chicago Press.

Hillyard, S. A., & Picton, T. W. (1979). Event-related brain potentials and selective information processing in man. In J. E. Desmedt (Ed.), *Cognitive components in cerebral event-related potentials and selective attention. Progress in clinical neurophysiology* (Vol. 6, pp. 1-52). Basel: Karger.

Ikema, A. (1988). Psychophysiological effects of self-regulation method: EEG frequency analysis and contingent negative variations. *Psychotherapy and Psychosomatics, 49,* 230-239.

Ikema, A., Tomita, S., Kuroda, M., Hayashida, Y., & Ikemi, Y. (1986). Self-regulation method: Psychological, physiological and clinical considerations: An overview. *Psychotherapy and Psychosomatics, 46,* 184-195.

Isaacson, R. L. (1982). *The limbic system.* New York: Plenum.

Isaacson, R. L., & Pribram, K. H. (Eds.). (1986). *The hippocampus. Volume 4.* New York: Plenum.

Jacobs, G. D., & Lubar, J. F. (1989). Spectral analysis of the central nervous system effects of the relaxation response elicited by autogenic training. *Behavioral Medicine, 16,* 125-132.

James, W. (1983). *Principles of psychology*. Cambridge, MA: Harvard University Press. (Original work published 1890)

Jones, A.K.P., Brown, W. D., Friston, K. R., Qi, L. J., & Frackowiak, R.S.J. (1991). Cortical and subcortical localization of response to pain in man using positron emission tomography. *Proceedings of the Royal Society of London, Series B, Biological Sciences, 244*, 39-44.

Kasamatsu, A., & Hirai, T. (1969). An EEG study on the Zen meditation (Zazen). In C. T. Tart (Ed.), *Altered states of consciousness* (pp. 489-501). New York: Wiley.

Kihlstrom, J. F. (1987). The cognitive unconscious. *Science, 237*, 1445-1552.

Kihlstrom, J. F., Diaz, W. A., McClellan, G. E., Ruskin, P. M., Pistole, D. D., & Shor, R. E. (1980). Personality correlates of hypnotic susceptibility: Needs for achievement and autonomy, self-monitoring, and masculinity-femininity. *American Journal of Clinical Hypnosis, 22*, 225-230.

Knebel, T. (1993). *EEG theta power during Necker Cube reversals*. Unpublished master's thesis, Virginia Polytechnic Institute and State University, Blacksburg, VA.

Kosslyn, S. M. (1988). Aspects of a cognitive neuroscience of mental imagery. *Science, 240*, 1521-1526.

Krippner, S., & Bindler, P. R. (1974). Hypnosis and attention: A review. *American Journal of Clinical Hypnosis, 26*, 166-177.

Kunzendorf, R. G. (1989-90). Posthypnotic amnesia: Dissociation of self-concept or self-consciousness? *Imagination, Cognition and Personality, 9*, 321-34.

Kunzendorf, R. G., & Boisvert, P. (in press). Presence vs absence of a 'hidden observer' during total deafness: The hypnotic illusion of subconsciousness vs the imaginal attenuation of brainstem evoked potentials. In R. G. Kunzendorf, N. Spanos, & B. Wallace (Eds.), *Imagination and hypnosis*. Amityville, NY: Baywood.

Lang, W., Lang, M., Kornhuber, A., Diekmann, V., & Kornhuber, H. H. (1988). Event related EEG spectra in a concept formation task. *Human Neurobiology, 6*, 295-330.

Larbig, W., Elbert, T., Lutzenberger, W., Rockstroh, B., Schneer, G., & Birbaumer, N. (1982). EEG and slow brain potentials during anticipation and control of painful stimulation. *Electroencephalography and Clinical Neurophysiology, 53*, 298-309.

Lubar, J. F. (1991). Discourse on the development of EEG diagnostics and biofeedback for attention-deficit/hyperactivity disorders. *Biofeedback and Self-Regulation, 16*, 201-225.

Lyons, L., & Crawford, H. J. (1991, October). *Attentional processing, arousal and hypnotizability*. Paper presented at the 42nd Annual Scientific Meeting of The Society for Clinical and Experimental Hypnosis, New Orleans, LA.

MacLeod, C. M. (1991). Half a century of research on the Stroop effect: An integrative review. *Psychological Bulletin, 109*, 163-203.

Martinot, J. L., Allilaire, J. F., Mazoyer, B. M., Hantouche, E., Huret, J. D., Deslauriers, A. G., Hardy, P., Pappata, S., Baron, J. C., & Syrota, A. (1990). Obsessive-compulsive disorder: A clinical, neuropsychological and positron emission tomography study. *Acta Psychiatrica Scandinavia, 82*, 233-242.

Mersky, H. (1986). Classification of chronic pain. *Pain, 3*, 215-217.

Mészáros, I., Bányai, E. I., & Greguss, A. C. (1981). Evoked potential, reflecting hypnotically altered state of consciousness. In G. Ádam, I. Mézáros, & E. I. Bányai (Eds.), *Brain and behaviour. Advances in physiological sciences, 17*, 467-475. Pergamon, Oxford, and Akadémiai: Kiadó, Budapest.

Mészáros, I., Crawford, H. J., Szabó, C., Nagy-Kovács, A., & Révész, M. A. (1989). Hypnotic susceptibility and cerebral hemisphere preponderance: Verbal-imaginal discrimination task. In V. Ghorghui, R. Netter, H. Eysenck, & R. Rosenthal (Eds.), *Suggestion and suggestibility: Theory and research* (pp. 191-204). New York: Springer-Verlag.

Meyer, H. K., Diehl, B. J., Ulrich, P. T., & Meinig, G. (1989). Änderungen der regionalen kortikalen Durchblutung unter Hypnose [Changes of the regional cerebral blood circulation under hypnosis]. *Zeitschrift fur Psychosomatische Medizin und Psychoanalyse, 35*, 48-58.

Michel, C. M., Lehmann, D., Henggeler, B., & Brandeis, D. (1992). Localization of the sources of EEG delta, theta alpha and beta frequency bands using the FFT dipole approximation. *Electroencephalography and Clinical Neurophysiology, 82*, 38-44.

Miller, M. E., & Bowers, K. S. (1986). Hypnotic analgesia and stress inoculation in the reduction of pain. *Journal of Abnormal Psychology, 95*, 6-14.

Miller, M. E., & Bowers, K. S. (1993). Hypnotic analgesia: Dissociated experience or dissociated control? *Journal of Abnormal Psychology, 102*, 29-38.

Miller, R. (1989). Cortico-hippocampal interplay: Self-organizing phase-locked loops for indexing memory. *Psychobiology, 17*, 115-128.

Miller, R. (1991). *Cortico-hippocampal interplay and the representation of contexts in the brain.* Berlin, Germany: Springer-Verlag.

Miller, R. J. (1975). Response to the Ponzo illusion as reflection of hypnotic susceptibility. *International Journal of Clinical and Experimental Hypnosis, 23*, 148-157.

Morin, F., Schwartz, H. G., & O'Leary, J. L. (1951). The experimental study of spino-thalamic and related tracts. *Acta Psychiatry et Neurologica Scandinavia, 26*, 3, 4.

Nadon, R., Laurence, J-R., & Perry, C. (1987). Multiple predictors of hypnotic susceptibility. *Journal of Personality and Social Psychology, 53*, 948-960.

Nakagawa, Y. (1988). Continuous observation of daytime EEG patterns in normal subjects under restrained conditions while sitting in armchair or on stool. Part 3. Awake state. *Japanese Journal of Psychiatry and Neurology, 42*, 247-264.

Perret, E. (1974). The left frontal lobe of man and the suppression of habitual responses in verbal categorical behavior. *Neuropsychologia, 12*, 323-330.

Posner, M. I., & Petersen, S. E. (1990). The attention span of the brain. *Annual Review of Neuroscience, 13*, 23-42.

Posner, M. I., Petersen, S. E., Fox, P. R., & Raichle, M. E. (1988). Localization of cognitive operations in the human brain. *Science, 240*, 1627-1631.

Pribram, K. H. (1991). *Brain and perception: Holonomy and structure in figural processing.* Hillsdale, NJ: Lawrence Erlbaum.

Pribram, K. H., & McGuinness, D. (1975). Arousal, activation, and effort in the control of attention. *Psychological Review, 82*, 116-149.

Pribram, K. H., & McGuinness, D. (1992). Attention and para-attentional processing: Event-related brain potentials as tests of a model. *Annals of the New York Academy of Sciences, 658*, 65-92.

Price, D. D. (1988). *Psychological and neural mechanisms of pain.* New York: Raven.

Priebe, F. A., & Wallace, B. (1986). Hypnotic susceptibility, imaging ability and the detection of embedded objects. *International Journal of Clinical and Experimental Hypnosis, 34*, 320-329.

Prince, M. (1910). The subconscious—Part 5. In H. Munsterberg, T. Ribot, P. Janet, J. Jastrow, B. Hart, & M. Prince (Eds.), *Subconscious phenomena* (pp. 71-101). Boston: Gorham.

Raichle, M. E. (1990). Exploring the mind with dynamic imaging. *Seminar in Neurosciences*, 2, 307-315.

Risberg, J. (1986). Regional cerebral blood flow in neuropsychology. *Neuropsychologia, 24*, 135-140.

Roche, S. M., & McConkey, K. M. (1990). Absorption: Nature, assessment, and correlates. *Journal of Personality and Social Psychology, 59*, 91-101.

Roland, P. (1992). Cortical representation of pain. *Trends in Neurosciences, 15*, 3-5.

Sabourin, M. E. Cutcomb, S. D., Crawford, H. J., & Pribram, K. (1990). EEG correlates of hypnotic susceptibility and hypnotic trance: Spectral analysis and coherence. *International Journal of Psychophysiology, 10*, 125-142.

Sack, S. A., & Rice, C. E. (1974). Selectivity, resistance to distraction and shifting as three attentional factors. *Psychological Reports, 34*, 1003-1012.

Saletu, B. (1987). Brain function during hypnosis, acupuncture and transcendental meditation. In B. Taneli, C. Perris, & D. Kemali (Eds.), *Advances in biological psychiatry:*

Neurophysiological correlates of relaxation and psychopathology (Vol. 16, pp. 18-20). Basel: Karger.

Schacter, D. L. (1977). EEG theta waves and psychological phenomena: A review and analysis. *Biological Psychology, 5*, 47-82.

Shallice, T. (1988). *From neuropsychology to mental structure*. Cambridge, England: Cambridge University Press.

Sharev, U., & Tal, M. (1989). Masseter inhibitory periods and sensations evoked by electrical tooth-pulp stimulation in subjects under hypnotic anesthesia. *Brain Research, 479*, 247-254.

Sheehan, P. W., Donovan, P., & MacLeod, C. M. (1988). Strategy manipulation and the Stroop effect in hypnosis. *Journal of Abnormal Psychology, 97*, 455-460.

Shiffrin, R. M., & Schneider, W. (1977). Controlled and automatic human information processing. II. Perceptual learning, automatic attending and a general theory. *Psychological Review, 84*, 127-190.

Skinner, B. F. (1989). The origins of cognitive thought. *American Psychologist, 44*, 13-18.

Skinner, J. E., & Yingling, C. D. (1977). Central gating mechanisms that regulate event-related potentials and behavior: A neural model for attention. In J. E. Desmedt (Ed.), *Attention, voluntary contraction and event-related cerebral potentials. Progress in clinical neurophysiology* (Vol. 1, pp. 28-68). Basel: Karger.

Spiegel, D., Bierre, P., & Rootenberg, J. (1989). Hypnotic alteration of somatosensory perception. *American Journal of Psychiatry, 146*, 749-754.

Stowell, H. (1984). Event related brain potentials and human pain: A first objective overview. *International Journal of Psychophysiology, 1*, 137-151.

Stuss, D. T., & Benson, D. F. (1986). *The frontal lobes*. New York: Raven.

Talbot, J. D., Marrett, S., Evans, A. C., Meyer, E., Bushnell, M. C., & Duncan, G. H. (1991). Multiple representations of pain in human cerebral cortex. *Science, 251*, 1355-1358.

Taneli, B., & Krahne, W. (1987). EEG changes of transcendental meditation practitioners. *Advances in biological psychiatry: Neurophysiological correlates of relaxation and psychopathology* (Vol. 16, pp. 41-71). Basel: Karger.

Tebecis, A. K., Provins, K. A., Farnbach, R. W., & Pentony, P. (1975). Hypnosis and the EEG: A quantitative investigation. *Journal of Nervous and Mental Disease, 161*, 1-17.

Tellegen, A. (1982). *Brief manual for the Multidimensional Personality Questionnaire*. Unpublished manuscript, University of Minnesota, Department of Psychology, Minneapolis.

Tellegen, A., & Atkinson, C. (1974). Openness to absorbing and self-altering experiences ("absorption"), a trait related to hypnotic susceptibility. *Journal of Abnormal Psychology, 83*, 268-277.

Treisman, A. (1964). Verbal cues, language and meaning in selective attention. *American Journal of Psychology, 77*, 205-219.

Ulett, G. A., Akpinar, S., & Itil, T. M. (1972). Quantitative EEG analysis during hypnosis. *Electroencephalography and Clinical Neurophysiology, 33*, 361-368.

Vogel, W., Broverman, D. M., & Klaiber, E. L. (1968). EEG and mental abilities. *Electroencephalography and Clinical Neurophysiology, 24*, 166-174.

Wallace, B. (1986). Latency and frequency reports to the Necker Cube illusion: Effects of hypnotic susceptibility and mental arithmetic. *Journal of General Psychology, 113*, 187-194.

Wallace, B. (1988). Hypnotic susceptibility, visual distraction, and reports of Necker Cube apparent reversals. *Journal of General Psychology, 115*, 389-396.

Wallace, B. (1990). Imagery vividness, hypnotic susceptibility, and the perception of fragmented stimuli. *Journal of Personality and Social Psychology, 58*, 354-359.

Wallace, B., & Garrett, J. B. (1973). Hypnotic susceptibility and autokinetic movement frequency. *Perceptual and Motor Skills, 36*, 1054.

Wallace, B., Garrett, J. B., & Anstadt, S. P. (1974). Hypnotic susceptibility, suggestion, and reports of autokinetic movement. *American Journal of Psychology, 87*, 117-123.

Wallace, B., Knight, T. A., & Garrett, J. B. (1976). Hypnotic susceptibility and frequency reports to illusory stimuli. *Journal of Abnormal Psychology, 85*, 558-563.

Wallace, B., & Patterson, S. L. (1984). Hypnotic susceptibility and performance on various attention-specific cognitive tasks. *Journal of Personality and Social Psychology, 47*, 175-181.

Walter, H. (1992). *Hypnose: Theorien, neurophysiologische Korrelate und praktische Hinweise zur Hypnosetherapie* [*Hypnosis: Theories, neurophysiological correlations and practical tips regarding hypnotherapy*]. Stuttgart, Germany: Georg Thieme Verlag.

Weitzenhoffer, A. M., & Hilgard, E. R. (1962). *Stanford Hypnotic Susceptibility Scale, Form C*. Palo Alto, CA: Consulting Psychologists Press.

Yamamoto, S., & Matsuoka, S. (1990). Topographic EEG study of visual display terminal (VDT) performance with special reference to frontal midline theta waves. *Brain Topography, 2*, 257-267.

Yanchar, R. J. (1983). *Hypnotic susceptibility and its relation to selective and divided attention*. Unpublished doctoral dissertation, Bowling Green State University, Bowling Green, OH.

Yanchar, R. J. (1984, October). *Hypnotic susceptibility and its relation to selective and divided attention*. Paper presented at the 36th Annual Scientific Meeting of The Society for Clinical and Experimental Hypnosis, San Antonio, TX.

Gehirnsdynamik und Hypnose: Aufmerksamkeits- und Unaufmerksamkeitsprozesse

Helen J. Crawford

Abstrakt: Diese Arbeit gibt einen Überblick über neuere Forschungsbefunde und damit ein entfaltendes, neuropsychophysiologisches Modell der Hypnose erweiternd (Crawford, 1989; Crawford & Gruzelier, 1992), das die Meinung unterstützt, daβ hoch hypnotisierbare Personen (die Hohen) stärkere aufmerksamkeitsfilternde Fähigkeiten besitzen als die schwach hypnotisierbaren Personen und daβ diese Unterschiede in der unterliegenden Gehirnsdynamik reflektiert werden. Der verhaltensmäβige, kognitive und neurophysiologische Nachweis wird untersucht, der andeutet, daβ die Hohen ihre Aufmerksamkeit besser fokussieren und aufrechterhalten können sowie auch unaufmerksamer auf irrelevante Stimuli in der Umgebung reagieren können. Es wird vorgeschlagen, daβ Hypnose ein Zustand der verstärkten Aufmerksamkeit ist, der ein Zwischenspiel zwischen kortikaler und subkortikaler Gehirnsdynamik während des Erlebens von dissoziierten, hypnotischen Phänomenen, wie hypnotische Analgesie, darstellt. Eine Sammlung von Forschungsbefunden ist untersucht, die andeutet, daβ Aufmerksamkeits- wie auch Unaufmerksamkeitsprozesse im Erleben der Hypnose und der hypnotischen Phänomene wichtig sind. Befunde aus Studien der elektrokortikalen Aktivität, geschehnisbezogen hervorgerufenen Potentialen und regionaler, zerebraler Blutzufuhr während des Wachzustandes und der Hypnose werden geboten, um anzudeuten, daβ diese Aufmerksamkeitsunterschiede in unterliegenden, neurophysiologischen Unterschieden im weiten fronto-limbischen Aufmerksamkeitssystem reflektiert sind.

Dynamiques cérébrales et hypnose: processus attentionnels et désattentionnels

Helen J. Crawford

Résumé: Cette étude examine les récentes découvertes, mettant de l'avant un modèle neuropsychophysiologique de l'hypnose (Crawford, 1989; Crawford &

Gruzelier, 1992), qui soutient le point vue que les individus à suggestibilité élevée possèdent des capacités de filtrage attentionnel plus élevées que n'en possèdent les individus à suggestibilité faible, et que ces différences sont reflétées dans les dynamiques cérébrales sous-jacentes. Les évidences béhaviorales, cognitives et neurophysiologiques revues suggèrent que les sujets fortement hypnotisables peuvent tout à la fois mieux se concentrer et maintenir leur attention aussi bien que de ne pas prêter attention aux stimuli non pertinents de l'environnement. Il est proposé que l'hypnose est un état d'attention accru qui active un processus interactionnel entre les dynamiques cérébrales corticales et sous-corticales durant l'expérience du phénomène de dissociation hypnotique telle l'analgésie hypnotique. Les nombreuses études recensées suggèrent que les deux processus, attentionel et désattentionel, sont importants dans l'expérience de l'hypnose et du phénomène hypnotique. Les résultats des études sur l'activité électrocorticale, les potentiels évoqués et le flot cérébral régional durant l'éveil et l'hypnose sont présentés pour suggérer que ces différences attentionelles sont reflétées dans les différences neurophysiologiques sous-jacentes au niveau du système d'attention fronto-limbique.

Dinámica cerebral e hipnosis: procesos de atención y distracción

Helen J. Crawford

Resumen: Este trabajo revisa recientes hallazgos de investigaciones que despliegan un modelo neurofisiológico desarrollado de la hipnosis (Crawford, 1989; Crawford y Gruzelier, 1992). Este modelo sostiene la idea que personas altamente hipnotizables poseen capacidades de filtrado de la atención más fuertes que aquellas personas de baja hipnotizabilidad, y que estas diferencias están reflejadas en la dinámica cerebral subyacente. Se revisaron evidencias conductuales, cognitivas y neurofisiológicas que sugieren que los sujetos altamente hipnotizables pueden focalizar y sostener su atención así como desatender estímulos irrelevantes del medio ambiente. Se propone que la hipnosis es un estado de atención incrementada que activa un interjuego entre la dinámica cerebral del fenómeno hipnótico, tal como la analgesia hipnótica. Se revisó un cuerpo de investigación que sugiere que los procesos de atención y de distracción son importantes en la experiencia del fenómeno hipnótico y de la hipnosis. Hallazgos provenientes de estudios de actividad electrocortical, de potenciales evocados y de flujo sanguíneo cerebral regional durante la vigilia y la hipnosis fueron presentados para indicar que estas diferencias atencionales están reflejadas en las diferencias neurofisiológicas subyacentes en el lejano sistema fronto-límbico de la atención.

[22]

Pain Affect Encoded in Human Anterior Cingulate But Not Somatosensory Cortex

Pierre Rainville, Gary H. Duncan, Donald D. Price, Benoît Carrier, M. Catherine Bushnell*

Recent evidence demonstrating multiple regions of human cerebral cortex activated by pain has prompted speculation about their individual contributions to this complex experience. To differentiate cortical areas involved in pain affect, hypnotic suggestions were used to alter selectively the unpleasantness of noxious stimuli, without changing the perceived intensity. Positron emission tomography revealed significant changes in pain-evoked activity within anterior cingulate cortex, consistent with the encoding of perceived unpleasantness, whereas primary somatosensory cortex activation was unaltered. These findings provide direct experimental evidence in humans linking frontal-lobe limbic activity with pain affect, as originally suggested by early clinical lesion studies.

Affective aspects of pain, such as perceived unpleasantness, have been classically considered to be distinct from the simple sensory dimensions of pain, which include the perception of location, quality, and intensity of noxious stimulation (*1*). Largely on the basis of indirect evidence, separate neuronal pathways have been postulated to underlie these different aspects of the pain experience (*2*). For example, involvement of frontal lobe regions, particularly the anterior cingulate cortex (ACC), in pain affect is suggested by clinical reports that patients with frontal lobotomies or cingulotomies sometimes still feel pain but report it as less distressing or bothersome (*3*). On the other hand, primary and secondary somatosensory cortices (SI and SII) have been considered plausible candidates for the processing of sensory-discriminative aspects of pain, on the basis of their anatomical connections to subcortical and spinal regions, which encode discriminative properties of somatosensory stimuli (*4*). Recent neuroimaging studies in humans documented pain-related activation in limbic sites, such as ACC and rostral insula (IC), and in the primary sensory regions SI and SII (*5*). In addition, anatomical and electrophysiological data show that these regions receive direct nociceptive input in the monkey (*6*). However, the extent to which these different cortical structures contribute to specific dimensions of the human pain experience is largely unknown and untested.

In the present study we used hypnosis as a cognitive tool to reveal possible cerebral mechanisms of pain affect in normal human volunteers. A perceptual dissociation of sensory and affective aspects of the pain experience was achieved with hypnotic suggestions to both increase and decrease pain unpleasantness, without changing the perceived intensity of the pain sensations (*7*).

Cerebral cortical activity related to this perceptual dissociation was measured by positron emission tomography (PET) (8).

PET scans were conducted during conditions of alert control, hypnosis control, and hypnotic suggestion for increased unpleasantness (↑UNP) or decreased unpleasantness (↓UNP) (9). During each scan tonic stimuli were presented to the left hand by passive immersion in "neutral" (35°C) or "painfully hot" (47°C) water (*10*). After each scan, the perceived intensity and unpleasantness of the stimulation were rated by the participant (*11*).

Regional cerebral blood flow (rCBF) was measured with three-dimensional high-resolution PET after $H_2{}^{15}O$ bolus injection (*12*). Each participant also received a high-resolution magnetic resonance imaging (MRI) anatomical brain scan that was used for alignment and transformation of PET volumes into the Talairach coordinate system (*13*). To obtain volumes of pain-related changes in rCBF for each participant, we subtracted normalized PET data recorded during the "neutral" condition from those of the "painfully hot" condition. Resulting volumes of pain-related changes in rCBF were averaged across sessions, and statistical activation maps were derived on the basis of the methods of Worsley *et al.* (*14*). Directed searches of rCBF increases were conducted on right (contralateral to stimulus) SI, SII, ACC, and IC to confirm pain-related activation of these structures and to test the hypothesis that changes in pain unpleasantness modulate activity only within limbic regions thought to be involved in affective processes. The threshold for statistical significance was corrected for multiple comparisons (*15*).

Results of "painfully hot" versus "neutral" subtractions from scans taken during the alert control condition support previous findings of significant pain-related activations in SI, SII, IC, and ACC (Table 1). After hypnotic induction, but before suggestions of increased or decreased unpleasantness, painful heat again activated these four cortical areas (Table 1), indicating little influence of hypnotic induction itself on pain-related activation. Similarly, the hypnotic induction had no significant effect on psychophysical ratings of either pain intensity or unpleasantness (alert control compared with hypnosis control: intensity, 77.6 ± 14.7 and 75.0 ± 14.0, and unpleasantness, 61.4 ± 28.8 and 54.8 ± 25.8, respectively).

Hypnotic suggestions for increased or decreased unpleasantness, on the other hand, altered both the perception of pain affect and the activation within some but not all of these pain-related cortical regions. A comparison of rCBF changes between hypnotic suggestion and hypnosis control conditions revealed significant pain-related activations in SI, ACC, and IC, during both ↑UNP and ↓UNP conditions. Within the vicinity of SII, however, no significant pain-evoked activity was observed in either the ↑UNP or ↓UNP conditions (Table 1). One possible explanation for this absence of pain-evoked activity in SII is that the mental effort or attention demanded by these suggestions may suppress such activation. Alternatively, there may have been an habituation of SII activity with repeated stimulation.

The effectiveness of hypnotic suggestions in selectively altering pain affect is demonstrated by the significant difference observed only in the participants' ratings of unpleasantness during the ↑UNP and ↓UNP conditions [unpleasantness: 81.4 ± 14.6 and 45.0 ± 25.8, respectively, analysis of variance (ANOVA) $P < 0.001$; intensity: 78.0 ± 14.6 and 71.2 ± 18.2, respectively, statistically not significant]. In parallel with this modulation in pain affect, direct volume-of-interest (VOI) comparisons (*16*) of the three pain sites activated during the hypnotic suggestion conditions revealed significantly greater activation during ↑UNP scans, compared with that observed during ↓UNP, only in ACC ($P < 0.02$; see Fig. 1). In SI, pain-related rCBF was actually lower (nonsignificantly) in the ↑UNP condition than in the ↓UNP condition, indicating no tendency for increased activation in this area related to increased unpleasantness.

To test the strength of the relation between pain affect and activation within the ACC, we did regression analyses of unpleasantness ratings and rCBF levels across all participants and all scans taken during the hypnotic suggestion condition for each pain activation site. After removing effects due to interperson variability, perceived intensity, and scan session, the residual variance in rCBF [analysis of covariance (ANCOVA)] demonstrates that only activation levels

Table 1. Pain-related activation sites within SI, SII, ACC, and IC. Coordinates are given in Talairach space (*13*); Lateral, anterior, and superior are relative to midline, anterior commisure, and commissural line, respectively (positive values are right, anterior, and superior). A *t* statistic of 2.55 is equivalent to $P = 0.05$ (*15*).

Region	Stereotaxic coordinates (mm)			
	Lateral	Anterior	Superior	
		Alert control		
SI	+42	−18	+40	3.01
SII	+44	−23	+20	4.18
ACC	+1	+5	+36	4.04
IC	+42	−6	+12	3.61
		Hypnosis control		
SI	+39	−21	+59	3.69
SII	+40	−18	+20	2.65
ACC	−8	−4	+34	3.86
	+7	+18	+32	2.52*
	+16	+18	+36	3.34
IC	+31	+10	+12	3.77
	+35	+2	+1	4.16
		Increased unpleasantness (↑UNP)		
SI	+31	−28	+57	3.84
SII	No peak with $t > 2.50$			
ACC	+3	+20	+30	6.11
IC	+34	+22	0	4.50
		Decreased unpleasantness (↓UNP)		
SI	+34	−19	+56	4.61
SII	No peak with $t > 2.50$			
ACC	−1	+25	+29	4.42
	+13	+18	+36	3.64
IC	+38	+8	+3	4.66

*$P = 0.053$

P. Rainville, Département de Psychologie and Centre de Recherche en Sciences Neurologiques, Université de Montréal, Montréal, Québec, Canada H3C 3J7, and McConnell Brain Imaging Center, Montreal Neurological Institute, Montréal, Québec, Canada H3A 2B4.
G. H. Duncan, Département de Stomatologie, Faculté de Médecine Dentaire, and Centre de Recherche en Sciences Neurologiques, Université de Montréal, Montréal, Québec, Canada H3C 3J7, and McConnell Brain Imaging Center, Montreal Neurological Institute, Montréal, Québec, Canada.
D. D. Price, Department of Anesthesiology, Medical College of Virginia, Richmond, VA 23298, USA.
B. Carrier, Département de Stomatologie, Faculté de Médecine Dentaire, Université de Montréal, Montréal, Québec, Canada H3C 3J7.
M. C. Bushnell, Centre de Recherche en Sciences Neurologiques, Université de Montréal, Montréal, Québec, Canada H3C 3J7, McConnell Brain Imaging Center, Montreal Neurological Institute, Montréal, Québec, Canada, and Department of Anesthesiology, McGill University, Montréal, Québec, Canada H3A 1A1.
*To whom correspondence should be addressed. E-mail: bushnellc@medcor.mcgill ca

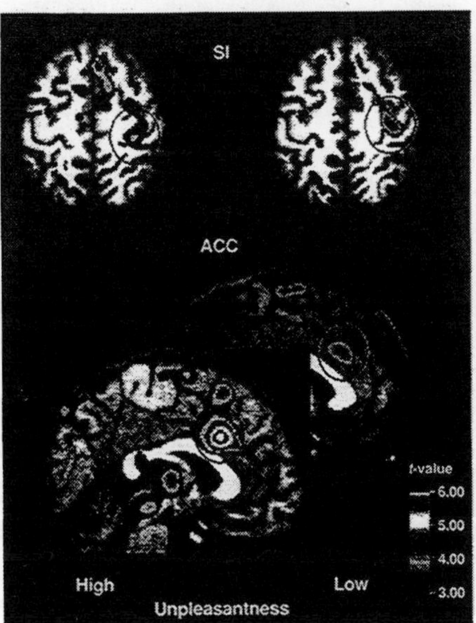

Fig. 1. Changes in pain-related activity associated with hypnotic suggestions of high and low unpleasantness (left and right images, respectively) are revealed by subtracting PET data recorded during the neutral/hypnosis control condition from those of the painfully hot/↑UNP and painfully hot/↓UNP conditions. PET data, averaged across 11 experimental sessions, are illustrated against an MRI from one person; horizontal and saggital slices through SI and ACC, respectively, are centered at the activation peaks observed during the relevant suggestion conditions; red circles indicate the location and size of VOIs used to analyze activation levels across the two conditions (*16*).

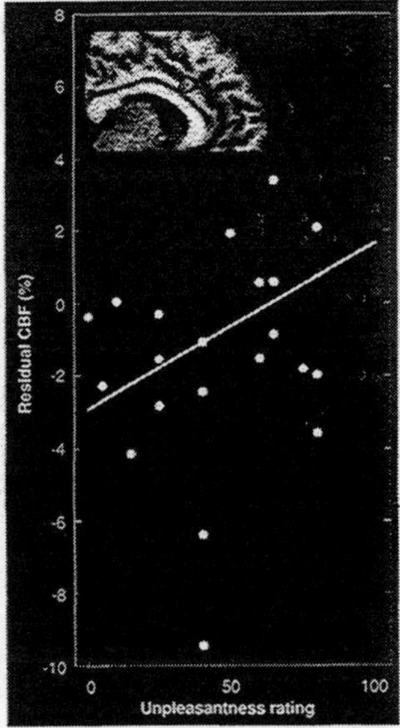

Fig. 2. Activation levels (as measured by residual rCBF) observed within the ACC during high (red) and low (yellow) unpleasantness conditions are significantly correlated with ratings of pain unpleasantness (ANCOVA: $r = 0.42$, $P = 0.005$). The coordinates of this r-value peak (inset: saggital section of PET regression volume—lateral, +7; anterior, +20; superior, +29) lie precisely within the region of ACC that was activated in both ↑UNP and ↓UNP conditions (see Fig. 1 and Table 1). Line shows linear best fit.

within the ACC (Fig. 2) are consistent with the encoding of the perceived unpleasantness of these noxious stimuli (ACC: Pearson's correlation coefficient, $r_s = 0.419$, $P = 0.005$; IC: $r = 0.245$, $P = 0.134$; SI: $r = -0.224$, $P = 0.149$).

These results demonstrate a modulation of pain-related activity in ACC that closely parallels a selective change in the perceived unpleasantness of painful stimuli. The absence of changes in the sensory component of pain perception and the lack of similar modulation within other pain-related cortical structures argue for a significant involvement of the ACC in the affective component of pain. Such findings support earlier proposals that the anterior cingulate gyrus is integrally involved in pain and emotions (*3*, *5*, *6*), but our findings go beyond these general ideas by providing direct evidence of a specific encoding of pain unpleasantness in the ACC.

We propose that pain-related activation in ACC reflects a nociceptive input from a highly modifiable pain pathway (*17*), and that the level of pain-evoked ACC activation is determinant in the individual's emotional and behavioral reactions to pain. The proximity of the nociceptive, motor, and attentional regions of ACC (*18*) suggests possible local interconnections that might allow the output of the ACC pain area to command immediate behavioral reactions. Similarly, the ACC pain area might participate in the substantial interconnections between the ACC and the "fight or flight" regions of the midbrain periaqueducal gray matter (*19*).

The anatomical connections between ACC, IC, SI, and SII (*20*) suggest that these regions do not function independently in encoding different aspects of pain but are highly interactive. Such interactions are reflected in the experiences of pain itself. For example, pain intensity, location, and quality (sensory features) are major factors in determining unpleasantness (*21*). Nevertheless, despite these associations, there appears to be at least a partial segregation of function between pain affect and sensation, with ACC activity possibly reflecting the emotional experience that provokes our reactions to pain.

REFERENCES AND NOTES

1. R. Melzack and K. L. Casey, in *The Skin Senses*, D. R. Kenshalo, Ed. (Thomas, Springfield, IL, 1968), pp. 423–443.
2. H. L. Fields, *Pain* (McGraw-Hill, New York, 1987).
3. E. L. Foltz and E. W. White, *J. Neurosurg.* **19**, 89 (1962); *Int. J. Neurol.* **6**, 353 (1968); R. W. Hurt and H. T. Ballantine Jr., *Clin. Neurosurg.* **21**, 334 (1973); S. Corkin and N. Hebben, *Pain* (suppl. 1) 150 (1981).
4. S. I. Gingold, J. D. Greenspan, A. V. Apkarian, *J. Comp. Neurol.* **308**, 467 (1991); R. T. Stevens, S. M. London, A V. Apkarian, *Brain Res.* **631**, 241 (1993).
5. J. D. Talbot *et al.*, *Science* **251**, 1355 (1991); A. K. P. Jones, W. D. Brown, K. J. Friston, L. Y. Qi, R. S. J. Frackowiak, *Proc. R. Soc. London Ser. B* **244**, 39 (1991); K. L. Casey *et al.*, *J. Neurophysiol.* **71**, 802 (1994); R. C Coghill *et al.*, *J. Neurosci.* **14**, 4095 (1994).
6. B. A. Vogt, D. L Rosene, D. N. Pandya, *Science* **204**, 205 (1979); R. W. Sikes and B. A. Vogt, *J Neurophysiol.* **68**, 1720 (1992); J. O. Dostrovsky and A. D. Craig, *Soc. Neurosci. Abstr.* **22**, 111 (abstr. 51.16) (1996); A. D. Craig and E.-T. Zhang, *ibid.*, (abstr. 51.18); E. Rausell and E. G. Jones, *J. Neurosci.* **11**, 226 (1991); D. R. Kenshalo Jr., E. H. Chudler, F. Anton, R. Dubner, *Brain Res.* **454**, 378 (1988).
7. Suggestions for increased and decreased unpleasantness were adapted from B. D. Kiernan, J. R. Dane, L H. Phillips, D. D. Price, *Pain* **60**, 39 (1995), validated for separating sensory and affective pain perception [B. Carrier, P. Rainville, G. H. Duncan, M C Bushnell, in abstracts of the *Eighth World Congress on Pain*, International Association for the Study of Pain, Vancouver, British Columbia, Canada, 17 to 22 August 1996 (IASP Press, Seattle, WA, 1996), abstr. 132, p. 478], and confirmed in the individuals chosen for these imaging experiments.
8. A preliminary report has appeared as an abstract [P. Rainville, G. H. Duncan, D. D. Price, M. C Bushnell, *Soc. Neurosci Abstr.* **22**, 117 (1996)].
9. Before the experiment a group of volunteers were tested with the noxious stimuli and hypnotic induction and suggestion procedures. From that group three female and five male participants, 19 to 53

years in age, who displayed moderate to high hypnotic suggestibility (Stanford Suggestibility Scale Form A) and robust modulation of pain unpleasantness were chosen for the PET study Experimental sessions (12 scans) were administered once to each of five participants and twice to three other participants. Because of possible residual effects of hypnotic suggestions, the alert control conditions were always presented first, followed by hypnotic control (without suggestions of altered perception), and finally suggestions for increased (↑UNP) or decreased (↓UNP) unpleasantness "Neutral" (35°C) and "painfully hot" (46 5° to 47.5°C) stimuli were counterbalanced across individuals within the alert and hypnotic control states, as were the blocks of two ↑UNP and two ↓UNP scans

10 This 75-s hand immersion stimulus was chosen on the basis of our previous findings that tonic pain has a stronger affective component than phasic pain [P Rainville, J S. Feine, M. C Bushnell, G H Duncan, *Somatosens. Mot Res.* **9**, 265 (1992)]. Temperatures were adjusted individually to obtain pain ratings of 40 to 80 on a scale of 0 to 100 [see (*11*)], resulting temperatures ranged from 46 5° to 47 5°C

11. Participants rated pain intensity and unpleasantness using separate numerical scales of 0 to 100 The intensity scale endpoints were "no burning, pricking, stinging sensation," the most frequently chosen words describing the sensory aspect of heat pain in an independent study [C Morin, L. TenBokum, M C Bushnell, *Soc. Neurosci. Abstr.* **20**, 127 (1994)], and "extremely intense sensation." The unpleasantness scale endpoints were "not at all unpleasant" and "extremely unpleasant." To avoid ceiling effects, we instructed participants that responses could surpass 100 if larger values were needed to describe sensations relative to those previously rated.

12 PET data (63 slices) were acquired with a Siemens ECAT HR+ camera Participants lay immobile in the scanner, eyes closed, with inserted earphones connected to a microphone through which they received instructions or hypnotic suggestions before each scan Stimulus onset was simultaneous with bolus injection (10 mCu of $H_2{}^{15}O$, half-life of 123 s, without arterial blood sampling) to synchronize the increase in pain sensation with brain uptake of $H_2{}^{15}O$. Scans began 15 s after the injection, and data were collected in two sequential frames of 40 and 20 s (data presented are derived from the 40-s frame, which yielded the better signal-to-noise ratio) Scans were separated by 12 to 15 min to allow tracer decay to background levels.

13 MRI scans (160 contiguous 1-mm-thick slices) were acquired on a Philips 1.5T Gyroscan system. Each participant's PET and MRI volumes were transformed into the Talairach coordinate system [J. Talairach and P. Tournoux, *Co-Planar Stereotaxic Atlas of the Human Brain* (Thieme, New York, 1988)] by using the automated methods of D. L Collins, P Neelin, T. M. Peters, and A C Evans, [*J Comput Assisted Tomogr.* **18**, 192 (1994)]. PET and MRI volumes were resampled to obtain voxels of 1.34 mm by 1 72 mm by 1.50 mm in the x, y, and z planes, respectively.

14 K J Worsley, A C Evans, S Marrett, P Neelin, *J Cereb Blood Flow Metab.* **12**. 900 (1992)

15. With four target foci, the search volume of 4 resels yields a threshold for statistical significance of t = 2.55 ($P < 0\ 05$, one-tailed t-test corrected for multiple comparisons).

16. VOIs were centered independently at the point of maximum pain-related increase in rCBF within each of the three pain sites identified in the two comparison conditions This procedure ensured that the maximum activation observed in ↑UNP was directly compared with the corresponding point of maximum activation obtained in ↓UNP To further verify the robustness of these comparisons, we tested different VOI radii (from 10 to 20 mm) for each structure, with similar results for all values.

17. In monkeys, responses of single neurons probably in the spino-thalamo-ACC pathway are modulated by cognitive factors that change both the perception of and reaction to pain [M C. Bushnell and G H Duncan, *Exp. Brain Res.* **78**, 415 (1989), ———, R Dubner, L F He, *J Neurophysiol* **52**, 170 (1984)]

18 M Corbetta, F M Miezin, S. Dobmeyer, G L Shulman, S E. Petersen, *J. Neurosci* **11**, 2383 (1991), J. V. Pardo, P J Pardo, K W Janer, M E. Raichle, *Proc. Natl. Acad. Sci. U S A.* **87**, 256 (1990), T. Paus, M. Petrides, A. C. Evans, E. Meyer, *J. Neurophysiol.* **70**, 453 (1993), T. Paus *et al.*, *Cereb. Cortex* **6**, 207 (1996), N Picard and P. L Strick, *ibid.*, p. 342.

19. R Bandler and M T. Shipley, *Trends Neurosci* **17** (no 9), 379 (1994).

20. D. P. Friedman, A. E Murray, J B O'Neill, M Mishkin, *J. Comp. Neurol.* **252**, 323 (1986); E J. Mufson and M -M Mesulam, *ibid.* **212**, 23 (1982), B. A. Vogt and D N Pandya, *ibid* **262**, 271 (1987)

21. D. D. Price, *Psychological and Neural Mechanisms of Pain* (Raven, New York, 1988)

14 April 197; accepted 24 June 1997

[23]

A WORKING MODEL OF THE NEUROPHYSIOLOGY OF HYPNOSIS: A REVIEW OF EVIDENCE

John Gruzelier

Imperial College of Science, Technology and Medicine, London, UK

Abstract

Neuropsychophysiological evidence is reviewed testing a three-stage, top-down working model of the traditional hypnotic relaxation induction involving: (1) a thalamocortical attentional network engaging a left frontolimbic focused attention control system underpinning sensory fixation and concentration on the induction; (2) instatement of frontolimbic inhibitory systems through suggestions of tiredness at fixation and relaxation whereby anterior executive functions are suspended and directed by the induction; (3) engagement of right-sided temporoposterior functions through passive imagery and dreaming. A selectivity of action in high susceptibles was a hallmark of the studies. Increased Stroop interference coincided with maintenance of error detection and abolition of error evaluation potentials, interpreted as dissociation of cognitive and affective executive systems of the anterior cingulate. Verbal, category and design fluency tasks were dissociated with hypnosis centring on left anterior processes as seen in left lateral and medial reduced EEG connectivity. Limbic modulated electrodermal orienting responses and frontal modulated mismatch negativity waves were inhibited. Asymmetries in electrodermal and electrocortical responses to tones shifted to favour the right hemisphere, an asymmetry also seen in visual sensitivity. Haptic processing and visual sensitivity disclosed more distributed changes in medium susceptibles, while low susceptibles were characterized by poorer attentional functions at baseline and improvements through the induction.

Key words: EEG, ERPs, attention laterality, frontal limbic cingulate

Introduction

This article provides a review of experiments, thematically rather than chronologically structured, that were carried out in the Charing Cross laboratory of Cognitive Neuroscience with the aim of understanding the neuropsychophysiological basis of hypnosis. Hypnosis was defined operationally on the basis of the traditional relaxation procedure, which began with eye fixation, suggestions of relaxation and eye closure, and was followed by imagery associated with deep relaxation and a dream. This was applied in all experiments except one where the active-alert procedure (Bányai and Hilgard, 1976) was compared. During the induction there were behavioural challenges to assess depth of hypnosis, and at the end questions about memory for the induction, a post hypnotic suggestion and subjective ratings. The purpose was to unravel some of the changes in brain activity that accompany the hypnotic induction in both high and low susceptible individuals, and features that may differentiate them in the baseline state.

4 *Gruzelier*

The history of localizing neurophysiological mechanisms in hypnosis began by likening hypnosis to sleep. Pavlov demonstrated the existence of hypnosis in his conditioned reflex studies in dogs and attributed this to a partial and spreading inhibition of the cortex, less extensive than occurs in sleep, though Heidenhain had reasoned earlier that more than the cortex was involved because animals did not behave as if they were decorticate (Windholz, 1996). Although sleep became an increasingly popular analogy, to date electroencephalographic (EEG) studies have not found similarities between hypnosis and sleep (for a review see Crawford and Gruzelier, 1992). At the same time sleep can be induced by instructions of hypnosis, but conventional procedures stop short of sleep induction. Hernandez-Peon (1977) proposed that hypnosis was closer to wakefulness than sleep, involving alterations in both consciousness and executive functions, which he localized to the midbrain, pons and medulla. Nevertheless, depending on the nature of the induction, dream-like features are close to the hypnotic experience of many high susceptibles.

Recordings from intracranial electrodes in epileptic patients have disclosed the importance of limbic structures in hypnosis. Craiselneck, McCranie and Jenkins (1956) reported anecdotally that hypnosis was terminated each time the hippocampus was electrically stimulated. De Benedittis and Sironi (1986) demonstrated in a high hypnotizable that there was a reduction in interictal focal abnormalities in the hippocampus during hypnosis and an increase in alpha activity. In a second patient they concluded that hypnosis was associated with functional inhibition of the amygdala, because stimulation of the amygdala aroused the patient from hypnosis unlike stimulation of the adjacent and reciprocally connected hippocampus. Electrical activity in the amygdala became synchronized with hypnosis whereas activity in the hippocampus became desynchronized (De Benedittis and Sironi, 1988).

In the 1960s parallels were drawn between hypnosis and right hemispheric processing and high hypnotic susceptibles were assumed to be characterized by right hemisphericity. This point of view has been popularized and has been found to be important in the clinical use of hypnosis (Pedersen, 1984). Aside from evidence from cognitive studies with putative hemisphere specific tasks, there were also neuropsychophysiological measures which took into account brain anatomy such as EEG, dichotic listening and conjugate lateral eye movements (Crawford and Gruzelier, 1992). Experimental evidence was, however, conflictual, but the methodologies of many studies were questionable (Gruzelier, 1988). Methods of inducing hypnosis were various and often poorly described. Often there was a failure to distinguish between high and low susceptibles or to attribute changes in low susceptibles that were absent in high susceptibles to the hypnotic process. Seldom was evidence cited of test-retest reliability, or of replication, or of validation of hypnotic level during the experimental procedure.

In integrating the results of a decade ago a three-stage working model of the induction process was proposed (Gruzelier, 1988, 1990).

- Stage I: The initial instructions of fixating on a small object and listening to the hypnostist's voice was posited to involve an attentional network including thalamocortical systems and parietofrontal connections with engagement of a left anterior focused attention control system. This underpins the focused, selective attention inherent in fixation and listening to the hypnotist's voice, processes that together require left hemispheric frontotemporal processing.
- Stage II: The first stage is then replaced by eye closure, suggestions of fatigue at continued fixation, and tiredness together with deep relaxation. This sets in

motion frontolimbic inhibitory processes underpinning the suspension of reality testing and critical evaluation, and the handing over of executive and planning functions to the hypnotist; the 'letting go' component of the hypnotic induction.

- Stage III: The third stage involves instructions of relaxed, passive imagery leading to a redistribution of functional activity and an augmentation of posterior cortical activity, particularly of the right hemisphere in high susceptibles. Simplifying the verbal content of the induction message may also facilitate right hemispheric processing, as does emphasizing past experience and emotion. In contrast, low susceptibles fail to show engagement of left frontal attentional control mechanisms, or if there is focal attentional engagement, low susceptibles fail to undergo the inhibitory, letting go process. This working model will serve to structure the review of findings. Here emphasis will be placed on the cognitive neuroscience of hypnosis; implications for socio-cognitive approaches will be found in a commentary (Gruzelier, 1998) on a theoretical paper by Wagstaff (1998).

Thalamo-frontal-limbic attentional processes

Electrodermal orienting, habituation, sensitization and tonic reactivity

We first investigated the basic attentional processes of orienting, which represents focusing of attention, and of habituation with stimulus repetition, which allows attention to be redirected, and which involve modulation by the limbic system, in particular the amygdala and hippocampus (e.g. Pribram and McGuinness, 1975; Gray, 1982). The electrodermal response was chosen because among physiological measures it has the advantage of indexing sympathetic nervous system activity unconfounded by competing parasympathetic influences. Using a standardized tone orienting and habituation paradigm (Gruzelier and Venables, 1972) the effects of hypnosis on orienting responses to tones that were interspersed with the hypnotic induction were monitored in normal and patient volunteers (Gruzelier and Brow, 1985). Subjects took part in three sessions separated by four weeks to avoid carryover effects on habituation. They were first monitored to provide a baseline measure and to equate groups for individual differences in rate of habituation. Then with session order counterbalanced they experienced a hypnosis session and one of two control conditions. The control conditions consisted of either a story read by the hypnotist, or relaxing listening to a story for a period equivalent in length to the hypnotic induction prior to the introduction of the tones, which were presented without any accompanying verbal message. Hypnotic susceptibility was monitored throughout the experimental session.

The outcome was clear and depended on level of susceptibility. As shown in Figure 1, in the group distributions of orienting and rate of habituation the hypnosis condition was distinguished from the three control conditions through a higher incidence of both non-responding and non-habituation, a bimodal distribution. It was the high susceptibles who showed a reduction in orienting and/or faster habituation with hypnosis, whereas low susceptibles showed retarded habituation with hypnosis, as can be seen in Figure 2.

Comparisons with other features of electrodermal activity shed light on arousal and attentional processes. In hypnosis for the group as a whole there was an absence of sensitization to a test tone presented towards the end of the session while throughout the induction there was an increase in electrodermal non-specific responses. It is important to note that both these effects were shared with the control story condition and did not vary with hypnotic susceptibility. From this it can be infered that listening to the story and to the hypnotic induction produced a similar degree of autonomic

6 *Gruzelier*

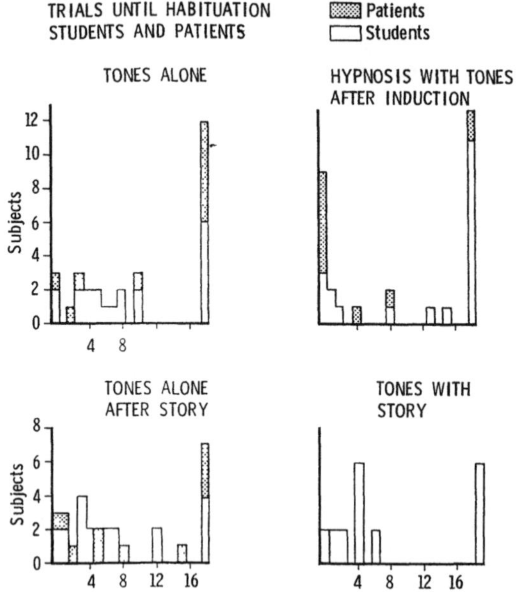

Figure 1. Electrodermal orienting response habituation in baseline (tones alone), hypnosis, relaxation after listening to a story, and story conditions.

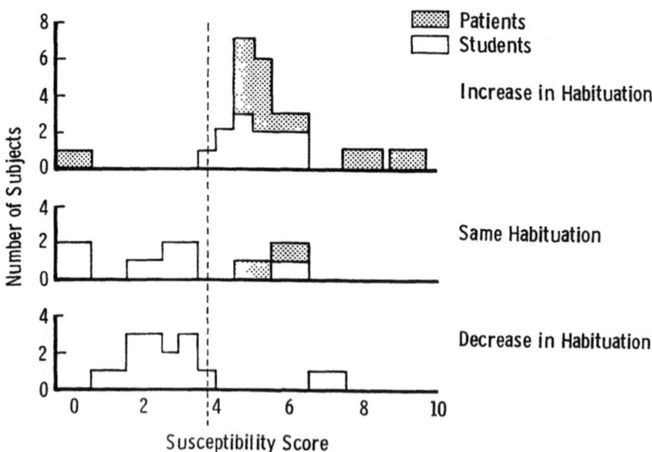

Figure 2. Subjects categorized according to increase, decrease or no change in habituation from baseline to hypnosis as a function of induction susceptibility score.

arousability and attentional engagement and these did not vary with susceptibility. Turning to the relaxation condition, this was insufficient to change either habituation (see also Teasdale, 1972) or sensitization, so that the facilitation of habituation could not be explained away as a function of relaxation. At the same time some components of arousal reduction were associated with hypnosis. This was shown by fewer non-specific responses during hypnosis both in the first half and second half of the hypnotic induction as well as by reductions in tonic levels of skin conductance. However, one high susceptible had levels of skin conductance two standard deviations above the control group mean, indicating that a reduction in tonic arousal is not a necessary part of the hypnotic process as will be confirmed later in an experiment with the active-alert induction procedure.

The facilitation of habituation with hypnosis was replicated in an experiment designed to compare hypnosis with *simulating hypnosis* in medium/high hypnotizables (Gruzelier et al., 1988). Subjects were examined first in a baseline session and then assigned with the Barber Suggestibility Scale (Barber, 1969) to the simulator or hypnosis groups matched for suggestibility, electrodermal reactivity and sex. Hypnotic susceptibility was monitored throughout the second session as in the former experiment. Levels of susceptibility all fell within the moderate to high range. As before, rate of habituation was faster with hypnosis in the susceptible subjects whereas in simulators habituation was slower. Simulators were more aroused during the induction prior to presentation of the tones ($p < 0.005$) but subsequently there was no difference in the number of non-specific electrodermal responses. Support was found for reports that simulators are characterized by exaggerated compliance (Williamsen et al., 1965; Hilgard et al., 1978), for in compliance with instruction by the hypnotist to forget about the tones, all but one simulating subject claimed at the end of the session not to have heard the tones, whereas all but one in the hypnosis group admitted to hearing the tones.

Neuroanatomically the influence on electrodermal orienting and habituation was compatible with the evidence of De Benedittis and Sironi (1988) arising from recordings of intracranial electrical activity. They found that hypnosis involved functional inhibition of the amygdala and activation of the hippocampus. The amygdala has been shown to exert mainly excitatory influences on orienting activity whereas the inhibitory action of the hippocampus facilitates the habituation of the orienting response with stimulus repetition (Gruzelier and Venables, 1972; Pribram and McGuinness, 1975).

Electrocortical event-related attentional components and frontal inhibition

Electrocortical procedures have also demonstrated alterations in attentional processing with the induction of hypnosis and, like electrodermal rates of habituation, these changed in opposite directions from baseline to hypnosis for high and low susceptibles (Gruzelier, 1996). Cortical evoked potentials were measured to infrequent tones mixed with frequent tones in a standard P300 paradigm with particular interest in a negative going (N2a) attentional component. The difference between the wave to the infrequent target or deviant when subtracted from the frequent non-target or standard belongs to the class of phenomena termed MisMatch Negativity (MMN). This is thought to involve a preattentive sensory specific process generated in the auditory cortex (superior temporal gyrus). Aside from bilateral temporal maxima it has a predominant single maximum over the frontal cortex suggestive of frontal involvement (Naatanen, 1992; Naatanen and Mitchie, 1979).

Before the topographical EEG recording session subjects were assigned with the Harvard Group scale (Shor and Orne, 1962) to high (9–12) and low (0–4) susceptibility groups. Baseline measures were first recorded and these were repeated following the hypnotic induction as in the electrodermal studies, and repeated a second time following an extended induction. Susceptibility was recorded throughout the session as in previous studies. As can be seen in Figure 3 high susceptibles showed a large magnitude difference wave at baseline and a progressive reduction in MMN with each stage of the induction and in keeping with frontal inhibition. By the later stage of the induction MMN was negligible in both the lateral frontal placements. Importantly opposite changes were manifested by the low susceptible group. Whereas at baseline their difference wave was absent, there was a progressive increase in MMN through the experiment, until in the last condition the magnitude of the difference wave was on a par with the results in high susceptibles at baseline, suggesting an increasing enhancement of attentional processing.

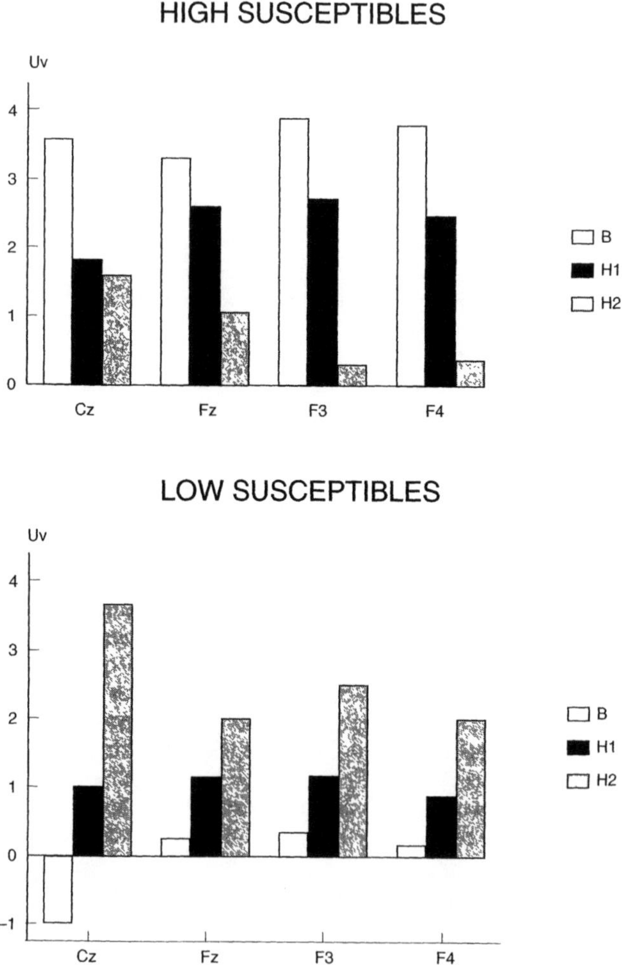

Figure 3. Mismatch negativity scores in baseline (B), induction (H1) and extended induction (H2) in high and low susceptible groups.

Summary
There was a consistency between the electrocortical MMN and electrodermal measures in depicting opposite changes from baseline to hypnosis in susceptible and unsusceptible subjects. Congruent opposing effects on attention have also been found in a recent Finnish study involving a computerized vigilance task. High susceptibles showed an increase in omission errors and greater variability in RTs from baseline to hypnosis, while low susceptibles showed a reduction in errors and RT variance (Kallio et al., 1998). Together these studies show that whereas susceptible subjects evinced inhibitory influences on attention with hypnosis, unsusceptible subjects improved attentional performance as the induction progressed.

Anterior inhibitory processes

Fronto-limbic supervisory attentional system
We went on to examine evidence of frontal inhibition in the context of contemporary models of anterior functions that focus on attentional control systems (Posner and Peterson, 1990; Shallice and Burgess, 1991). A supervisory attentional system that involves the frontal lobes and limbic system monitors ongoing activity and modulates behaviour in response to novelty, as in orienting, and when environmental stimuli convey conflicting information. We tested this with a behavioural and electrophysiological paradigm that required the monitoring of errors in performance (Kaiser et al., 1997). We utilized a Stroop-like task involving a simple two-choice reaction time task in which a button was pressed according to the side in which a green arrow was pointing (congruent condition). This was contrasted with a complex four-choice task where in addition to the green arrow condition red arrows were randomly presented, in which case the button must be pressed in the opposite direction to the arrow (incongruent condition). Electrophysiological evidence has shown that following an erroneous response in a reaction time task there is a large negative going wave at about 100 ms, referred to as error-related negativity and termed an *error detection wave*, which is not elicited following correct responses (Falkenstein et al., 1990; Gehring et al., 1993). This negative wave is followed by a positive wave that varies with a range of task-related factors and may represent context updating, error evaluation and adjustment of response strategies, an *error evaluation wave* (Falkenstein et al., 1995).

With hypnosis the medium/high susceptibility group showed an increase in errors on incongruent trials – the stroop interference effect – but no change in errors on congruent trials, whereas the performance of low susceptibles remained constant. Reaction times were not influenced by hypnosis in either group. Therefore in medium/high susceptibles there was a failure to inhibit the automatic response in keeping with an inhibition of frontal attentional control. However, the large negative going error detection waves that were elicited were non-significantly *larger* in the medium/high than the low susceptibility group, and these waves were unaltered by hypnosis. In other words an error detection system which operates at an early and possibly pre-conscious stage of processing was not compromised by hypnosis; to wit the unconscious hidden observer of Hilgard, Morgan and McDonald (1975). In contrast we found that the positive going error evaluation wave following the error detection wave was reduced in amplitude with hypnosis but only in medium/high susceptibles. Results for the susceptible subjects are found in Figure 4. This was in keeping with inhibition of a frontal error evaluation process and was compatible with the behavioural data showing a higher error rate on incongruous trials in the medium/high susceptibles with hypnosis.

The error detection wave has been localized to a midline anterior cingulate generator (Dehaene et al., 1994), a promising candidate for involvement in hypnosis. The anterior cingulate performs executive functions that have been subdivided into affective and cognitive components (Devinsky et al., 1995). The cognitive executive component is involved in response selection in advance of any movement and in cognitively demanding information processing such as Stroop interference, localized by blood flow imaging and lesion studies to the anterior cingulate (Pardo et al., 1990; George et al., 1993; Vendrell et al., 1995), and by some to the right anterior cingulate (Bench et al., 1993). The affective executive functions are involved in regulation of autonomic and endocrine functions, assessment of motivational context and significance of sensory stimuli and emotional valence. These are mediated through extensive connections with the amygdala and periaqueductal grey and autonomic brainstem nuclei. Our results have indicated that the monitoring of motor performance carried out by the cognitive executive component remained intact, for the error detection wave and RTs were unchanged by hypnosis. Rather it would appear that the affect system involving connections with the rostral limbic system including the amygdala was unresponsive, as shown by the absence of the error evaluation wave and apparently motivational influences on performance. This interpretation is also in keeping with the reduced electrodermal orienting activity reflecting a reduction in amygdaloid excitatory modulatory influences. Dissociation between cognitive and affective anterior cingulate executive systems would explain the increase in the Stroop interference effect with hypnosis.

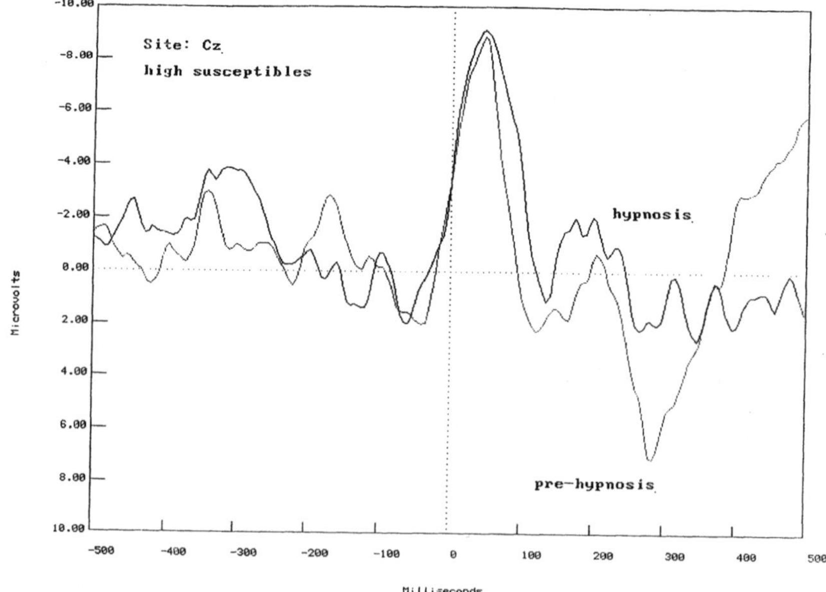

Figure 4. Error detection and error evaluation waves in medium/high susceptibles in hypnosis and pre-hypnosis baseline.

Left anterior inhibition

Some evidence has suggested that the anterior inhibition may be laterally asymmetrical and biased towards the left hemisphere. This was disclosed by measuring right and left hemisphere processing times in dextral subjects with a haptic object sorting task comparing left and right hands (Gruzelier et al., 1984). This was planned initially to validate asymmetries disclosed by the bilateral monitoring of electrodermal orienting and habituation processes described in the next section; in the haptic task the mediation of hemispheric influences is unambiguously contralateral. Subjects sorted objects by class with each hand separately while blindfolded. Hand order was counterbalanced and there was control for movement time. The task was done prior to hypnosis and again after the hypnotic induction, with susceptibility monitored through the experiment. As shown in Figure 5 high susceptibles showed an increase in right hand processing times with hypnosis while there was no change in their left hand times, nor were there bilateral changes in low susceptibles. The increase in the processing times of the right hand (indexing the left hemisphere) correlated positively with the hypnotic susceptibility score. We replicated the slowing of left hemispheric processing with hypnosis in high susceptibles in contrast to low susceptibles in a follow-up experiment with middle aged subjects, which was performed away from the laboratory and which included a non-hypnosis control group, (Gruzelier et al., 1984). The combining of both experiment samples disclosed evidence of a left hemispheric preference in high susceptibles at baseline as had been shown in the electrodermal study outlined in the next section.

Left-sided inhibition of somatosensory functions was replicated further by examining haptic processing with an *active-alert induction* (Cikurel and Gruzelier, 1990). Following Bányai and Hilgard (1976) subjects pedalled a stationary exercise bicycle against a load and with instructions of mental alertness in the hypnotic induction. Dextral subjects were selected with the Barber scale to form groups of high and medium susceptibles. Each subject participated in two sessions, one involving the conventional relaxation induction and the other the active-alert induction. In both conditions a baseline measure was obtained either while seated or while pedalling. Session order was counterbalanced and in each session hypnotic susceptibility was monitored to validate the group designation and to compare the induction procedures, which in the event produced similar influences on susceptibility (r = 0.79,

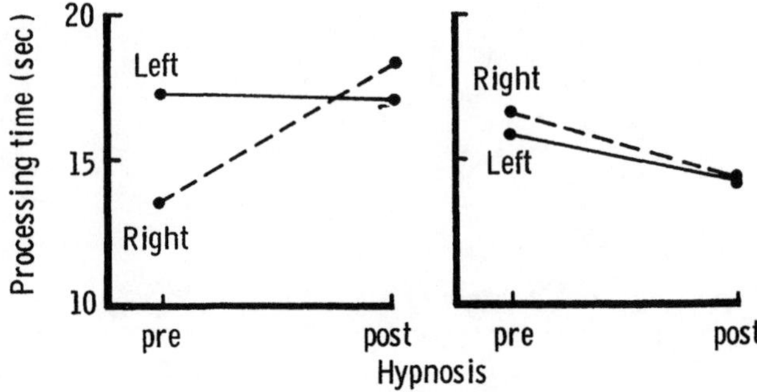

Figure 5. Haptic processing times for right and left hands for pre-hypnosis baseline and with hypnosis in high (left figure) and low (right figure) susceptibles.

$p < 0.001$). As in previous experiments there was a hypnosis x hand interaction such that for the group as a whole there was a slowing of right hand processing times with hypnosis and no change with the left hand. Subdivision of the subjects into high and medium groups showed that whereas both groups shared the right hand slowing with hypnosis, the left hand of high susceptibles gave faster sorting times with hypnosis, whereas in medium susceptibles there was a bilateral slowing of processing. Comparing induction procedures, the active-alert induction shared with the conventional procedure the slowing of left hemispheric processing but the active-alert induction was solely responsible for the improvement in right hemispheric processing.

Lateralized anterior inhibitory functions were examined further with a small battery of neuropsychological tasks (Gruzelier and Warren, 1993). These included word and category fluency, which are both left hemisphere tasks with word fluency left frontal and category fluency left temporal. Design fluency was included to index right anterior processing. Left and right hand finger tapping was included to examine motor and pre-motor functions. Dextral subjects were first selected with the Barber scale and divided into high and low susceptibility groups. Susceptibility level was also monitored throughout the experiment. The influence of hypnosis on word fluency differed substantively between the groups. While low susceptibles showed an increase in fluency from the pre-hypnosis baseline with hypnosis, high susceptibles showed a decrease. While the groups did not differ at baseline in word fluency (although there was a mean advantage to high susceptibles) with hypnosis there was a highly significant difference between them. The semantic category test showed similar mean changes but did not disclose significant effects. These results are contrasted in Figure 6. With design fluency both groups showed an improvement with hypnosis whereas in finger tapping only the low susceptibles showed improvement in finger tapping – the high susceptibles showed an impairment. The word versus category fluency effects have now been replicated in the Finnish study mentioned above (Kallio et al., 1998), which has brought together in one investigation opposite changes in susceptible and unsusceptible subjects, first in vigilance performance involving a thalamo-cortical (parieto-frontal) attentional network mentioned above and second in word generation involving the left prefrontal cortex.

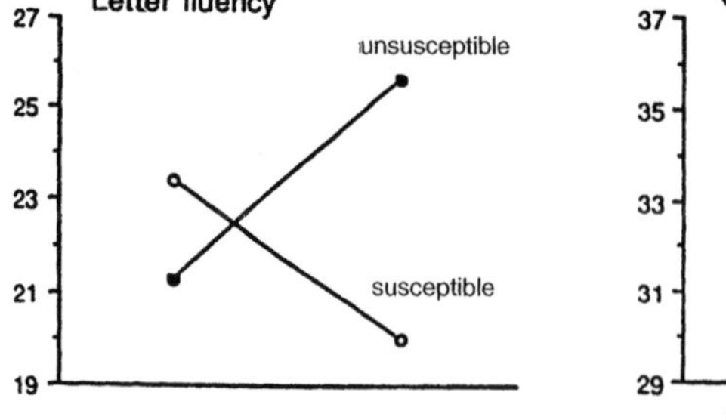

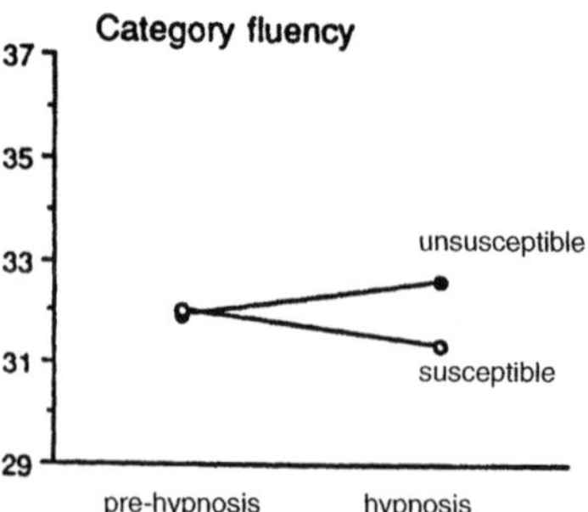

Figure 6. Word fluency for letters and categories in high and low susceptibles in pre-hypnosis baseline and with hypnosis.

Patterns of correlations between the fluency tasks supported an inhibitory influence of hypnosis centring on the left anterior word fluency performance. First, the three fluency tests did not correlate at baseline implying an independence of function. Second, correlations between baseline and hypnosis conditions were significant for category fluency and design fluency but not for word fluency, in support of the word fluency test alone being altered by hypnosis. In contrast, significant correlations were obtained with hypnosis between word fluency and both design fluency and category fluency, but not between design and category fluency. This could be interpreted as showing that an underlying process such as distributed inhibition was most at work with word fluency, and while centring on left anterior processes was also having some impact on design and category fluency which involved right anterior and left temporal processing respectively. Correlations also showed that the significant relation between left and right hand finger tapping dexterity before hypnosis was reduced with hypnosis in keeping with a tendency towards lateral dissociation.

Anterior disconnection with hypnosis in susceptible subjects was recently disclosed by Kaiser in an unpublished experiment involving EEG topographical mapping with a 32 electrode array in which we examined regional connectivity with EEG coherence. EEG coherence, a putative measure of connectivity, was examined between bipolar pairs of electrodes. This disclosed a significant hypnosis x group x condition interaction in high alpha activity, as shown in Figure 7. In high susceptibles with hypnosis there was a reduction in connectivity within the left prefrontal region – specifically between left lateral (FP1 and F7) and medial (F3 and FTC1) placements – whereas the opposite effect, namely an increase in connectivity was found in low susceptibles. In baseline there was also a highly significant difference between susceptibility groups in the direction of greater left anterior connectivity in high rather than low susceptibles.

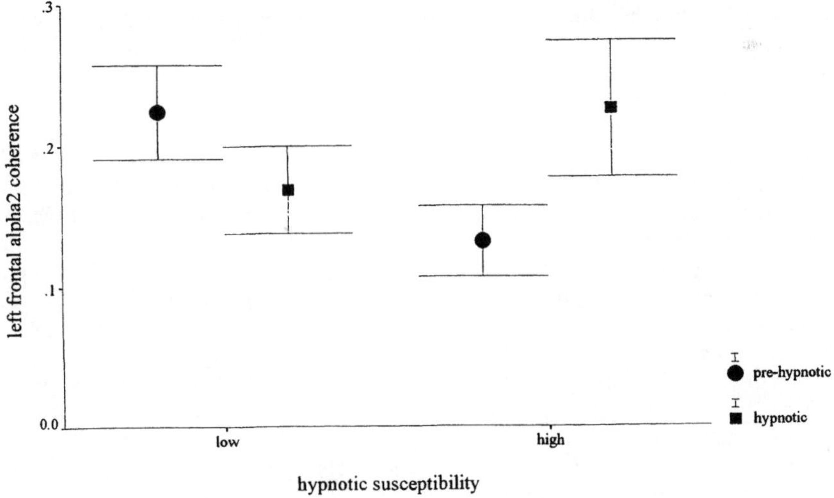

Figure 7. Left anterior EEG coherence in baseline and hypnosis for medium/high and low susceptibles (high short distance coherence represents low connectivity and vice versa).

Importantly the coherence result did not generalize to all bands but was restricted to high alpha activity. This represents an EEG band that relates to cognitive as distinct from connative processing, variously described as indexing high workload, sustained motor control and long-term memory (Mecklinger and Bosel, 1989; Sterman et al., 1994; Klimesche, 1996; Burgess and Gruzelier, 1998). The importance of selectivity in narrow band EEG power has also been demonstrated by our differentiating hypnosis from baseline in high and low susceptibles (Williams and Gruzelier, 1998).

Summary

Further evidence of a selectivity of neurophysiological action of hypnosis was shown through examination of anterior inhibitory influences:

- the dissociation between error detection and error evaluation waves;
- the left lateralized influences on haptic processing, and the improvement in right-sided processing that was specific to the active-alert induction;
- the specificity within the left hemisphere for the effects on verbal fluency that were restricted to letter and not semantic designated categories;
- the localization of the changes in EEG coherence to within the left frontal lobe;
- the restriction of the EEG coherence changes to the high alpha band.

These factors serve to introduce a note of caution in attempts to interpret changes in brain blood flow and metabolism in hypnosis, which do not permit such fine grained interpretation, nor do they discriminate between facilitatory and inhibitory functional systems.

Right-sided processing

Focal versus distributed influences of hypnosis have also been demonstrated in experiments investigating the popular view of right hemispheric involvement in hypnosis (Pedersen, 1984). Firstly, in our original experiment on electrodermal orienting and habituation processes (Gruzelier and Brow, 1985) bilateral recording disclosed an asymmetry in the amplitude of orienting responses favouring the right hand in hypnosis in high susceptibles whereas there was no reliable asymmetry in low susceptibles. This was in contrast to the baseline session where after the initial tones there was an asymmetry favouring the left hand in high susceptibles and again no reliable asymmetry in low susceptibles; the initial stage of orienting is thought to involve the right hemisphere, which governs states of broadened attention, after which the focal and selective attentional abilities of left hemisphere take over as would be exemplified in the high suseptibles with their left preference after the initial trials (see Figure 8). At the time the psychophysiological experiment was undertaken the mediation of hemispheric influences on electrodermal activity was considered controversial. Subsequently the influence of limbic modulation has been clarified by intracranial stimulation studies (Mangina and Beuzeron-Mangina, 1996), which have supported the original interpretation of the dominance of ipsilateral limbic modulatory influences on the passive orienting processes (Gruzelier, 1973). Therefore the results may be interpreted as showing a left hemispheric preference in high susceptibles at baseline. While this result was not predicted and ran counter to right hemisphericity theories of hypnotic susceptibility, support was forthcoming from the subsequent investigation of lateralized haptic processing described above (Gruzelier et al., 1984). Such baseline left hemispheric advantages may simply reflect greater cognitive agility

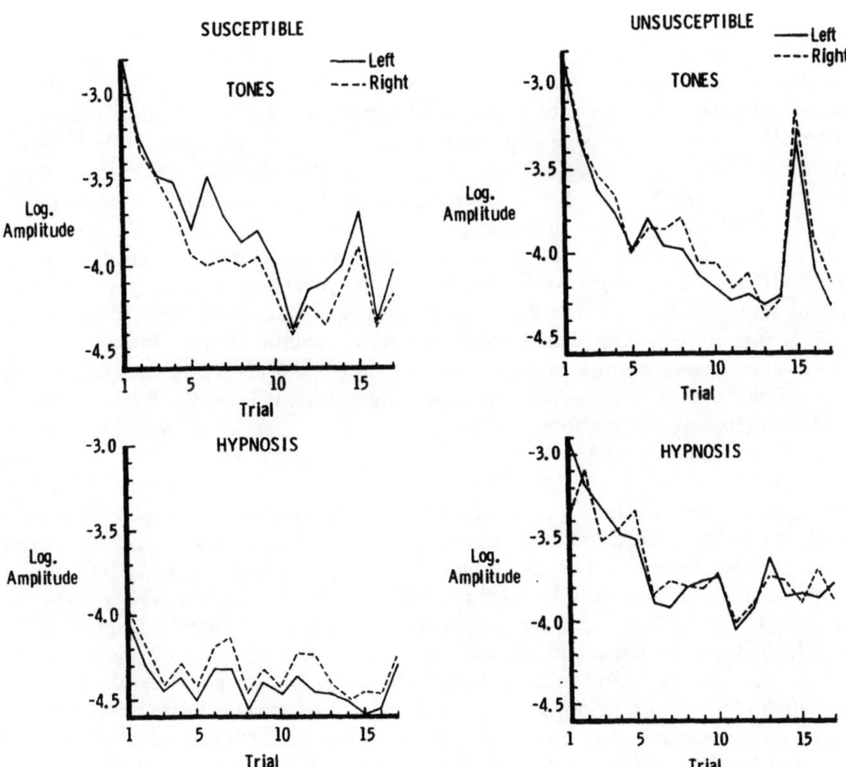

Figure 8. The amplitude of bilateral electrodermal orienting responses showing reversal of asymmetry from baseline (tones) to hypnosis in high susceptibles and no consistent changes in low susceptibles.

in line with task demands by high susceptibles (Crawford, 1989). Accordingly it would appear that it was the hypnotic induction that instated the right hemispheric functional preference in susceptible subjects.

An enhancement of right posterior functions was found in an experiment involving the divided visual field presentation of flashes requiring brightness judgements. The experiment involved three sessions in the order baseline, hypnosis, baseline. It was conducted with eyes open with sufficient trials to perform signal detection analysis to give estimates of perceptual sensitivity independent of cognitive bias (McCormack and Gruzelier, 1993). Blocks of trials were interspersed with a live hypnotic induction. Susceptibility was monitored throughout the experiment with subjects divided into medium and high susceptibles. Results are shown in Figure 9. Perceptual sensitivity was found to be enhanced in the hypnosis condition compared with the control conditions. Comparison of the susceptibility groups indicated a bilateral increase in perceptual sensitivity in medium susceptibles whereas in high susceptibles there was no change in susceptibility in the left hemisphere (right visual field) in contrast to a focal right hemispheric enhancement (left visual field). An improvement in perceptual sensitivity is according to signal detection theory indicative of an increase in signal to noise ratio as will occur with a reduction in central levels of arousal. Analysis of the cognitive bias variable showed that judgements were more conservative for the right hemisphere than the left for the group as a whole (p <0.05). However, there was no effect of group, providing no evidence for the possibility that the influence of hypnosis may be due to a shift in attitude such as an adoption of a lax response criterion leaving perceptual sensitivity unaffected (Naish, 1985). The demonstrable changes in perceptual sensitivity with hypnosis were consistent with other reports (Segal and Fusella, 1970; Miller and Leibowitz, 1976; Farthing et al., 1982). Thus the results, which disclosed an enhancement of right posterior processing with hypnosis, showed that only in high susceptibles was this strictly lateralized. It was more widely distributed in medium susceptibles to include a bilateral processing enhancement and was of lesser magnitude. A similar conclusion was reached in the haptic sorting task experiment above (Cikurel and Gruzelier, 1990).

Turning to central and temporal regions, an electrophysiological study was performed measuring evoked potentials to tone probes presented simultaneously with the hypnotic induction and compared with their presentation during a story read by the hypnotist. Event-related potentials in both conditions were referred to a baseline condition giving three conditions in all (Jutai et al., 1993). Bilateral electrode placements included central and temporal sites and the analysis centred on the N100 attentional component. According to assessment of hypnotic susceptibility monitored throughout the study subjects were categorized as low or medium/high susceptibles. Specific to the hypnosis condition there was a right>left asymmetry at the temporal location (electrodes T3/4) in the medium/high group. In contrast there was an opposite left>right asymmetry in the story condition of medium/high susceptibles, as well as in both the conditions of the low susceptibles. This reversal of asymmetry to favour the right hemisphere in susceptible subjects did not extend to the lateral central (C3/4) placements. The results demonstrated that right anterior temporal lobe activity was raised in medium/high susceptibles with hypnosis.

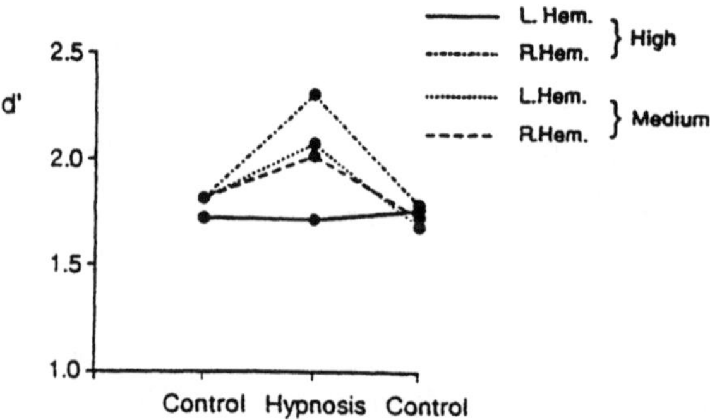

Figure 9. Visual sensitivity in baseline control conditions and hypnosis in high and medium susceptibles for left and right hemispheres.

Summary
The asymmetries in electrodermal orienting responses and the cortical evoked potential N100, both to auditory stimuli presented during the latter part of the induction (Gruzelier and Brow, 1985; Jutai et al., 1993), indicate a shift in the balance of temporal-limbic activity to favour the right hemisphere. In contrast the asymmetry of visual sensory sensitivity assessed with signal detection analysis (McCormack and Gruzelier, 1993) depicted an enhancement of right hemispheric processing in high susceptibles and no change in the left hemisphere whereas medium susceptibles showed bilateral improvement.

Conclusion

This series of experiments has shown a number of reproducible changes in brain function that distinguished medium/high susceptibles after instructions of hypnosis both from their baseline state and from low susceptibles. The attempts were modest in scope and must be confined to the traditional hypnotic relaxation induction. Continuing support was provided for associations between hypnosis and:

- activation of anterior fronto-limbic inhibitory processes,
- anterior inhibition or disconnection, either lateralized to left hemispheric regions or bilateral depending on the processes examined,
- involvement of right temporoposterior processing,
- evidence of superior attentional abilities in high susceptibles,
- evidence of poor attentional abilities in unsusceptible subjects with progressive improvement through the induction, and
- no evidence of right hemisphericity in the baseline state in susceptible subjects.

Across electrodermal, electrocortical and behavioural domains susceptible subjects evinced inhibitory influences on attention with hypnosis whereas unsusceptible subjects improved attentional performance as the induction progressed. Evidence was also found for bilateral alterations of function in medium susceptibles in situations where changes in high susceptibles were lateralized, suggesting more diffuse or distributed changes in medium susceptibles and more focal changes in high susceptibles. Together these results indicate the importance of stratifying groups into low, medium and high susceptibles.

In our neuropsychological translation of the traditional hypnotic induction, hypnosis was initiated by engaging anterior executive control systems. Aside from alterations in cortical functions along anterior-posterior and lateral axes, these will orchestrate top down changes influencing thalamic and brain stem mechanisms. Currently there is renewed interest in the electrophysiology of thalamocortical mechanisms in perceptual binding, conscious perception and altered states of awareness (Llinas and Pare, 1991; Singer, 1993). Llinas, Ribary, Joliot and Wang (1994) have proposed that consciousness is a noncontinuous event determined by simultaneity of activity in specific thalmocortical nuclei, which provide the content of experience, and the non-specific diffuse thalamic projection system that provides the context and alertness. In this regard the anterior and posterior cingulate appear of particular promise in the top down control of thalamic activity relevant to hypnosis. Devinsky, Morrell and Vogt (1995) have remarked 'One of the unique features of anterior cingulate cortex circuitry is its diverse thalamic afferents and consequent ability to sample inputs from more thalamic nuclei than any other cortical region.

The ability to sample from a wide range of thalamic inputs may be crucial for its contributions to motor response selection functions. p 280.' The same could be said for conative functions and the limbic thalamus (Bentivoglio et al., 1993). Hypnosis research would benefit from examining the interplay between cortical and thalamocortical systems, for which the methodology of fast frequency EEG transients holds much promise.

In Llinas's model dreaming is regarded as a state of hyperattentiveness to intrinsic activity without the registration of sensory input, a state with an obvious affinity with hypnosis. This serves to acknowledge that the dream analogy remains appealing for aspects of the hypnotic experience. Consider Fuster's (1995) description of cognitive features of dreaming, which include the altered sense of time and absence of temporality, the lack of guiding reality and critical judgement, the anchoring in personal experience, affective colouring, dissociation from sensory input and context. 'The fragmented networks activated in the dream seem to lack the associative links to a time frame, anchored as they are in the present, without time tags and references.' This could equally be a description of the hypnotic state as high susceptibles experience it.

As the studies unfolded a selectivity of central action increasingly became a hallmark of hypnosis providing undeniable evidence of neurophysiological changes in susceptible subjects, which distinguished them from unsusceptible subjects. As Schopenhauer remarked 'All truth passes through three stages. First it is ridiculed. Second it is violently opposed. Third it is accepted as being self-evident'. Application of the rapid advances in cognitive neuroscience to hypnosis research may make the reality of the third stage ever more likely.

Acknowledgements

The research was suppported by the Saugstad Fund, the Institut für Grenzgebiete der Psychologie und Psychohygiene and studentships from the Medical Research Council and the Wellcome Trust.

References

Bányai EI, Hilgard ER. A comparison of active-alert hypnotic induction with traditional relaxation induction. Journal of Abnormal Psychology 1976; 85: 218–224.

Barber TX. Hypnosis: A Scientific Approach. New York: Von Nostrand, 1969.

Bench CJ, Frith CD,Grasby PM, Friston KJ, Paulescu E, Frackowiack RSJ, Dolan RJ. Investigations of the functional anatomy of attention using the Stroop test. Neuropsychologia 1993; 31: 907–922.

Bentivoglio M, Kultas-Ilinsky K, Ilinsky I. In: Vogt BA, Gabriel M, eds. Neuurobiology of Cingulate Cortex and Limbic Thalamus: A Comprehensive Handbook. Boston: Birkhauser, 1993; 71–122.

Burgess A, Gruzelier JH. Short duration power changes in the EEG during recognition memory for words and faces. Submitted, 1998.

Cikurel K, Gruzelier J. The effect of an active-alert hypnotic induction on lateral asymmetry in haptic processing. British Journal of Experimental and Clinical Hypnosis 1990; 7: 17–25

Craiselneck HB, McCranie EJ, Jenkins MT. Special indications for hypnosis as a method anaesthesia. Journal of the American Medical Association 1956; 162: 1606–1608.

Crawford HC. Cognitive and physiological flexibility: Multiple pathways to hypnotic responsieness. In: Ghorghiu V, Netter P, Eysenck H, Rosenthal R, eds. Suggestion and Suggestibility: Theory and Research. Berlin: Springer-Verlag, 1989; 155–168.

Crawford HJ, Gruzelier J. A midstream view of the neuropsychophysiology of hypnosis: Recent research and future directions. In: Fromm W, Nash M, eds. Hypnosis; Research Developments and Perspectives, 3rd edn. New York: Guildford Press, 1992; 227–266.

De Benedittis G, Sironi VA. Deep cerebral electrical activity in man during hypnosis. International Journal of Clinical and Experimental Hypnosis 1986; 34: 63–70.

De Benedittis G, Sironi VA. Arousal effects of electrical deep brain stimulation in hypnosis. International Journal of Clinical and Experimental Hypnosis 1988; 36: 96–106.

Dehaene S, Posner MI, Tucker DC. Localisation of a neural system for error detection and compensation. Psychological Science 1994; 5: 303–305.

Devinsky O, Morrell MJ, Vogt BA. Contributions of anterior cingulate cortex to behaviour. Brain 1995; 118: 279–306.

Falkenstein M, Hohnbein J, Hoorman J, Blanke L. Effects of errors in choice reaction time tasks on the ERP under focussed and divided attention. In: Brunia CHM, Gaillard AWK, Koh A, eds. Psychophysiological Brain Research. Tilburg: Tilburg University Press, 1990; 192–195.

Falkenstein, M., Hohnsbein, J. and Hoorman, J. Event-related potential correlation of errors in reaction time tasks. In: Kamas G, Molnar M, Csepe V, Czigler I, Desmedt JE, eds. Perspectives of Event-Related Potentials Research (EEG supplement 44). Amsterdam: Elsevier, 1995; 287–296.

Farthing GW, Brown SW, Venturio M. Effects of hypnotisability and mental imagery on signal detection sensitivity and response bias. International Journal of Clinical and Experimental Hypnosis 1982; 30: 289–305.

Fuster JM. Memory in the Cerebral Cortex. Boston: MIT Press, 1995.

Gehring WJ, Goss B, Coles MGH, Meyer DE, Donchin E. A neural system for error detection and compensation. Psychological Science 1993; 4: 385–390.

George MS, Ketter TA, Gill DS, Haxby JV, Ungerleider LG, Herschovitch P. Brain regions involved in recognising facial emotion or identity: an oxygen-15 PET study. Journal of Neuropsychiatry and Clinical Neuroscience 1993; 5: 384–394.

Gray JA. The Neuropsychology of Anxiety. Oxford: Oxford University Press, 1982.

Gruzelier JH. Bilateral asymmetry of skin conductance orienting activity and levels in schizophrenics. Biological Psychology 1973; 1: 21–41.

Gruzelier JH. The neuropsychology of hypnosis. In: Heap M, ed. Hypnosis: Current Clinical, Experimental and Forensic Practices. London: Croom Helm, 1988; 68–76.

Gruzelier JH. Neuropsychological investigations of hypnosis: Cerebral laterality and beyond. In: Van Dyck R, Spinhoven Ph, Van der Does AJW, eds. Hypnosis: Theory, Research and Clinical Practice. Free University Press, 1990; 38–51.

Gruzelier JH. The state of hypnosis: Evidence and applications. Quarterly Journal of Medicine 1996; 89: 313–317.

Gruzelier JH, Venables PH. Skin conductance orienting activity in a heterogeneous sample of schizophrenics. Journal of Nervous and Mental Disease 1972; 155: 277–287.

Gruzelier JH, Brow TD. Psychophysiological evidence for a state theory of hypnosis and susceptibility. Journal of Psychosomatic Research 1985; 29: 287–302.

Gruzelier JH, Warren K. Neuropsychological evidence of left frontal inhibition with hypnosis. Psychological Medicine 1993; 23: 93–101.

Gruzelier JH, Brow TD, Perry A, Rhonder J, Thomas M. Hypnotic susceptibility: A lateral predisposition and altered cerebral asymmetry under hypnosis. International Journal of Psychophysiology 1984; 2: 131–139.

Gruzelier JH, Allison J, Conway A. A psychophysiological differentiation between hypnosis and the simulation of hypnosis. International Journal of Psychophysiology1988; 6: 331–338.

Hernandez-Peon R. Las bases neurofisiologicas de la hipnosis. Neurologia Neurocirugia Psiquiatria (Mexico) 1977; 18: 7–26.

Hilgard ER, Morgan AH, MacDonald H. Pain and dissocaition in the cold pressor test: A study of hypnotic analgesia with 'hidden reports' through automatic key pressing and automatic talking. Journal of Abnormal Psychology 1975; 84: 280–289.

Hilgard ER, McDonald H, Morgan AH, Johnson LS. The reality of hypnotic analgesia: a comparison of highly hypnotisables with simulators. Journal of Abnormal Psychology 1978; 87: 239–246.

Jutai J, Gruzelier JH, Golds J, Thomas M. Bilateral auditory-evoked potentials in conditions of hypnosis and focused attention. International Journal of Psychophysiology 1993; 15: 167–176.

Kaiser J, Barker R, Haenschel C, Baldeweg T, Gruzelier J. Hypnosis and event-related potential correlates of error processing in a stroop-type paradigm: a test of the frontal hypothesis. International Journal of Psychophysiology 1997; 27: 215–222.

Kallio S, Revonsuo A, Hamalainen H, Markela J, Gruzelier J. Changes in anterior attentional functions and word fluency associated with hypnosis. Submitted, 1998.

Klimesche W. Memory processes, brain oscillations and EEG synchronisation. International Journal of Psychophysiology 1996; 24: 61–100.

Llinas RR, Pare D. Of dreaming and wakefulness. Neuroscience 1991; 44: 521–535

Llinas R, Ribary U, Joliot M, Wang XJ. Content and context in temporal thalamocortical binding. In: Buzsaki G, ed. Temporal Coding in the Brain. Berlin: Springer-Verlag, 1994; 251–273.

Mangina CA, Beuzeron-Mangina JH. Direct electrical stimulation of specific human brain structures and bilateral electrodermal activity. International Journal of Psychophysiology 1996; 22: 1–8.

McCormack K, Gruzelier JH. Cerebral asymmetry and hypnosis: A signal detection analysis of divided visual field stimulation. Journal of Abnormal Psychology 1993; 102: 352–357.

Mecklinger A, Bosel R. Veraenderungen im EEG-Frequenzspektrum bei verscheiden Phasen mentaler belastung. Z. Exp. U. Angew. Psychologie 1989; 36: 453–475.

Miller RJ, Leibowitz HK. A signal detection analysis of hypnotically induced narrowing of peripheral vision. Journal of Abnormal Psychology 1976; 85: 446–454.

Naatanen R. Attention and Brain Function. New York: Erlbaum, 1992.

Naatanen R, Mitchie PT. Early selective attention effects on the evoked potential. A critical review and reinterpretation. Biological Psychology 1979; 8: 81–136.

Naish P. The trance described in signal detection terms. British Journal of Experimental and Clinical Hypnosis 1985; 2: 133–138.

Pardo JV, Pardo PJ, Janer KW, Raichle ME. The anterior cingulate mediated processing selection in the Stroop attentional conflict paradigm. Proceedings of the National Academy of Science 1990; USA 87: 256–259.

Pedersen D. Hypnosis and the right hemisphere. Proceedings of the British Society of Medical and Dental Hypnosis 1984; 5: 2–14.

Posner M, Peterson S. The attention system of the human brain. Annual Review of Neuroscience 1990; 13: 25–42.

Pribram KH, McGuinness D. Arousal, activation and effort in the control of attention. Psychological Review 1975; 82: 116.

Segal SV, Fusella V. Influence of imaged pictures and sounds on detection of visual and auditory signals. Journal of Psychology 1970; 83: 458–464.

Shallice T, Burgess P. Deficits in strategy application following frontal lobe damage in man. Brain 1991; 114: 727–741.

Shor RE, Orne EC. The Harvard Group Scale of Hypnotic Susceptibility. Form A. Palo Alto: Consulting Psychologists' Press, 1962.

Singer W. Synchronisation of cortical activity and its putative role in information processing and learning. Annual Review of Physiology 1993; 55: 349–374.

Sterman MB, Mann CA, Kaiser DA, Suyenobu BY. Multiband topographic EEG analysis of a simulated visuomotor aviation task. International Journal of Psychophysiology 1994; 16: 49–56.

Teasdale JD. Relaxation and habituation: A theoretical and experimental analysis. PhD thesis, University of London, 1972.

Vendrell P, Junque C, Pujol J, Jurando MA, Molet J, Grafman J. The role of prefrontal regions in the Stroop task. Neuropsychologia 1995; 33: 341–352.

Wagstaff G. The semantics and physiology of hypnosis as an altered state: Towards a definition of hypnosis. Contemporary Hypnosis, 1998, in press.

Williams JD, Gruzelier JH. Differentiation of hypnosis and relaxation by analysis of narrow band theta and alpha frequencies. Submitted, 1998.

Williamsen JA, Johnson HJ, Eriksen CE. Some characteristics of post-hypnotic amnesia. Journal of Abnormal Psychology 1965; 74: 123–131.

Windholz G. Hypnosis and inhibition as viewed by Heidenhain and Pavlov. Integrative Physiological and Behavioural Science 1996; 31: 155–162.

Address for correspondence:

Professor John Gruzelier,
Department of Behavioural and Cognitive Sciences,
Imperial College School of Medicine,
St Dunstans Road,
London W6 8RF, UK

[24]

PSYCHOPHYSIOLOGICAL CORRELATES OF HYPNOSIS AND HYPNOTIC SUSCEPTIBILITY[1]

VILFREDO DE PASCALIS[2]

University of Rome

Abstract: This article reviews and summarizes electroencephalographic (EEG)-based research on physiological and cognitive indicators of hypnotic responding and hypnotic susceptibility, with special attention to the author's programmatic research in this area. Evidence that differences in attention levels may account for hypnotic depth and individual differences in hypnotizability is provided with traditional EEG rhythms, event-related potentials, and 40-Hz EEG activity. The alteration of stimulus perception may be a secondary effect with respect to allocation of attentional resources. In both nonhypnosis and hypnosis conditions, high hypnotizables appeared to show greater task-related EEG hemispheric shifts than did low hypnotizables. Findings concerning cognitive and physiological correlates of hypnotic analgesia are discussed with respect to hemispheric functioning in the apparent control of *focused* and *sustained* attention. The conclusion is that although a definitive EEG-based signature for hypnosis and hypnotizability is not yet established, there are a number of promising leads.

Since the 1980s, the Department of Psychology at the University of Rome has carried out a series of psychophysiological studies investigating the relationship between electroencephalographic (EEG) rhythms and hypnotic behavior. These investigations were informed by the theory of E. R. Hilgard, often referred to as neodissociation theory, which views hypnotic phenomena as involving a shift in cognitive processing. The main focus of this work was the search for specific and reliable physiological signatures of hypnotizability and hypnosis. This article surveys the EEG research regarding hypnotic responding and hypnotic susceptibility and summarizes the programmatic research on this question.

In their reviews of the current status of hypnotic research, Kirsch and Lynn (1995) and Nadon (1997) noted the search for an EEG-based

Manuscript submitted January 21, 1996; final revision received August 7, 1998.

[1]A portion of this article was presented at the 46th annual meeting of the Society for Clinical and Experimental Hypnosis, San Antonio, Texas, November 9-11, 1995.

[2]Address correspondence to Vilfredo De Pascalis, Ph.D., Dipartimento di Psicologia, Via Dei Marsi 78, 00185 Roma, Italy or depascal@giannutri.caspur.it.

physiological signature of hypnosis and hypnotizability. As these authors state, there are three tasks faced by the researcher. The first is to identify the physiological substrate of general hypnotic response, the second is to search for correlates of hypnotizability, and the third is to find physiological concomitants of specific hypnotic suggestions.

Early psychophysiological research failed to identify a reliable EEG signature of hypnosis and found little evidence for EEG indices that could distinguish between low and high hypnotizable subjects (Dixon & Laurence, 1992; Perlini & Spanos, 1991). The problem here may reflect a lack of sophisticated recording equipment.

Recent work with nonlinear (chaotic) dimensional estimations of hypnotic processes has also apparently failed to clearly show differences between waking and hypnosis conditions (Ray, Wells, Elbert, Lutzenberger, & Birbaumer, 1991) but has been more successful in distinguishing individual differences in hypnotic susceptibility (Ray, 1997). This article will discuss several productive theory-based lines of research.

EVENT-RELATED POTENTIALS AND ALTERATIONS OF THE PERCEPTUAL FIELD

One approach to this issue examines hypnotic responses for specific hypnotic suggestions as opposed to more global state conditions. In this vein, Weitzenhoffer (1980) suggested that hypnotized individuals are capable of alterations in subjective experience and that they demonstrate a special ability to alter perception via hypnotically induced hallucinations.

> The primary underlying premise is not to seek to characterize the hypnotic state, per se, by some unique brain activity [hypnotic signature] but rather to show that highly hypnotizable individuals in a hypnotic state should show ERP changes that correspond to their subjective experience of perceptual alteration. (Barabasz et al., 1999, p. 6)

Event-related potentials (ERPs) have been shown to be useful for studying attentional and cognitive processes in humans (Barabasz & Lonsdale, 1983; Hillyard & Picton, 1987; Naatanen, 1992). It follows then that examination of ERP shifts during hypnotically induced hallucinations may reveal something about the physiological concomitants of hypnosis during suggestion of perceptual alterations. Using ERPs, Barabasz, Barabasz, and Jensen (1995) and Barabasz, Barabasz, Jensen, and Calvin (1996a, 1996b) demonstrated reliable alterations in ERP responses for high but not low hypnotizable patients following suggested hallucinations during hypnosis. By comparing the ERPs with reports of subjective hallucination experiences, it is possible to determine whether highly hypnotizable individuals during hypnosis show parallel changes on both the subjective and electrocortical level. Because of limited design and technical considerations, earlier studies often presented unclear and confusing results. Some of these early studies seemed to find a reduction in the evoked response during a hypnotic procedure (i.e., negative hallucinations), which, in fact, suggests ablation of perception (Galbraith, Cooper, & London, 1972; Hernandez-Peon & Donoso, 1959; Wilson, 1968), whereas other studies failed to detect such a shift (e.g., Andreassi, Balinsky, Gallichio, De Simone, & Mellers, 1976; Beck & Barolin, 1965; Beck, Dustman, & Beier, 1966). These mixed findings are probably due to at least three factors: (a) differences in subject selection, (b) inconsistent ERP measurements, and (c) the nature of the hypnotic instructions.

In what was to become a model for this line of research, Barabasz and Lonsdale (1983) conducted the first ERP study that sought to distinguish high and low hypnotizables by using a real-simulator controlled design (Orne, 1959). Olfactory-evoked responses to strong, weak, and odorless stimuli were measured. High, but not low, hypnotizable subjects showed, for both strong and weak odors, a significant increase in P300 peak amplitude in response to the anosmia instruction, "You can no longer smell anything at all" (Item 9, negative hallucination, of the Stanford Hypnotic Susceptibility Scale: Form C, SHSS:C; Weitzenhoffer & Hilgard, 1962). Spiegel, Cutcomb, Ren, and Pribram (1985) reported the opposite effect with visual ERPs in response to light flashes on a video display. In this study, the high hypnotizables showed a *decrease* in P300 amplitude during suggestion of an obstructive hallucination. Individuals were given the suggestion of an imaginary cardboard box blocking the view of the screen. To better understand these differences, Spiegel and Barabasz (1988) collaborated in a comprehensive evaluation of their data and speculated that the differences were due to different hypnosis suggestions and instructions. These authors hypothesized that in the Barabasz and Lonsdale (1983) study, instructing subjects that they would not smell anything at all produced a surprise effect when any smell was present. This is known to increase rather than decrease ERP peak amplitudes (see, e.g., Hillyard, Picton, & Regan, 1978).

De Pascalis (1994) confirmed Spiegel et al.'s (1985) study, showing decreases in P1 and N1 peak amplitudes for high hypnotizables during a hypnotic obstructive hallucination. Furthermore, Barabasz, Barabasz, and Jensen (1995) suggest that when hypnotic instructions are accounted for, independent laboratories (e.g., Barabasz, De Pascalis, and Spiegel) show consistent results in which ERP peak amplitude is reduced during a hypnotic visual obstructive hallucination and increased when a negative hypnotic hallucination instruction is given.

40-Hz EEG Activity and Hemisphere Functioning

Theoretical foundation. It is generally accepted that one purpose of a hypnotic induction procedure is to assist the subject in eliminating sources of irrelevant stimulation and focusing attentional resources to the most relevant source of information. Tellegen and Atkinson (1974) defined the construct of *absorption* as the individual's disposition to experience episodes of "total" attention on a certain type of event that becomes particularly relevant. Absorption in no way fully explains hypnotizability, but this ability may still be relevant to the facilitation of dissociation.

A number of investigations were conducted in our laboratory to test how hypnotic ability might covary with individual differences in focusing attention on relevant stimuli. In addition, we studied how altered attention induced by hypnotic procedures is reflected in cerebral hemisphere functioning. In this respect, particular relevance has been given to a high-frequency EEG signal centered at 40 Hz, which we view as a physiological marker of focused arousal. This high-frequency, low-amplitude EEG signal, centered at 40 Hz within the 36-44 Hz frequency band, has been suggested as the physiological signature of focused arousal (Makeig & Inlow, 1993; Sheer, 1970, 1976, 1984; Steriade, Gloor, Llinas, Lopes da Silva, & Mesulam, 1990; Tiitinen et al., 1993). Sheer (1976, 1989) developed the psychophysiological construct of "focused arousal" as a first-order functional component in attention, specifying its brain circuitry and its direct electrical measurement operationalized as 40-Hz EEG activity. Task-dependent lateralizations of 40-Hz EEG rhythm and its independence from alpha and beta EEG activities have been found with a variety of cognitive tasks (Loring & Sheer, 1984; Sheer, 1989; Spydell, Ford, & Sheer, 1979; Spydell & Sheer, 1982). More recently, a number of studies have shown a neuronal resonance phenomenon within the gamma band EEG (25-90 Hz), which can be induced by auditory stimuli (e.g., Basar, Rosen, Basar-Eroglu, & Greitschus, 1987; Jokeit & Makeig, 1994; Makela & Hari, 1987; Tiitinen et al., 1993), coherent visual stimuli (Basar-Eroglu, Struber, Kruse, Basar, & Stadler, 1996; Lutzenberger, Pulvermuller, Elbert, & Birbaumer, 1995; Tallon-Buadry, Bertrand, Bouchet, & Pernier, 1995; Tallon, Bertrand, Delpuech, & Pernier, 1996), or motor behavior (Pfurtscheller, Flotzinger, & Neuper, 1994; Pfurtscheller & Neuper, 1992; Pfurtscheller, Neuper, & Kalcher, 1993). Common to these studies is the view that 40-Hz EEG activity serves as an operator on attentional sensory and motor functions to allow single elements in the central nervous system to be linked or bound into functional states that represent and integrate external stimuli and motor sets into a unified whole.

Likewise, our EEG-hypnosis research assumes that 40-Hz EEG activity is an indicator of focused arousal. If we also assume that hypnosis is usually characterized by a condition of narrowly focused attention and that one aspect of individual differences in hypnotizability may be the ability to focus attention on task requirement, we would expect to find an increased level of 40-Hz EEG activity during hypnosis. Further, when compared with low hypnotizables, highly hypnotizable subjects should manifest distinct 40-Hz EEG hemispheric activation patterns in relation to task requirements.

Empirical Findings on 40-Hz EEG, Emotionality, and Hemispheric Functioning

Research on emotionality has taken two very different directions. One direction, based on behavioral and physiological observations of emotional states, assumes that there is a small number of primary emotions such as happiness, sadness, and anger that have distinguishable physiological patterns (e.g., Ekman, Friesen, & Ellsworth, 1972; Ekman, Levenson, & Friesen, 1983; Izard, 1977). The other direction, based on self-report of cognitive and emotional states, posits two primary dimensions of emotionality: the valence dimension (e.g., pleasantness vs. unpleasantness) and the arousal dimension (e.g., high vs. low arousal) (cf. Nyklicek, Thayer, & van Doornen, 1997; Osgood, Suci, & Tannenbaum, 1957; Russell, 1979; Thayer & Miller, 1988). These two directions can be seen as complementary rather than antagonistic.

Levenson (1988) suggested a discrete model that includes the arousal dimension and that might be the most productive for explorations of emotional processing. Starting from the attentional model of Pribram and McGuinness (1975), Tucker and Williamson (1984) differentiated the activity of a tonic activation system, which is thought to control preparatory mechanisms for action, from that of a phasic activation system (arousal), which supports perceptual processes. These two systems are seen to reflect the activity of different cortical systems. For example, the left hemisphere has been considered to be an important part of the attentional characteristics of the tonic activation system. This hemisphere is mainly engaged in the production of focused attention required in sequential processing and analytical thinking. The activity of the right hemisphere is coherent with the phasic activation system (arousal), which is engaged in the orienting response to novel stimuli. According to this model, the right hemisphere should be more engaged in emotional processing, whereas the left hemisphere should control emotional stability by inhibiting the affective response of the right hemisphere.

Study 1. Given our assumption that 40-Hz EEG activity is a physiological expression of focused arousal (Sheer, 1976), our first study (De Pascalis, Marucci, Penna, & Pessa, 1987) was based on two main hypotheses: (a) emotional valence may affect interhemispheric activity in the direction suggested by Tucker's (1987) model, and (b) even outside hypnosis, highly hypnotizable subjects, as compared to low hypnotizables, should display more pronounced task-related 40-Hz EEG hemispheric shifts in accordance with attentional requirements of the task. The aim of this study was also to determine whether highly hypnotizable subjects, compared to low hypnotizables, have a greater capacity to access affect in the nonhypnotic condition. This greater ability should be reflected in task-related hemispheric shifts of 40-Hz EEG activity during recall of events with positive and negative emotional valence in a nonhypnotic condition. In this early study, we were limited to two EEG recording channels, which did not allow us to evaluate the role of the frontal region (Barabasz & Barabasz, 1995, 1996) during self-generated emotional events. Twenty-two high and 21 low hypnotizable right-handed women were selected with the Harvard Group Scale of Hypnotic Susceptibility: Form A (HGSHS:A; Shor & Orne, 1962). We used only females because there is some evidence indicating that gender may affect both hypnotic susceptibility and EEG symmetry (Bowers, 1971; Glass, Butler, & Carter, 1984; Ray, Morrel, Frediani, & Tucker, 1976; Trotman & Hammond, 1979; but see Hilgard, 1965). Because subject selection was based only on a single group screening, some sampling noise was likely introduced into this study. Only subjects with one standard deviation (*SD*) above and one *SD* below the group mean ($N = 99$, $M = 6.5$, $SD = 2.4$) were selected in this study. They were required to remember three positive (gladness, happiness, satisfaction) and three negative (fear, sadness, anger) situations of personal life events in a nonhypnotic, eyes-closed condition. Hypnosis was not induced or otherwise suggested. All tasks were preceded by a 1-min eyes-closed rest period. Each task was of 2-min duration. Self-report rating scores for vividness of visual imagery and emotional feelings of the recalled material were obtained. The time periods in which 40-Hz EEG activity was present over 2-sec epochs were recorded during each 2-min eyes-closed emotional task and then expressed in seconds/minutes. The EEG activity was considered to be present when 40-Hz EEG amplitude was greater than an averaged amplitude level, measured during a 7-min eyes-closed rest period preceding each group of positive and negative emotional tasks. During each emotional task, the 40-Hz EEG hemispheric activity was compared to the resting 40-Hz EEG level obtained during the rest period preceding each group of tasks. This was done by subtracting the 40-Hz EEG density during an eyes-closed rest period from that obtained during a task.

The relationship between 40-Hz EEG asymmetry and emotional processing was found to be moderated by hypnotizability. High hypnotizables showed an increase of 40-Hz EEG density over both left and right hemispheres during positive emotions, whereas they showed a depressed activity over the left and an increased activity over the right during negative emotions. Low hypnotizables, in contrast, did not exhibit differential hemispheric patterns that could be attributed to different emotional valences. High hypnotizable individuals also had a lower 40-Hz EEG density compared to the lows in eyes-closed rest and task conditions.

No differences in vividness of visual material were found between groups. High hypnotizables, in contrast to lows, were more able to access affective events and, perhaps because of this, showed greater task-related hemispheric shifts (hemispheric specificity) compared to the lows. This greater hemispheric specificity exhibited by the highs is consistent with most previous findings (e.g., Karlin, Goldstein, Cohen, & Morgan, 1980; MacLeod-Morgan, 1979; MacLeod-Morgan & Lack, 1982; Meszaros, Banyai, & Greguss, 1986).

Study 2. Of the 43 individuals who took part in the first experiment, 32 participated in a second hypnosis study (De Pascalis, Marucci, & Penna, 1989). The study sought to replicate and extend previous work (De Pascalis et al., 1987). In particular, based on a functional link between focused arousal and 40-Hz EEG activity and assuming that hypnosis is characterized as a condition of selective attention to monotonous stimulation (Hilgard, 1965), we expected an increase of 40-Hz EEG in hypnosis in contrast to the nonhypnosis condition. In addition, given that high hypnotizable subjects should experience affective states as more intense during hypnosis, it was predicted that these experiences would be associated with more pronounced hemispheric asymmetries.

Low hypnotizables ($N = 13$) scored between 0 and 4 and high hypnotizables ($N = 16$) scored between 10 and 12 on the HGSHS:A and SHSS:C scales of hypnotizability. After a hypnotic induction, suggestions to "relive" four of the six emotional life situations reported by the subject in the first study were administered to that same subject. From the original pool, two positive emotional events (gladness and happiness) and two negative emotional events (anger and fear) were selected. These tasks displayed the most marked hemispheric differences. Subjects also used two separate 5-point scales to rate the vividness of visual imagery and the level of emotional feeling of the material recalled. The data of three subjects were excluded from statistical analyses because their level of hypnotizability was significantly different between the first (with HGSHS: A) and the second administration of hypnotic induction (1 year later with SHSS:C), harkening back to the problem of measurement error in Study 1. Of these three subjects, two changed from low to high and one changed from high to low.

We found the following differences between subjects:

1. High hypnotizables reported greater emotional feeling than did lows;
2. High hypnotizable subjects during rest conditions in hypnosis produced significantly lower 40-Hz density in both hemispheres than did lows;

3. High hypnotizables during positive emotions (gladness and happiness) showed a left and right increase of 40-Hz EEG density, whereas during negative affects (anger and fear) they showed a density increase in the right and a density decrease in the left—low hypnotizables did not show differential hemispheric patterns among emotional types; and
4. The differential hemispheric activity across emotional types described above for highs were more pronounced in the hypnotic condition than in the nonhypnotic condition.

The evidence of 40-Hz EEG differences between highs and lows and between nonhypnosis and hypnosis conditions confirmed our previous findings that EEG indices of absorption differentiates high and low hypnotizables and that hypnosis might be fairly characterized as a condition of narrowly focused attention. The greater ability to access affects and the greater hemispheric specificity found for high hypnotizable subjects even when not hypnotized suggest that the differences in physiological flexibility between highs and lows exist independent of hypnosis per se. Finally, despite different methodologies, our results of right hemisphere activation during negative emotions appear similar to those of Davidson, Schwartz, Saron, Bennett, and Goleman (1979); Karlin, Weinapple, Rochford, and Goldstein (1979); and Tucker, Stenslie, Roth, and Shearer (1981). However, we also observed that right-hemisphere activation was paralleled by left-hemisphere inhibition. During positive emotions, the activation of both hemispheres was present in high hypnotizable subjects. A significant relationship between hypnotizability, hypnosis, and 40-Hz EEG density was also observed in this study. High hypnotizable subjects produced less 40-Hz EEG density than did low hypnotizable subjects. Another characteristic of high hypnotizables was that in the hypnosis condition they showed greater 40-Hz EEG density increases than did lows.

Congruent results on 40-Hz EEG hemispheric asymmetries during emotional processing were obtained in our recent study (De Pascalis, Ray, Tranquillo, & D'Amico, 1998) using highly hypnotizable subjects. During the experience of happiness, these subjects showed an increased production of 40-Hz activity in the left frontal and central region of the scalp, whereas during sadness they showed an increased activity in the right central and posterior regions. Low hypnotizable subjects failed to evidence significant task-related hemispheric shifts.

Because the responsiveness to hypnotic suggestion is not a unitary phenomenon even among highly hypnotizable subjects, the quality and extent of response varies considerably (Balthazard & Woody, 1992; Barabasz & Barabasz, 1992; Bowers, 1971). For example, Schnyer and Allen (1995) divided (a) high hypnotizable subjects into two groups based on those who did and did not pass a word-recognition amnesia test and (b) low hypnotizables into two groups, one of simulators and one of nonsimulators, on the recognition amnesia test. The N1-P1 peak amplitude of the ERPs and 40-Hz EEG spectral amplitudes were used as predictors of hypnotizability in a contrast regression analysis. The analysis indicated that high hypnotizables showing recognition amnesia may be a separate group from all other subjects. The analysis also showed that the N1-P1 peak and resting eyes-open 40-Hz spectral amplitude recorded over the right parieto-temporal region accounted for 58% of the total variance. High hypnotizable participants who demonstrated recognition amnesia had a greater spectral amplitude than did other subjects. Results from this study appear in the same direction as those obtained in an early study by Akpinar, Ulett, and Itil (1971), who found greater 40-Hz spectral amplitudes in high hypnotizables as compared to lows.

However, for a variety of reasons the result of these studies cannot be compared with those obtained in our previous investigations in which we found lower temporal 40-Hz EEG density in high hypnotizable persons. First, we measured 40-Hz EEG density, that is, the time production of 40-Hz over an eyes-closed baseline amplitude (threshold obtained as the mean value of the amplitude variation over 7-min baseline preceding each group of tasks). Second, the subjects were grouped into hypnotic categories using different scales (Barber Suggestibility Scale in Akpinar et al.'s [1971] study) and selection criteria (HGSHS:A, SHSS:C, and word recognition amnesia scores in the Schnyer and Allen [1995] study). And third, 40-Hz temporal density and 40-Hz spectral amplitudes are different measures. Temporal density is derived from a threshold baseline measure (i.e., the amount of time the amplitude of a 40-Hz burst persists over an averaged baseline threshold) that varies among subjects. Spectral amplitude is in the frequency domain.

In conclusion, the dual attentional model of Tucker and Williamson (1984) and the Gruzelier (Gruzelier, Brow, Perry, Rhonder, & Thomas, 1984; Gruzelier & Warren, 1993) model of attentional asymmetry can explain the observed task-related hemispheric asymmetries. According to these models, the left hemisphere is more involved in maintaining selective or focal attention and the right in maintaining "sustained" attention. Our results can be explained assuming that the memories of positive affects may require the enhancement of activity in both hemispheres: the left to recall from memory and to analyze the positive emotional material and the right to monitor if the left has received information. The recollection of negative emotional experiences may produce a decrease in the left hemisphere activity because the negative connotation of the recollected material per se tends to reduce the focus of attention that is mainly under the control of the left hemisphere. It is noteworthy that differences in hypnotic ability are associated with the patterning of EEG hemispheric response to affect.

40-Hz EEG Activity Dissociation, Hypnosis, and Hypnotizability

Dissociated Control

The theory of dissociated control (Bowers, 1990, 1992) explains hypnotic behavior as spontaneous deviations from planned behavior that convey impressive parallels with explanatory models of frontal lobe disorders (e.g., Shimamura, 1995). This suggests that hypnosis may be characterized by changes in frontal lobe functions. This view, supported by a number of research findings, prompted researchers to examine left hemisphere activity during hypnosis (e.g., Cikurel & Gruzelier, 1990; Gruzelier, 1996; Gruzelier & Warren, 1993). Parallel with frontal inhibition, right posterior brain functions may become enhanced as the subject enters a condition of receptivity and vivid imagery. Enhancement of posterior functions in hypnosis has some modest experimental support (e.g., Crawford, 1990; Gruzelier, 1990; Jutai, Gruzelier, Golds, & Thomas, 1993; McCormack & Gruzelier, 1993). Less work has been directed at decreases in frontal function (Barabasz & Barabasz, 1995, 1996; Gruzelier, 1996; Gruzelier & Warren, 1993). Guided by these neurophysiological and dissociated control models of hypnosis, we evaluate our EEG findings regarding hypnosis per se. Furthermore, the validity of the assumption that a characteristic of the highly hypnotizable subject is greater cognitive and physiological flexibility in the allocation of processing resources is examined (i.e., highly hypnotizable individuals exhibiting a greater ability to shift from one strategy to another in response to task requirements).

The association of hypnotic induction and hypnotizability on left and right 40-Hz EEG activity was evaluated in our laboratory in two separate investigations (De Pascalis, 1993; De Pascalis & Penna, 1990). Only the most recent study is reported below.

Study 3. The aim of this study was to evaluate EEG hemispheric activity during hypnotic induction and hypnotic testing using the Stanford Hypnotic Clinical Scale (SHCS; Morgan & Hilgard, 1978-1979) with high and low hypnotizable subjects. Six electrode sites were used and spectral amplitudes of 7 Hz bands (theta1: 4-6 Hz; theta2: 6-8 Hz; alpha1: 8-10 Hz; alpha2: 10-13 Hz; beta1: 13-16 Hz; beta2: 16-20 Hz; beta3: 20-36 Hz) were obtained using Fast-Fourier Transform (FFT). EEG was recorded monopolarly at frontal (F3, F4), central (C3, C4), and posterior (in the middle of O1-P3-T5 and O2-P4-T6 triangles) sites during the hypnotic induction and during hypnotic dream and age-regression items of the SHCS. Spectral amplitude (FFTs) of EEG frequency bands including 40-Hz EEG activity (36-44 Hz), which was corrected for EMG artifacts, was recorded from anterior and posterior regions. Ten low hypnotizable (0-4 on both HGSHS:A and SHSS:C scales) and 10 high hypnotizable (10-12 on both

HGSHS:A and SHSS:C scales) right-handed women participated in a single experimental session consisting of the administration of the SHCS. EEG was recorded during the following periods: nonhypnosis-rest eyes-open and eyes-closed conditions; early (eyes open), middle (eyes closed), and late (1 to 20 counting period, eyes closed) periods of hypnotic induction; and hypnotic dream and age-regression suggestions. The following results were obtained: In waking eyes-open and eyes-closed conditions preceding hypnotic induction and during hypnotic induction, highly hypnotizable subjects produced a greater 40-Hz EEG amplitude than did low hypnotizable subjects at frontal, central, and posterior locations. High hypnotizables during the hypnotic dream instruction displayed a greater 40-Hz EEG amplitude in the right hemisphere with respect to the left hemisphere. This difference was even more pronounced over posterior scalp recordings.

Mainly at the onset of hypnotic induction, highly hypnotizables displayed a significantly greater amount of beta3 than did low hypnotizables, and this difference was even more pronounced in the left hemisphere. On posterior scalp recordings, during hypnotic dream and age regression items, high hypnotizables displayed a decrease in alpha1 and alpha2 amplitudes compared to a rest-hypnosis condition. This effect was not observed for low hypnotizables. Beta1, beta2, and beta3 amplitudes increased in the left hemisphere during age regression in high hypnotizables. Low hypnotizables, in contrast, displayed an hemispheric balance across rest, imaginative, and age-regression conditions.

The 40-Hz EEG results from this study have also showed that the level of 40-Hz EEG spectral amplitude increases as a function of hypnotizability and hypnosis and is consistent with the Schnyer and Allen (1995) findings.

This study failed to show a significant relationship between hypnotizability or hypnosis and theta1 and theta2 amplitudes. This negative result is in contrast to a number of previous findings, suggesting that theta-band activity increases as a function of hypnotizability (for a review, see Crawford & Gruzelier, 1992; De Pascalis & Imperiali, 1984; Graffin, Ray, & Lundy, 1995; Sabourin, 1982; Sabourin, Cutcomb, Crawford, & Pribram, 1990). The apparent discrepancy in results may be due to the interpretation of theta activity with respect to attentional level (Crawford, 1994).

Finally, one of the most interesting findings of this study was that among high hypnotizables, beta3 amplitude in the early hypnotic induction was greater in the left hemisphere as compared to the right, and as the induction proceeded, the activity of this hemisphere was inhibited, resulting in the hemispheres becoming similar. This significant, although post hoc, finding appears to be in agreement with the frontal inhibition model proposed by Gruzelier et al. (1984). In general, our findings support those of other researchers who posit a relationship between hypnosis and frontal inhibition (Gruzelier, 1996; Gruzelier &

Warren, 1993; Jutai et al., 1993) as well as other studies in which beta activity was found to discriminate task performance between high and low hypnotizable subjects (Meszaros et al., 1986; Meszaros, Crawford, Szabo, Nagy-Kovacs, & Revesz, 1989; Sabourin et al., 1990).

The Obstructive Hallucination

Dramatic perceptual alterations (e.g., positive and negative hallucinations) are some of the most compelling experiences of highly hypnotizable subjects. Yet, there are only a handful of studies examining the neurological concomitants of this experience. Some of the most impressive results were obtained in the study of Spiegel et al. (1985), which examined the influence of obstructive hypnotic hallucination over ERPs. The authors reported that among high hypnotizable subjects, there were significant reductions in P300 amplitude to visual stimuli during obstruction hallucination.

Study 4. In order to replicate and extend these findings, a study on the effect of visual obstructive hallucination in hypnosis was carried out in our laboratory (De Pascalis, 1994). High ($N = 7$) and low ($N = 9$) hypnotizable (HGSHS:A and SHSS:C) right-handed women participated in the experiment. Eight medium hypnotizable right-handed women served as a control group. A trial consisted of a sequence of three flash trains, a series of lights intended to elicit an ERP, in which one of the flash trains was the target stimulus. Peak amplitudes and latencies of P1, N1, P2, N2, and P3 ERP components to target stimuli were compared across two hypnotic suggestion conditions: (a) suggestion of stimulus enhancement and (b) suggestion of stimulus elimination. In the stimulus enhancement condition, the subject was told that the target stimulus would appear unusually bright and it would be easily recognized among a sequence of less bright stimuli. In the obstructive hallucination condition, the subject was told to visualize a cardboard box that would surround the circular stimulation light spot. High hypnotizable subjects displayed a significant attenuation of P1 and N1 ERP amplitudes while experiencing stimulus elimination. The effect for the P1 component was greater at the posterior sites as compared to that found at the anterior and central sites. Similar findings across conditions were also observed for P3 peak amplitude, even though the Group × Condition effect was only marginally significant. P3 peak latency also showed a significant effect, including hypnotizability. During negative hallucination, highly hypnotizable subjects showed a significantly shorter P3 latency as compared to the stimulus enhancement condition. This effect was more pronounced across the right hemisphere.

The results of this study support the notion that highly hypnotizable subjects exhibit task-related changes in the amplitudes of visual ERP responses. A relative increase of P1 and N1 ERP peaks was also observed for the stimulus enhancement condition. No hemispheric asymmetries in the peak amplitude of these ERP components were related to the obstructive hallucination or the stimulus enhancement suggestions. Such task-related differences were not found among low hypnotizable subjects. These data indicate that hypnosis-induced subjective changes in perception are paralleled by congruent changes in ERP amplitude. The findings of ERP peak amplitudes observed in this and the Spiegel et al. (1985) study were similar to work by Barabasz et al. (1995, 1996b).

The results of the De Pascalis (1994) study are also consistent with the few existing studies of hypnotic phenomena that demonstrate alterations in the attention-related ERP components during perception-related hypnotic suggestions. Significantly smaller amplitudes for N1, P1, and late positive component (after 400 ms) elicited by word stimuli in high hypnotizables who reported hypnotic word recognition amnesia were found by Allen, Iacono, Lavaruso, and Dunn (1995). Spiegel, Bierre, and Rootenberg (1989) reported enhanced P100 amplitudes in highly hypnotizable participants during hypnosis with suggestions to intensify attention to somatosensory stimuli and reduced P100 and P300 amplitudes during a hypnotic suggestion to block the perception of the stimulus. Reduced P1 and N1 components of the visual ERP in highly hypnotizable subjects was found by Jasiukaitis, Nouriani, Hillyard, and Spiegel (1993). In a more recent study, Jasiukaitis, Nouriani, and Spiegel (1996) found that suggestions for hypnotic obstruction reduced the P200 component to visual stimuli in the right hemifield but did not affect P200 for stimulation in the left hemifield. This result was discussed by the authors as a left hemisphere mechanism for image generation. Another research group (Perlini, Lorimer, Campbell, & Spanos, 1992/1993; Perlini, Spanos, & Jones, 1996) reported that hypnotic hallucinations did not alter visual ERPs over baseline in highly hypnotizable subjects. However, post hoc analyses more appropriate to the study indicated amplitude attenuations in both the P2 and P3 components of the parietal ERP in the obstructive hallucination condition. Furthermore, this hallucination condition was accompanied by a significant attenuation of the P1 component at the left temporo-parieto-occipital region.

The difference in P1 and N1 peak amplitudes between high and low hypnotizable subjects found in this study was unexpected. How can these P1 and N1 changes among highly hypnotizable subjects be explained? It is conceivable that these are trait differences that reflect different styles of visual information processing, with high hypnotizables being more able to experience mental imagery.

Systematic augmentation in the amplitude of the P1 component has been related to sustained attention to stimuli appearing within a particular visual field (Heinze, Luck, Mangun, & Hillyard, 1990; Hillyard & Picton, 1987; Luck, Heinze, Mangun, & Hillyard, 1990). This augmentation has been assumed to reflect a facilitation of early sensory processing that follows from a tuning or facilitation of the visual pathways. These findings suggest that at the earliest stages of informational processing, highly hypnotizable individuals may attenuate or amplify the stimulus input in a way that low hypnotizable individuals can not.

It is known that the N1 component is also sensitive to attention (for a review see Naatanen, 1992). The N1 peak is larger when subjects recruit attentional resources to attend to a target stimulus. In relation to the present findings, this model suggests that high hypnotizables who passed a hypnotic obstructive hallucination suggestion apply fewer attentional resources to the stimuli as compared to the same subjects who experienced a hallucination stimulus enhancement. Previously, early technology studies of 20 to 30 years ago were unable to show changes in either the amplitude or latency of the ERPs between hypnotic and baseline conditions (Andreassi et al., 1976; Beck & Barolin, 1965; Beck et al., 1966).

Hypnotic Analgesia

There is still little consensus regarding the physiological mechanisms involved in hypnotic analgesia (Price, 1988). This is in part because the hypnotic situation is often structured in such a manner that the subject is pressured to inhibit overt signs of pain and in part because any neural substrate mediating the pain response to noxious stimuli in humans is still poorly understood. A study using functional information derived from positron emission tomography (PET) and anatomical information derived from magnetic resonance imaging (MRI) (Talbot et al., 1991) showed that painful heat applied to an arm caused the activation of three cortical foci contralateral to the stimulated arm: anterior cingulate, primary somatosensory, and secondary somatosensory cortices. Another PET study (Jones, Brown, Friston, Qi, & Frackowiak, 1991) failed to find increased blood flow to painful heat in the somatosensory cortex, whereas significant increases were detected in the contralateral cingulate cortex, thalamus, and lenticular nucleus. Using frontoparietal bipolar EEG recordings, Chen, Dworkins, and Bloomquist (1981) found, in a patient undergoing dental surgery, that the production of total spectral power decreased during hypnotic analgesia with a more pronounced decrease in the left hemisphere for theta and alpha bands. Karlin et al. (1980), with bipolar parieto-occipital EEG recordings, found that cold-pressor pain produced a right-hemisphere engagement. Using unipolar recordings at frontal temporal, parietal, and occipital leads with references to earlobes, Crawford (1990) reported that highly hypnotizable subjects, in hypnosis, generated more theta power than lows during pain and hypnotic analgesia across all locations. Especially in the temporal regions, high hypnotizables showed greater theta power in the left hemisphere during the experience of pain, whereas they showed a shift toward a greater theta power in the right hemisphere during hypnotic analgesia. Higher theta power during analgesia in a fakir was also reported by Larbig et al. (1982). Hilgard and Hilgard (1975) observed that the physiological reactivity to painful stimulation is still evidenced in cases in which highly hypnotizable subjects can completely eliminate the perception of pain. In this respect, there are a number of reports that cardiovascular responses are not inhibited during hypnotic analgesia (Evans & Paul, 1970; Hilgard & Hilgard, 1975). More recent studies using spectral analysis of beat-to-beat variability (DeBenedittis, Panerai, & Villamira, 1989; Hautkappe & Bongartz, 1992) have shown that hypnosis affects heart rate variability, shifting the sympathovagal balance toward an enhanced parasympathetic activity in parallel with a reduction in sympathetic activity.

Study 5. Taking into account previous EEG and heart rate findings, we examined the effects of hypnotic analgesia and hypnosis on interhemispheric EEG activity and heart rate (HR) during painful stimulations of the left median nerve (De Pascalis & Perrone, 1996). Painful stimuli consisted of unipolar electric pulses delivered on the left wrist. The painful stimulation was delivered in three experimental conditions: (a) nonhypnotic, (b) hypnosis with no analgesia, and (c) hypnosis with analgesia suggestions that the stimuli were less intense without including images designed to help subjects reduce pain. EEG signal was recorded from frontal (F3, F4), central (C3, C4), and posterior (in the middle of O1-P3-T5 and O2-P4-T6 triangles) scalp sites and then processed using FFT. Measures of cardiac activity, including cardiac interbeat interval (ms), midfrequency, and high-frequency peak powers (MFP in the 0.06-0.14 Hz range and HFP in the 0.15-0.32 Hz range), were obtained. The State-Trait Anxiety (Spielberger, Gorsuch, & Lushene, 1970) and pain and distress tolerance rating scores were also administered.

The results of this study showed that pain and distress scores for high hypnotizables were smaller during hypnotic analgesia, as compared to a nonhypnotic and hypnotic no analgesia condition, with the reduction observed for distress scores being more pronounced than that for pain scores. This result was generally consistent with previous findings of a hypnotically induced dissociation between the sensory-discriminative and affective-motivational dimensions of the pain experience (DeBenedittis et al., 1989; Hilgard & Hilgard, 1975; Knox, Morgan, & Hilgard, 1974). There were no significant differences in state and trait anxiety between groups.

Highly hypnotizable subjects also exhibited significantly lower total EEG amplitude (0.50-31.75 Hz) and beta1 (13-15.75 Hz) amplitude than did low hypnotizables. These results indicate that generally high hypnotizables had a lower level of cortical arousal/arousability to painful stimulation than did lows. Results from separate ANOVAs on the high and low groups also indicate that hypnosis during painful stimulation reduces overall cortical functioning as reflected by a decrease in total spectral amplitude across central and posterior recording areas. A reduction in total spectral amplitude in highly hypnotizable subjects during hypnosis was observed, but it did not occur symmetrically across hemispheres. High hypnotizable subjects, both in hypnosis/no analgesia and hypnosis/analgesia compared to a waking control condition, displayed considerable amplitude reductions for total and delta (0.50-3.75 Hz) spectral amplitudes in both hemispheres. Moreover, for total, delta, and beta1 amplitudes, during hypnosis/analgesia compared to hypnosis/no analgesia, the amplitude reductions were more pronounced in the right hemisphere, resulting in a more pronounced hemispheric asymmetry in favor of the left hemisphere. In contrast, low hypnotizable subjects showed no significant changes in the hemispheric asymmetry across conditions. The ANOVA on low hypnotizables displayed, for posterior recordings, a significant reduction in delta amplitude during both hypnosis/no analgesia and hypnosis/analgesia conditions. These subjects also showed a significant reduction in theta1 (4-5.75 Hz) amplitude across all the recording sites during hypnosis/no analgesia as compared to a waking condition. However, low subjects failed to show significant amplitude differences between the two hypnosis conditions. No significant effects involving hypnotizability for 40 Hz EEG (36-44 Hz) activity were detected.

Due to the fact that during hypnotic analgesia, pain reductions correlated significantly with right-hemisphere decreases in total EEG amplitude, it was deduced that the inhibition of the right hemisphere may play an important role in the relief of pain.

The analysis of variance did not evidence significant effects on cardiac interbeat intervals. The analysis of covariance on MFP scores with HFP scores as covariates indicated that high hypnotizables had lower MFPs as compared to low hypnotizables and that during hypnosis/analgesia as compared to waking and hypnosis/no analgesia, high hypnotizables displayed a reduction in the MFP. In lows, no significant differences were observed.

The reduced sympathetic activity found during hypnotic analgesia in the present study does not contradict previous observations supporting the lack of inhibition in cardiovascular responses during hypnotic analgesia (Evans & Paul, 1970; Hilgard et al., 1974). In fact, we observed a relatively small reduction in sympathetic activity. In this condition, the sympathetic activity was still prevalent as compared to the parasympathetic activity. Therefore, our opinion is that the reduced sympathetic activity is a secondary effect of how attentional resources are allocated in the experience of analgesia.

By comparing EEG and HR variability findings, we excluded a possible hypothesis for a centrifugal inhibition of nociceptive transmission (for a clear introduction to psychophysiological mechanisms of pain inhibition, see Price, 1988). If a centrifugal inhibition of nociceptive transmission had been operative, we should have observed, in parallel with the reduced sympathetic activity during hypnotic analgesia, a reduced EEG spectral amplitude in the hypnosis/analgesia versus hypnosis/no analgesia condition. EEG patterns between the two hypnosis conditions differed only in that during hypnosis/analgesia the right-hemisphere amplitude was smaller as compared to the left-hemisphere amplitude. Thus, during analgesia, the reduction in right hemisphere activity may be responsible for the reduction in sympathetic activity. This association is supported by a number of psychophysiological studies in which manipulations devoted to selectively activating the right hemisphere evoked an acceleration of heart rate (Hugdahl, Franzon, Andersson, & Walldebo, 1983; Lane, Novelly, Cornell, Zeitlin, & Schwartz, 1988; Rosen, Gur, Sussman, Gur, & Hurtig, 1982; Weisz, Szilagyi, Lang, & Adam, 1992). Perhaps the reduction in pain perception during hypnotic analgesia can be explained as a reduction of right hemisphere activity that is reflected in a reduced activity of the sustained attentional component responsible for the negative emotional state. Arendt-Nielsen, Zachariae, and Bjerring (1990) and Zachariae and Bjerring (1994) report ERP findings that are consistent with this explanation of hypnotic analgesia. These authors found that both pain reports and event-related brain potentials elicited by laser stimuli can be reduced with suggestions of hypnotic analgesia. Focusing and defocusing attention has been cited as a possible explanation for the observed hypnotically induced changes.

Kropotov, Crawford, and Polyakov (1997) studied the neurophysiological correlates of pain control by recording somatosensory ERPs to painful cutaneous stimuli from intracranial electrodes. A hypnotically responsive patient who reduced pain perception during suggested hypnotic analgesia showed a significant reduction of a positive ERP component in the range of 140-160 ms in the left-anterior cingulate cortex and a significant enhancement of a negative ERP component in the range of 200-260 ms in the left-anterior temporal cortex (Brodman area 21). ERP findings from a recent study carried out in our lab (De Pascalis & Carboni, 1997) also evidenced, in high hypnotizable subjects, a reduced P300 peak to electric somatosensory target stimuli in the left frontal and posterior scalp sites during hypnotic obstructive hallucination as compared to a normal attention condition. In this condition, P300 suppression was paralleled by a smaller anticipatory HR deceleration response to target stimuli. These findings indicate that obstructive hallucinations to somatosensory stimuli may involve alterations in neural and autonomic activities consistent with a trait conception of hypnotizability.

Conclusion

Psychophysiological results from our laboratory appear to support Hilgard's (1986, pp. 147-153) hypothesis that highly hypnotizable persons differ from lows in their ability to focus attention on task-relevant stimuli. The 40-Hz EEG rhythm, which, according to Sheer (1976), is the physiological representation of focused arousal, appears to discriminate high and low hypnotizables both in and outside hypnosis.

High hypnotizables, who seem more able to access affective events during negative and positive emotions, also show a greater 40-Hz EEG hemispheric specificity in both nonhypnotic and hypnotic conditions. Our EEG rhythm findings support the greater physiological flexibility (i.e., the subjective capacity to shift from one "state" to another) of high in contrast to low hypnotizables, which is consistent with Barabasz and Lonsdale (1983) as well as Spiegel et al. (1985). High hypnotizables, during the recollection of happy experiences, showed a 40-Hz EEG increase on posterior regions of both hemispheres, a density increase in the posterior right, and a density reduction in the posterior left during recollection of anger and fearful experiences. The hemispheric patterns observed in high hypnotizables in the nonhypnotic condition were significantly more pronounced in hypnosis.

High hypnotizables, in the early stage of hypnotic induction, produced a significantly greater amount of fast beta activity (20-36 Hz) than did lows, and this difference was even more pronounced in the left hemisphere. At a later stage of hypnotic induction, the prevalent inhibition of left-hemisphere activity produced a hemispheric balancing. This finding supports Gruzelier's (1988, 1996) model of hypnosis. In sensory distortion and ideomotor items of the SHSS:C, highly hypnotizable subjects showed a significant increase of 40-Hz EEG density in the left hemisphere as compared to the right and a relative right hemisphere increase in imaginative items.

Our ERP study, showing a significant reduction of P1 and N1 peak amplitudes following obstructive hallucination, can not adequately be explained as individual differences in goal-directed strategies. The P1 peak occurred at about 80 ms from stimulus onset. The automaticity of the process generating this early ERP component makes it difficult to reconcile these findings with the sociocognitive interpretation of hypnosis as noted by Dixon and Laurence (1992). The effect of increases in amplitude of the ERP components in the early latency ranges as a function of the rated confidence of signal detection has been observed in a number of studies (Chapman, Chen, Colpitts, & Martin, 1981; Hillyard & Picton, 1987; Parasuraman, Richer, & Beatty, 1982; Paul & Sutton, 1972). This suggests that the earlier exogenous components, such as P1 and N1 waves, may be indices of the perceived sensory magnitude of the signal, that is, they reflect more the effect of signal detection. Our findings are entirely consistent with those of Barabasz, Barabasz et al. (1996b), showing that hypnotic alteration of stimulus perception operates early at the level of the detection of the signal as well as later at the level of response bias.

Finally, the evidence regarding physiological shifts during hypnotic analgesia is as follows: High hypnotizables, experiencing hypnotic analgesia, showed significantly smaller total, delta, and beta1 amplitudes in the right hemisphere across all frontal, central, and posterior recordings so that a significantly more pronounced hemispheric asymmetry in favor of the left hemisphere was displayed. In contrast, low hypnotizables showed no significant changes in hemispheric asymmetry during hypnotic analgesia. The hemispheric asymmetry in highly hypnotizable subjects experiencing hypnotic analgesia was parallel to a reduced sympathetic activity. This reduction may be explained as a product of the reduced right hemisphere activity because there is experimental evidence supporting the idea that right hemisphere activation increases heart rate (Hugdahl et al., 1983; Weisz et al., 1992).

In sum, although a definitive physiological "signature" for hypnosis and hypnotizability is not yet available, there are some productive lines of research that are moving toward this end. Programmatic research in a number of sophisticated neurophysiological laboratories has yielded promising leads as to the neurological and physiological shifts associated with hypnosis as condition, hypnotizability as trait, and hypnotizability in interaction with task. But the findings span across a host of sampling, measurement, and instrumentation methodologies, thus rendering cross-study comparisons difficult and sometimes impossible. As it stands now, it is essential for neurophysiological researchers to rectify this situation by careful replication, with an eye to connecting these findings not only to the physiological literature but to theories of hypnosis and cognitive science more generally.

References

Akpinar, S., Ulett, G. A., & Itil, T. M. (1971). Hypnotizability predicted by digital computer-analyzed EEG pattern. *Biological Psychiatry, 3*, 387-392.

Allen, J. J., Iacono, W. G., Lavaruso, J. J., & Dunn, L. (1995). An event-related potential investigation of posthypnotic recognition amnesia. *Journal of Abnormal Psychology, 104*, 421-430.

Andreassi, J. L., Balinsky, B., Gallichio, J. A., De Simone, J. J., & Mellers, B. W. (1976). Hypnotic suggestion of stimulus change and visual cortical evoked potential. *Perceptual and Motor Skills, 42*, 371-378.

Arendt-Nielsen, L., Zachariae, R., & Bjerring, P. (1990). Quantitative evaluation of hypnotically suggested hyperaesthesia and analgesia by painful laser stimulation. *Pain, 42*, 243-251.

Balthazard, C. G., & Woody, E. Z. (1992). The spectral analysis of hypnotic performance with respect to "absorption." *International Journal of Clinical and Experimental Hypnosis, 40*, 21-43.

Barabasz, A. F., & Barabasz, M. (1992). Research designs and considerations. In E. Fromm & M. R. Nash (Eds.), *Contemporary hypnosis research* (pp. 173-226). New York: Guilford.

Barabasz, A. F., & Barabasz, M. (1995). Attention deficit hyperactivity disorder: Neurological basis and treatment alternatives. *Journal of Neurotherapy, 1*, 1-10.

Barabasz, A. F., & Barabasz, M. (1996, November). *Hypnosis in unusual places.* Paper presented at the 47th annual Scientific Program of the Society for Clinical and Experimental Hypnosis, Tampa, FL.

Barabasz, A. F., Barabasz, M., & Jensen, S. (1995, November). *Effects of hypnosis on cortical event-related potentials during visual and olfactory hypnotic hallucinations.* Paper presented at the 46th annual meeting of the Society for Clinical and Experimental Hypnosis, San Antonio, TX.

Barabasz, A. F., Barabasz, M., Jensen, S., & Calvin, S. (1996a, August). *Alternative hypnotic suggestions alter EEG event-related potentials: The clinicians had it right.* American Psychological Association Convention, Toronto, Canada.

Barabasz, A. F., Barabasz, M., Jensen, S., & Calvin, S. (1996b, November). *Alternative hypnotic suggestions alter visual and auditory EEG event-related potentials.* Paper presented at the 47th annual Scientific Program of the Society for Clinical and Experimental Hypnosis, Tampa, FL.

Barabasz, A., Barabasz, M., Jensen, S., Calvin, S., Trevisan, M., & Warner, D. (1999). Cortical event-related potentials show the structure of hypnotic suggestions is crucial. *International Journal of Clinical and Experimental Hypnosis, 47,* 5-22.

Barabasz, A. F., & Lonsdale, C. (1983). Effects of hypnosis on P300 olfactory evoked potential amplitudes. *Journal of Abnormal Psychology, 92,* 520-523.

Basar, E., Rosen, B., Basar-Eroglu, C., & Greitschus, F. (1987). The associations between 40 Hz EEG and the middle latency response of the auditory evoked potential. *International Journal of Neuroscience, 33,* 103-117.

Basar-Eroglu, C., Struber, D., Kruse, P., Basar, E., & Stadler, M. (1996). Frontal gamma-band enhancement during multistable visual perception. *International Journal of Psychophysiology, 24,* 113-125.

Beck, E. C., & Barolin, G. S. (1965). The effect of hypnotic suggestion on evoked potentials. *Journal of Nervous and Mental Disease, 140,* 154-160.

Beck, E. C., Dustman, R., & Beier, E. G. (1966). Hypnotic suggestions and visually evoked potentials. *Electroencephalography and Clinical Neurophysiology, 20,* 397-400.

Bowers, K. S. (1971). Sex and susceptibility as moderator variables in the relationship of creativity and hypnotic susceptibility. *Journal of Abnormal Psychology, 78,* 93-100.

Bowers, K. S. (1990). Unconscious influences and hypnosis. In J. L. Singer (Ed.), *Repression and dissociation: Implications for personality theory, psychopathology and health* (pp. 143-178). Chicago: University of Chicago Press.

Bowers, K. S. (1992). Imagination and dissociation in hypnotic responding. *International Journal of Clinical and Experimental Hypnosis, 40,* 253-275.

Chapman, C. R., Chen, A.C.N., Colpitts, Y. M., & Martin, R. W. (1981). Sensory decision theory describes evoked potentials in pain discrimination. *Psychophysiology, 18,* 114-120.

Chen, A. C. N., Dworkins, S. F., & Bloomquist, D. S. (1981). Cortical power spectrum analysis of hypnotic pain control in surgery. *International Journal of Neuroscience, 13,* 127-136.

Cikurel, K., & Gruzelier, J. (1990). The effect of an active-alert hypnotic induction on lateral asymmetry in haptic processing. *British Journal of Experimental and Clinical Hypnosis, 7,* 17-25.

Crawford, H. J. (1990). Cognitive and psychophysiological correlates of hypnotic responsiveness and hypnosis. In M. L. Fass & D. P. Brown (Eds.), *Creative mastery in hypnosis and hypnoanalysis: A festschrift for Erika Fromm* (pp. 155-168). Hillsdale, NJ: Lawrence Erlbaum.

Crawford, H. J. (1994). Brain dynamics and hypnosis: Attentional and disattentional processes. *International Journal of Clinical and Experimental Hypnosis, 42,* 204-232.

Crawford, H. J., & Gruzelier, J. H. (1992). A midstream view of the neuropsychophysiology of hypnosis: Recent research and future directions. In E. Fromm & M. Nash (Eds.), *Contemporary hypnosis research.* New York: Guilford.

Davidson, R. J., Schwartz, G. E., Saron, C., Bennett, J., & Goleman, D. J. (1979). Frontal versus parietal EEG asymmetry during positive and negative affect. *Psychophysiology, 16,* 202-203.

DeBenedittis, G., Panerai, A. A., & Villamira, M. A. (1989). Effects of hypnotic analgesia and hypnotizability on experimental ischemic pain. *International Journal of Clinical and Experimental Hypnosis, 37,* 55-69.

De Pascalis, V. (1993). EEG spectral analysis during hypnotic induction, hypnotic dream and age-regression. *International Journal of Psychophysiology, 15,* 153-166.

De Pascalis, V. (1994). Event-related potentials during hypnotic hallucination. *International Journal of Clinical and Experimental Hypnosis, 42,* 39-55.

De Pascalis, V., & Carboni, G. (1997). P300 event-related-potential amplitudes and evoked cardiac responses during hypnotic alteration of somatosensory perception. *International Journal of Neuroscience, 92,* 187-208.

De Pascalis, V., & Imperiali, M. C. (1984). Personality, hypnotic susceptibility and EEG responses: Preliminary study. *Perceptual and Motor Skills, 59,* 371-378.

De Pascalis, V., Marucci, F. S., & Penna M. P. (1989). 40-Hz EEG asymmetry during recall of emotional events in waking and hypnosis: Differences between low and high hypnotizables. *International Journal of Psychophysiology, 7,* 85-96.

De Pascalis, V., Marucci, F. S., Penna, M. P., & Pessa, E. (1987). Hemispheric activity of 40-Hz EEG during recall of emotional events: Differences between low and high hypnotizables. *International Journal of Psychophysiology, 5,* 167-180.

De Pascalis, V., & Penna M. P. (1990). 40-Hz EEG activity during hypnotic induction and hypnotic testing. *International Journal of Clinical and Experimental Hypnosis, 38,* 125-138.

De Pascalis, V., & Perrone, M. (1996). EEG asymmetry and heart rate during experience of hypnotic analgesia in high and low hypnotizables. *International Journal of Psychophysiology, 21,* 163-175.

De Pascalis, V., Ray, W. J., Tranquillo, I., & D'Amico, D. (1998). EEG activity and heart rate during recall of emotional events in hypnosis: Relationships with hypnotizability and suggestibility. *International Journal of Psychophysiology, 29,* 255-275.

Dixon, M., & Laurence, J. -R. (1992). Two hundred years of hypnosis research: Questions resolved? Questions unanswered! In E. Fromm & M. R. Nash, *Contemporary hypnosis research* (pp. 34-66). New York: Guilford.

Ekman, P., Friesen, W. V., & Ellsworth, P. C. (1972). *Emotion in the human face: Guidelines for research and an integration of findings.* New York: Pergamon.

Ekman, P., Levenson, R. W., & Friesen, W. V. (1983). Autonomic nervous system activity distinguishes among emotions. *Science, 221,* 1208-1210.

Evans, M. B., & Paul, G. L. (1970). Effects of hypnotically suggested analgesia on physiological and subjective responses to cold stress. *Journal of Consulting and Clinical Psychology, 35,* 362-371.

Galbraith, G. C., Cooper, L. M., & London, P. (1972). Hypnotic susceptibility and the sensory evoked response. *Journal of Comparative and Physiological Psychology, 80,* 509-514.

Glass, A., Butler, S. R., & Carter, J. C. (1984). Hemispheric asymmetry of EEG alpha activation: Effects of gender and familial handedness. *Biological Psychology, 19,* 169-187.

Graffin, N. F., Ray, W. J., & Lundy, R. (1995). EEG concomitants of hypnosis and hypnotic susceptibility. *Journal of Abnormal Psychology, 104,* 123-131.

Gruzelier, J. H. (1988). The neuropsychology of hypnosis. In M. Heap (Ed.), *Hypnosis: Current clinical, experimental and forensic practices* (pp. 68-86). London: Croom Helm.

Gruzelier, J. H. (1990). Neuropsychophysiological investigations of hypnosis: Cerebral laterality and beyond. In R. Van Dyck, P. H. Spinhoven, A. J. W. Van der Does, Y. R. Van Rood, & W. De Moor (Eds.), *Hypnosis: Current theory, research and practice* (pp. 37-51). Amsterdam: VU University Press.

Gruzelier, J. H. (1996). The state of hypnosis: Evidence and applications. *Quarterly Journal of Medicine, 89,* 313-317.

Gruzelier, J. H., Brow, T., Perry, A., Rhonder, J., & Thomas, M. (1984). Hypnotic susceptibility: A lateral predisposition and altered cerebral asymmetry under hypnosis. *International Journal of Psychophysiology, 2,* 131-139.

Gruzelier, J. H., & Warren, K. (1993). Neuropsychological evidence of reductions on left frontal tests with hypnosis. *Psychological-Medicine, 23,* 93-101.

Hautkappe, H. J., & Bongartz, W. (1992). Heart rate variability as an indicator for posthypnotic amnesia in real and simulating subjects. In W. Bongartz, V. A. Gheorghiu, & B. Bongartz (Eds.), *Hypnosis: 175 years after Mesmer—recent developments in theory and application* (pp. 75-83). Konstanz, Germany: Univ.-Verl. Konstanz.

Heinze, H. J., Luck, S. J., Mangun, G. R., & Hillyard, S. A. (1990). Visual event-related potentials index focused attention within bilateral stimulus arrays. I. Evidence for early selection. *Electroencephalography and Clinical Neurophysiology, 75,* 511-527.

Hernandez-Peon, R., & Donoso, M. (1959). Influence of attention and suggestion upon subcortical evoked electrical activity in the human brain. In L. van Bogaert & J. Radermecker (Eds.), *Proceedings of the First International Congress of Neurological Sciences* (Vol. 3, pp. 385-396). London: Pergamon.

Hilgard, E. R. (1965). *Hypnotic susceptibility.* New York: Harcourt, Brace & World.

Hilgard, E. R. (1986). *Divided consciousness: Multiple controls in human thought and action.* New York: John Wiley.

Hilgard, E. R., & Hilgard, J. R. (1975). *Hypnosis in the relief of pain.* Los Altos, CA: William Kaufmann.

Hilgard, E. R., Ruch, J. C., Lange, A. F., Lenox, J. R., Morgan, A. H., & Sachs, L. B. (1974). The psychophysics of cold pressor pain and its modification through hypnotic suggestion. *American Journal of Psychology, 87,* 17-31.

Hillyard, S. A., & Picton, T. W. (1987). Electrophysiology of cognition. In V. B. Mountcastle, F. Plum, & S. R. Geiger (Eds.), *Handbook of physiology: Section 1. The nervous system.* Bethesda, MD: American Physiological Society.

Hillyard, S. A., Picton, T. W., & Regan, D. (1978). Sensation, perception, and attention: Analysis using ERPs. In E. Callaway, P. Tueting, & S. H. Koslow (Eds.), *Event-related brain potentials in man.* New York: Academic Press.

Hugdahl, K., Franzon, M., Andersson, B., & Walldebo, G. (1983). Heart-rate responses (HRR) to lateralized visual stimuli. *Pavlovian Journal of Biological Science, 18,* 186-198.

Izard, C. E. (1977). *Human emotion.* New York: Plenum.

Jasiukaitis, P., Nouriani, B., Hillyard, S., & Spiegel, D. (1993). The effects of hypnotic obstruction on the visual ERP. *Psychophysiology, 30,* S37.

Jasiukaitis, P., Nouriani, B., & Spiegel, D. (1996). Left hemisphere superiority for event-related potential effects of hypnotic obstruction. *Neuropsychologia, 34,* 661-668.

Jokeit, H., & Makeig, S. (1994). Different event-related patterns of gamma-band power in brain waves of fast- and slow-reacting subjects. *Proceedings of National Academy of Sciences, USA, 91,* 6339-6343.

Jones, A. K. A., Brown, W. D., Friston, K. J., Qi, L. Y., & Frackowiak, S. J. (1991). Cortical and subcortical localization of response in pain in man using positron emission tomography. *Proceedings of the Royal Society London, Series B., Biological Sciences, 244,* 39-44.

Jutai, J., Gruzelier, J. H., Golds, J., & Thomas, M. (1993). Bilateral auditory-evoked potentials in conditions of hypnosis and focused attention. *International Journal of Psychophysiology, 15,* 167-176.

Karlin, R. A., Goldstein, L., Cohen, A., & Morgan, D. (1980). *Hypnotizability, attention, and hemispheric EEG activity during verbal and nonverbal tasks.* Unpublished manuscript.

Karlin, R. A., Weinapple, M., Rochford, J., & Goldstein, L. (1979). Quantitated EEG features of negative affective states: Report of some hypnotic studies. *Research Communications in Psychology, Psychiatry and Behavior, 4,* 397-413.

Kirsch, I., & Lynn, S. J. (1995). The altered state of hypnosis: Changes in theoretical landscape. *American Psychologist, 50,* 846-858.

Knox, V. J., Morgan, A. H., & Hilgard, E. R. (1974). Pain and suffering in ischemia: The paradox of hypnotically suggested anesthesia as contradicted by reports from the "hidden observer." *Archives of General Psychiatry, 30,* 840-847.

Kropotov, J. D., Crawford, H. J., & Polyakov, Y. I. (1997). Somatosensory event-related potential changes to painful stimuli during hypnotic analgesia: Anterior cingulate cortex and anterior temporal cortex intracranial recordings. *International Journal of Psychophysiology, 27,* 1-8.

Lane, R. D., Novelly, R., Cornell, C., Zeitlin, S., & Schwartz, G. (1988). Asymmetric hemispheric control of heart rate. *Psychophysiology, 25,* 464.

Larbig, W., Elbert, T., Lutzenberger, W., Rockstroh, B., Schnerr, G., & Birbaumer, N. (1982). EEG and slow brain potentials during anticipation and control of painful stimulation. *Electroencephalography and Clinical Neurophysiology, 53,* 298-309.

Levenson, R. W. (1988). Emotion and the autonomic nervous system: A prospectus for research on autonomic specificity. In H. L. Wagner (Ed.), *Social psychophysiology and emotion: Theory and clinical applications* (pp. 17-42). Chichester, UK: Wiley.

Loring, D. W., & Sheer, D. E. (1984). Laterality of 40-Hz EEG and EMG during cognitive performance. *Psychophysiology, 21,* 34-38.

Luck, S. J., Heinze, H. J., Mangun, G. R., & Hillyard, S. A. (1990). Visual event-related potentials index focused attention within bilateral stimulus arrays. II. Functional dissociation of P1 and N1 components. *Electroencephalography and Clinical Neurophysiology, 75,* 528-542.

Lutzenberger, W., Pulvermuller, F., Elbert, T., & Birbaumer, N. (1995). Visual stimulation alters local 40-Hz responses in humans: An EEG-study. *Neuroscience Letters, 83,* 39-42.

MacLeod-Morgan, C. (1979). Hypnotic susceptibility, EEG theta and alpha waves, and hemispheric specificity. In G. D. Burrows, D. R. Collinsos, & L. Dennerstein (Eds.), *Hypnosis 1979.* Amsterdam: Elsevier North-Holland.

MacLeod-Morgan, C., & Lack, L. (1982). Hemispheric specificity: A physiological concomitant of hypnotizability. *Psychophysiology, 19,* 687-690.

Makeig, S., & Inlow, M. (1993). Lapses in alertness: Coherence of fluctuations in performance and EEG spectrum. *Electroencephalography and Clinical Neurophysiology, 86,* 23-35.

Makela, J. P., & Hari, R. (1987). Evidence for cortical origin of the 40 Hz auditory evoked response in man. *Electroencephalography and Clinical Neurophysiology, 66,* 539-546.

McCormack, K., & Gruzelier, J. H. (1993). Cerebral asymmetry and hypnosis: A signal detection analysis of divided visual-field stimulation. *Journal of Abnormal Psychology, 102,* 352-357.

Meszaros, I., Banyai, E., & Greguss, A. C. (1986, July). *Enhanced right hemisphere activation during hypnosis: EEG and behavioral task performance evidence.* Paper presented at the meeting of the Third International Conference of the International Organization of Psychophysiology, Vienna, Austria.

Meszaros, I., Crawford, H. J., Szabo, C., Nagy-Kovacs, A., & Revesz, M. A. (1989). Hypnotic susceptibility and cerebral hemisphere preponderance: Verbal-imaginal discrimination task. In V. Gheorghiu, P. Netter, H. Eysenck, & R. Rosenthal (Eds.), *Suggestion and suggestibility: Theory and research* (pp. 191-204). Heidelberg, Germany: Springer-Verlag.

Morgan, A. H., & Hilgard, J. R. (1978-1979). The Stanford Hypnotic Clinical Scale for Adults. *American Journal of Clinical Hypnosis, 21,* 134-147.

Naatanen, R. (1992). *Attention and brain function.* Hillsdale, NJ: Lawrence Erlbaum.

Nadon, R. (1997). What this field needs is a good nomological network. *International Journal of Clinical and Experimental Hypnosis, 45,* 314-323.

Nyklicek, I., Thayer, J. F., & van Doornen, J. P. (1997). Cardiorespiratory differentiation of musically-induced emotions. *Journal of Psychophysiology, 11,* 304-321.

Orne, M. T. (1959). The nature of hypnosis: Artifact and essence. *Journal of Abnormal and Social Psychology, 58,* 277-299.

Osgood, C., Suci, G., & Tannenbaum, P. (1957). *The measurement of meaning*. Urbana: University of Illinois.

Parasuraman, R., Richer, F., & Beatty, J. (1982). Detection and recognition: Concurrent processes in perception. *Perception and Psychophysics, 31*, 1-12.

Paul, D. D., & Sutton, S. (1972). Evoked potential correlates of response criterion in auditory signal detection. *Science, 177*, 362-364.

Perlini, A. H., Lorimer, A. L., Campbell, K. B., & Spanos, N. P. (1992-1993). An electrophysiological and psychophysical analysis of hypnotic visual hallucinations. *Imagination, Cognition and Personality, 12*, 301-312.

Perlini, A. H., & Spanos, N. P. (1991). EEG alpha methodologies and hypnotizability: A critical review. *Psychophysiology, 28*, 511-530.

Perlini, A. H., Spanos, N. P., & Jones, B. (1996). Hypnotic negative hallucinations: A review of subjective, behavioral, and physiological methods. In R. G. Kunzendorf, N. Spanos, & B. Wallace (Eds.), *Hypnosis and imagination* (pp. 199-221). Amityville, NY: Baywood.

Pfurtscheller, G., Flotzinger, D., & Neuper, C. (1994). Differentiation between finger, toe and tongue movement in man based on 40 Hz EEG. *Electroencephalography and Clinical Neurophysiology, 90*, 456-460.

Pfurtscheller, G., & Neuper, C. (1992). Simultaneous EEG 10 Hz desynchronization and 40 Hz synchronization during finger movements. *Neuro Report, 3*, 1057-1060.

Pfurtscheller, G., Neuper, C., & Kalcher, J. (1993). 40-Hz oscillations during motor behavior in man. *Neuroscience Letters, 164*, 179-182.

Pribram, K. H., & McGuinness, D. (1975). Arousal, activation, and effort in the control of attention. *Psychological Review, 82*, 116-149.

Price, D. D. (1988). *Psychological and neural mechanisms of pain*. New York: Raven.

Ray, W. J. (1997). EEG concomitants of hypnotic susceptibility. *International Journal of Clinical and Experimental Hypnosis, 45*, 301-313.

Ray, W. J., Morrel, M., Frediani, A. W., & Tucker, D. (1976). Sex differences and lateral specialization of hemispheric functioning. *Neuropsychologia, 14*, 391-394.

Ray, W. J., Wells, R., Elbert, T., Lutzenberger, W., & Birbaumer, N. (1991). EEG and chaos: Dimensional estimation of sensory and hypnotic processes. In D. Duke & W. Pritchard (Eds.), *Measuring chaos in the human brain* (pp. 199-215). Cleveland, OH: World Scientific.

Rosen, A. D., Gur, R. C., Sussman, R., Gur, R. E., & Hurtig, H. (1982). Hemispheric asymmetry in the control of heart rate. *Neuroscience Abstracts, 8*, 917.

Russell, J. A. (1979). Affective space is bipolar. *Journal of Personality and Social Psychology, 37*, 345-356.

Sabourin, M. (1982). Hypnosis and brain function: EEG correlates of state trait differences. *Research Communications in Psychology, Psychiatry and Behavior, 7*, 149-168.

Sabourin, M. E., Cutcomb, S. D., Crawford, H. J., & Pribram, K. (1990). EEG correlates of hypnotic susceptibility and hypnotic trance: Spectral analysis and coherence. *International Journal of Psychophysiology, 10*, 125-142.

Schnyer, D. M., & Allen, J. J. (1995). Attention-related electroencephalographic and event-related potential predictors of responsiveness to suggested posthypnotic amnesia. *International Journal of Clinical and Experimental Hypnosis, 43*, 295-315.

Sheer, D. E. (1970). Electrophysiological correlates in memory consolidation. In G. Ungar (Ed.), *Molecular mechanisms in memory and learning* (pp. 177-211). New York: Plenum.

Sheer, D. E. (1976). Focused arousal and 40-Hz EEG. In R. M. Knight & D. J. Bakker (Eds.), *The neuropsychology of learning disorders* (pp. 71-87). Baltimore: University Park Press.

Sheer, D. E. (1984). Focused arousal, 40-Hz EEG, and disfunction. In T. Elbert (Ed.), *Self-regulation of the brain and behavior* (pp. 69-84). Berlin, Germany: Springer-Verlag.

Sheer, D. E. (1989). Sensory and cognitive 40-Hz EEG event-related potentials: Behavioral correlates, brain function and clinical application. In E. Basar & T. H. Bullock (Eds.), *Brain dynamics* (pp. 339-374). Berlin, Germany: Springer-Verlag.

Shimamura, A. P. (1995). Memory and frontal lobe function. In M. S. Gazzaniga (Ed.), *The cognitive neurosciences* (pp. 803-813). Cambridge, MA: MIT Press.

Shor, R. E., & Orne, E. C. (1962). *Harvard Group Scale of Hypnotic Susceptibility: Form C*. Palo Alto, CA: Consulting Psychologists.

Spiegel, D., & Barabasz, A. F. (1988). Effects of hypnotic instructions on P300 event-related-potential amplitudes: Research and clinical implications. *American Journal of Clinical Hypnosis, 31*, 11-17.

Spiegel, D., Bierre, P., & Rootenberg, J. (1989). Hypnotic alteration of somatosensory perception. *American Journal of Psychiatry, 146*. 749-754.

Spiegel, D., Cutcomb, S., Ren, C., & Pribram, K. (1985). Hypnotic hallucination alters evoked potentials. *Journal of Abnormal Psychology, 94*, 249-255.

Spielberger, C. D., Gorsuch, R., & Lushene, R. (1970). *The State-Trait Anxiety Inventory (STAI) Test Manual*. Palo Alto, CA: Consulting Psychologists.

Spydell, J. D., Ford, M. R., & Sheer, D. E. (1979). Task dependent cerebral lateralization of the 40-Hertz EEG rhythm. *Psychophysiology, 16*, 347-350.

Spydell, J. D., & Sheer, D. E. (1982). Effect of problem solving on right and left hemisphere 40-Hertz EEG activity. *Psychophysiology, 19*, 20-25.

Steriade, M., Gloor, P., Llinas, R. R., Lopes da Silva, F. H., & Mesulam, M. M. (1990). Basic mechanisms of cerebral rhythmic activities. *Electroencephalography and Clinical Neurophysiology, 76*, 481-508.

Talbot, J. D., Marrett, S., Evans, A. C., Meyer, E., Bushnell, M. C., & Duncan, G. H. (1991). Multiple representations of pain in human cerebral cortex. *Science, 251*, 1355-1358.

Tallon-Buadry, C., Bertrand, O., Bouchet, P., & Pernier, J. (1995). Gamma-range activity evoked by coherent visual stimuli in humans. *European Neuroscience Association, 7*, 1285-1291.

Tallon, C., Bertrand, O., Delpuech, C., & Pernier, J. (1996). Stimulus specificity of phase-locked and nonphase-locked 40 Hz visual responses in human. *European Journal of Neuroscience, 16*, 4240-4249.

Tellegen, A., & Atkinson, G. (1974). Openness to absorbing and self-altering experiences ("absorption"), a trait related to hypnotic susceptibility. *Journal of Abnormal Psychology, 83*, 268-277.

Thayer, J. F., & Miller, M. L. (1988). Further evidence for the independence of hedonic level and emotional intensity. *Personality and Individual Differences, 9*, 425-426.

Tiitinen, H., Sinkkonen, J., Reinikainen, K., Alho, K., Lavikainen, J., & Naatanen, R. (1993). Selective attention enhances the auditory 40-Hz transient response in humans. *Nature, 364*, 59-60.

Trotman, S. C., & Hammond, G. R. (1979). Sex differences in task-dependent EEG asymmetries. *Psychophysiology, 16*, 429-431.

Tucker, D. M. (1987). Substrati neuronali del pensiero e disordini affettivi [Neuronal substrates of thought and affective disorders]. In C. Caltagirone & G. Gainotti (Eds.), *Emozioni e specializzazione emisferica* [Emotions and hemispheric specialization] (pp. 179-187). Roma: Istituto della Enciclopedia Italiana.

Tucker, D. M., Stenslie, C. E., Roth, R. S., & Shearer, S. L. (1981). Right frontal lobe activation and right hemisphere performance decrement during a depressed mood. *Archives of General Psychiatry, 38*, 169-174.

Tucker, D. M., & Williamson, P. A. (1984). Asymmetric neural control systems in human self-regulation. *Psychological Review, 91*, 185-215.

Weisz, J., Szilagyi, N., Lang, E., & Adam, G. (1992). The influence of monocular viewing on heart period variability. *International Journal of Psychophysiology, 12*, 11-18.

Weitzenhoffer, A. M. (1980). Hypnotic susceptibility revisited. *American Journal of Clinical Hypnosis, 22*, 130-146.

Weitzenhoffer, A. M., & Hilgard, E. R. (1962). *Stanford Hypnotic Susceptibility Scale, Form C*. Palo Alto, CA: Consulting Psychologists.

Wilson, N. J. (1968). Neurophysiologic alterations with hypnosis. *Diseases of the Nervous System, 29*, 618-620.

Zachariae, R., & Bjerring, P. (1994). Laser-induced pain-related brain potentials and sensory pain ratings in high and low hypnotizable subjects during hypnotic suggestions of relaxation, dissociated imagery, focused analgesia, and placebo. *International Journal of Clinical and Experimental Hypnosis, 42*, 56-80.

Psycho-physiologische Korrelate von Hypnose und hypnotischer Suggestibilität

Vilfredo De Pascalis

Zusammenfassung: Wir geben einen Überblick und eine Zusammenfassung der auf EEG basierenden Forschung über physiologische und kognitive Indikatoren der hypnotischen Reaktion und der Hypnose-Suggestibilität, unter besonderer Berücksichtigung unserer programmatischen Forschung auf diesem Gebiet. Der Nachweis, daß Unterschiede im Aufmerksamkeitsgrad möglicherweise für Hypnose und individuelle Unterschiede in Hypnotisierbarkeit verantwortlich sind, wird mit traditionellen EEG-Rhythmen, ereigniskorrelierten Potentialen und 40-Hz EEG-Aktivität erbracht. Die Veränderung der Stimuluswahrnehmung ist möglicherweise ein sekundärer Effekt im Hinblick auf Verteilung der Aufmerksamkeitsressourcen. Sowohl unter wachenden als auch unter Hypnosebedingungen schienen hoch-suggestible Vpn größere aufgabenbezogene Hemisphärenverschiebungen zu zeigen als niedrig-suggestible. Befunde bezüglich der kognitiven und physiologischen Korrelate von hypnotischer Analgesie werden in bezug auf hemisphärisches Funktionieren in der scheinbaren Kontrolle von fokussierter und anhaltender Aufmerksamkeit diskutiert. Wir schließen, daß es eine Anzahl weiterzuverfolgender Anhaltspunkte gibt, obwohl eine definitive, auf EEG basierende Signatur für Hypnose und Hypnotisierbarkeit noch nicht etabliert ist.

ROSEMARIE GREENMAN
University of Tennessee, Knoxville, USA

Corrélations psychophysiologiques de l'hypnose et de la sensibilité hypnotique

Vilfredo De Pascalis

Résumé: Nous avons passé en revue et résumé la recherche basée sur l'EEG et les indicateurs physiologiques et cognitifs de la réponse hypnotique et de la sensibilité hypnotique, avec une attention toute spéciale sur notre recherche de programmation dans ce secteur. L'évidence que les différences dans les niveaux d'attention puisse compter dans l'hypnose et les différences individuelles d'hypnotisabilité est montrée par les rythmes traditionnels d'EEG, les potentiels d'évènements relatés, et l'activité de 40-Hz. L'altération d'une perception de stimulation peut être un effet secondaire avec toutefois respect de l'attribution de la ressource d'attention. Dans les deux cas de condition d'éveil ou d'hypnose, les sujets hautement hypnotisables montrèrent des changements plus importants dans les tracés EEG des hémisphères où une tache était en cours, par rapport au sujet faiblement hypnotisables. Les

découvertes concernant les corrélations cognitives et physiologiques de l'analgésie hypnotique sont discutées en respectant les fonctionnement hémisphérique au cours du contrôle apparent de l'attention "concentrée" et l'attention "soutenue." Notre conclusion est que tant qu'une signature définitive basée sur l'EEG concernant l'hypnose et l'hypnotisablité n'est pas établie, il y a encore un certain nombre de voies prometteuses.

Victor Simon
Psychosomatic Medicine & Clinical Hypnosis Institute, Lille, France

Correlatos psicofisiológicos de la hipnosis y la susceptibilidad hipnótica

Vilfredo De Pascalis

Resumen: En este artículo reseño y resumo la investigación basada en EEGs sobre los indicadores fisiológicos y cognitivos de la respuesta y susceptibilidad hipnóticas, con especial atención a mi investigación programática en esta área. La evidencia de que diferencias en niveles de atención pueden explicar a la hipnosis y las diferencias individuales en hipnotizabilidad se basa en los ritmos tradicionales del EEG, potenciales evocados y la actividad de EEG de 40-Hz. La alteración en la percepción de estímulos puede ser un efecto secundario de la distribución de las reservas de atención. Tanto en la condición de vigilia como de hipnosis, las personas muy hipnotizables parecen exhibir mayores cambios hemisféricos de EEG que personas poco hipnotizables. Analizo también los hallazgos sobre los correlatos cognitivos y fisiológicos de la analgesia hipnótica con respecto al funcionamiento hemisférico en el control aparente de la atención "enfocada" y "mantenida." Concluyo que aunque no se ha establecido una señal definitiva de la hipnosis y la hipnotizabilidad en el EEG, hay varias direcciones prometedoras.

Etzel Cardeña
Uniformed Services University of the Health Sciences, Bethesda, Maryland, USA

Part VII
Clinical Applications

[25]

Hypnosis: practical applications and theoretical considerations in normal labour

Mary W. Jenkins *Medical Hypnotherapist*, M. H. Pritchard, *Consultant Rheumatologist*

ABSTRACT

Objective To assess the effects of hypnotherapy on the first and second stages of labour in a large group of pregnant women.

Design A semi-prospective case control study in which women attending antenatal clinics were invited to undergo hypnotherapy.

Subjects One hundred twenty-six primigravid women with 300 age matched controls, and 136 parous women having their second baby with 300 age matched controls. Only women who had spontaneous deliveries were included.

Setting Aberdare District Maternity Unit, Mid Glamorgan, Wales.

Intervention Six sessions of hypnotherapy given by a trained medical hypnotherapist during pregnancy.

Outcome measures Analgesic requirements, duration of first and second stages of labour.

Results The mean lengths of the first stage of labour in the primigravid women was 6·4 h after hypnosis and 9·3 h in the control group ($P<0{\cdot}0001$); the mean lengths of the second stage were 37 min and 50 min, respectively ($P<0{\cdot}001$). In the parous women the corresponding values were 5·3 h and 6·2 h ($P<0{\cdot}01$); and 24 and 22 min (ns). The use of analgesic agents was significantly reduced ($P<0{\cdot}001$) in both hypnotised groups compared with their controls.

Conclusion In addition to demonstrating the benefits of hynotherapy, the study gives some insight into the relative proportions of mechanical and psychological components involved in the longer duration of labour in primigravid women.

It is a widely held belief, supported by large scale studies, (Friedman 1967) that women having their first baby have a longer, more difficult and more painful labour than those having subsequent babies. Although this is usually attributed to a combination of relative uterine inefficiency and increased soft tissue tension, the explanation remains controversial. Since the work of Grantly Dick-Read in the 1930s and 1940s (Dick-Read 1944) drawing attention to the importance of emotional factors, several authors have attempted to modify these using hynotherapeutic techniques (Abramson & Heron 1950; Michael 1952; Clark 1956; Winklestein 1958; August 1960; Davidson 1962; Tom 1960; Schibly & Aanonson 1966; Freeman *et al*, 1986; Brann & Guzvica 1987). Although results were generally encouraging, there has been little interest in this topic over the past 30 years.

Correspondence: Dr M. W. Jenkins, 60 Cathedral Road, Cardiff CF1 9LL, UK.

This study demonstrates that in addition to important practical benefits, the use of simple hypnotic techniques could be used to give new insight into the psychological aspects of labour.

Subjects and methods

The study was carried out over a period of five years, from 1984 to 1989, at the Aberdare General Hospital Maternity Unit, Mid Glamorgan. This is a satellite district maternity unit run by three consultants, used for approximately 800 low risk deliveries per annum in a population predominantly of social class 3, 4 and 5. There is no routine epidural analgesia and women needing caesarean sections and those with multiple pregnancies or other predictable obstetric complications are transferred to the Prince Charles Hospital, Merthyr Tydfil (Merthyr General Hospital until 1990). The caesarean section rate remained steady at between 11% and 12% over the five year period, and the pre-eclampsia rate remained at 7%. Ventouse or forceps assisted deliveries averaged 6% of all women, both in the unit as a whole and in the women initially in the hypnosis group.

Five hundred women of all parities, or approximately 10% of those attending the antenatal clinics during this period, expressed an interest in the hypnotherapy service. However, there were two factors that made this group atypical compared with the clinic attenders as a whole; firstly, there was a very high dropout rate through lack of interest or inability to co-operate fully, and secondly, the average age of those completing the course was approximately four years older than unselected women in the antenatal clinic of the same parity. This reduced the proportion of single women in the study, most of whom were under 20. These figures have been averaged for the duration of the study, as the proportion of single women attending the antenatal clinic increased markedly over the five years (Table 1). The overall smoking prevalence was 35% among the married women and 49% among the single women, but information on smoking recorded in the antenatal clinic notes was not considered reliable by the midwifery staff. Data on perineal trauma (episiotomy or tears requiring suturing) were recorded, together with maternal height and birth weight (Table 1).

Although it is normal practice to subject any new therapy to a double blind randomised controlled trial, this is clearly not possible in a study of hypnotherapy. The subject must not only know she is being hypnotised, but must be prepared to co-operate fully, and it was therefore decided that inviting women to volunteer was the only practical way of selecting a workable study group. We also considered that as this was a preliminary study, the analysis of the effects of hynotherapy on labour could only be made if the latter was as normal as possible; thus, all women who needed therapeutic intervention (caesarean section, ventouse or forceps) were excluded.

For analysis of the data, the women in the study were divided into two groups: women having their first baby (primigravid group) and women having their second baby (parous group). Other parities were excluded. Each of these groups had a control group chosen by selecting for each woman in the study who achieved a successful delivery without assistance or intervention, the next two or three women in the labour ward register of the same parity and age (± 2 years), who were also delivered without assistance or intervention.

The hypnotherapy was carried out by M.J. who was not present at the labour. The data were recorded in the routine labour ward notes by the midwifery staff on duty who were not aware of the study. The women were also unaware that their performance was being monitored and recorded. The data were analysed at the end of the study. The study involved 126 primigravid and 136 parous women, both groups having control groups of 300 women each. There were no exclusions on the grounds of previous obstetric history or performance, and there was no rejection or selection by the medical hypnotherapist of any woman for any other reason, medical or non-medical. Ethical approval was not thought necessary at the time the study was initiated.

Although every effort was made to exclude bias, doubts must remain that the women volunteering for hypnotherapy were different in some way from those who did not. It was not possible to stratify for all possible confounding variables but, as Table 1 shows, the two groups were well matched for all the important physical characteristics. The only unexpected finding was that in both groups the hypnotised women had heavier babies than their respective

Table 1. Obstetric data for the two study groups and their controls. *t=3·71, P<0·001; †t=2·79, P<0·001; SD=standard deviation and Student's t test was used.

	Primigravid women		Parous women	
Physical characteristics	Hypnotised	Controls	Hypnotised	Controls
n	126	300	136	300
Mean age (years)	26·5	26·2	29·7	28·8
SD	4·5	4·3	4·6	4·4
Range	17–41	18–38	20–41	21–41
Mean height (cm)	159·5	159·0	158·8	159·0
SD	4·1	5·0	4·4	5·0
Range	145–70	145–72	147–70	145–72
Single	15 (12%)	50 (17%)	2 (2%)	15 (5%)
Birth weight	3390*	3159*	3472†	3296†
SD (g)	417	475	380	310
Range	2420–4426	1750–4200	2660–4210	2390–4060
Episiotomy	45 (33%)	99 (35%)	19 (14%)	48 (16%)
Tears	51 (39%)	117 (41%)	65 (48%)	132 (44%)
No trauma	30 (28%)	84 (24%)	50 (37%)	120 (40%)

controls. There was no obvious reason for this, as the mean maternal heights were the same as the clinic means, but we could not stratify adequately for smoking habits, and this may have been relevant. Social class was also difficult to define, as Aberdare is an ex-mining area of relatively high unemployment, and the pregnant woman may often have been better educated than her husband.

Following the request for hypnotherapy, each woman received six individual half hour sessions with the medical hypnotherapist. The methods used were classical techniques taught by the British Medical and Dental Hypnosis Society for auto-relaxation and auto-analgesia. The subject was encouraged to learn and practice the techniques for auto-hypnosis during labour when the therapist would not be present. Approximately one third of the subjects dropped out after the first session due to lack of interest but of those who successfully completed the course several have been able to re-use the technique for subsequent pregnancies.

Two outcome measurements were used: the analgesic requirements and the duration of first and second stages of labour which was recorded routinely in the labour ward register by the midwifery staff on duty. Nitrous oxide/oxygen was self-administered. Further analgesia (100 mg pethidine, repeated as necessary) was given by the midwife according to her assessment of the analgesic requirement at the time. Oxytocin infusions were given in approximately 12% of control and 11% of hypnotised primigravid women and in 6% of control and 7% of hypnotised parous women for induction of labour when the pregnancy was considered to be two weeks post term, or when labour was taking excessively long to become established. The onset of labour was taken as the start of regular contractions.

The χ^2 test was used to compare the proportion of women who required no analgesia and the proportion who did not require pethidine in the hypnotised and control groups. The durations of the first and second stages of labour in the hypnotised and control groups were compared using student's *t* test.

Results

Analgesic requirements

The comparative analgesic requirements for all groups are shown in Fig. 1. All forms of analgesia were used by fewer women in the hypnotised groups compared with controls. Significantly more hypnotised primigravid women required no analgesia compared with controls (33/126 versus 13/300, respectively; χ^2=42, P<0·001). Also, significantly more hypnotised primigravid women did not require pethidine compared with controls 66/126 versus 49/300, respectively; χ^2=42, P<0·001).

The analgesic requirement differences in the parous groups were less marked, and both these groups required less analgesia than the equivalent groups of primigravid women. Significantly more hypnotised parous women required no analgesia compared with controls (50/136 versus 33/300, respectively; χ^2=32, P<0·001). Also, significantly more hypnotised parous women did not require pethidine compared with controls (80/136 versus 99/300, respectively; χ^2=15, P<0·001).

Duration of first stage of labour

Figure 2 shows cumulative percentage data on times taken to complete the first stage of labour (latent and active phases combined), for both primigravid and parous groups. There was a highly significant difference between the performance of the controls and hypnotised primigravid women, the latter having labour times similar to the parous control group. Mean, standard deviation (SD) and median data are shown in Table 2 together with the figures for normal labour published by Friedman (1967) for comparison. There was a small difference between the two parous groups, with a mean shortening of labour of about 14%, statistically but not clinically significant.

Duration of second stage of labour

Figure 3 shows the cumulative percentage data for the second stage of labour for the four groups. There were marked differences between primigravid and parous women, and whereas hypnosis was associated with a 25% shorter mean second stage in the primigravid women, there was no difference between the two parous groups. In spite of the improvement, the mean duration of the second stage in the hypnotised primigravids remained longer than the parous groups, although by one hour the percentage delivered was the same.

The results presented in Table 2 show that the control group results are similar to published normal data, but that hypnotherapy has been associated with almost complete elimination of the difference in duration of the first stage of labour normally seen between primigravidae and parous women. By contrast, although there was an improvement, the performance of primigravid women in the second stage did not reach that of the parous group, except in the percentage completed in one hour.

Discussion

There is little doubt that the main effect of hypnotherapy is to induce a high level of relaxation in a tense and emotionally charged atmosphere. In this respect it is the ultimate placebo. There was considerable interest in the use of this technique in the 1950s, but the results of studies were conflicting and, in addition, the overall view was that hypnosis was likely to be more trouble than it was worth.

Comparative analysis of these studies reveals the probable cause of this disagreement. Some, such as those reported by Clark (1956) and Schibley & Aanonson (1966) were mainly anecdotal, being carried out by individual enthusiastic obstetricians without enough scientific data to enable the value of hypnosis to be analysed. The controlled studies carried out by Abramson (1950) and August (1960) also found hypnotherapy to be beneficial, but these studies were relatively unstructured and thus difficult to evaluate. Of the other controlled studies, some

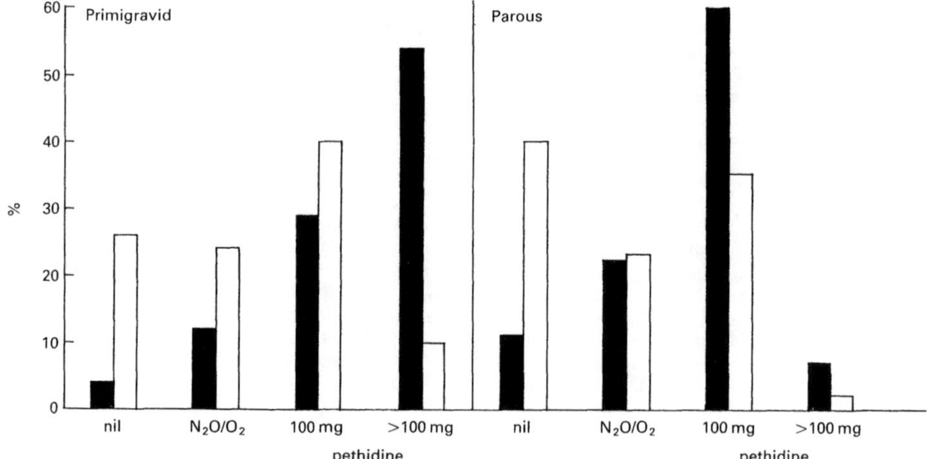

Fig. 1. Analgesic requirements for the two study groups and their controls (126 primigravid, 136 parous women and two control groups of 300 each). ■, control group; □ hypnotised group.

involved random allocation of women to hypnosis or control groups, or used consecutive women attending the clinic. These studies generally found hypnotherapy to be of little benefit (Winklestein 1958; Tom 1960; Freeman *et al.* 1986). Tom (1960), while finding that hypnosis was useful, considered it too time consuming to be worthwhile. On the other hand, those studies whose design was similar to this one, in which pregnant women were told that a hypnosis service was available if they so wished, reported favourable results (Michael 1952; Davidson 1962; Brann & Guzvica 1987).

The reason for these contradictions may be found in the review by Hilgard & Hilgard (1975) who pointed out that the range of individual susceptibility to hypnosis in an unselected population varied from nil to extreme, and could be scored on a 1–12 scale (The Stanford Hypnotic Clinical Scale). In randomly selected groups, many will be predictably resistant to hypnosis, so disappointing results should not be surprising, whereas a volunteer group would be more likely to contain a high proportion of motivated and susceptible people, and so better results should be expected. Surprisingly, Venn (1987), in a small study, found that motivation made no difference to hypnosis susceptibility, and a group of pregnant women scored the same as a group of volunteer college students, but the skill of the individual hypnotherapist must be taken into account in any of these studies.

Hilgard and Hilgard (1975) suggested that assessing the usefulness of hypnosis is only valid if the subject's individual susceptibility to this was known, and that perception

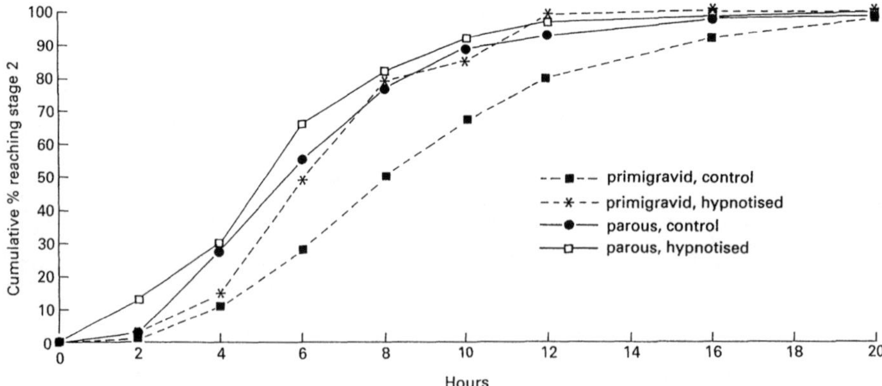

Fig. 2. Cumulative graph of duration of second stage of first stage for primigravid, parous women and their control groups.

Table 2. Comparative labour data for the two study groups, controls and published 'ideal' performances. Friedman (1967) refers to published delivery times. Values derived from Student's *t* test.

	Primigravid women			Parous women		
Stage	Hypno	Control	Friedman	Hypno	Control	Friedman
First (h)						
Mean	6·4***	9·3***	10·5	5·3*	6·2*	7·5
SD	3·2	4·2	5·5	3·2	3·3	5·6
Median	6·0	8·3	10·3	5·1	5·6	6·3
Second (mins)						
Mean	37**	50**	46	22†	24†	14
SD	19	24	35	20	18	20
Median	36	43	30	18	18	12

*t=3·0, P<0·01; **t=3·74, P<0·001; ***t=11·4, P<0·0001; †t=1 (not significant).

of pain was a more useful measure than duration of labour or analgesic requirements. The latter are, however, of more practical importance to both pregnant women and obstetricians, and have the advantage that statistical analysis is possible.

In practice, hypnotherapy is undoubtedly time consuming, but it is considerably more effective than relaxation classes which, both in the opinion of our subjects and in the study of Brann & Guzvica (1987), achieve little. It is also probable that the baby benefits from reduced exposure to drugs and shorter second stage times (Moya & James 1960) with greater maternal satisfaction.

Although this paper confirms the studies of 30 years ago by demonstrating the practical benefits of hypnotherapy in reduced analgesic requirement and shortening of labour, the large numbers and defined groups also allow these two benefits to be analysed separately. Since hypnotherapy is a purely psychological technique, it is possible to speculate about the role of emotional factors in labour.

Inspection of the data shows that the reduction of analgesic requirement applies to a greater or lesser extent to all women in labour; on the other hand the changes in first and second stage labour duration are highly specific. Analgesic requirement must be to some extent a voluntary decision on the part of the woman, who may decide to give auto-hypnosis a try before resorting to nitrous oxide/oxygen, but the performance during labour has no obvious voluntary component. Yet this study, as did earlier ones, seems to demonstrate that a nontherapeutic technique can have a profound effect on a process over which an individual has apparently no voluntary control. It is important to emphasise that these results have been obtained from normal, unassisted labour in volunteer subjects treated by an experienced medically qualified therapist and, although accurately matched to control groups, they are clearly not necessarily relevant to pregnancies in general, particularly when there has been mechanical, surgical or medical intervention. Nevertheless, the object of the argument is to establish a principle: if the duration of labour, especially in primigravid women, is due to a mixture of mechanical and emotional factors, it may be possible substantially to eliminate the latter with hypnotherapy, with consequent improvement in performance.

The results show that for primigravid women the duration of the first stage of labour was apparently shortened

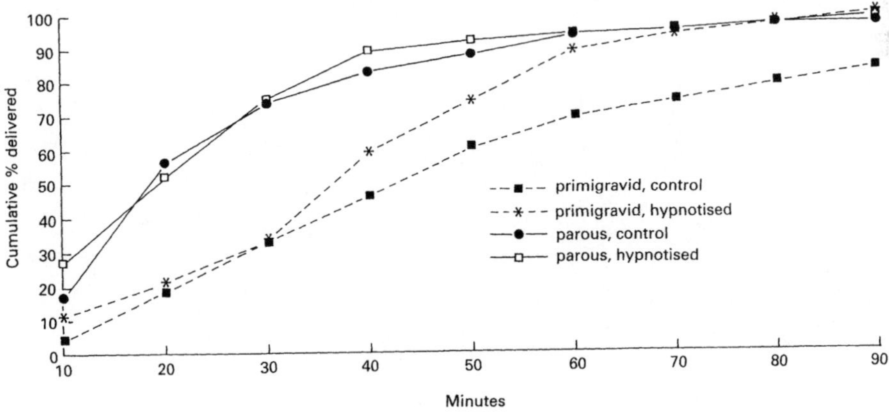

Fig. 3. Cumulative graph of duration of second stage of labour for the two study groups and their controls.

in the hypnotised group to become almost indistinguishable from that of the parous controls. There was a small improvement in the parous study group, with reduction of the mean duration but no change in the percentage completing in 8 h. All other things being equal, it would seem that, in this idealised group, once emotional factors have been eliminated by hypnotherapy, primigravid women may be capable of performing as well in the first stage of labour as parous women. This conclusion brings the argument full circle, since this is what Dick-Read was proposing 50 years ago.

On the other hand, the data for the second stage are different, with the performance of all groups being either relatively or completely unaffected by hypnotherapy. Although there is a significant improvement in the performance of primigravid women, this does not approach the delivery times of the parous women. This suggests that in the second stage the differences in performance are likely to be mechanical rather than psychological.

This study is the first of its kind for several decades, and having shown both practical benefits and the possibilities of a new approach to the analysis of the physiology of labour, it clearly needs further studies with a wider range of variables being considered prospectively, and more efficient hypnotherapy in terms of time spent with each pregnant woman. Such studies are already under consideration. Hypnotherapy seems to have several useful roles in obstetrics; as well as resulting in a reduction in analgesic requirements and shorter labour in primigravid women, it may also have the potential to be a research tool.

Acknowledgments

We would like to thank the consultants, nursing staff and clerical officers of Aberdare District Maternity Unit and Prince Charles Hospital, Merthyr Tydfil, for their help and co-operation in the collection of the data in this study.

References

Abramson M. & Heron W. T. (1950) An objective study of hypnosis in childbirth. *Am J Obs Gynecol* **59,** 1069–1074.

August R. V. (1960) Obstetric hypnoanaesthesiae. *Am J Obs Gynecol* **79,** 1131–1138.

Brann L. R. & Guzvica S. A. (1987) Comparison of hypnosis with conventional relaxation for antenatal and intrapartum use: a feasability study in general practice. *J Roy Coll Gen Pract* **37,** 437–440.

Clark R. N. (1956) A training method for childbirth using hypnosis. *Am J Obs Gynecol* **72,** 1302–1304.

Davidson J. A. (1962) An assessment of the value of hypnosis in pregnancy and labour. *Brit Med J* **2,** 951–953.

Dick-Read G. (1944) *Childbirth Without Fear.* Harper & Brothers, New York.

Freeman R. M., Macauley A. J., Eve L. & Chamberlain G. V. P. (1986) Randomised trial of self-hypnosis for analgesia in labour. *Brit Med J* **292,** 657–658.

Friedman E. A. (1967) Normal labor. In *Labor, Clinical Evaluation and Management* Appleton Century Crofts, New York.

Hilgard E. R. & Hilgard J. R. (1975) Hypnotic responsiveness. In *Hypnosis in the Relief of Pain.* Kaufman, Los Altos, California.

Michael A. M. (1952) Hypnosis in childbirth. *Brit Med J* **1,** 734–737.

Moya F. & James L. S. (1960) Medical hypnosis for obstetrics. *JAMA* **174,** 2026–2032.

Schibly W. J. & Aanonsen G. A. (1966) Hypnosis—practical in obstetrics? *Medical Times* **94,** 340–343.

Tom K. S. (1960) Hypnosis in obstetrics and gynaecology. *Obstet Gynecol* **16,** 222–226.

Winklestein L. B. (1958) Routine hypnosis for obstetrical delivery. *Am J Obs Gynecol* **76,** 152–160.

Venn J. (1987) The Stanford hypnotic clinical scale and a group of obstetrical patients. *Am J Clin Hypnosis* **30,** 66–70.

Received 29 October 1991
Final revised version received 1 June 1992
Accepted 2 September 1992

[26]

Hypnosis as an Adjunct to Cognitive–Behavioral Psychotherapy: A Meta-Analysis

Irving Kirsch, Guy Montgomery, and Guy Sapirstein
University of Connecticut

A meta-analysis was performed on 18 studies in which a cognitive–behavioral therapy was compared with the same therapy supplemented by hypnosis. The results indicated that the addition of hypnosis substantially enhanced treatment outcome, so that the average client receiving cognitive–behavioral hypnotherapy showed greater improvement than at least 70% of clients receiving nonhypnotic treatment. Effects seemed particularly pronounced for treatments of obesity, especially at long-term follow-up, indicating that unlike those in nonhypnotic treatment, clients to whom hypnotic inductions had been administered continued to lose weight after treatment ended. These results were particularly striking because of the few procedural differences between the hypnotic and nonhypnotic treatments.

Once relegated to the realm of the supernatural, hypnosis is increasingly accepted as a legitimate therapeutic procedure (Rhue, Lynn, & Kirsch, 1993). A century ago, hypnotherapy often consisted of a hypnotic induction, followed by the administration of suggestions for symptom removal. Consequently, hypnotherapy has been viewed by some writers as a mode of therapy that might be compared with psychodynamic, cognitive–behavioral, or other therapeutic approaches (e.g., Smith, Glass, & Miller, 1980). However, suggestions for symptom relief play a relatively minor role in contemporary hypnotherapy. Instead, hypnotherapy generally consists of the addition of hypnosis to some recognized form of psychotherapy (Rhue et al., 1993). As a result, the question to be asked is not whether hypnosis works better than another treatment but rather whether it enhances the effectiveness of a treatment.

Before 1980, research on the efficacy of hypnotherapy was largely confined to psychodynamic hypnotherapy (Smith et al., 1980). More recently, empirical studies have focused on the use of hypnosis in behavior therapy, cognitive therapy, and cognitive–behavior therapy (Spinhoven, 1987). The distinction between these latter modes of therapy is not entirely clear. Cognitive processes (e.g., imagery) are a component of many behavior therapies, and behavioral tasks are a component of virtually all cognitive therapies. In this article, we use the term *cognitive–behavioral psychotherapy* to refer to treatment procedures described as behavioral, cognitive, or cognitive–behavioral.

Irving Kirsch, Guy Montgomery, and Guy Sapirstein, Department of Psychology, University of Connecticut.

The research reported in this article was supported by a grant from the University of Connecticut Research Foundation.

Correspondence concerning this article should be addressed to Irving Kirsch, Department of Psychology, U-20, Room 107, University of Connecticut, 406 Babbidge Road, Storrs, Connecticut 06269-1020.

Clinical hypnosis is a procedure in which a therapist suggests that a client experience changes in sensation, perception, thought, and behavior. The hypnotic context is established by an induction procedure that usually includes instructions for relaxation. Hypotheses about how this procedure might enhance therapy vary with theoretical conceptions of hypnosis. Most therapists believe that hypnotic inductions produce an altered state of consciousness in susceptible individuals (see Kirsch, 1993). Among the presumed characteristics of the hypothesized hypnotic state are hypersuggestibility, more vivid imagery, more primary process thinking, greater availability of childhood memories, and a tolerance of logical incongruities often referred to as "trance logic" (Fromm, 1992; Hilgard, 1965; Orne, 1959). From a traditional state perspective, the benefits of adding hypnosis to treatment are due to these characteristics of the hypothesized trance state.[1]

In contrast to this view, cognitive–behavioral theorists have rejected the hypothesis that there is a distinctly hypnotic state of consciousness (Barber, 1969; Kirsch, 1990; Sarbin & Coe, 1972; Spanos & Chaves, 1989). From a nonstate perspective, hypnosis has been hypothesized to augment therapy outcome through its effects on clients' beliefs and expectations (Barber, 1985; Coe, 1993; Fish, 1973; Kirsch, 1985, 1990). Thus, state theorists and cognitive-behavioral theorists agree that hypnosis can enhance treatment effects, albeit for different reasons. The purpose of this review is to assess the empirical data bearing on this question of whether cognitive-behavioral psychotherapies are enhanced by the addition of hypnosis.

[1] Some hypnosis theorists use the terms *state* and *trance* in a purely descriptive sense, without ascribing any causal properties to the concept (Hilgard, 1969; Kihlstrom, 1985). With respect to the altered state issue, this view is virtually identical to the cognitive–behavioral conception of hypnosis.

There are a number of reasons for supposing that if hypnosis enhances psychotherapy outcome, its effects are likely to be relatively modest. First, most of the procedures conducted in hypnotherapy are the same as those conducted in nonhypnotic psychotherapy. This is a consequence of the fact that hypnosis is an adjunct to therapy rather than a mode of therapy. Second, clients vary in their responsiveness to hypnosis. From a traditional state viewpoint, only those with sufficient hypnotic talent or ability are likely to benefit substantially from the addition of hypnosis to a treatment (Levitt, 1993). Third, clients vary in their attitudes and expectancies regarding hypnosis. Enhancement of outcome should be limited to clients with positive attitudes and expectations, whereas a degradation of treatment outcome might be expected among clients with negative attitudes (Kirsch, 1990, 1993). Finally, typical hypnotic inductions closely resemble conventional relaxation training. In fact, all that is needed to convert relaxation training into a hypnotic induction is the addition of the word hypnosis. Instead of saying "more and more deeply relaxed," the therapist says "more and more deeply hypnotized." Because relaxation training is a frequent component of behavior therapy, the addition of hypnosis to behavior therapy may consist of little more that the use of the word "hypnosis."

The small magnitude of anticipated mean effects, combined with the relatively small samples used in many therapy outcome studies, are likely to lead to inconsistent outcomes, in which some studies show significant effects and others do not. In situations of this sort, meta-analyses can provide more definitive answers than individual studies, narrative reviews, or box scores of significant results (Hunter & Schmidt, 1990). Meta-analysis allows comparison of outcomes across studies by the calculation of effect sizes, defined as the standardized mean difference between the experimental group and the control group. The meta-analysis reported here assesses the effect of adding hypnosis to cognitive-behavioral psychotherapy. Because hypnosis is not a treatment in its own right, we limited our sample of studies to those in which a cognitive-behavioral treatment administered in a hypnotic context was compared to the same treatment administered without hypnosis. In calculating effect sizes, the nonhypnotic treatment was treated as the control condition.

Method

Studies of cognitive-behavioral hypnotherapy were obtained from previous reviews (Rhue et al., 1993; Spanos, 1991; Spinhoven, 1987) and a computer search of the PsycLIT database from 1974 to 1993 using the search terms, *cognitive-behavioral hypnotherapy, hypnosis and psychotherapy, hypnosis and behavior therapy,* and *hypnotherapy or hypnosis and adjunct to therapy.* Inclusion criteria were as follows: (a) A cognitive-behavioral psychotherapy was administered to at least one group of participants in a hypnotic context; (b) the same therapy was administered to at least one group of clients in a nonhypnotic context; and (c) sufficient data were reported to allow calculation of effect sizes.

These criteria resulted in a sample of 18 studies in which 20 hypnotic treatments were compared with identical nonhypnotic treatments and from which we were able to calculate the magnitude of 90 effects. These comparisons involved 577 participants. Fourteen treatment comparisons were derived from data of clinical patients as participants, 5 used college students as participants, and 1 involved a mix of clinical patients and college students. Participants were assigned to treatment randomly in 16 of these comparisons and sequentially in 2 (Edelson & Fitzpatrick, 1989; Lazarus, 1973). Method of participant assignment was unclear in two of the reports (Howard & Reardon, 1986; O'Brien, Cooley, Ciotti, & Henninger, 1981).

Effect sizes (*d*) were calculated for each outcome variable as the standardized mean difference between the hypnosis group and the corresponding no-hypnosis group. Where sufficient data were not provided for direct calculation of effect sizes, they were estimated using the procedures described by Smith et al. (1980).

Three different units of analysis can be used in calculating mean effect sizes, individual dependent variables (e.g., Smith et al., 1980), treatments (e.g., Barker, Funk, & Houston, 1988), or studies (e.g., Lyons & Woods, 1991). In the latter two methods, effect sizes are averaged across dependent variables. Using individual dependent variables as the unit of analysis results in substantial violations of the assumption of statistical independence when standard inferential statistical tests are applied to the results. In contrast, statistical independence is assured when only one effect size is used from each study (Hunter & Schmidt, 1990).

Some studies contain evaluations of more than one treatment. In such cases, the use of a single effect size for each study obscures differences between these treatments. In the present sample, there were two studies in which more than one hypnotic treatment were compared with a comparable nonhypnotic treatment. Goldstein (1981) included two hypnosis groups, in one of which the participants were given an arm levitation suggestion as a means demonstrating the effects of hypnosis and thereby enhancing the participants' treatment outcome expectations. Barabasz and Spiegel (1989) also used two hypnosis groups, one in which the same hypnotic suggestions were used for all participants and another in which suggestions were individualized on the basis of participant characteristics.

Treatment was chosen as the unit of analysis in this meta-analysis because it avoids shortcomings associated with other options. Using studies as the unit of analysis would not have allowed complete assessment of variations in cognitive-behavioral hypnotherapy, thereby impeding the search for moderator variables. Using individual effects as the unit of analysis would have biased the results in the direction of studies with large numbers of dependent variables. Calculating a mean effect for each treatment avoided both of these shortcomings. Also, because there were only two studies in which more than one hypnotic treatment was included, the use of treatment as the unit of analysis affected statistical independence only minimally. As a further precaution, standard inferential statistics were replaced by the calculation of confidence intervals calculated as 1.96 times the standard deviation of the sampling error (i.e., 1.96 times the standard deviation of the observed effect sizes divided by the number of effects; Hunter & Schmidt, 1990, pp. 437–438).

Results

Presenting problems, treatments, sample sizes, and effect sizes are presented in Table 1. The mean effect size across studies was .87 standard deviations. This effect differed significantly from zero, indicating that hypnosis enhanced the efficacy of cognitive-behavioral treatments. Inspection of Table 1 reveals a wide range in sample size, which is a source of potential bias. Calculation of the correlation between sample size and effect size indicated that significantly larger effects were reported in studies with larger samples ($r = .50, p < .05$). To correct for this bias, we weighted effects by the size of the samples from which they were obtained and calculated the mean weighted effect size

Table 1
Description of Studies and Mean Effect Sizes

Study	Presenting problem	Cognitive–behavioral treatment	*n*	*d*
McAmmond et al. (1971)	Pain	Relaxation	18	−0.20
Borkovec & Fowles (1973)	Insomnia	Relaxation	18	−0.10
Deabler et al. (1973)	Hypertension	Relaxation	30	0.51
Lazarus (1973)	Mixed	Varied	20	1.45
Sullivan et al. (1974)	Anxiety	Relaxation	16	1.40
Graham et al. (1975)	Insomnia	Relaxation	22	−0.01
Bornstein & Devine (1980)	Obesity	Covert modeling	18	0.83
Deyoub & Wilkie (1980)	Obesity	Imagery + coping suggestions	48	−0.17
Goldstein (1981) (Hypnosis with arm levitation)	Obesity	Self-monitoring + stimulus control + self-reinforcement	40	5.57
Goldstein (1981) (hypnosis without arm levitation)	Obesity	Self-monitoring + stimulus control + self-reinforcement	40	−0.08
O'Brien et al. (1981)	Snake phobia	Systematic desensitization	18	0.73
Wadden & Flaxman (1981)	Obesity	Covert modeling	22	−0.22
Bolocofsky et al. (1985)	Obesity	Self-monitoring + goal setting + stimulus control	109	3.65
Howard & Reardon (1986)	Self-concept & athletic performance	Cognitive restructuring	16	0.02
Barabasz & Spiegel (1989 [standard suggestions])	Obesity	Self-monitoring + goal setting	30	0.62
Barabasz & Spiegel (1989 [individualized suggestions])	Obesity	Self-monitoring + goal setting	29	0.75
Edelson & Fitzpatrick (1989)	Chronic pain	Cognitive strategy	18	0.16
Tosi et al. (1989)	Duodenal ulcer	Cognitive restructuring	12	0.93
Tosi et al. (1992)	Hypertension	Cognitive restructuring	21	1.11
Schoenberger (1993)	Public speaking anxiety	Relaxation + imagery + cognitive restructuring + in vivo practice	32	0.40

(*D*) following the procedures described by Hunter and Schmidt (1990). This revealed a significant effect of 1.36 standard deviations resulting from the addition of hypnosis to cognitive-behavioral psychotherapy. This indicates that the average client receiving cognitive-behavioral hypnotherapy showed more improvement than 90% of clients receiving nonhypnotic treatment.[2]

Inspection of Table 1 reveals two effects that might be classified as outliers (Bolocofsky, Spinler, & Coulthard-Morris, 1985; Goldstein, 1981). To provide conservative estimates of effect sizes, we winsorized with $g = 1$ and $g = 2$, which resulted in weighted mean effect sizes of 1.23 and .66, respectively. The more conservative of these estimates indicates that the average client receiving therapy with hypnosis was better off at the end of it than 75% of clients receiving the same therapy without hypnosis.

Besides calculating overall effects, we examined effect size as a function of type of dependent variable. Physiological variables were assessed in 12 studies, behavioral measures in 5 studies, and self-report measures in 9 studies. Mean unweighted (*d*) and weighted (*D*) effect sizes for each category of dependent variable are reported in Table 2, along with the variances of the weighted estimates of the population effect sizes. Neither weighted nor unweighted effect sizes differed significantly as a function of type of measure, and each was significantly greater than zero.

Although the mean effect for the addition of hypnosis to cognitive-behavioral psychotherapy was significantly greater than zero, the variance of the overall population effect sizes and that of physiological measures were very large, indicating the presence of a moderator variable. Although the variances of population effect sizes suggested the presence of a moderator only for physiological outcomes, we were also interested in examining theoretically predicted potential moderators. Therefore, we began assessing possible moderating variables using the treatment effect sizes listed in Table 1.

The use of hypnosis in psychotherapy entails the provision of a hypnotic induction followed by therapeutic suggestions. Most hypnotic inductions (including all of those described in the studies reviewed here) contain relaxation instructions that are very similar to those used in relaxation training. In some of the studies reviewed here, the only difference between the hypnotic induction and the relaxation instructions used in the nonhypnotic condition was the use of the term *hypnosis* (e.g., Lazarus, 1973; Schoenberger, 1993). Because relaxation training was used in only some of the nonhypnotic cognitive-behavioral treatments described in this review, the enhancement of treatment outcome that we observed may have been due to relaxation instructions rather than to other aspects of hypnosis.

In many of the studies, suggestions other than those contained in the nonhypnotic treatment were included in the hypnotic treatment. As noted earlier, a hand levitation suggestion was included in one of the hypnotic conditions in the Goldstein (1981) study. Similarly, Schoenberger (1993) added brief direct suggestions for symptom improvement to her treatment when

[2] Because of the exceptional magnitude of this effect, we recalculated the weighted effect using the procedure described by Hedges & Olkin (1985) for $d_+^{(1)}$. This yielded the same mean weighted effect as that obtained using the Hunter and Schmidt (1990) procedure.

Table 2
Population Effect Sizes as a Function of Type of Variable

Type of measure	*n*	*d*	*D*	Variation of *D*
Physiological	12	0.95	1.42	3.15
Behavioral	5	0.73	0.73	0.08
Self-report	9	0.60	0.58	0.10
Combined	20	0.87	1.36	2.94

it was conducted in a hypnotic context. Thus, a second potential moderating variable is the addition of suggestions not included in the nonhypnotic treatment.

Hypnosis may enhance the effectiveness of treatment for some problems but not for others. Wadden and Anderton (1982), for example, hypothesized that hypnosis might have special value in the treatment of "nonvoluntary" disorders (i.e., pain, warts, asthma) but not in the treatment of disorders of "self-initiated" behavior (i.e., obesity, cigarette smoking, alcoholism). Although a variety of presenting problems were treated in the studies we found, in most instances the number of studies per presenting problem was too small for meaningful comparison of effect sizes. However, obesity was the presenting problem in eight of the treatment comparisons under review, allowing a comparison of the effectiveness of adding hypnosis to the treatment obesity with that of adding it to the treatment of various other problems (e.g., pain, insomnia, hypertension, and anxiety).

Participants for half of the treatment comparisons were solicited by advertisements or from college student bodies. Those for the other comparisons consisted of patients who had sought or were referred for treatment. Patients seeking treatment might be more distressed and more motivated for change, and these characteristics might interact with type of treatment, leading to differential outcomes.

Finally, direct calculation of effect sizes from means and standard deviations was possible in only nine treatment comparisons. In the remaining 11, standard deviations were estimated using the methods described by Smith et al. (1980). It is possible that these indirect procedures produced effect sizes that were different from those produced by calculation from exact data.

The results of analyses of these potential moderating variables are displayed in Table 3. They indicate that hypnotic enhancement of therapeutic outcome is not due to the addition of relaxation instructions nor to the addition of therapeutic suggestions. Nature of the participant population also did not affect outcome. There was considerable variance in population effect sizes regardless of whether relaxation was included in the control treatment, whether additional therapeutic suggestions were added to the hypnotic treatment or whether the participants had sought treatment or were solicited. This indicates that none of these variables was the source of the variation in the estimated population effect sizes.

Estimation of standard deviations resulted in significantly greater effects than those calculated from studies in which the standard deviations were reported, although both effect sizes differed significantly from zero. There was also substantial variation in estimated effect sizes, indicating that this methodological difference did not fully account for the observed lack of homogeneity in effect sizes. Similarly, the mean weighted effect size for treatments of obesity was more than triple that of treatments for other disorders, and both effect sizes differed significantly from zero. However, the variance in effect sizes in studies of obesity was so large that the difference was not statistically significant. In contrast, the variance in effect sizes for treatments of presenting problems other than obesity was negligible, and the variance in exactly calculated effect sizes was relatively low.

The data indicate that the as-yet undiscovered moderating variable affected only physiological variables and studies in which obesity was the focus of treatment. Also, it was more evident in estimated effect sizes than in exactly calculated effects. The pattern of overlap between these variables suggested to us that presenting problem was central to the as yet undiscovered moderating variable. The dependent variables of studies on obesity were limited to a single physiological measure (weight). Similarly, all but two of the effects for obesity were estimated. Our suspicion was confirmed by separate analyses of the six estimated obesity effects and the five estimated effects involving other presenting problems, which indicated inflated effect sizes and substantial variance for estimated obesity effects ($D = 2.53$, variance = 4.27), but not for estimated effects for other presenting problems ($D = .13$, variance = .07).

In a narrative review of the use of hypnosis in weight reduction treatments, Levitt (1993) noted that participants in one hypnotic treatment program (Bolocofsky et al., 1985) continued to lose weight over a 2-year period after the end of the program, whereas participants in nonhypnotic treatment did not. Examination of obesity studies in this meta-analysis revealed a wide range in the length of time during which follow-up data

Table 3
Population Effect Sizes as a Function of Hypothesized Moderators

Potential moderator	No. of treatments in comparison	*d*	*D*	Variation in *D*
Relaxation				
In both treatments	11	0.77	1.51	2.21
In hypnotic treatment only	9	0.99	1.15	3.84
Suggestions				
Same in both treatments	14	0.63	1.20	2.21
More in hypnotic treatment	6	1.42	1.74	4.50
Presenting problem				
Obesity	8	1.37	1.96	4.14
Other	12	0.53	0.52	0.06
Participant population				
Sought or referred for treatment	10	1.24	1.42	3.19
Solicited	10	0.49	1.31	2.74
Effect calculation method				
Exact	9	0.62	0.47	0.20
Estimate	11	1.07	1.87	3.79

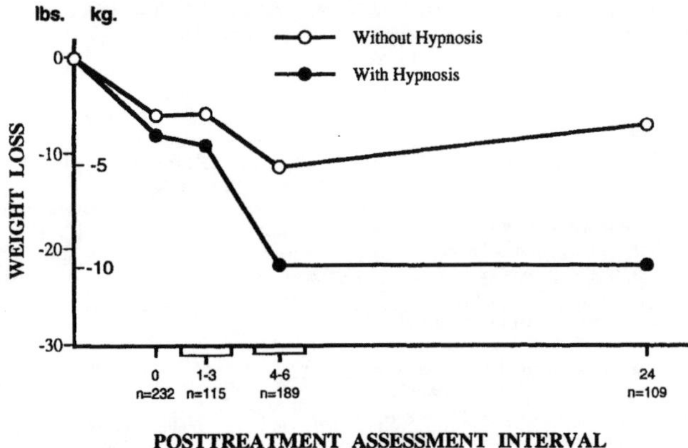

Figure 1. Weight loss as a function of assessment interval and inclusion of hypnosis in treatment.

were collected (2–24 months). To determine if effect size was influenced by duration of the follow-up period, we calculated the correlation between time of assessment and magnitude of effect, using individual assessments as the unit of analysis. This revealed that after treatment ended, the effect of hypnosis increased over time ($r = .59, p < .02$). Thus, the observed effect of adding hypnosis to treatments of obesity was moderated by the length of the follow-up assessment interval. The association between assessment interval and effect of treatment is graphically displayed in Figure 1. By using mean weight loss in place of effect size, the problems associated with estimating standard deviations are avoided and the clinical significance of the difference can be judged more accurately.

Discussion

The results of this meta-analysis indicates a fairly substantial effect as a result of adding hypnosis to cognitive-behavioral psychotherapies. Effect sizes were consistent for behavioral and self-report measures of change and for all measures of change in studies of presenting problems other than obesity. This indicates that hypnosis enhances the effects of cognitive-behavioral psychotherapy across a broad range of problems. Our most conservative estimates of this effect approximate 0.5 standard deviations, indicating that the average client receiving cognitive-behavioral hypnotherapy benefitted more than at least 70% of clients receiving the same treatment without hypnosis.

There are two factors that appear to account for the variance in physiological effects: presenting problem and length of follow-up. For problems other than obesity, the variance in weighted effect sizes was negligible, thus allowing clear interpretation. We found a reliable effect of just over one half standard deviation caused by the addition of hypnosis to these treatments. Weight reduction treatments showed even larger effects that were due to the addition of hypnosis, although the exact magnitude of this effect is uncertain because of the failure to report standard deviations in most of the weight reduction studies. For the sake of future meta-analyses, we strongly advocate the reporting of exact means (or adjusted means, if pretreatment scores are available) and standard deviations as a precondition for publication of outcome studies.

In contrast to treatments of other presenting problems, the effect of adding hypnosis to cognitive-behavioral treatment of obesity did not become apparent until some time after treatment had ended. Differences between hypnotic and nonhypnotic treatment of obesity increased up to 6 months after treatment ended and remained intact at 2-year follow-up. Furthermore, this phenomenon was independent of the effect size estimation problem resulting from missing standard deviations. It should be noted, however, that long-term follow-up data were reported only for obesity studies. Therefore, at least two interpretations of these data are possible. First, it is possible that the effects of hypnosis are particularly pronounced in the treatment of obesity, which is largely due to the failure of nonhypnotic treatments to produce lasting change. Alternately, it is possible that the advantages of adding hypnosis to cognitive-behavioral treatment increases over time, regardless of presenting problem. Resolution of this issue will require studies with long-term follow-up data for problems other than obesity.

Many scholars maintain that if treatment effects are due to hypnosis, rather than a function of nonspecific variables, they ought to be correlated with hypnotizability. Unfortunately, few of the studies considered in this review reported correlations of outcome with hypnotizability scores. In any case, correlations between hypnotizability and treatment outcome do not provide much information about hypothesized causal mechanisms, regardless of whether hypnotizability is assessed before or after treatment. If hypnotizability is assessed before treatment, the person's response to hypnosis should affect his or her outcome expectations for a "hypnotic" treatment. If hypnotizability is assessed after treatment, the effects of treatment could influence their subsequent responses to a test of hypnotizability (Council, Kirsch, & Grant, in press; Kirsch & Council, 1992). Thus, correlations between hypnotizability and treatment outcome might be indicators of expectancy effects, rather than effects of some special hypnotic process.[3]

In summary, the results of this meta-analysis indicate that hypnosis can be a useful adjunct to cognitive behavior therapy for a wide variety of problems, and it may be particularly effective in treating obesity. The data indicating that hypnosis promotes long-term weight loss is particularly important, given the finding that most obese individuals who lose weight in nonhypnotic treatments soon regain it (Stunkard, 1972). Research is needed to establish the range of treatments and conditions that can be enhanced by the addition of hypnosis and to investigate participant variables that might predict when hypnosis would be helpful and when it might be harmful. Nevertheless, the current data suggest that training in hypnosis should be included routinely as a part of training in cognitive-behavioral treatments.

[3] Note that the variance in effect sizes is probably not related to differences in hypnotizability, because individual difference variables of this sort would be more likely to affect within-study variance than between-study variance.

References

References preceded by an asterisk were included in the meta-analysis.

*Barabasz, M., & Spiegel, D. (1989). Hypnotizability and weight loss in obese subjects. *International Journal of Eating Disorders, 8,* 335–341.

Barber, T. X. (1969). *Hypnosis: A scientific approach.* New York: Van Nostrand Reinhold.

Barber, T. X. (1985). Hypnosuggestive procedures as catalysts for psychotherapies. In S. J. Lynn & J. P. Garske (Eds.), *Contemporary psychotherapies: Models and methods* (pp. 333–375). Columbus, OH: Merrill.

Barker, S. L., Funk, S. C., & Houston, B. K. (1988). Psychological treatment versus nonspecific factors: A meta-analysis of conditions that engender comparable expectations for improvement. *Clinical Psychology Review, 8,* 579–594.

*Bolocofsky, D. N., Spinler, D., & Coulthard-Morris, L. (1985). Effectiveness of hypnosis as an adjunct to behavioral weight management. *Journal of Clinical Psychology, 41,* 35–41.

*Borkovec, T. D., & Fowles, D. C. (1973). Controlled investigation of the effects of progressive and hypnotic relaxation on insomnia. *Journal of Abnormal Psychology, 82,* 153–158.

*Bornstein, P. H., & Devine, D. A. (1980). Covert modeling-hypnosis in the treatment of obesity. *Psychotherapy: Theory, Research, and Practice, 17,* 272–276.

Coe, W. C. (1993). Expectations and hypnotherapy. In J. W. Rhue, S. J. Lynn, & I. Kirsch (Eds.), *Handbook of clinical hypnosis* (pp. 73–93). Washington, DC: American Psychological Association.

Council, J. R., Kirsch, I., & Grant, D. L. (in press). Imagination, expectancy and hypnotic responding. In R. G. Kunzendorf, N. K. Spanos, & B. J. Wallace (Eds.), *Imagination and Hypnosis.* Amityville, NY: Baywood.

*Deabler, H. L., Fidel, E., & Dillenkoffer, R. I. (1973). The use of relaxation and hypnosis in lowering high blood pressure. *American Journal of Clinical Hypnosis, 16,* 75–83.

*Deyoub, P. L., & Wilkie, R. (1980). Suggestion with and without hypnotic induction in a weight reduction program. *International Journal of Clinical and Experimental Hypnosis, 28,* 333–340.

*Edelson, J., & Fitzpatrick, J. L. (1989). A comparison of cognitive-behavioral and hypnotic treatments of chronic pain. *Journal of Clinical Psychology, 45,* 316–323.

Fish, J. M. (1973). *Placebo therapy.* San Francisco: Jossey-Bass.

Fromm, E. (1992). An ego-psychological theory of hypnosis. In E. Fromm & M. Nash (Eds.), *Contemporary hypnosis research* (pp. 131–148). New York: Guilford.

*Goldstein, Y. (1981). The effect of demonstrating to a subject that she is in a hypnotic trance as a variable in hypnotic interventions with obese women. *International Journal of Clinical and Experimental Hypnosis, 29,* 13–23.

*Hedges, L. V., & Olkin, I. (1985). *Statistical methods for meta-analysis.* Orlando, FL: Academic Press.

Hilgard, E. R. (1965). *Hypnotic susceptibility.* New York: Harcourt, Brace & World.

Hilgard, E. R. (1969). Altered states of awareness. *Journal of Nervous and Mental Disease, 149,* 68–79.

*Howard, W. L., & Reardon, J. P. (1986). Changes in the self-concept and athletic performance of weight lifters through a cognitive-hypnotic approach: An empirical study. *American Journal of Clinical Hypnosis, 28,* 248–257.

Hunter, J. E., & Schmidt, F. L. (1990). *Methods of meta-analysis: Correcting error and bias in research findings.* Newbury Park, CA: Sage.

Kihlstrom, J. F. (1985). Hypnosis. *Annual Review of Psychology, 36,* 385–418.

Kirsch, I. (1985). Response expectancy as a determinant of experience and behavior. *American Psychologist, 40,* 1189–1202.

Kirsch, I. (1990). *Changing expectations: A key to effective psychotherapy.* Pacific Grove, CA: Brooks/Cole.

Kirsch, I. (1993a). Cognitive–behavioral hypnotherapy. In J. W. Rhue, S. J. Lynn, & I. Kirsch (Eds.), *Handbook of clinical hypnosis* (pp. 151–171). Washington, DC: American Psychological Association.

Kirsch, I. (1993b). Professional opinions about hypnosis: Results of the APA Division 30 survey. *Psychological Hypnosis, 2,* 4–5.

Kirsch, I., & Council, J. R. (1992). Situational and personality correlates of suggestibility. In E. Fromm & M. Nash (Eds.), *Contemporary hypnosis research* (pp. 267–292). New York: Guilford.

*Lazarus, A. A. (1973). "Hypnosis" as a facilitator in behavior therapy. *International Journal of Clinical and Experimental Hypnosis, 21,* 25–31.

Levitt, E. E. (1993). Hypnosis in the treatment of obesity. In J. W. Rhue, S. J. Lynn, & I. Kirsch (Eds.), *Handbook of clinical hypnosis* (pp. 511–532). Washington, DC: American Psychological Association.

Lyons, L. C., & Woods, P. J., (1991). The efficacy of rational-emotive therapy: A quantitative review of the outcome research. *Clinical Psychology Review, 11,* 357–369.

*McAmmond, D. M., Davison, P. O., & Kovitz, D. M. (1971). A comparison of the effects of hypnosis and relaxation training on stress reactions in a dental situation. *American Journal of Clinical Hypnosis, 13,* 233–242.

*O'Brien, R. M., Cooley, L. E., Ciotti, J., & Henninger, K. M. (1981). Augmentations of systematic desensitization of snake phobia through posthypnotic dream suggestion. *American Journal of Clinical Hypnosis, 23,* 231–238.

Orne, M. T. (1959). The nature of hypnosis: Artifact and essence. *Journal of Abnormal Psychology, 58,* 277–299.

Rhue, J. W., Lynn, S. J., & Kirsch, I. (1993). *Handbook of clinical hypnosis.* Washington, DC: American Psychological Association.

Sarbin, T. R., & Coe, W. C. (1972). *Hypnosis: A social psychological analysis of influence communication.* New York: Holt, Rinehart & Winston.

Schoenberger, N. E. (1993). *Effectiveness of a cognitive–behavioral hypnotherapy for public speaking anxiety.* Unpublished doctoral dissertation, University of Connecticut.

Smith, M. L., Glass, G. V., & Miller, T. I. (1980). *The benefits of psychotherapy.* Baltimore: John Hopkins University Press.

Spanos, N. P. (1991). Hypnosis, hypnotizability, and hypnotherapy. In C. R. Snyder & D. R. Forsyth (Eds.), *Handbook of clinical and social psychology.* New York: Pergamon Press.

Spanos, N. P., & Chaves, J. F. (Eds.). (1989). *Hypnosis: The cognitive-behavioral perspective.* Buffalo, NY: Prometheus Press.

Spinhoven, P. (1987). Hypnosis and behavior therapy: A review. *International Journal of Clinical and Experimental Hypnosis, 35,* 8–31.

Stunkard, A. J. (1972). Foreword. In R. B. Stuart & B. Davis, *Slim chance in a fat world: Behavioral control of obesity.* Champaign, IL: Research Press.

*Sullivan, D. S., Johnson, A., & Bratkovitch, J. (1974). Reduction of behavioral deficit in organic brain damage by use of hypnosis. *Journal of Clinical Psychology, 30,* 96–98.

*Tosi, D. J., Judah, S. M., & Murphy, M. A. (1989). The effects of a cognitive experiential therapy utilizing hypnosis, cognitive restructuring, and developmental staging on psychological factors associated with duodenal ulcer disease: A multivariate experimental study. *Journal of Cognitive Psychotherapy, 3,* 272–290.

*Tosi, D. J., Rudy, D. R., Lewis, J., & Murphy, M. A. (1992). The psychobiological effects of cognitive experiential therapy, hypnosis, cognitive restructuring, and attention placebo control in the treatment of essential hypertension. *Psychotherapy, 29,* 274–284.

Wadden, T. A., & Anderton, C. H. (1982). The clinical use of hypnosis. *Psychological Bulletin, 91,* 215–243.

*Wadden, T. A., & Flaxman, J. (1981). Hypnosis and weight loss: A preliminary study. *International Journal of Clinical and Experimental Hypnosis, 29,* 162–173.

Received November 15, 1993
Revision received February 2, 1994
Accepted February 6, 1994 ■

Correction to Frick et al. (1991)

The article "Academic Underachievement and the Disruptive Behavior Disorders," by Paul J. Frick, Randy W. Kamphaus, Benjamin B. Lahey, Rolf Loeber, Mary Anne G. Christ, Elizabeth L. Hart, and Lynne E. Tannenbaum (*Journal of Consulting and Clinical Psychology,* 1991, Vol. 59, No. 2, 289–294), contained an error.

On page 290, in the formula to calculate the discrepancy score between IQ and academic achievement, Step 3 should appear as follows:

3. Differences between achievement and full-scale intelligence were expressed in z-score units adjusting for the standard error of estimate. For example, reading discrepancy = $(Z^{READ} - r \cdot Z^{FSIQ})/SE^{R}$.

[27]

Long term benefits of hypnotherapy for irritable bowel syndrome

W M Gonsalkorale, V Miller, A Afzal, P J Whorwell

Gut 2003;**52**:1623–1629

See end of article for authors' affiliations

Correspondence to: Dr W M Gonsalkorale, Hypnotherapy Unit, Withington Hospital, Nell Lane, Manchester M20 2LR, UK; wgonsalkorale@compuserve.com

Accepted for publication 23 July 2003

Background and aims: There is now good evidence from several sources that hypnotherapy can relieve the symptoms of irritable bowel syndrome in the short term. However, there is no long term data on its benefits and this information is essential before the technique can be widely recommended. This study aimed to answer this question.
Patients and methods: 204 patients prospectively completed questionnaires scoring symptoms, quality of life, anxiety, and depression before, immediately after, and up to six years following hypnotherapy. All subjects also subjectively assessed the effects of hypnotherapy retrospectively in order to define their "responder status".
Results: 71% of patients initially responded to therapy. Of these, 81% maintained their improvement over time while the majority of the remaining 19% claimed that deterioration of symptoms had only been slight. With respect to symptom scores, all items at follow up were significantly improved on pre-hypnotherapy levels ($p<0.001$) and showed little change from post-hypnotherapy values. There were no significant differences in the symptom scores between patients assessed at 1, 2, 3, 4, or 5+ years following treatment. Quality of life and anxiety or depression scores were similarly still significantly improved at follow up ($p<0.001$) but did show some deterioration. Patients also reported a reduction in consultation rates and medication use following the completion of hypnotherapy.
Conclusion: This study demonstrates that the beneficial effects of hypnotherapy appear to last at least five years. Thus it is a viable therapeutic option for the treatment of irritable bowel syndrome.

Irritable bowel syndrome (IBS) is a functional bowel disorder, the symptoms of which include abdominal pain, distension, and altered bowel habit. Patients also commonly complain of associated extra-colonic symptoms, such as nausea, lethargy, and backache.[1] This is a common condition and, although the majority of sufferers do not seek medical help, those who do account for up to half of the gastroenterologist's workload.[2 3] Symptoms can be sufficiently severe and troublesome in some individuals as to impair their quality of life.[1 4] It is not uncommon for patients to have repeated consultations and investigations and patients tend to consult their own general practitioner for other minor ailments more frequently than other people.[5] The socioeconomic impact of IBS is therefore considerable and patients account for significant healthcare resources.[6]

Treatment of IBS by conventional means is often unsatisfactory, with symptoms failing to respond to an array of currently available medications. Gut directed hypnotherapy, however, has been shown previously to be extremely effective in the treatment of IBS, with the majority of patients showing improvement in symptoms, associated extra-colonic features and quality of life,[7–9] findings which have been confirmed by independent studies.[10–12]

Gut directed hypnotherapy comprises a course of up to 12 weekly 1 hr sessions.[7 13] Each session consists of induction of the hypnotic state and deepening procedures, followed by "ego strengthening" suggestions relevant to the individual. These are accompanied by further suggestions and interventions, such as inducing warmth in the abdomen using the hands and imagery, directed towards controlling and normalising gut function.

This work led to the establishment of the first hypnotherapy unit in the National Health Service in the UK devoted to the treatment of IBS patients. We have recently published an audit on the first 250 patients treated at this unit,[13] confirming the beneficial effects of hypnotherapy in a large number of patients. However, outcome was measured immediately after patients completed the course of hypnotherapy. The aim of this present study, therefore, was to establish follow up on a large number of patients treated, to determine the longer term effects of therapy, in terms of symptom improvement, consultation rates, and use of medication.

METHODS

Patients and procedure

The following set of questionnaires was mailed to 273 patients with IBS who had completed a course of gut directed hypnotherapy (HT) at least one year previously. The patients were asked to complete and return:

(i) A validated IBS questionnaire,[14] rating IBS symptoms, extra-colonic features, and quality of life measures by visual analogue scale (0–100 mm) (Appendix 1);

(ii) The Hospital Anxiety and Depression (HAD) Scale[15];

(iii) A subjective assessment questionnaire (SAQ), rating the effects of hypnotherapy on symptoms, consultation rates, and use of medication through Likert-type responses, and other information, for example, continued practice of HT techniques (Appendix 2).

All patients had already completed the IBS Questionnaire and HAD Scale both immediately before and after the course

Abbreviations: HAD, Hospital Anxiety and Depression Scale; HT, hypnotherapy; IBS, irritable bowel syndrome; SAQ, subjective assessment questionnaire of HT, and therefore data were available for three different time points—that is, pre-HT, post-HT, and follow up.

Statistical analysis

Mean values (with SEM) were calculated for all scores in the IBS questionnaire and HAD Scale completed pre- and post-HT and at follow up. Intra-individual differences in scores between these time points, with positive and negative values denoting improvement or deterioration in scores, respectively, relative to the earlier time point, were compared by paired t test. Comparison between individual groups was performed using independent t test (two groups) or analysis of variance (more than two groups). For each item in the SAQ, data are given as the proportion (%) of patients rating each response category. Intra-individual comparisons were made using McNemar's test and independent groups compared using χ^2 test. Spearman (ρ) correlation coefficients were calculated to assess relationships between variables. For further analysis, patients were subdivided into responders and non-responders, based on the response to SAQ(i), with responders defined as patients rating their symptoms either "very much better" or "moderately better" at the end of the course of HT and non-responders as those rating symptoms "slightly better" or less. Patients were also grouped according to the number of years that had lapsed since completing treatment.

Binary logistic regression analysis was performed to identify factors affecting "responder" status. In order to limit the number of variables examined at any one time, a stepwise analysis was carried out using a series of variable blocks, with blocks relating to pre-HT measures for all symptoms, quality of life, and HAD scores as well as age, gender, and bowel habit.

Overall scores for IBS symptoms and extra-colonic features were treated as the primary outcomes. For the purpose of comparing secondary endpoints—that is, the individual measures making up these overall scores—only differences at the 0.1% ($p<0.001$) were interpreted as showing reasonable evidence of a true difference, instead of adjusting for multiple comparisons.

RESULTS

Return rate

Of the 273 questionnaires 204 were returned, representing a 75% return rate. These were reasonably equally distributed according to the time since completing treatment (1<2 years ago: 22.4%; 2<3 years: 18.4%; 3<4 years: 27.8%; 4<5 years: 21.4%; ⩾5: 10.0%).

Subjective assessment questionnaire

Improvement after hypnotherapy (SAQ(i))

There were 106 (52.0%) patients who reported their symptoms as "very much better" at the end of the course of HT, 39 (19.1%) as "moderately better", 32 (15.7%) as "slightly better", while 27 (13.2%) reported no change in symptoms. No patients reported worsening of symptoms. Patients in whom symptoms were very much or moderately better (71.1% of total) were then defined as "responders", and those with only slight improvement or no change as "non-responders".

Progress in symptoms since completing HT (SAQ(ii))

Subdividing according to responder status as above, 81.3% of responders maintained the improvement gained, with the majority stating that their symptoms had improved even further (29.2% improved "much more", 24.3% "moderately more", 11.1% "slightly more", and 16.7% "about the same as at the end of HT"). The remaining 18.7% had experienced mostly slight deterioration in symptoms. More responders than non-responders stated that symptoms had continued to improve after finishing HT (responders (R) *v* non-responders (NR): 64.6% *v* 35.0%, $\chi^2 = 13.54$, $p<0.001$) and symptom improvement was mainly rated as slight for these non-responders. The majority of non-responders, therefore, had no improvement in symptoms during the follow up period, with 49.1% being about the same as at the end of treatment (that is, about the same or only slightly improved compared with before HT) and 15.8% slightly worse.

IBS questionnaires

IBS symptoms

Scores from pre- and post-HT IBS questionnaires were compared in patients returning and not returning follow up questionnaires, in order to ensure that those returning these questionnaires were representative of the patient group as a whole. No differences in symptom severity before treatment or in initial improvement after HT emerged. Questionnaires returned (n = 204) *v* not returned (n = 69): pre-HT (mean, SEM): pain severity 56.1 (1.9) *v* 60.1 (2.6); pain frequency 55.0 (2.4) *v* 64.1 (3.3); bloating 61.0 (1.9) *v* 61.8 (2.9); bowel habit dissatisfaction 71.6 (1.8) *v* 73.0 (2.4); life interference 72.5 (1.4) *v* 75.1 (1.7); overall score 314.2 (6.1) *v* 330.4 (8.6), all $p>0.05$. Pre-HT/post-HT intra-individual differences (mean, 95% confidence interval (CI)): pain severity 25.5 (21.5 to 29.5) *v* 27.2 (22.0 to 32.4); pain frequency 23.8 (19.1 to 28.6) *v* 35.3 (28.5 to 42.1); bloating 29.4 (25.5 to 33.4) *v* 31.9 (26.7 to 37.2); life interference 33.2 (29.4 to 36.9) *v* 31.1 (25.7 to 36.6); overall score 144.1 (128.8 to 159.4) *v* 151.3 (129.2 to 173.5), all $p>0.05$, except pain frequency where $p = 0.005$.

Intra-individual differences in scores between the three different time points (that is, pre-HT, post-HT, and follow up) in the 204 patients for whom follow up data were obtained (figure 1) showed that all symptoms as well as the overall score had improved immediately after HT and remained better at follow up (pre-HT/post-HT and pre-HT/follow up intra-individual differences, all $p<0.001$). Symptoms had increased slightly at follow up compared with post-HT levels but this was significant only for bloating and bowel habit

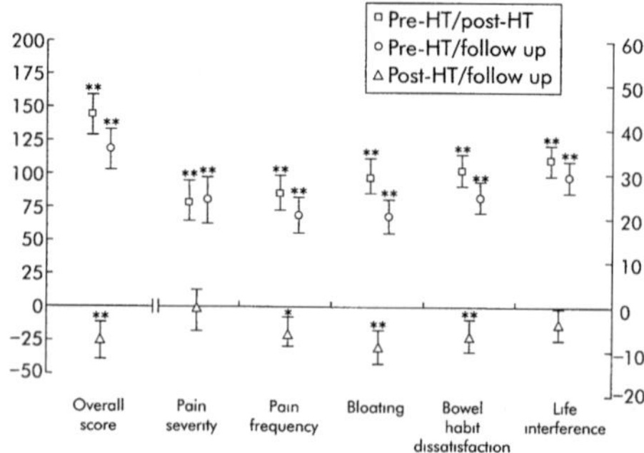

Figure 1 Intra-individual differences in IBS symptom scores for all patients (n = 204) between the different time points—that is, pre-HT post-HT, pre-HT/follow up, and post-HT/follow up. Data expressed as mean (95% confidence interval (CI)), with positive and negative values denoting reduction (improvement) and increase (deterioration) in score relative to earlier time point. (Mean values of scores at these time points are given in the text.) Overall score treated as the primary outcome and therefore no adjustment is made for multiple comparisons. "Unadjusted" comparisons for individual symptoms significant at the 0.1% level are assumed significant at the 5% level if multiple comparison adjustment is made. *p<0.01, **p<0.001.

dissatisfaction (post-HT/follow up intra-individual differences, both p<0.001).

Patients' rating of improvement in the SAQ was reflected in the IBS questionnaire scores with a direct correlation, firstly, between rating of improvement after HT, SAQ(i), and intra-individual differences in pre-HT/post-HT overall IBS scores ($\rho = 0.433$, p<0.001), and, secondly, between rating of symptom progress since completing HT, SAQ(ii), and differences in post-HT/follow up overall IBS scores ($\rho = 0.488$, p<0.001).

Analysis according to responder status

As shown in table 1, severity of IBS symptoms prior to HT was no different between the responders and non-responders (R *v* NR: all p>0.05). However, mean scores for responders were significantly lower than those for non-responders both immediately after HT (all p<0.001) and at follow up (all p<0.001, except pain severity (p<0.5) and bloating (p<0.01). Intra-individual differences in scores between the different time points (figure 2) shows that while some symptom measures were also significantly improved in the non-responder group post-HT and at follow up (bowel habit dissatisfaction and life interference p<0.001 at both time points), these changes were small compared with those in responders. Indeed, responders had greater reduction in symptom scores than non-responders both immediately after HT (pre-HT/post-HT intra-individual differences, R *v* NR: all p<0.001) and at follow up (pre-HT/follow up intra-individual differences, R *v* NR: all p<0.001 except pain frequency, p<0.005). Furthermore, no significant intra-individual differences between post-HT and follow up symptom scores occurred for non-responders (all p>0.05), showing that symptoms did not improve with the course of time.

Analysis according to time lapsed since completing treatment

There was no association between the time, in years, since responders had completed treatment and intra-individual differences in post-HT and follow up overall IBS score ($\rho = -0.027$, p = 0.752), suggesting that those with a longer gap since treatment had maintained improvement just as well as those who had finished more recently. In addition, there were no marked differences in overall IBS scores (table 2) between the different time intervals either before HT (p = 0.310) or at follow up (p = 0.458) or in the pre-HT/follow up intra-individual differences in this score (p = 0.781).

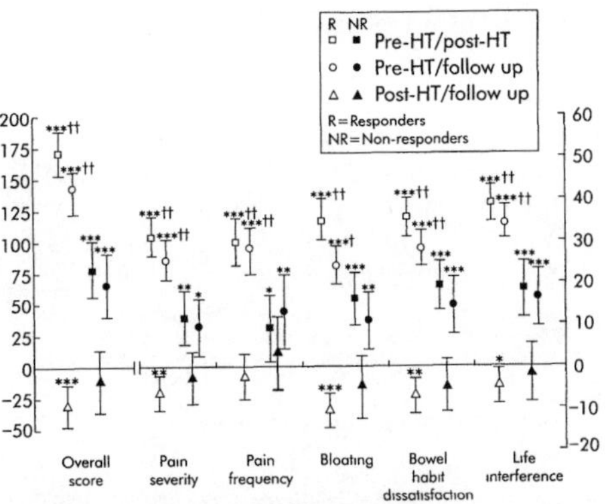

Figure 2 Intra-individual differences in IBS symptom scores for responders and non-responders between the different time points shown. Data expressed as mean (95% confidence interval (CI)), with positive and negative values denoting reduction and increase in score relative to earlier time point. (Mean values of scores at these time points are given in table 1.) Overall score treated as the primary outcome and therefore no adjustment is made for multiple comparisons. "Unadjusted" comparison for individual symptoms significant at the 0.1% level are assumed to be significant at the 5% level if multiple comparison adjustment made. *p<0.05, **p<0.01, ***p<0.001 (intra-individual difference); †p<0.005, ††p<0.001 (responders *v* non-responders).

Extra-colonic symptoms

Severity of extra-colonic symptoms before HT was similar for both responders and non-responders (table 3). Responders had significant improvement in individual symptoms and overall score after HT (pre-HT/post-HT intra-individual differences, all p<0.001) and most of these remained better than pre-HT levels at follow up (pre-HT/follow up intra-individual differences all p<0.001, except urinary symptoms, thigh pain, and bodily aches, p<0.05). Although non-responders had significant improvement in overall extra-colonic score and some individual symptoms immediately after HT (pre-HT/post-HT intra-individual differences: overall score, nausea, excess wind, lethargy all p<0.001), this had deteriorated at follow up. Responders had more pronounced improvement in overall score than non-responders, both post-HT and at follow up (intra-individual differences, R *v* NR: pre-HT/post-HT p<0.001; pre-HT/follow up: p<0.005) and for a number of individual symptoms after HT, including excess wind (pre-HT/follow up intra-individual differences, R *v* NR: p<0.001), lethargy, backache, and

Table 1 IBS symptom scores

	Pre-HT		Post-HT		Follow up	
Symptom	**R**	**NR**	**R**	**NR**	**R**	**NR**
Pain severity	58.0 (2.2)†	51.4 (3.6)	26.4 (1.9)***	39.9 (3.3)	32.2 (2.1)*	42.0 (3.6)
Pain frequency	53.1 (2.8)†	59.3 (4.5)	22.8 (2.6)***	50.2 (4.6)	25.2 (2.4)***	45.7 (5.1)
Bloating	61.0 (2.2)†	60.8 (3.8)	27.1 (2.1)***	44.0 (4.1)	36.9 (2.1)**	49.0 (4.2)
BH dissatisfaction	71.1 (2.1)†	72.6 (3.4)	35.6 (1.8)***	53.9 (3.4)	42.5 (1.8)***	58.0 (3.7)
Life interference	71.4 (1.6)†	75.2 (2.7)	32.2 (1.9)***	57.1 (3.1)	37.0 (1.9)***	58.4 (3.3)
Overall score	312.2 (7.4)†	318.2 (11.0)	143.6 (8.3)***	241.7 (13.1)	173.7 (8.0)***	251.3 (14.8)

Irritable bowel syndrome (IBS) symptom scores (mean, SEM) shown for responders (R) and non-responders (NR), as measured in IBS questionnaire (VAS 0–100 mm), completed at the time points shown. For data in this table (and similarly in all tables), overall score is treated as the primary outcome and therefore no adjustments are made for multiple comparisons. "Unadjusted" comparisons for individual symptoms significant at the 0.1% level (p<0.001) assumed significant at the 5% level if multiple comparison adjustments were made.
*p<0.05; **p<0.01; ***p<0.001; †p>0.05 (R *v* NR).
BH, bowel habit; HT, hypnotherapy.

Table 2 Overall IBS scores for responders according to time since treatment

Years since HT	N	Pre-HT*	Follow up*	Pre-HT/follow up†
1<2	37	283.8 (13.9)‡	161.2 (16.1)§	122.7 (95.5 to 149.8)¶
2<3	25	330.8 (18.2)	197.6 (21.4)	133.2 (94.3 to 172.1)
3<4	36	328.4 (14.1)	183.8 (16.8)	145.1 (105.8 to 184.5)
4<5	32	319.5 (16.6)	168.5 (16.9)	151.0 (107.5 to 194.5)
⩾5	15	298.8 (23.3)	147.5 (18.0)	151.3 (93.1 to 209.6)

Data shown as: *overall IBS scores (mean (SEM)) and †intra-individual differences (mean, 95% CI) for time points shown for responders, subdivided according to time since completing treatment. Intra-individual differences having positive value denote reduction (improvement) in score relative to earlier time point.
‡p=0.310; §p=0.458; ¶p=0.781 (all ANOVA).

heartburn (all p<0.005), although this was not evident at follow up (intra-individual pre-HT/follow up differences, R *v* NR: excess wind, lethargy, backache all p<0.05; heartburn p>0.05).

Quality of life, anxiety, and depression

Quality of life measures before HT were no different for responders and non-responders (table 4). Although there was some improvement in the non-responder group immediately after HT (pre-HT/post-HT intra-individual differences, all p<0.005, physical well being and control p<0.001), this was significant at follow up only for mood (p<0.005). Improvement occurred in responders both after HT and at follow up compared with pre-HT levels (intra-individual differences: pre-HT/post-HT all p<0.001; pre-HT/follow up all p<0.001, social/relationships p<0.005) and this was more marked than in non-responders, particularly for psychic and physical well being (R *v* NR: pre-HT/post-HT p<0.001; pre-HT/follow up p<0.01).

HAD scores for anxiety and depression were similar in both patient groups before HT (R *v* NR: HAD "A" anxiety (mean (SEM)): 10.7 (0.4) *v* 9.8 (0.6), p = 0.184; HAD "D" depression: 6.7 (0.3) *v* 6.8 (0.4), p = 0.798). Scores had improved in both groups post-HT and were still better than pre-HT levels at follow up (intra-individual differences (mean (95%CI)): pre-HT/post-HT: anxiety, R: 4.1 (3.5 to 4.7), NR: 2.4 (1.4 to 3.3); depression, R: 3.4 (2.8 to 4.0), NR: 1.7 (0.9 to 2.6), all p<0.001; pre-HT/follow up: anxiety, R: 2.7 (2.0 to 3.3), p<0.001; NR: 1.5 (0.5 to 2.5), p = 0.003; depression, R: 2.5 (1.9 to 3.2), NR: 1.4 (0.7 to 2.2), both p<0.001). Improvement was overall greater in the responder group, particularly post-HT (R *v* NR: anxiety and depression, both p = 0.002) but less evident at follow up (R *v* NR: anxiety: p = 0.068; depression, p = 0.031). Fewer responders were significantly anxious or depressed (HAD scores >9) after HT and at follow up, while fewer non-responders were anxious post-HT only (HAD "A" >9 (anxious): Pre-HT *v* post-HT: R: 59.0% *v* 24.4%, p<0.001; NR: 48.3% *v* 28.1%, p = 0.008; versus follow up: R: 31.9%, p<0.001; NR: *v* 37.3%, p = 0.210; HAD "D" >9 (depressed): Pre-HT *v* post-HT: R: 20.7% *v* 5.5%, p<0.001; NR: 18.6% *v* 11.9%, p = 0.424; versus follow up: R: 9.0%, p = 0.002; NR: 13.6%, p = 0.549, McNemar's test).

Consultation rates

The majority of responders compared with around half of non-responders stated they had seen their GP and the hospital consultant less often about IBS symptoms since HT, and more responders had seen their GP less often about other symptoms (consulted "less often", "about same", "more often": R *v* NR (%): GP/IBS symptoms: 87.9%, 10.7%, 1.4% *v* 50.9%, 45.6%, 3.5%, $\chi^2 = 31.75$, p<0.001; Consultant/IBS symptoms: 83.3%, 13.7%, 3.7% *v* 54.8%, 40.5%, 4.8%, $\chi^2 = 13.41$, p = 0.001; GP/other symptoms: 61.2%, 32.6%, 6.2% *v* 21.8%, 63.6%, 14.5%, $\chi^2 = 24.10$, p<0.001).

Use of medication

Medication taken before HT included antispasmodics (42.0% of all patients on medication), antidiarrhoeals (23.2%), laxatives (12.3%), bulking agents (9.4%), antidepressants (21.0%), and anxiolytics (10.9%), with 27.5% taking at least two types of medication. A similar proportion of responders and non-responders were taking medication before HT but fewer responders were on medication during follow up (R *v* NR: Pre-HT: 67.6% *v* 67.8%, $\chi^2 = 0.03$, p = 0.856; during follow up: 36.6% *v* 55.9%, $\chi^2 = 6.27$, p = 0.012). Of those patients continuing to take medication, more responders stated they had taken it less often than before ("less often", "about same", "more often", R *v* NR: 62.3%, 26.4%, 11.3% *v* 9.1%, 69.7%, 21.2%, $\chi^2 = 23.91$, p<0.001).

While proportionately more non-responders than responders with low anxiety and depression scores (HAD scores <10) at follow up were taking antidepressants and/or anxiolytics (NR *v* R: 21.1% *v* 6.0%, p<0.001) these represented only a minority of non-responders with low scores, since 63% and 80% of this group had low HAD "A" and "D" scores, respectively.

Factors influencing initial response to hypnotherapy

There were no differences between responders and non-responders in any baseline measures of symptoms, quality of life, or HAD scores (tables 1, 3, and 4 and HAD results section) but more males than females were non-responders

Table 3 Extra-colonic symptom scores

Symptoms	Pre-HT§ R	Pre-HT§ NR	Pre-HT/Post-HT¶ R	Pre-HT/Post-HT¶ NR	Pre-HT/follow up¶ R	Pre-HT/follow up¶ NR
Nausea/vomiting	28.5 (2.3)‡	27.8 (3.8)	13.9 (10.4 to 17.4)***	11.4 (6.1 to 16.7)***	13.0 (9.5 to 16.5)***	11.5 (4.9 to 18.0)**
Early satiety	29.1 (2.3)‡	23.8 (3.8)	10.1 (6.8 to 13.4)***	6.5 (1.8 to 11.2)**	10.1 (5.8 to 14.5)***	6.9 (2.3 to 11.5)**
Heartburn	31.7 (2.4)‡	26.5 (3.9)	15.9 (11.7 to 20.2)*** ††	5.1 (−0.9 to 11.1)	10.5 (5.9 to 15.2)***	7.8 (1.9 to 13.7)*
Backache	49.7 (2.6)‡	41.6 (4.2)	16.9 (12.8 to 21.1)*** ††	4.5 (−1.7 to 10.7)	14.2 (9.7 to 18.6)*** †	3.7 (−3.7 to 11.0)
Headaches	41.6 (2.4)‡	35.7 (4.0)	13.3 (9.6 to 17.0)***	8.9 (3.5 to 14.3)**	9.4 (5.6 to 13.2)***	3.9 (−1.4 to 9.2)
Excess wind	74.2 (1.9)‡	74.6 (3.5)	33.7 (28.9 to 38.5)*** †††	19.2 (13.4 to 25.0)***	18.7 (14.1 to 23.3)*** †	9.6 (2.5 to 16.6)**
Lethargy	67.2 (2.3)‡	67.2 (3.6)	29.0 (24.5 to 33.5)*** ††	15.1 (7.7 to 22.5)***	16.4 (11.8 to 21.0)*** †	5.4 (−1.9 to 12.6)
Urinary	48.0 (2.8)‡	38.7 (4.4)	15.9 (11.5 to 20.4)*** ††	2.2 (−5.1 to 9.4)	6.2 (1.1 to 11.3)* †	−4.6 (−13.8 to 4.5)
Thigh pain	24.3 (2.5)‡	24.9 (4.6)	10.3 (6.1 to 14.5)***	7.6 (1.1 to 14.1)*	4.5 (−0.5 to 9.4)*	3.2 (−4.4,10.8)
Bodily aches	47.9 (2.7)‡	46.4 (4.6)	16.6 (12.0 to 21.3)*** †	6.9 (−0.6 to 13.9)	6.5 (1.4 to 11.6)*	0.4 (−7.2 to 8.0)
Overall score	219.5 (7.6)‡	201.1 (11.5)	80.4 (65.1 to 95.6)*** †††	40.1 (24.5 to 55.6)***	53.7 (41.1 to 66.2)*** ††	21.6 (7.6 to 35.5)**

Data shown for responders (R) and non-responders (NR) as §mean scores (SEM); ¶intra-individual differences (mean (95% CI)) between time points shown, with positive and negative values denoting reduction and increase in scores, respectively, relative to earlier time point.
*p<0.05, **p<0.005, ***p<0.001 (versus pre-HT); †††p<0.001; ††p<0.01; †p<0.05; ‡p>0.05 (R *v* NR).

Table 4 Quality of life measures

	Pre-HT§		Pre-HT/Post-HT¶		Pre-HT/follow up¶	
	R	NR	R	NR	R	NR
Psychic well being	50.3 (1.8)‡‡	55.1 (3.1)	27.6 (23.9 to 31.4)*** †††	10.3 (4.4 to 16.2)**	18.7 (14.2 to 23.2)*** ††	6.2 (−0.4 to 12.8)‡
Physical well being	47.2 (1.7)‡‡	45.1 (2.7)	21.8 (18.6 to 25.0) *** †††	12.0 (7.4 to 16.6)***	12.5 (8.9 to 16.0)*** †	4.9 (−0.1 to 10.0)‡
Mood	48.9 (1.6)‡‡	47.4 (2.6)	19.9 (16.4 to 23.4) *** ††	10.6 (4.4 to 16.8)**	12.8 (9.0 to 16.5)*** ‡‡	10.2 (4.2 to 16.3)**
Control	53.8 (1.9)‡‡	59.2 (3.4)	18.2 (14.8 to 21.5)*** †	11.0 (5.2 to 16.8)***	13.0 (8.8 to 17.3)*** †	4.7 (−2.5 to 11.8)‡
Social/relationships	68.6 (1.6)‡‡	67.1 (2.9)	10.8 (8.6 to 18.6)*** ††	5.0 (1.7 to 8.3)**	7.4 (4.3 to 10.4)* ‡‡	3.9 (−1.3 to 7.6)‡

Data shown for responders (R) and non-responders (NR) as §mean scores (SEM) and ¶intra-individual differences (mean (95% CI)) between time points.
Note: In contrast with other symptom scores, higher values in quality of life measures signify improvement; positive and negative values in intra-individual differences denote reduction (deterioration) and increase (improvement) in scores, respectively, relative to earlier time point.
*p<0.05; **p<0.005; ***p<0.001; ‡p>0.05 (versus pre-HT); †††p<0.001; ††p<0.01; †p<0.05; ‡‡p>0.05 (R *v* NR).

(males *v* females: R: 57.5% *v* 74.7%; NR: 42.5% *v* 25.3%, $\chi^2 = 4.63$, p = 0.031). Although more males had diarrhoea predominant bowel habit (males *v* females, bowel habit type: constipation 12.8% *v* 25.5%, diarrhoea 51.3% *v* 24.8%, alternating 35.9% *v* 49.7%, $\chi^2 = 10.77$, p = 0.005), no more non-responders were found with this or any other bowel habit type, either for patients as a whole or for males (constipation *v* diarrhoea *v* alternating: all patients, R: 69.6% *v* 73.3% *v* 71.3%; NR 30.4% *v* 26.7% v 28.7%, $\chi^2 = 0.19$, p = 0.911; males: R: 40.0% *v* 60.0% *v* 57.1%; NR: 60.0% *v* 40.0% *v* 42.9%, $\chi^2 = 0.66$, p = 0.721). Non-responders were also overall slightly older than responders (mean age (SEM), years: R *v* NR: 45.1 (1.2) *v* 50.3 (1.8), p = 0.017). However, binary logistic regression analysis identified only gender as having a significant relationship with responder status (OR (95% CI): 0.30 (0.16 to 0.97), p = 0.042).

Continued practice of hypnotherapy techniques during follow up

More responders than non-responders continued to practise HT techniques after treatment (R (% patients): 85% *v* 58%, p<0.001), although both groups had a similar pattern of practice (R *v* NR: with tape only: 38.7% *v* 36.4%; without tape: 42.4% *v* 42.5%; both with/without tape: 18.9% *v* 21.1%; $\chi^2 = 0.24$, p = 0.970). There was no difference in symptom change during follow up between patients who still practised and those who did not (intra-individual difference in post-HT/follow up overall IBS score (mean (SEM)), practice *v* no practice: all patients: −19.5 (16.6) *v* −27.4 (7.8), p = 0.392; R only: −24.8 (32.6) *v* −31.9 (8.7), p = 0.628). Similarly, there was no correlation between symptom change and frequency of practice (all patients: $\rho = 0.027$, p = 0.777; R only: $\rho = 0.067$, p = 0.572).

Other considerations

The continued improvement seen in responders cannot be explained by the use of other treatments after finishing HT. Only 14 (9.7%) of responders had tried other treatments, including dietary changes, alternative medicines, yoga, and reflexology and found these helpful. Of all patients, 93.1% considered that the course of HT had been worthwhile, which included all of the responders and 76.3% of non-responders.

DISCUSSION

This study presents the first long term follow up of a large number of patients who have undergone hypnotherapy for IBS symptoms. Immediately after HT, 71% of patients considered their symptoms very much or moderately better and these patients were defined as "responders". Of these initial responders, 81% maintained the benefit of treatment or reported further improvement. In contrast, non-responders, with only slight or no improvement in symptoms with HT, had little or no change in symptoms over the follow up period.

There was a good correlation between the SAQ ratings and the objective symptom scores. IBS symptom scores were significantly improved after HT and remained so at follow up, with only a slight deterioration compared with post-HT levels. The beneficial effects did not appear to decline with time since patients who had finished treatment more than five years ago maintained symptom improvement just as well as those who had completed only a year ago. Similarly, extracolonic features, quality of life, anxiety, and depression scores were still better at follow up compared with pre-HT levels. Interestingly, all patients reported taking less medication and had consulted less often for IBS and other symptoms, but this was particularly striking for the responder group.

The subdivision of patients into "responders" and "non-responders", based on the SAQ rating of symptom change, was undertaken in order to concur with the current practice of using a subjective global assessment as a primary outcome in clinical trials in functional bowel disorders.[16] It also facilitated further analysis of the data, and indeed revealed that there were clear differences between responders and non-responders in terms of IBS and other symptom scores, consultation rates, and use of medication after treatment.

The SAQ was only completed at follow up, hence requiring patients to assess the effects of HT retrospectively and therefore the reliability of their reports could be called into question. However, the fact that the SAQ correlated with changes in symptom rating from the IBS questionnaires would indicate that the SAQ assessments are a reliable reflection of treatment outcome. Similarly, patients' reports of consultation rates and use of medication must be interpreted with some caution. However, one could determine the number of patients who had stopped medication after HT, since medication was recorded at the start of HT and at follow up. Reports in terms of fewer consultations and less medication were markedly different between responders and non-responders, suggesting that these cannot be explained entirely by recall bias.

The return rate in this study was 75%. These patients can be considered to be representative of all patients contacted since their pre-HT IBS symptom scores and improvement immediately after HT were similar to the patients who did not return the follow up questionnaires. This study was an audit of patients who had undergone hypnotherapy and hence there was no control group, which may be considered a weakness to the study, although it is difficult to conceive how one could have been included. There is known to be a high level of placebo response in IBS patients which can last for at least three months.[17] However, the improvement seen in this study lasted at least one year and was at the same level in patients after five or more years, making a placebo effect very unlikely. In addition, the fact that non-responders did not exhibit significant improvement during the follow up period makes it very unlikely the improvements observed in the responder group were due to the natural course of the condition. The favourable response to HT reported here is unlikely to be influenced to any great extent by the fact that treatment was at a specialist centre providing this treatment, since independent studies at other centres have also shown beneficial results with HT.[10–12] Therefore, we believe our results could be generalised to the treatment of IBS patients in general. Out of all the pre-HT measures and demographic features examined with regression analysis, only gender was significantly associated with responder status, with males being more likely to be non-responders and this is in keeping with our previous observations.[13]

Very little deterioration occurred in IBS symptoms over time, although some of the other measures, such as certain extra-colonic symptoms, quality of life, and scores for anxiety and depression, did show some attrition, but most of these were still better at follow up than before treatment. Quality of life and psychological well being are influenced by many other factors such as life events, irrespective of gastrointestinal problems and it is possible that any of these could have been operating within an individual since treatment, thus contributing to the change in these scores. Anxiety and depression scores were significantly lower both post-HT and at follow up in both responders and non-responders, although the proportion of patients who could be classified as significantly anxious or depressed was only lower in responders. This would suggest that even though non-responders did not improve in terms of IBS symptoms, they did derive some benefit psychologically. This is unlikely to be an effect of taking anxiolytics or antidepressants, since only a relatively small proportion of these non-responders were taking such medication after treatment. It is also interesting to note that nearly all patients considered the hypnotherapy to have been worthwhile, so that even non-responders felt that they had benefited in some way even though their symptoms had not altered with treatment.

Maintained improvement of symptoms did not appear to have any association with whether or not or how often responders continued to practise hypnotherapeutic techniques following treatment, although only 15% of responders discontinued practice. The reason for this somewhat unexpected finding is not readily apparent and does raise the question whether continued practice is necessary for any particular individual to maintain benefit. It may suggest that those who did well with HT yet did not continue to practise overtly have developed the ability to continue using their hypnotic skills at a subconscious level.

In conclusion, this study confirms that the beneficial effects of HT are long lasting, with continued improvement in symptoms, thus giving patients better control over their condition, although it may be less useful for male patients. A potential criticism for the use of hypnotherapy as a treatment for IBS has been that it is costly to provide because of the demands on therapists' time. However, because of its sustained effects in the majority of patients, costs of treatment could be rapidly offset by the ensuing reduction in cost of medication and other healthcare demands.

APPENDIX 1

IBS QUESTIONNAIRE[14]

Items in the questionnaire were scored using a visual analogue scale of 0–100 mm. Increased severity of IBS symptoms and extra-colonic features was indicated by a higher score, whereas increased impairment of quality of life measures was denoted by a lower score. Overall scores were calculated as the sum of the following individual items, adjusted as necessary to give a maximum score as indicated:

Overall IBS score (maximum 500; sum of 5 items): pain severity, pain frequency, distension, bowel habit dissatisfaction, life interference

Overall extra-colonic score (maximum 500; sum of 10 items ÷2): nausea/vomiting, early satiety, headaches, backache, excess wind, heartburn, bodily pains, urinary symptoms, thigh pain, lethargy.

QUALITY OF LIFE

The value of each quality of life measure was derived from the mean of the individual items shown indicated in parentheses, to give a maximum score of 100.

- Psychic well being (coping with problems, confidence, usefulness, security)
- Physical well being (sleep, energy levels, aches and pains, feeling physically well)
- Mood (irritability, worrying, hopefulness, enjoyment of life)
- Locus of control (feeling in control of life, helplessness, ability to make decision)
- Social/relationship (relationships with family/partner, ability to maintain friendships, inferiority, feeling wanted, enjoyment of leisure).

APPENDIX 2

SUBJECTIVE ASSESSMENT QUESTIONNAIRE (SAQ)

This is a simple questionnaire devised in the Unit asking patients to rate the effects of HT on symptoms, consultation rates and use of medication etc, using Likert-type responses, as shown below.

IBS symptoms

(i) Compared with how you felt before HT, how would you rate your symptoms were at the end of the course of HT?

- very much better, moderately better, slightly better, about the same, slightly worse, moderately worse, very much worse

(ii) Compared with how your symptoms were at the end of the course of HT, would you say that since completing treatment your symptoms have:

- continued to: improve much more, moderately more, a little more; remained about same as at end of HT;
- gone: slightly worse, moderately worse, much worse.

Consultation rates

Since HT, have you had to consult:

(a) your GP (b) a hospital consultant about IBS symptoms:

- more often, about the same, less often (than before)

(c) your GP about other symptoms:

- more often, about the same, less often (than before).

Use of medication

(a) Do you currently take medication for IBS symptoms? Yes, No (If yes, please specify)

(b) Do you take medication:

- more often, about the same, less often (than before)

(Information on any medication taken before starting the course of HT was recorded at the time.)

4. Continued practice

Do you still practise HT techniques? Yes, No If so, do you practise:

(a) using tape, on own

(b) daily, several times/week, several times/month, rarely

5. Did you consider the course of HT to be worthwhile? Yes, No

6. (a) Have you tried any other treatment/therapy since HT to relieve IBS symptoms? Yes, No

(b) If so, what?

(c) Did you find this to be helpful? Yes, No

ACKNOWLEDGEMENTS

We wish to thank the other staff of the Hypnotherapy Unit who treated some of the patients used in this study: Mrs P Cooper, Mrs P Cruickshanks, Mrs J Randles, and Mrs V Whelan. We also thank Mrs Julie Morris, Head of Medical Statistics, University Hospital of South Manchester, for help with statistical analysis.

....

Authors' affiliations

W M Gonsalkorale, V Miller, A Afzal, P J Whorwell, Department of Medicine, University Hospital of South Manchester, Manchester, UK

REFERENCES

1 **Whorwell PJ**, McCallum M, Creed FH, *et al* Non-colonic features of irritable bowel syndrome. *Gut* 1986;**27**:37–40.

2 **Switz DM**. What the gastroenterologist does all day. A survey of a state society's practice. *Gastroenterology* 1976;**70**:1048–50.

3 **Harvey RF**, Salih SY, Read AE. Organic and functional disorders in 2000 gastroenterology outpatients. *Lancet* 1983;i:632–4.

4 **Drossman DA**, Li Z, Andruzzi E, *et al.* U.S. householder survey of functional gastrointestinal disorders: prevalence, sociodemography and health impact. *Dig Dis Sci* 1993;**38**:1569–80.

5 **Maxton DG**, Whorwell PJ. Use of medical resources and attitudes to health care of patients with 'chronic abdominal pain'. *Br J Med Econ* 1992;**2**:75–9.

6 **Talley NJ**, Gabriel SE, Harmsen WS, *et al.* Medical costs in community subjects with irritable bowel syndrome. *Gastroenterology* 1995;**109**:1736–41.

7 **Whorwell PJ**, Prior A, Faragher EB. Controlled trial of hypnotherapy in the treatment of severe refractory irritable bowel syndrome. *Lancet* 1984;**ii**:1232–4.

8 **Whorwell PJ**, Prior A, Colgan SM. Hypnotherapy in severe irritable bowel syndrome: further experience. *Gut* 1987;**28**:423–5.

9 **Houghton LA**, Heyman DJ, Whorwell PJ. Symptomatology, quality of life and economic features of irritable bowel syndrome—the effect of hypnotherapy. *Aliment Pharmacol Ther* 1996;**10**:91–5.

10 **Harvey R**, Hinton RA, Gunary RM, *et al.* Individual and group hypnotherapy in the treatment of refractory irritable bowel syndrome. *Lancet* 1989;i:424–5.

11 **Galovski TE**, Blanchard EB. The treatment of irritable bowel syndrome with hypnotherapy. *Appl Psychophysiol Biofeedback* 1998;**23**:219–32.

12 **Palsson OS**, Turner MJ, Johnson DA, *et al.* Hypnosis treatment for severe irritable bowel syndrome—investigation of mechanisms and effects on symptoms. *Dig Dis Sci* 2002;**47**.2605–14.

13 **Gonsalkorale WM**, Houghton LA, Whorwell PJ. Hypnotherapy in irritable bowel syndrome: a large-scale audit of a clinical service with examination of factors influencing responsiveness. *Am J Gastroenterol* 2002;**97**:954–61.

14 **Francis CY**, Morris J, Whorwell PJ. The irritable bowel severity scoring system: a simple method of monitoring irritable bowel syndrome and its progress. *Aliment Pharmacol Ther* 1997;**11**:395–402.

15 **Zigmond AS**, Snaith RP. The Hospital Anxiety and Depression scale. *Acta Psychiatr Scand* 1983;**67**:361–70.

16 **Veldhuzen van Zanten S**, Talley N, Bytzer P, *et al.* Design of treatment trials for functional bowel disorders. *Gut* 1999;**45**:1169–77.

17 **Spiller RC**. Problems and challenges in the design of irritable bowel syndrome clinical trials: experience from published trials. *Am J Med* 1999;**107**:91–7S.

[28]

Hypnosis and Clinical Pain

David R. Patterson and Mark P. Jensen
University of Washington School of Medicine

Hypnosis has been demonstrated to reduce analogue pain, and studies on the mechanisms of laboratory pain reduction have provided useful applications to clinical populations. Studies showing central nervous system activity during hypnotic procedures offer preliminary information concerning possible physiological mechanisms of hypnotic analgesia. Randomized controlled studies with clinical populations indicate that hypnosis has a reliable and significant impact on acute procedural pain and chronic pain conditions. Methodological issues of this body of research are discussed, as are methods to better integrate hypnosis into comprehensive pain treatment.

After varying in popularity for the past century, interest in hypnosis has more recently been on the upswing. Evidence for a greater recent interest in hypnosis in psychology and health care is demonstrated in two trends in the literature. First, there has been an increased focus on hypnosis as interest in alternative, cost-saving therapies has grown. Although the notion that hypnosis is an alternative therapy can be disputed (Crasilneck, Stirman, & Wilson, 1955), recent evidence suggests that it can have an effective and cost-saving role in medicine. For example, Lang et al. (2000) demonstrated substantial cost savings in the operating room with hypnotic procedures. A second source of evidence for a resurgence of interest in hypnosis is the increasing presence of brain and neuroimaging studies of hypnosis. Studies of this nature have increased both in number and sophistication, as evidenced by Rainville, Duncan, Price, Carrier, and Bushnell's (1997) report on brain activity in response to hypnotic analgesia in *Science*.

Clinical pain is a problem that causes substantial suffering (Melzack, 1990) as well as billions of dollars in costs to society in areas such as health care and unemployment (Turk & Okifuji, 1998). Numerous studies have demonstrated the efficacy of hypnotic analgesia for reducing pain in the laboratory setting (E. R. Hilgard & Hilgard, 1975), and many case reports (e.g. J. Barber, 1977; B. Finer & Graf, 1968) have indicated significant reductions in clinical pain. However, relatively few randomized clinical studies on hypnotic analgesia have been published, and the extant reviews of this literature, although making important contributions to the understanding of hypnotic analgesia, are limited. For example, J. Holroyd (1996) published a review on the use of clinical hypnosis for pain that included theoretical discussion of modulation, management, and hypnotizability, but her work included only a small sample of the randomized controlled studies available.

Chaves's writings have questioned the uncritical acceptance of some of the more dramatic claims that have been made about hypnosis over the past 2 centuries (Chaves, 1994; Chaves & Dworkin, 1997). He has also championed a cognitive–behavioral theoretical explanation for hypnotic analgesia and challenged many assumptions that are common to the field (Chaves, 1993). Although the writings of J. Holroyd (1996), Chaves, and others have raised many important hypotheses concerning hypnotic analgesia, none has included a systematic review of controlled trials of this treatment. In a recent meta-analysis, Montgomery, DuHamel, and Redd (2000) calculated 41 effect sizes from 18 published studies including hypnosis for pain control in both the laboratory and clinical settings. Eight of the 18 studies reviewed by Montgomery and his colleagues included patient populations—the majority of effect sizes came from studies of experimentally induced pain. Their findings indicate that hypnosis provided substantial pain relief for 75% of the populations studied. Montgomery et al. also concluded that the majority of the population (excluding those scoring in the low hypnotic suggestibility range) should obtain at least some benefit from hypnotic analgesia.

In conducting the present review, we sought to build on this previous body of research in a number of ways. Montgomery et al.'s (2000) meta-analysis looked at the hypnotic analgesia studies in aggregate and demonstrated that hypnosis reduces pain in most people under both clinical and experimental settings. Our review focuses primarily on the randomized, controlled clinical studies.

For the purposes of this review, we used Kihlstrom's (1985) definition of hypnosis as "a social interaction in which one person, designated the subject, responds to suggestions offered by another person, designated the hypnotist, for experiences involving alterations in perception, memory, and voluntary action" (p. 385). This definition is sufficiently broad to incorporate those studies which purport to examine the effects of hypnotic analgesia as well as specific enough to include a primary component of hypnosis, that is, suggestion. We specifically avoided studies that examined interventions that were not defined as hypnosis by the investigators even though they might have included suggestions (e.g., relaxation

David R. Patterson and Mark P. Jensen, Department of Rehabilitation Medicine, University of Washington School of Medicine.

This work was supported by National Institutes of Health Grants R01 GM42725-09A1 and R01 HD42838 and by the National Institutes of Health, National Institute of Child Health and Human Development, National Institute of Neurological Disorders and Stroke Grant P01 HD/NS33988. We gratefully acknowledge the substantial contributions of Sally Boeve, Carina Morningstar, Alison Schultz, Jennifer Tininenko, and Anne Schmidt in preparing this article, as well as the presubmission review of Pierre Rainville. Authorship order for this publication was determined by coin toss

Correspondence concerning this article should be addressed to David R. Patterson, Department of Rehabilitation Medicine, University of Washington School of Medicine, Box 359740, 325 Ninth Avenue, Seattle, Washington 98104. E-mail: davepatt@u.washington.edu

and biofeedback training often includes verbal suggestions for relaxation; "autogenic" training often includes verbal suggestions for comfort and pain-competitive experiences and sensations; imagery or distraction interventions often include suggestions for becoming absorbed in either external stimuli or internally generated images and sensations) unless these interventions were a control condition for a hypnotic intervention or were included as part of the hypnotic intervention and labeled as such by the investigator. The analysis of relaxation training, autogenic training, or imagery studies is beyond the scope of this review, particularly because there is not yet consensus that these interventions fit into the realm of hypnosis. In this review, we also examine the studies along such parameters as the type of pain treated (e.g., acute vs. chronic), study design, and the nature of the control group. In critically examining the studies in this area, we hope to determine the utility of hypnosis in clinical settings as well as the circumstances in which it seems to be most effective.

The article begins with a brief summary of the research on the effects of hypnosis on induced pain in the laboratory setting and theoretical explanations for hypnotic analgesia. The bulk of the review focuses on the controlled trials of hypnotic analgesia for clinical pain problems, including both acute (mostly procedural) pain and chronic pain. We end with a discussion of how hypnosis and hypnotic analgesia may be more effectively applied to chronic pain problems.

Laboratory Studies of Hypnotic Analgesia

Although there are important differences between pain induced in the laboratory in otherwise healthy volunteers and that associated with clinical conditions, analogue studies can provide an important theoretical foundation for understanding hypnotic analgesia. It is useful to discuss the findings of such analogue studies in terms of the general hypnotic theory that drove the investigator's work. For example, E. R. Hilgard and Hilgard (1975) described a number of studies that showed an association between standard measures of hypnotizability and response to hypnotic analgesia (e.g., Greene & Reyher, 1972). From this perspective, E. R. Hilgard and Hilgard's seminal work can be viewed in terms of the trait theory of hypnotizability that they were espousing at that time (M. B. Evans & Paul, 1970; Greene & Reyher, 1972). Specifically, through their work and that of subsequent investigators, hypnotic suggestibility[1] has been demonstrated to be a measurable construct that is highly stable in subjects even over a period of many years (i.e., .80–.90 test–retest correlations after 10 years; E. R. Hilgard & Hilgard, 1975). This body of research supports the view that there is great individual variability in responsiveness to hypnotic suggestions.

The trait theory of hypnosis has spawned numerous laboratory studies demonstrating an association between analgesia and hypnotic suggestibility. E. R. Hilgard and others have demonstrated that reduction in cold pressor pain (R. Freeman, Barabasz, Barabasz, & Warner, 2000; E. R. Hilgard, 1969; Miller, Barabasz, & Barabasz, 1991) and ischemic muscle pain perception (E. R. Hilgard & Morgan, 1975; Knox, Morgan, & Hilgard, 1974) are both related to suggestibility as measured by standardized scales. McGlashan, Evans, and Orne (1969) also demonstrated an interaction between suggestibility and pain control, whereas those high in suggestibility show analgesia in response to hypnosis but not to placebo, and those low in suggestibility show the same (minimal) response to hypnosis as they do to a placebo. This study was consistent with E. R. Hilgard and Hilgard's (1975) assertion that hypnotic analgesia is not solely a function of placebo analgesia and that different mechanisms underlie responses to placebos and hypnosis (see also Stern, Brown, Ulett, & Sletten, 1977). M. B. Evans and Paul (1970) reported that suggestibility was such an important variable that waking suggestions for laboratory pain relief given without a hypnotic induction were as successful as those given within the context of an induction for subjects with high suggestibility scores. As mentioned above, Montgomery et al. (2000) recently reported a meta-analysis of the effects of hypnosis on pain. Consistent with the earlier findings of E. R. Hilgard and colleagues, they found that the effect size of hypnotic analgesia in the laboratory was associated with suggestibility across studies; subjects who scored high on measures of suggestibility during experimental pain paradigms (e.g., cold pressor tasks, painful heat stimuli) across a wide variety of settings tended to demonstrate larger responses to analgesia suggestions than subjects who scored low.

A second line of laboratory pain studies were conducted within the realm of social–cognitive views of hypnosis (T. X. Barber, Spanos, & Chaves, 1974; Chaves, 1989; Chaves & Barber, 1976; Spanos & Chaves, 1989a, 1989b, 1989c). Social–cognitive models include theories of hypnosis that suggest that the operative variables in hypnosis include contextual cues in the social environment, patient and subject expectancies, demand characteristics of the setting or situation, and role enactment (Kirsch & Lynn, 1995). Consistent with this view, experimental hypnotic analgesia has been found to be associated with contextual variables (Spanos, Kennedy, & Gwynn, 1984), instructional set (Spanos & Katsanis, 1989), and compliance (Spanos, Perlini, Patrick, Bell, & Gwynn, 1990). According to such social–cognitive models, neither hypnotic induction nor the existence of an altered state of consciousness are necessary for hypnotic responding, including responses to suggestions for pain relief (Chaves, 1993). Hypnotic analgesia is thought to reduce pain instead through cognitive–behavioral mechanisms, in which changes in cognitions are thought to alter the affective states associated with pain (Chaves, 1993). This conceptualization is consistent with the plethora of evidence that cognitive–behavioral interventions reduce both acute (Tan, 1982) and chronic clinical pain (Bradley, 1996; Holzman, Turk, & Kerns, 1986).

Theoretical approaches that maintain that hypnosis represents a unique or special cognitive process distinct from normal day-to-day cognitive processes have generated a different series of laboratory pain studies. Two such approaches are the neodissociative (E. R. Hilgard & Hilgard, 1975) and, more recently, "dissociated control" views (Bowers & LeBaron, 1986; E. R. Hilgard & Hilgard, 1975). The neodissociative model, originally proposed by E. R. Hilgard and Hilgard (1975), regards hypnosis as a state in which one or more forms of consciousness is split off from the rest

[1] Recent work by Braffman and Kirsch (1999) indicates that the term *hypnotic suggestibility* more accurately describes the concept of hypnotizability and is henceforth used in this review. Because we limit our discussion primarily to the field of hypnosis, the terms *hypnotic suggestibility* and *suggestibility* are used interchangeably.

of mental processing. Although the neodissociative model is a general one used to describe multiple hypnotic phenomena, it was the work of E. R. Hilgard and Hilgard on pain control that largely fueled this theoretical approach. Earlier studies consistent with the neodissociation theory suggested that voluntary responses to induced pain, such as verbal reports of intensity, showed reduction with hypnosis, whereas involuntary indicators (e.g., heart rate) did not always change (T. X. Barber & Hahn, 1962; E. R. Hilgard, 1967, 1969; Shor, 1962; Sutcliffe, 1961). Such findings were also central to E. R. Hilgard and Morgan's (1975) hidden observer concept—that a part of consciousness can be split off from executive cognitive control and can respond to hypnotic suggestion.

The more recent dissociated control theory stresses the perceived automaticity of response under hypnosis. Bowers's (1992) dissociated control theory differs somewhat from neodissociation theory in that the former views dissociation as a process of keeping cognitive processes out of consciousness through amnesia or other means. Bowers and his colleagues maintained that subsystems of control in the brain can be activated directly rather than through higher level executive control. For example, Hargadon, Bowers, and Woody (1995) reported that consciously evoked pain strategies were not necessary for subjects to experience a reduction in laboratory induced pain. Similarly, Eastwood, Gaskovski, and Bowers (1998) reported that analgesia in the laboratory involved cognitive mechanisms that were effortlessly engaged. In other words, the strategies subjects used to reduce pain were evoked automatically without any type of conscious, thought-out strategy (Bowers, 1990, 1992). A number of investigators (Barabasz, 1982; Barabasz & Barabasz, 1989; R. Freeman et al., 2000; Miller et al., 1991; J. T. Smith, Barabasz, & Barabasz, 1996) have reported laboratory pain findings consistent with the theories of E. R. Hilgard and Hilgard (1975) or Bowers (1992).

More recent theorists have suggested that attempting to explain the effects of hypnosis solely in terms of one school of thought presents distinctions that are too arbitrary (Kihlstrom, 1992) and that, at the same time, seeming disparate theoretical orientations about hypnosis have a surprising degree of commonality in many cases (Kirsch & Lynn, 1995). However, the findings from these studies that were originally designed to test different theories of hypnosis raise important hypotheses concerning the conditions under which pain control might be optimized in the clinical situation. For example, studies supporting a trait model of hypnotic suggestibility indicate that highly suggestible patients would be more likely to respond to suggestions for analgesia. As we discuss later, there are several studies that support an association between suggestibility and clinical hypnotic analgesia (Harmon, Hynan, & Tyre, 1990; J. T. Smith et al., 1996; ter Kuile, Spinhoven, Linssen, Zitman, Van Dyck, & Rooijmans, 1994). The findings from studies testing social–cognitive models suggest that, because the patient's expectations for pain relief is a critical variable, treatment effects can be maximized by capitalizing on this element of the social interaction. Such theoretical work also suggests that identifying the patient's cognitive style and his or her thoughts about pain and then targeting hypnotic suggestions to alter these cognitions should facilitate hypnotic analgesia (Chaves, 1993). Supporting the potential benefit of suggestions that target cognitions in hypnotic analgesia are studies in which subjects have been shown to engage in self-generated cognitive strategies to reduce pain even in the absence of specific suggestions for this (Chaves & Barber, 1974; Chaves & Brown, 1987). Furthermore, Chaves (1989) has pointed out that "catastrophizing" subjects tend to amplify the negative effects of pain. Whereas social–cognitive models might indicate that patients obtain pain relief by concentrating on their thoughts and restructuring them, dissociated control models are more useful in explaining those instances in which hypnotic pain relief seems to come effortlessly to patients. Subjects or patients that appear to respond easily to the hypnotist's suggestions, often perhaps with amnesia for the experience, would be showing the types of behaviors consistent with this model (Patterson, 2001).

Physiological Correlates of Laboratory Pain Reduction

Hypnosis researchers have long sought specific physiological indicators of the hypnotic state. Much of the early research in this area was fueled by investigators seeking to confirm that the identification of a specific physiological indicator of hypnosis would lend support to the view that hypnosis is a state of consciousness distinct from other states, such as waking or sleep (Dixon & Laurence, 1992). Although some findings from this research have been helpful to determine what hypnosis is not (e.g., cortical activity during hypnosis is unlike cortical activity during sleep; Dynes, 1947), no physiological indicator has been identified that consistently shows characteristics unique to hypnosis. However, some of this research has identified interesting and consistent physiological correlates of hypnotic analgesia. The physiological responses to hypnotic analgesia that have been studied include sympathetic responses (heart rate and blood pressure), electrocortical activity (including the assessment of brain wave patterns at various sites and cortical evoked potentials), possible hypnotic analgesia-related release of endorphins, and regional brain blood flow.

Sympathetic Responding

Some of the first physiological responses to be studied in hypnosis research were sympathetic in nature such as heart rate and galvanic skin responses. However, although decreases in heart rate and blood pressure are sometimes found with hypnosis (De Pascalis & Perrone, 1996; E. R. Hilgard & Morgan, 1975; Lenox, 1970), more often involuntary sympathetic responses to pain are not altered by hypnotic analgesia (T. X. Barber & Hahn, 1962; E. R. Hilgard, 1967, 1969; Shor, 1962; Sutcliffe, 1961; but see Rainville, Carrier, Hofbauer, Bushnell, & Duncan, 1999, for evidence suggesting a possible link between heart rate and *pain unpleasantness,* or the affective component of pain). Because physiological responses to painful stimuli may be less influenced by subject bias than self-report, some might conclude from the lack of consistent effect on heart rate and blood pressure that hypnosis does not affect actual experienced pain but only a person's willingness to report that pain. However, as E. R. Hilgard and Hilgard (1975) made clear, the effects of hypnosis on heart rate and blood pressure only speak to the effects of hypnosis on a subset of physiological responses to pain; they say nothing about the effects of hypnosis on pain experience.

Endogenous Opioid and Acupuncture Studies

Given the ability of humans to modulate pain experience through endogenous opioids (Melzack & Wall, 1973), it would be reasonable to test whether hypnotic analgesia might operate by influencing endogenous opioid levels. This hypothesis has been tested in at least two studies in which the opioid antagonist naloxone was introduced after hypnotic analgesia was initiated (J. Barber & Mayer, 1977; Goldstein & Hilgard, 1975). In both studies, naloxone failed to reverse the effects of hypnotic analgesia. These findings suggest that endogenous opioids may not be responsible for hypnotic analgesia. However, with only two studies, it may be premature to rule out a role for endogenous opioids in hypnotic analgesia. Research has also shown that response to hypnosis does not correlate with response to acupuncture (Knox, Gekoski, Shum, & McLaughlin, 1981; Knox, Handfield-Jones, & Shum, 1979; Knox & Shum, 1977), suggesting that the underlying mechanisms for these two forms of analgesia may be different.

Evoked Potential Studies

The findings from electrocortical studies have shown some specific physiological correlates of hypnotic analgesia. For example, the late evoked potential (roughly 300–400 ms after the stimulation), measured at the scalp, has been shown to be associated with the level of reported pain intensity and, like perceived pain intensity, is influenced by cognitive factors such as attention and degree to which the stimuli are expected (Chen, Chapman, & Harkins, 1979; Stowell, 1984). A number of studies have shown reductions in late somatosensory potentials evoked by nociceptive stimuli after hypnosis (Arendt-Nielsen, Zachariae, & Bjerring, 1990; Barabasz & Lonsdale, 1983; Crawford et al., 1998; Danziger et al., 1998; De Pascalis, Magurano, & Bellusci, 1999; Halliday & Mason, 1964; Meier, Klucken, Soyka, & Bromm, 1993; Meszaros, Banyai, & Greguss, 1980; D. Spiegel, Bierre, & Rootenberg, 1989; Zachariae & Bjerring, 1994). Thus, these studies support an effect of hypnotic analgesia on a physiological response that is both (a) linked to perceived pain intensity and (b) not under conscious control. Unfortunately, however, these studies do not identify the specific physiological substrates involved in hypnotic analgesia. Also, these studies on evoked potentials, indeed many studies on hypnotic analgesia, do not disentangle the influence of suggestion from the hypnotic context—it is possible that these same effects on evoked potential could be obtained with analgesia suggestions alone (e.g., not only when suggestions are made after an induction or in a situation when the suggestions are not labeled as hypnosis).

Electroencephalogram (EEG) Studies

Surface EEG recordings made during hypnotic analgesia have also yielded some interesting findings. Crawford (1990) assessed EEG correlates of cold pressor pain under conditions of waking and hypnosis in persons with high versus low hypnotic suggestibility scores. She found significantly greater theta activity (5.5–7.5 Hz) among those subjects with high suggestibility scores than among those with low scores during the hypnotic analgesia condition, especially in the anterior temporal region. Although those with low scores showed little hemispheric differences during the experimental conditions, the highly suggestible subjects showed greater left hemisphere dominance during the pain condition and a reversal in hemispheric dominance during hypnotic analgesia (see also De Pascalis & Perrone, 1996). Crawford (1994) has maintained that persons who are highly suggestible demonstrate greater cognitive flexibility and abilities to shift from left to right anterior functioning than do those who are less suggestible. She concluded that hypnosis may operate via attention filtering and that the fronto-limbic system is central to this process. However, the fact that suggestions for focused analgesia are as effective (or more effective) than dissociative imagery to reduce pain (De Pascalis, Magurano, Bellusci, & Chen, 2001) poses a problem for the interpretation that hypnotic analgesia operates solely via attention mechanisms and suggests that the specific mechanisms involved may depend on the specific type of suggestion given.

Brain Imaging Studies

Although EEG studies of evoked potentials and brain wave patterns do not provide information about the specific neuroanatomical sites at which the modulation of pain experience occurs (Price & Barrell, 2000), studies using positron emission tomography (PET) can provide a more precise analysis of these physiological substrates. Rainville et al. (1997) used PET scans to study brain activity of subjects exposed to hot water pain before, during, and after hypnotically induced analgesia for the unpleasantness, but not the intensity, of a noxious stimulus. Their results indicated that hypnosis-related changes in the affective dimension of pain were associated with changes in cortical limbic regional activity (anterior cingulate cortical area 24) but not with changes in the primary somatosensory cortex. In a second study using PET methodology, Hofbauer, Rainville, Duncan, and Bushnell (2001) demonstrated that suggestions for sensory analgesia resulted, at least in part, in a reduction in activity in the somatosensory cortex. In review, Price and Barrell (2000) concluded that hypnotic analgesia can produce both an inhibition of afferent nociceptive signals arriving at the somatosensory cortex and a modulation of pain affect by producing changes in the limbic system (e.g., anterior cingulate cortex; see also Kroptov, 1997).

Possible Inhibition at the Spinal Cord Level

There is evidence that hypnotic analgesia may also operate, at least to some degree, through inhibition at the level of the spinal cord. Support for this mechanism comes from a variety of research studies that demonstrate hypnotically induced reductions in skin reflex on the arm (Hernandez-Peon, Dittborn, Borlone, & Davidovich, 1960), nerve response in the jaw (Sharav & Tal, 1989), and muscle response in the ankle (J. Holroyd, 1996; Kiernan, Dane, Phillips, & Price, 1995). The study by Kiernan and colleagues (1995) has received particular attention because it demonstrates that suggestions for analgesia were correlated with the spinal nociceptive (R-III) reflex, a response that has little to do with higher order central nervous system processing. More recently, Danziger and colleagues (1998) found two distinct patterns of R-III reflex associated with hypnotic analgesia. Using a methodology similar to that of Kiernan et al., these investigators found that 11 subjects showed strong inhibition, and 7 showed strong facilitation of the R-III reflex with hypnosis. Although the reasons for such differences in response are not easily explained, they do indicate that highly suggestible individuals show a marked change in R-III reflex when given hypnotic analgesia suggestions. As pointed out by J. Holroyd (1996), hypnotic effects on nervous system inhibition at the level of the spinal cord have also been demonstrated by alterations in galvanic skin response (Gruzelier, Allison, & Conway, 1988; West, Niell, & Hardy, 1952). Unfortunately, however, these are limited by the absence of control groups with nonhypnotized patients, as are many studies on the physiological effects of hypnosis. This limits the inferences that can be drawn about the effects of hypnosis (vs. suggestions made outside of a hypnotic context) on physiological responses to hypnotic analgesia.

Sensory Versus Affective Pain Effects

Several recent studies have focused on whether hypnotic analgesia has a greater effect on sensory or affective components of pain. It is understandable that there has been speculation that affective components of pain, which are thought to have a greater cognitive–evaluative component, might be more responsive to hypnosis than sensory components, which are presumably more closely associated with nociceptive input. In one of the earlier studies that examined this question, Price, Harkins, and Baker (1987) reported that affective components of pain showed a greater reduction with hypnosis than did sensory ones. However, another study by Price and Barber (1987), showed that both components could show a reduction, and that the amount of change depended on the nature of suggestion. Further support for the hypothesis that the effects of hypnotic analgesia on pain sensation versus pain affect depend on the specific suggestions given comes from Rainville et al.'s (1999) brain imaging work, which shows that brain activity also varies as a function of the nature of analgesic suggestion. In short, the recent evidence does not support the hypothesis that hypnotic analgesia necessarily impacts affective pain to a greater extent than sensory pain. However, this research has demonstrated the importance of the wording of the analgesic suggestions and that subjects can respond to suggestions that are targeted toward distinct elements of pain.

In summary, the research on neurophysiological correlates of hypnotic analgesia suggests that highly suggestible subjects show different patterns of cortical responding than do those who score low on measures of suggestibility. Research also shows that individuals engaged in successful hypnotic analgesia invoke physiological inhibitory processes in the brain. Suggestions for sensory reductions in pain show corresponding changes in activity in the somatosensory cortex, whereas suggestions for affective pain reduction are reflected in the part of the brain that corresponds to processing emotional information. Another line of research suggests that successful inhibition of pain through hypnosis may also occur, at least in part, through descending (spinal) inhibitory mechanisms. However, the lack of nonhypnotic control conditions in much of this research prohibits conclusions regarding the impact of hypnosis versus nonhypnotic suggestions on physiological responding. Perhaps what can best be concluded from this body of research is that neurophysiological changes are associated with hypnotic analgesia in receptive subjects and that multiple physiological mechanisms appear to play a role in the pain reduction associated with hypnotic suggestions for pain relief.

Anecdotal and Clinical Reports

There are many anecdotal reports and case studies that support the use of hypnosis for a wide variety of clinical pain conditions. Perhaps the most time honored of these are those of Esdaile (1957), a Scottish physician, who reported on 345 major operations performed in India in the nineteenth century with hypnosis (termed *mesmerism* at that time) as the sole anesthetic. Similarly, E. R. Hilgard and Hilgard (1975) listed at least 14 different types of surgeries (cited by multiple investigators) for which hypnosis was used as the sole anesthetic, including appendectomies, gastrostomies, tumor excisions, and vaginal hysterectomies. Rausch (1980) reported undergoing a cholecystectomy using self-hypnosis and being able to walk consciously back to his room immediately after the procedure. Burn injuries are another source of severe pain for which there are multiple reports of good patient response to hypnosis (Patterson, Questad, & Boltwood, 1987; Gilboa, Borenstein, Seidman, & Tsur, 1990), and B. L. Finer and Nylen (1961) reported bringing a patient through several extensive burn surgeries with hypnosis as the sole anesthetic. Other case studies have described a wide variety of problems that have responded to hypnosis, including pain associated with dental work (J. Barber, 1977; J. Barber & Mayer, 1977; Hartland, 1971), cancer (J. R. Hilgard & LeBaron, 1984), reflex sympathetic dystrophy (Gainer, 1992), acquired amputation (Chaves, 1986; Siegel, 1979), childbirth (Haanen et al., 1991), spinal cord injury (M. Jensen & Barber, 2000), sickle cell anemia (Dinges et al., 1997), arthritis (Appel, 1992; Crasilneck, 1995), temporomandibular joint disorder (Crasilneck, 1995; Simon & Lewis, 2000), multiple sclerosis (Dane, 1996; Sutcher, 1997), causalgia (B. Finer & Graf, 1968), lupus erythematosus (S. J. Smith & Balaban, 1983), postsurgical pain (Mauer, Burnett, Ouellette, Ironson, & Dandes, 1999), and unanesthetized fracture reduction (Iserson, 1999). Other types of pain problems reported to respond to hypnotic analgesia include low back pain (Crasilneck, 1979, 1995), headaches (Crasilneck, 1995; Spinhoven, 1988), and mixed chronic pain (F. J. Evans, 1989; Jack, 1999; Sacerdote, 1978). Even this long list of pain etiologies is by no means exhaustive. In short, hypnosis has been reported to be useful for virtually every clinical pain problem imaginable.

However, the many limitations of case reports are well known, including potential subjective bias from the clinician and patient, potential spontaneous remission, placebo effects, and selective reporting of only the most successful cases (Campbell & Stanley, 1963). All of these drawbacks severely limit any conclusions that may be drawn from the anecdotal reports and case studies of hypnotic analgesia. Even the frequently cited findings of Esdaile (1957) and the hypnotic analgesia–surgery literature have been called into question (T. X. Barber et al., 1974; Chaves, 1993; Dingwall, 1967; Spanos, 1986). Furthermore, Chaves and Dworkin (1997) have argued that patients can also demonstrate extraordinary pain control without hypnosis and that contentions that such patients show no pain under hypnosis are often false.

A number of other additional methodological problems are specific to published hypnosis case reports, including the failure to include validated measures of pain, hypnotic suggestibility, and levels of pain medication used by the patients. Another shortcoming is that consecutive patients often are not subjected to hypnotic treatment; patients often appear to be selectively treated and reported on without a description of the decision rules used to select the cases. Because of these limitations, the best and only conclusion we can make from these clinical case studies is that there appear to be some individuals with clinical pain problems who may benefit from hypnotic analgesia. Unfortunately, however, the available case study evidence does not allow us to determine whether this group of responders represents an exception or the norm.

Controlled Clinical Studies

Acute Pain

As mentioned above, randomized controlled studies have largely been absent from the clinical hypnosis literature, although a welcome increase has occurred over the past 2 decades. A difficulty in this literature is that the nature of the pain problems treated are rarely discussed in detail. Of particular concern, the important distinction between acute and chronic pain is seldom mentioned. When the research is considered with this distinction in mind, it becomes clear that the two types of pain represent dramatically different treatment issues.

Acute pain may be defined as that which occurs in response to tissue damage (Melzack & Wall, 1973; Williams, 1999). In most of the reports in this area, hypnosis is applied to acute pain associated with a medical procedure. Table 1 summarizes the findings, and Table 2 describes the hypnotic interventions that were used in the 19 controlled studies that have been published on the effects of hypnosis on acute pain, organized by the type of pain. We have indicated in Table 1 whether the study included an adult or child sample, whether a measure of hypnotic suggestibility was included, the nature of the control group (or comparison groups), whether the subjects were randomly assigned to treatment condition, the outcome dimensions assessed, and the findings concerning any differences found between the hypnosis and control conditions.

Through MEDLINE and PsycINFO searches using the key words *hypnotic analgesia*, *hypnosis*, and *pain*, and through a careful review of the citations of previous review articles and the articles themselves, we were able to identify the published studies listed in Tables 1 and 2 that examined the effects of hypnosis on acute pain, including pain from invasive medical procedures (included in this category is one study [Syrjala, Cummings, & Donaldson, 1992] that examined the effects of hypnosis for painful oral mucositis, which is one of the results of chemotherapy and total body irradiation done in preparation for marrow transplantation in some persons with cancer), burn care, and childbirth.

Invasive medical procedure pain. Weinstein and Au (1991) compared 16 patients who received presurgery hypnosis and then underwent angioplasty with 16 patients who received standard care. The hypnotic intervention was based on a modification of the induction reported by J. Barber (1977). Relative to the control group, patients in the hypnosis group showed a (statistically insignificant, $p = .10$) 25% increase in the time that they allowed the cardiologist to keep the balloon catheter inflated during the surgery and a statistically significant reduction in the opioid analgesics required during the procedure. The hypnosis group also showed a significant decrease in catecholamine blood levels relative to the control group. However, the experimental group did not demonstrate changes in other physiological variables measured including blood pressure or pulse.

Lambert (1996) randomly assigned 52 children (matched for age, sex, and diagnosis) to either an experimental group that received both hypnosis and guided imagery or a control group in which each child spent an equal amount of time discussing the surgery and topics related to the child's interests. The experimental treatment involved a single 30-min session 1 week before the surgery that included suggestions for relaxation based on an image selected by the child followed by suggestions for positive surgical outcomes and minimal pain. The therapist was not present during the surgery. The experimental group rated their pain as significantly lower than the control group did. However, although anxiety scores decreased in the experimental group and increased in the control group, mean postsurgery anxiety scores did not differ between groups. The experimental group also showed shorter hospital stays, but the groups did not differ on length of surgery, anesthesia, or time in postanesthesia care.

Faymonville et al. (1997) randomly assigned a group of patients undergoing elective plastic surgery while sedated to receive either hypnosis ($n = 31$) or a stress-reducing physiological technique ($n = 25$) by the treating anesthesiologist. According to the authors, "a hypnotic state was . . . induced using eye fixation, muscle relaxation, and permissive and indirect suggestions. The exact words and details of the induction technique . . . depended on the anesthesiologist's observation of patient behavior" (Faymonville et al., 1997, p. 362). However, the authors stated that the word *hypnosis* was never used to describe that treatment to the study participants. Patients in the control group received continuous stress reduction strategies including "deep breathing and relaxation . . ., positive emotional induction . . . and cognitive coping strategies (imaginative transformation of sensation or imaginative inattention)" (Faymonville et al., 1997, p. 362). Patients in the hypnosis group required significantly less analgesia (alfentanil) and sedation (midazolam), reported better perioperative pain and anxiety relief, higher levels of satisfaction, greater perceived control, lower blood pressure, heart rate, and respiratory rate, and lower postoperative nausea and vomiting. Surgeons of patients in the experimental condition also reported observing higher levels of satisfaction in patients than surgeons of patients in the control condition. Despite the positive effects of the hypnosis intervention reported, there are several aspects of this study that make the interpretation of the findings difficult. First, because the hypnosis intervention was never defined as such to the patients, this intervention differs from most others tested in which the intervention was presented as hypnosis. It is not entirely clear what effect, if any, labeling the intervention as hypnosis might have had on the outcome. In addition, the differences between the hypnosis and the stress-reducing intervention are not entirely clear in this study. Patients in both conditions appear to have been given suggestions (although the specific suggestions given to each group did differ). Finally, the findings are further complicated by the fact that the treating anesthesiologist provided all interventions and was aware of the study conditions.

Lang and her colleagues have reported two studies on hypnosis for invasive medical procedures. In the first (Lang, Joyce, Spiegel, Hamilton, & Lee, 1996), 16 patients were randomized to an experimental group that received "combined elements of relaxation training and guided imagery for induction of a self-hypnotic process" (p. 109). Relative to 14 patients in a standard treatment control, hypnosis patients used less pain medication, reported less maximal pain (but not average pain), and showed more physiologic stability during the procedures (primarily diagnostic arterio-

(*text continues on p. 505*)

Table 1
Description of Controlled Studies of Acute and Procedural Pain Hypnotic Treatment

Study and type of acute pain	Hypnotizability assessed?	*N*	Randomized?	Control conditions	Adult or child?	Outcome dimensions	Findings
Zeltzer & LeBaron (1982) Bone marrow aspiration pain	No	33	Yes	Deep breathing and distraction (DBD)	Child (6–17 years)	Patient-rated pain intensity	H > DBD
						Patient-rated anxiety	H > DBD
						Observer-rated pain intensity	H > DBD
						Observer-rated anxiety	H > DBD
Katz et al. (1987) Bone marrow aspiration pain	No	36	Yes	Nondirected play (NDP)	Child (6–11 years)	Observed distress; PBRS–R	H = NDP
						Nurse-rated anxiety	H = NDP
						Patient-rated fear	H = NDP
						Patient-rated pain	H = NDP
						Therapist-rated rapport	H = NDP
						Therapist-rated response to hypnosis	H = NDP
Kuttner (1988) Bone marrow aspiration pain	No	25	Yes	Standard care (SC), distraction (D)	Child (3–6 years)	Observed distress; PBRS–R	H > SC; H > D
						Observer-rated pain	H > SC; H > D
						Observer-rated anxiety	H > SC; H > D
						Patient-rated pain	H = SC = D
						Patient-rated anxiety	H = SC = D
Liossi & Hatira (1999) Bone marrow aspiration pain	Yes; Stanford Hypnotic Clinical Scale for Children	30	Yes	Cognitive–behavioral therapy (CBT), SC	Child (5–15 years)	Observed distress; PBCL	H > CBT > SC
						Patient-rated pain intensity	(H = CBT) > SC
						Patient-rated anxiety	H > CBT > SC
Wakeman & Kaplan (1978) Burn wound dressing change and debridement pain	No	42	No	Attention control (AC)	Both (7–70 years)	Percentage of allowable medication use during study participation	H > AC
Patterson et al. (1989) Burn wound dressing change and debridement pain	No	13	No	SC	Adult	Patient-rated pain intensity	H > SC
Patterson et al. (1992) Burn wound dressing change and debridement pain among burn patients	No	30	Yes	SC, AC	Adult	Morphine equivalents for administered pain medications	H = SC = AC
						Patient-reported pain	H > (SC = AC)
						Nurse-rated pain	H > (SC = AC)
Everett et al. (1993) Burn wound dressing change and debridement pain	No	32	Yes	AC, lorazepam (L)	Adult	Patient-rated pain intensity	(H + L) = (H) = (AC + L) = (L)
						Patient-rated anxiety	(H + L) = (H) = (AC + L) = (L)
						Nurse-rated patient pain intensity	(H + L) = (H) = (AC + L) = (L)
						Nurse-rated patient pain anxiety	(H + L) = (H) = (AC + L) = (L)
Patterson & Ptacek (1997) Burn wound dressing change and debridement pain	No	61	Yes	AC	Adult	Self-reported worst pain intensity	H = AC (among subjects with high pain, H > AC)
						Nurse-reported worst patient pain intensity	H > AC
						Patient-rated effectiveness of hypnosis	H = AC
						Opioid intake	H = AC

(table continues)

Table 1 (*continued*)

Study and type of acute pain	Hypnotizability assessed?	*N*	Randomized?	Control conditions	Adult or child?	Outcome dimensions	Findings
Wright & Drummond (2000) Burn wound dressing change and debridement pain	No	30	Yes	SC	Both (16–48 years)	Medication consumption	H > SC
						During-procedure pain intensity	H > SC
						During-procedure pain unpleasantness	H > SC
						Post-procedure pain intensity	H > SC
						Post-procedure pain unpleasantness	H > SC
						Pre- to postprocedure change in patient-rated relaxation	H > SC
Davidson (1962) Labor pain	No	210	No	SC, relaxation training (RT)	Adult	Duration of labor	H > (RT = SC)
						Patient-rated pain in the first stage	H > (RT = SC)
						Patient-rated pain in the second stage	H > (RT = SC)
						Analgesia intake	H > (RT = SC)
						Patient-rated pleasantness of labor	H > (RT = SC)
R. M. Freeman et al. (1986) Labor pain	Yes; Stanford Hypnotic Clinical Scale for Adults	65	Yes	SC	Adult	Duration of pregnancy	H longer than SC by 0.06 weeks
						Duration of labor	H longer than SC by 2.7 hr
						Analgesic intake	H = SC
						Mode of delivery	H = SC
						Pain relief	H = SC
						Satisfaction with labor	H > SC (p = .08)
Harmon et al. (1990) Labor pain	Yes; Harvard Group Scale of Hypnotic Susceptibility, Form A	60	Yes	Breathing and relaxation exercises (BR)	Adult	Length of Stage 1 labor	H > BR
						Length of Stage 2 labor	H = BR
						Newborn Apgar, 1 min	H > BR
						Newborn Apgar, 5 min	H > BR
						Spontaneous delivery (%)	H > BR
						Percent given medications	H > BR
						MMPI Depression Scale score	H = BR (among subjects with high pain, H > BR)
						Pain intensity; MPQ	H > BR
						Sensory pain; MPQ	H > BR
						Affective pain; MPQ	H > BR
						Evaluative pain; MPQ	H > BR
						Miscellaneous pain; MPQ	H > BR
Weinstein & Au (1991) Pain during angioplasty	No	32	Yes	SC	Adult	Pulse	H = SC
						Systolic blood pressure (BP)	H = SC
						Diastolic BP	H = SC
						Total time of balloon inflation during procedure	H = SC
						Requests for additional medicine	H > SC
						Catecholamine levels	H > SC
Syrjala et al. (1992) Pain following chemotherapy for cancer	No	45	Yes	CBT, AC, SC	Adult	Oral pain	H > (AC = CBT)
						Nausea	H = AC = CBT = SC
						Presence of emesis	H = AC = CBT
						Opioid intake	H = AC = CBT

Table 1 (*continued*)

Study and type of acute pain	Hypnotizability assessed?	*N*	Randomized?	Control conditions	Adult or child?	Outcome dimensions	Findings
Lang et al. (1996) Mixed invasive medical procedures—primarily diagnostic arteriograms	Yes; Hypnotic Induction Profile	30	Yes	SC	Adult	Self-administration of analgesics	H > SC
						BP increase	H = SC
						Heart rate increase	H = SC
						Oxygen desaturation during procedure	H > SC
						Procedural interruptions due to hemodynamic instability	H > SC
						Patient-rated pain intensity	H = SC
						Patient-rated maximal pain	H > SC
						Patient-rated anxiety; BAI	H = SC
Faymonville et al. (1997) Elective plastic surgery	No	56	Yes	Emotional support (ES)	Adult	Analgesic requirements	H > ES
						Perioperative patient-rated anxiety	H > ES
						Patient-rated pain intensity	H > ES
						Patient-rated level of control	H > ES
						Observed complaints during surgery	H > ES
						Diastolic BP	H > ES
						Maximum decrease in SpO2	H > ES
						Maximum increase in heart rate	H > ES
						Maximum increase in respiratory rate	H > ES
						Maximum increase in systolic BP	H > ES
						Maximum increase in cutaneous temperature	H = ES
						Patient-rated surgery satisfaction	H > ES
						Observer-rated surgical comfort	H > ES
						Postoperative nausea and vomiting	H > ES
						Surgeon's satisfaction	H > ES
Lambert (1996) Variety of surgical procedures	No	52	Yes	AC	Child (7–19 years)	Patient-rated pain	H > AC
						Patient-rated postoperative anxiety; STAIC	H = AC
						Length of surgery	H = AC
						Length of hospital stay	H > AC
						Length of anesthesia	H = AC
						Time in postanesthesia care unit	H = AC
						Medication consumption	H = AC
Lang et al. (2000) Variety of surgical procedures including arterial and venous surgery and nephrostomy	No	241	Yes	SC, AC	Adult	Patient-rated pain intensity	H > (AC = SC)
						Patient-rated anxiety	H > SC; H = AC; AC = SC
						Medication use	(H = AC) > SC
						Time needed for procedure	H > SC; H = AC; AC = SC
						Hemodynamic stability	H > (AC = SC)

Note. H = hypnosis alone; PBRS–R = Procedural Behavior Rating Scale—Revised; PBCL = Procedural Behavior Checklist; MMPI = Minnesota Multiphasic Personality Inventory; MPQ = McGill Pain Questionnaire; BAI = Beck Anxiety Inventory; SpO2 = Oxygen saturation; STAIC = State–Trait Anxiety Inventory for Children.

Table 2
Description of Hypnotic Treatment: Acute and Procedural Pain Studies

Study	Manualized?	Described as hypnosis to subjects?	Audiotaped?	Description of intervention
Zeltzer & LeBaron (1982)	No	Unclear	No	Suggestions to become increasingly involved in interesting and pleasant imagery. Therapist present during procedures.
Katz et al. (1987)	No	Unclear	No	Two sessions prior to the procedures plus 20-min sessions immediately before each of three procedures. Sessions began with eye fixation, which was followed by suggestions for relaxation, pain reduction, reframing pain, distraction, positive affect, and mastery. Posthypnotic suggestions for practicing and reentering hypnosis with a cue from the therapist during the procedure. Therapist was present during procedures, but interactions were limited to the provision of the cue (hand on shoulder) and brief encouraging statements.
Kuttner (1988)	No	Unclear	No	Suggestions to become involved with a favorite story that incorporated reinterpretations of the procedural noxious experience. Therapist present and provided intervention during procedure.
Liossi & Hatira (1999)	No	Unclear	No	Suggestions for relaxation, well-being, self-efficacy, and comfort followed by suggestions for numbness, topical anesthesia, local anesthesia, and glove anesthesia transferred to the low back were finished with posthypnotic suggestions that the hypnotic experience would be repeated during the procedure. Therapist was present during procedure, but interactions were limited to cue for subject to use the skills learned and to brief verbal encouragements.
Wakeman & Kaplan (1978)	No	Yes	No	Procedures varied. They typically included initial eye fixation and eye roll followed by suggestions for relaxation and other suggestions tailored for individual subjects such as analgesia, anesthesia, dissociation, and reduction of anxiety. Subjects were instructed to use self-hypnosis when therapist was not present. Therapist was present during procedures and other regularly scheduled times until "self-hypnosis was mastered" (p. 4)
Patterson et al. (1989)	No	Yes	No	J. Barber's (1977) rapid induction analgesia, which includes suggestions for relaxation, imagining 20 stairs for deepening, and posthypnotic suggestions for comfort, relaxation, analgesia, and anesthesia, was used during the procedures. Intervention was performed 10 min to 3 hr prior to wound debridement, and therapist was not present during procedure.
Patterson et al. (1992)	No	Yes	No	J. Barber's (1977) rapid induction analgesia was used during the procedures. Intervention was performed prior to wound debridement, and therapist was not present during procedure.
Everett et al. (1993)	No	Yes	No	J. Barber's (1977) rapid induction analgesia was used during the procedures. Intervention was performed prior to wound debridement, and therapist was not present during procedure.
Patterson & Ptacek (1997)	No	Yes	No	J. Barber's (1977) rapid induction analgesia was used during the procedures. Intervention was performed prior to wound debridement, and therapist was not present during procedure.
Wright & Drummond (2000)	No	Yes	No	J. Barber's (1977) rapid induction analgesia was used during the procedures. Intervention was performed immediately prior to wound debridement, and therapist was not present during procedure.
Davidson (1962)	No	Unclear	No	Six sessions of group training, which included eye fixation followed by suggestions for relaxation, normality of pregnancy and labor, diminished awareness of pain and need for analgesics, ability to produce anesthesia of the perineum at birth, and satisfaction and pleasure after childbirth. Therapist was sometimes present to provide intervention during labor.
R. M. Freeman et al. (1986)	No	Yes	No	Weekly group sessions prior to labor providing suggestions for relaxation, pain relief, and transfer of warmth from hand to abdomen. Subjects were also seen individually weekly from 32 weeks after gestation until birth. Therapist was not present during labor.
Harmon et al. (1990)	No	Yes	Yes	Suggestions for relaxation, heaviness, deep breathing, backward counting, enjoyment of childbirth delivery, and numbness. Sessions were taped, and subjects were asked to listen to tapes daily prior to delivery (average number of listenings = 23).
Weinstein & Au (1991)	No	Yes	No	Suggestions for relaxation followed by posthypnotic suggestions for relaxation during angioplasty the next morning. Suggestions were based on J. Barber's (1977) scripted induction. Clinician available to assist with relaxation during procedure if necessary.

Table 2 (*continued*)

Study	Manualized?	Described as hypnosis to subjects?	Audiotaped?	Description of intervention
Syrjala et al. (1992)	No	Yes	Yes	Two pre-inpatient training sessions that included suggestions for relaxation and imagery tailored to patient's preference (visual, auditory, kinesthetic) and suggestions for analgesia, nausea reduction, well-being, and self-control. Initial sessions were followed by 10 inpatient sessions provided following chemotherapy. All sessions were taped, and subjects were encouraged to listen to the tapes daily through the 20 days following chemotherapy.
Lang et al. (1996)	No	No	No	Relaxation followed by suggestions for imagery of self in nature and for pain competitive sensations. Therapist spent varying amounts of time with patients during procedures.
Faymonville et al. (1997)	No	No	No	Eye fixation followed by suggestions for relaxation and additional indirect suggestions to relive a pleasant life experience (no analgesic suggestions were given). Therapist present during surgery.
Lambert (1996)	No	Unclear	No	One 30-min session 1 week prior to surgery that included suggestions for relaxation using imagery to rehearse impending operation followed by suggestions for positive surgical outcomes and minimal pain. Therapist was not present during surgery.
Lang et al. (2000)	Yes	No	No	Suggestions for relaxation or (for the final 53 hypnosis patients) eye roll, eye closing, and deep breathing followed by suggestions of the sensation of floating followed by self-generated imagery of a safe and pleasant experience. Intervention performed during surgery.

grams). Differences in anxiety ratings were not statistically significant, nor were differences in blood pressure or heart rate increases during the procedures. In addition, treatment benefits did not correlate with suggestibility as measured by the Hypnotic Induction Profile (H. Spiegel & Spiegel, 1978). A limitation of the study is that the clinicians were aware of the patients' group assignments.

More recently, Lang et al. (2000) randomly assigned 241 patients undergoing cutaneous vascular and renal procedures to standard care (n = 79), structured attention (n = 80), or self-hypnotic relaxation (n = 82). Structured attention involved eight key components described in a treatment manual cited by the authors, and hypnosis involved these key components plus a hypnotic induction followed by suggestions for the patients to imagine themselves in a safe and pleasant environment during the procedure. Procedure times were shorter and hemodynamic stability was greater in the hypnosis group relative to the attention control group. Both the attention and hypnosis treatments showed less drug use than did the standard care condition. This study is remarkable because it is one of the few studies in this area that used manualized treatment. Moreover, fidelity of the treatment intervention was established through a video coding system, and the multiple outcome measures included one that demonstrated cost savings (i.e., length of procedures).

As part of preparation for bone marrow transplantation, patients receive supralethal doses of chemotherapy often followed by supralethal doses of total body irradiation. This treatment often results in severe nausea and vomiting and pain from oral mucositis that can last from several days to 3 weeks. Syrjala et al. (1992) reported a randomized controlled study of the effects of hypnosis and a cognitive–behavioral intervention, relative to two control conditions, on these symptoms during 20 days after chemotherapy and irradiation. The cognitive–behavioral intervention included cognitive restructuring, information, goal development, and exploration of the meaning of the disease. Hypnosis involved relaxation and suggestions for pain control. Rather than standardized inductions, interventions were tailored to the needs of the patient and were then placed on audiotapes for the patient's benefit. Patients were asked to listen to the hypnosis daily for 20 days following chemotherapy and irradiation. The control conditions were therapist contact and standard care (although through randomization, the standard care group had a preponderance of men, making the investigators choose to eliminate this condition from most analyses because of the potential biasing impact this might have). Patients in the hypnosis group reported significantly less pain following chemotherapy and irradiation than patients in the attention control or cognitive–behavioral therapy groups. However, no significant differences emerged between the conditions in nausea, presence of emesis, or medication use.

Burn care pain. Burn-related pain is similar in many ways to that associated with invasive medical procedures. Typical care of burn wounds often involves daily dressing changes and wound debridements, that is, procedures that clearly produce significant nociception. As mentioned earlier, there are numerous case reports of the utility of hypnosis for burn pain (Patterson et al., 1987), starting with Crasilneck et al.'s (1955) report in the *Journal of the American Medical Association.* Of additional note are Ewin's (1983, 1984, 1986) reports that the early application of hypnosis in the emergency room can not only prevent the development of burn-related pain but can also facilitate wound healing. However, these findings must be considered preliminary as they were case reports and did not include control conditions. We were able to identify six controlled trials of hypnosis for burn wound care pain in the literature.

Wakeman and Kaplan (1978) reported that patients with burns who received hypnosis used significantly less analgesic drugs over a 24-hr period than did a group of patients randomly assigned to receive attention only from a psychologist. Treatment included a variety of therapist and audio-induced hypnotic techniques and suggestions were given for hypnoanalgesia, hypnoanesthesia or dissociation, and reduction of anxiety and fear. The control group received verbally supportive time from the therapist without interventions for pain control. In this study, the therapist was present during the wound care procedures.

In a series of studies, using the rapid induction analgesia technique reported in detail by J. Barber (1977), Patterson and colleagues have reported that hypnosis reduces patient reports of severe pain. In the first study, Patterson, Questad, and DeLateur (1989) found that patients who received hypnotic analgesia prior to their wound care (the therapist was not present during wound care) who also reported high initial levels of burn pain at baseline showed a significant drop in pain ratings relative to a control group. This initial study did not involve random assignment to treatment condition, but in a subsequent study by Patterson, Everett, Burns, and Marvin (1992), patients randomized to a hypnosis group reported a greater drop in pain scores than did a control group of patients who only received attention from the psychologist. It is interesting to note that Patterson et al. (1992) found this significant effect even though the control intervention was labeled and presented as hypnosis. However, Everett, Patterson, Burns, Montgomery, and Heimbach (1993) did not find that posthypnotic suggestions for comfort, relaxation, and analgesia resulted in reduced pain ratings when compared with an attention control group or to the tranquilizer lorazepam in a subsequent study. One possible explanation for the inconsistent findings is that the initial pain ratings may not have been high enough in the sample of burn patients examined in the Everett et al. study. This explanation has been supported in a subsequent replication, in which Patterson and Ptacek (1997) found that posthypnotic suggestions had a large effect, but only for patients with high levels of initial pain. We should note that Wright and Drummond (2000) showed positive effects of the rapid induction analgesia technique (J. Barber, 1977) and posthypnotic suggestions for analgesia during burn wound care, even when initial levels of pain were not considered. These findings with burn wound care pain led the authors to suspect that motivation (to avoid high levels of pain), increased compliance (from a natural dependence of patients on trauma health care personnel through the course of intensive and acute hospital care), and dissociation (from the acute stress associated with the burn injury) all might play a role in the apparent impact of hypnosis among patients with burns (Patterson, Adcock, & Bombardier, 1997). Unfortunately, none of the six studies on burn wound care included measures of suggestibility and therefore do not allow for examination of the association between this variable and outcome, a particular weakness in this series of investigations.

Labor pain. Labor pain represents another type of acute pain that is a candidate for hypnotic intervention. Moya and James (1960) and Flowers, Littlejohn, and Wells (1960) reported earlier studies on the clinical benefits of hypnosis for pregnancy. Davidson (1962) also published an earlier successful trial of hypnosis for labor, although this study did not feature a randomized assignment to study groups. Mothers in this study that received six sessions of posthypnotic suggestions for relaxation and pain relief during labor prior to giving birth showed shorter Stage 1 labor, reported that analgesia was more effective, reported less labor pain, and indicated that labor was a more pleasant experience.

R. M. Freeman, Macaulay, Eve, Chamberlain, and Bhat (1986) compared 29 women who received hypnosis before labor with 36 women who received standard care (both groups participated in weekly prenatal classes). Hypnosis involved suggestions for relaxation, pain relief and for transferring anesthesia in the hand to the abdomen. The Stanford Hypnotic Clinical Scale for Adults (Morgan & Hilgard, 1978–1979a) was administered to patients in the hypnosis group. No differences were found in analgesia intake, pain relief during labor, or mode of delivery, and the hypnosis group actually had longer duration of labor (by 2.7 hr, on average). Patients with good to moderate hypnotic suggestibility reported that hypnosis reduced their anxiety and helped them cope with the labor, though specific statistical analyses comparing high and low suggestible patients were not reported.

Harmon et al. (1990) divided 60 pregnant women into two groups on the basis of high and low hypnotic suggestibility scores, who then received six sessions of childbirth education and skill mastery. Half of the women were randomly assigned to receive a hypnotic induction and suggestions as part of this session; the other half received breathing and relaxation exercises. The hypnosis treatment involved a number of suggestions for relaxation and analgesia, is carefully described in the article, and was audiotaped for the patients to listen to daily prior to delivery. Control subjects listened to a commercial prebirth relaxation tape that had several suggestions that may have been similar to hypnosis. The benefits of hypnosis, relative to childbirth education alone, were demonstrated across several variables. The women that received hypnosis had shorter Stage 1 labor, used less pain medication, gave birth to children with higher Apgar scores, and had a higher rate of spontaneous deliveries than did women in the control group. Women receiving hypnosis also reported lower labor pain across a number of scales of the McGill Pain Questionnaire (Melzack & Perry, 1975). In examining the data, it appears that all women in the hypnosis group benefited to some degree but that the women with high hypnotic suggestibility scores showed more benefit in both treatment conditions across all of the outcome domains than did women with low hypnotic suggestibility scores. The women with high suggestibility scores who received hypnosis also showed lower depression scores after birth than did the women with low suggestibility scores in the hypnosis group or women in the control group. An interesting feature of this study is that the participating women were subjected to an ischemic pain task during the training sessions leading up to childbirth. High suggestible women reported lower ischemic pain than did those with low suggestibility scores, and women in the hypnosis group reported lower pain than those in the control group.

Bone marrow aspiration pain. Another type of acute pain that has shown good response to hypnosis in controlled studies is pain associated with bone marrow aspirations. At least five studies have shown positive findings with such procedures (Katz, Kellerman, & Ellenberg, 1987; Kuttner, 1988; Liossi & Hatira, 1999; Syrjala et al., 1992; Zeltzer & LeBaron, 1982). Zeltzer and LeBaron (1982) randomly assigned 33 children (ages 6–17 years) undergoing either lumbar punctures or bone marrow aspirations to either hypnosis or control (deep breathing, distraction, and practice sessions) groups. Hypnosis, as described by the investigators, involved helping children become increasingly involved in interesting and pleasant images. Interventions were unique to each child and involved story telling, fantasy, imagery, and deep breathing. Both groups demonstrated a reduction in pain, but lower ratings of pain were reported in the hypnosis group, and hypnosis subjects reported a reduction of anxiety that was not seen in control subjects.

Katz et al. (1987) randomly assigned 36 children (ages 6–11 years) undergoing lymphoblastic leukemia related bone marrow aspirations to hypnosis or play comparison groups. Children in the hypnosis condition received relaxation—imagery and suggestions for pain control and distraction—and posthypnotic suggestions for reentering hypnosis following a cue from the therapist. Although the therapist was present during the procedure, interactions during the procedure were limited to the provision of the cue (hand on shoulder) and brief encouraging statements. The control condition involved nondirected play for an equivalent amount of time spent in the hypnosis condition. Children in both the hypnosis and play groups showed decreases in self-reports of pain and fear relative to baseline. Hypnosis was not found to be superior to the play group comparison intervention.

Kuttner (1988) randomly assigned children (ages 3–6 years) with leukemia to three groups: a control group (standard medical intervention including information, reassurance and support; $n = 8$), a distraction treatment (pop up books, bubbles; $n = 8$), and a hypnotic intervention in which the child's favorite story became the vehicle to create pleasant imaginative involvement ($n = 9$). The therapist was present to provide both the distraction and experimental (hypnosis) interventions during the procedure. On a behavioral checklist completed by external observers, the hypnotic intervention had an immediate impact on observed distress, pain and anxiety; however, this effect was not found in the patient self-report measures.

Liossi and Hatira (1999) compared hypnosis, cognitive–behavioral coping skills training, and standard treatment (lidocaine injection alone) in 30 children (ages 5–15 years) undergoing bone marrow aspirations. Children in both the hypnosis and cognitive–behavioral interventions reported less pain and pain-related anxiety than did controls, relative to their own baseline. Children in the cognitive–behavioral group showed more behavioral distress and reported more anxiety than the hypnosis group, but the authors concluded that both treatments are effective in preparing pediatric patients for bone marrow aspirations. Suggestibility scores were obtained with the Stanford Hypnotic Clinical Scale for Children (Morgan & Hilgard, 1978–1979b). Hypnotic suggestibility showed a strong association with outcome among the hypnosis group ($rs = .69$, .63, and .60 for pain, anxiety, and observed distress, respectively) but were less consistent in the cognitive–behavioral therapy group ($rs = .54$, .13, and .36) and the control group ($rs = .30$, .00, and .06).

Summary of acute pain studies. In summary, there is a substantial amount of anecdotal evidence and there are several well-designed controlled studies to support the efficacy and use of hypnosis with acute pain problems. Most studies in this area have focused on pain produced by invasive medical procedures (e.g., surgery, burn wound care pain, bone marrow aspirations) or childbirth. Across these domains, out of 17 studies that included self-report measures of pain, 8 studies showed hypnosis to be more effective than no treatment, standard care, or an attention control condition. Three studies showed hypnosis to be no better than such control conditions (in one of these, significant effects for hypnosis were found among subjects scoring high in suggestibility), and one study showed mixed results (this study showed significant effects for one pain measure but not another). Out of eight comparisons with other viable treatments (e.g., cognitive–behavioral therapy, relaxation training, distraction, emotional support), hypnosis was shown to be superior four times. In no case was any condition superior to hypnosis for reducing patient-rated pain severity. In short, treatments described as hypnosis by investigators, and often those involving suggestions for focused attention and for pain relief, are at least as, and about half the time even more, effective than other treatments for reducing the pain associated with invasive medical procedures in both children and adults.

There are a number of important variables that could potentially play a role in the beneficial effects of hypnosis found in these studies. Acute procedural pain is time limited and generally predictable in onset and duration. Both the transient and predictable nature of acute procedural pain makes it possible for hypnotic interventions and skills to be taught to patients in a preparatory manner. In several studies the beneficial effects of hypnosis were obtained even when the therapist was not present during the medical procedure. It is also possible that the severity of acute pain in many of these procedures may contribute to the motivation of patients to participate in treatment, which may, in turn, actually increase the effectiveness of hypnotic analgesia (Patterson & Ptacek, 1997). What is yet to be determined is whether such benefits as reductions in pain and anxiety and improved medical status are worth the cost of clinician time needed to train patients in the use of hypnosis (i.e., whether other studies will demonstrate the cost-effectiveness seen in Lang et al., 2000).

Chronic Pain

Whereas acute pain is that associated with a specific injury and is expected to be short lived, resolving once the injury heals, chronic pain may be defined as pain that persists beyond the healing time needed to recover from an injury (often operationalized as pain that has lasted for more than 3 months) or as pain associated with an ongoing chronic disease or degenerative process (Chapman, Nakamura, & Flores, 1999). The location, pattern, and description of acute pain usually provides information about an underlying acute disease process, and the description of the pain often matches well with what is known about the cause of the pain (Gatchel & Epker, 1999). Chronic pain, on the other hand, usually communicates little about an underlying disease process. Moreover, psychosocial factors, such as patient cognitions, patient pain-coping responses, and social and environmental factors come to play an increasingly important role in the experience and expression of chronic pain over time (Fordyce, 1976; Turk & Flor, 1999). Treatments known to have strong effects on acute pain, such as rest and immobility or opioid analgesics, may have limited usefulness for persons with chronic pain conditions (Fordyce, 1976).

These important differences between acute and chronic pain may have significant implications concerning the manner in which effective hypnotic analgesia is provided, as well as the duration of effect of hypnotic treatments. For example, the likelihood that cognitive factors such as beliefs and cognitive coping responses play a larger role in the experience of chronic pain than the experience of acute pain could make the effects of a psychological intervention such as hypnosis more pronounced. On the other hand, the fact that chronic pain tends to be generally less severe than procedural pain suggests the possibility that persons with chronic pain may feel less urgency or motivation to put effort into

Table 3
Controlled Studies of Chronic Pain Hypnotic Treatment

Study and type of chronic pain problem	Hypnotizability assessed?	*N*	Randomized?	Control conditions	Adult or child?	Follow-up	Outcome dimensions	Findings
Spiegel & Bloom (1983) Cancer-related pain	No	54	Yes	Standard care (SC), support group without hypnosis (SG)	Adult	None	Patient-rated pain intensity	H > SG > SC
Haanen et al. (1991) Fibromyalgia pain	No	40	Yes	Physical therapy (PT)	Adult	3 months	Morning stiffness	H = PT
							Muscle pain	H > PT
							Fatigue	H > PT
							Sleep disturbance	H > PT
							Self-reported global assessment of outcome	H > PT
							Physician reported global assessment of outcome	H = PT
							FM point tenderness	H = PT
							Symptoms (HSCL–90)	H > PT
Anderson et al. (1975) Headache	No	47	Yes	Medication (M; prochlorperazine)	Adult	None	Number of headaches	H > M
							Number of Grade 4 headaches	H > M
							Frequency of being headache free	H > M
Andreychuk & Skriver (1975) Headache	Yes; Hypnotic Induction Profile	33	Yes	Hand temp biofeedback (HTB), alpha enhancement biofeedback (AEB)	Adult	None	Headache Index (Daily Headache Duration × Headache Severity)	H = HTB = AEB
Schlutter et al. (1980) Headache	No	48	Yes	Biofeedback (BF), biofeedback + relaxation (BFR)	Adult	10–14 weeks	Number of headache hours per week	H = BF = BFR
							Pain intensity	H = BF = BFR
							Pain intensity during submaximum effort tourniquet technique	H = BF = BFR
Friedman & Taub (1984) Headache	Yes; Stanford Hypnotic Susceptibility Scale, Form A	66	No	H (without thermal suggestion), hypnosis with thermal suggestion (HT), BF, relaxation (R), wait list (WL)	Adult	1 year	Highest headache intensity	(H = HT = BF = R) > WL
							Number of headaches	(H = HT = BF = R) > WL
							Medication use	(H = HT = BF = R) > WL
Melis et al. (1991) Headache	Yes, but used for descriptive purposes only; Stanford Hypnotic Clinical Scale for Adults	26	Yes	WL	Adult	4 weeks	Number of headache days per week	H > WL
							Number of headache hours per week	H > WL
							Headache intensity	H > WL
Spinhoven et al. (1992) Headache	Yes, but used for description purposes only; Stanford Hypnotic Clinical Scale for Adults	56	Yes	Autogenic training (AT), baseline control (BC)	Adult	6 months	Headache intensity	(H = AT) > BC
							Psychological distress; CSQ	(H = AT) > BC
							Headache relief	(H = AT) > BC
Zitman et al. (1992) Headache	No	79	Yes	AT, hypnosis not presented as hypnosis (HN)	Adult	6 months	Headache intensity	H > AT; H = HN; HN = AT
							Headache relief	H = HN = AT
							Medication use	H = HN = AT
							Anxiety; STAI	H = HN = AT
							Depression; SDS	H = HN = AT

Table 3 (*continued*)

Study and type of chronic pain problem	Hypnotizability assessed?	*N*	Randomized?	Control conditions	Adult or child?	Follow-up	Outcome dimensions	Findings
ter Kuile et al. (1994) Headache	Yes; Stanford Hypnotic Clinical Scale for *Adults*	146	Yes	WL, AT	Adult	6 months	Headache Index (intensity and duration) Medication use Psychological distress; SCL–90	(H = AT) > WL H = AT = WL H = AT = WL
Melzack & Perry (1975) Various chronic pain problems including back, nerve injury, cancer-related, and arthritis pain	No	24	Yes	Alpha feedback alone (A), H, Hypnosis + alpha feedback (HA)	Adult	4–6 months	Sensory pain; MPQ Affective pain; MPQ Pain severity; MPQ	HA > (H = A) HA > (H = A) HA > (H = A)
Edelson & Fitzpatrick (1989)	No	27	No	Cognitive–behavioral therapy (CBT), attention control (AC)	Adult	1 month	Walking Sitting Reclining Pain intensity; MPQ Pain severity; MPQ	CBT > (H = AC) CBT > (H = AC) H = CBT = AC H = CBT = AC H > AC; H = CBT; CBT =AC

Note. H = hypnosis alone; FM = fibromyalgia; HSCL–90 = Hopkins Symptom Checklist—90; CSQ = Coping Strategy Questionnaire; STAI = State–Trait Anxiety Inventory; SDS = Self-Rating Depression Scale; SCL–90 = Symptom Checklist—90; MPQ = McGill Pain Questionnaire.

making hypnotic treatment effective. Another potential challenge to the success of hypnosis is the fact that the pain is chronic. To the extent that effective blocking or ignoring of pain facilitated by hypnosis requires psychological resources of the patient, maintaining a reduced pain awareness may prove to be challenging over the long term.

In earlier reviews, efficacy of hypnosis with chronic pain did not fare well. Turner and Chapman (1982) identified many case studies reporting success for hypnosis in alleviating a wide variety of chronic pain syndromes. Yet, at that time, they were unable to identify a single controlled trial that compared hypnosis with a credible placebo condition. They concluded:

> Remarkably, even though hypnosis has been used for longer than any other psychological method of analgesia, the clinical research in this area is sparse, appallingly poor, and has failed to convincingly demonstrate that hypnosis has more than a placebo effect in relieving chronic pain. (Turner & Chapman, 1982, p. 30)

Six years later, Malone and Strube (1988) performed a meta-analysis of nonmedical treatments for chronic pain. Out of 109 published studies, they identified 48 that provided sufficient information to calculate effect size. Fourteen of these studies included hypnosis, with the types of pain problems treated described as mixed group, nonspecific, cancer, headache, back/neck, and lupus. However, only one of these studies of hypnosis provided enough detailed outcome data for Malone and Strube to calculate an effect size and an average percentage of improvement. The mean rate of improvement in this one study was only 13%, which did not compare favorably with that of autogenic training (68%) or of biofeedback-assisted relaxation training (84%). In fact, none of these compared that well with the average 77% improvement rate they found for no-treatment conditions.

Although hypnosis did not fare well in earlier reviews with chronic pain, there were very few randomized controlled studies available at the time these reviews were written from which to base conclusions about the effects of hypnosis on chronic pain. However, a number of controlled trials of. hypnosis for chronic pain have been published since these reviews were written. As we describe below, these studies show hypnosis as a potentially helpful treatment for reducing the pain associated with chronic pain conditions.

Headache pain. Far more studies have focused on the use of hypnosis for headache than for any other etiology of chronic pain. We identified nine such studies that are listed in Table 3 along with other chronic pain etiologies; the nature of the hypnotic interventions used in these studies are described in Table 4. Andreychuk and Skriver (1975) randomly assigned 33 patients with migraine headaches to groups in which they received biofeedback training for hand warming, alpha enhancement biofeedback, or self-training in hypnosis. Hypnosis treatment lasted 10 weeks and was provided during the weekly sessions through audiotapes that included suggestions for relaxation, visual imagery techniques, verbal reinforcers, and suggestions for pain reduction. Patients were also asked to listen to the tapes outside of the sessions twice every day. Patients in the biofeedback conditions also listened to a tape that included suggestions for relaxation and were asked to listen to this tape twice daily throughout treatment. Outcome was measured with the Headache Index (the product of Daily Headache Dura-

Table 4
Description of Hypnotic Treatment: Chronic Pain Studies

Study	Length of treatment (no. and length of sessions)	Audiotaped?	Description of intervention
D. Spiegel & Bloom (1983)	1 year (5–10 min of hypnosis after weekly 90-min group therapy sessions)	No	Suggestions to "filter the hurt out of the pain" (p. 338) by imagining competing sensations in affected areas.
Haanen et al. (1991)	3 months (eight 1-hr sessions)	Yes	Suggestions for arm levitation, deepening, ego strengthening, control of muscle pain, relaxation, and improvement of sleep disturbance. Third session was taped, and subjects were asked to listen to tape daily.
Anderson et al. (1975)	1 year (six or more sessions)	No	Unstandardized trance induction followed by suggestions for ego strengthening, relaxation, and decreased tension and anxiety. Patients asked to give themselves similar suggestions with autohypnosis daily.
Andreychuk & Skriver (1975)	10 weeks (ten 45-min sessions)	Yes	Listening to a tape (two listenings per session) that included suggestions for relaxation and visual imagery and "direct suggestions for dealing with pain" (p. 177), which included relaxation instructions and verbal reinforcers. Subjects were encouraged to practice twice daily between sessions.
Schlutter et al. (1980)	4 weeks (four 1-hr sessions)	No	Eye fixation followed by suggestions for relaxation, analgesia or numbness, and visualization of an enjoyable situation.
Friedman & Taub (1984)	3 weeks (three 1-hr sessions)	No	Induction only or induction plus thermal imagery, which included suggestions for imagery involving placing hands in warm water and experiencing hand warmth. Subjects were asked to practice self-hypnosis daily for 3–5 min.
Melis et al. (1991)	4 weeks (four 1-hr sessions)	Yes	Eye fixation followed by suggestions for relaxation and the flow off technique (expressing headache as visual image and changing). Each session was taped, and patients were asked to listen to the tape daily between sessions.
Spinhoven et al. (1992)	8 weeks (four 45-min sessions) and three booster sessions at 2, 4, and 6 months after treatment	Yes	Suggestions for relaxation, imaginative inattention, pain displacement, transformation, and imagining self in the future without pain. In Session 4, a tape was made for self-practice, and subjects were instructed to listen to tape twice daily.
Zitman et al. (1992)	8 weeks (four 45-min sessions) and three booster sessions at 2, 4, and 6 months after treatment	Yes	Suggestions for relaxation and for imagining self in a future situation in which pain control has been achieved. Subjects were asked to practice with tape twice daily.
ter Kuile et al. (1994)	7 weeks (seven 1-hr sessions) and then three 1-hr booster sessions at 2, 4, and 6 months after treatment	Yes	Suggestions for relaxation, imaginative, pain displacement, transformation, hypnotic analgesia, and altering maladaptive cognitive responses. The suggestions of the last session were taped, and subjects were asked to listen to tapes twice daily for 15 min.
Melzack & Perry (1975)	6–12 sessions (2 hr for hypnosis + alpha feedback group, 1–1.5 hr for alpha feedback alone and hypnosis alone groups)	Yes	Taped 20-min suggestions for relaxation, feeling stronger and healthier, having greater alertness and energy, less fatigue, less discouragement, feeling greater tranquility and ability to overcome things that are ordinarily upsetting, being able to think more clearly, to concentrate and remember things, be more calm, less tense, more independent, and less fearful.
Edelson & Fitzpatrick (1989)	2 weeks (four 1-hr sessions)	No	Hypnosis condition was identical to cognitive–behavioral control condition, except that the hypnotic condition was preceded by a "hypnotic induction"; any specific suggestions made were not described.

Note. None of the studies were manualized.

tion × Headache Severity), and suggestibility was measured with the Hypnotic Induction Profile (H. Spiegel & Bridger, 1970). Reduction in headaches was seen in all three groups, with no significant differences. However, patients with high hypnotizability scores showed larger treatment effects than patients with low hypnotizability scores, independent of treatment.

Anderson, Basker, and Dalton (1975) randomly assigned 47 patients with migraines to hypnosis or medication (prochlorperazine) groups. Hypnosis patients received six or more sessions over the course of 1 year and were asked to practice autohypnosis daily (without the assistance of an audiotape) and to give self-suggestions for relaxation, ego strengthening, decreased tension, and aversion of migraine attacks. Patients receiving hypnotherapy showed fewer headaches per month, fewer Grade 4 headaches, and a higher frequency of remission than those who received prochlorperazine.

Schlutter, Golden, and Blume (1980) randomly assigned 48 patients to groups that received hypnosis, electromyograph (EMG) biofeedback alone, or EMG feedback plus progressive relaxation. Patients in the hypnosis condition received four 1-hr sessions over the course of 4 weeks, and hypnosis consisted of eye fixation followed by suggestions for relaxation, analgesia or numbness, and visualization of an enjoyable experience (Greene & Reyher, 1972). Patients in each of the treatment conditions reported similar reductions in number of headache hours per week and average headache pain.

Friedman and Taub (1984) also failed to find differences among treatments including a hypnotic induction-only condition, an induction plus thermal imagery condition, a thermal biofeedback condition (which included the provision of standard autogenic phrases eliciting feelings of warmth), and a relaxation condition in 66 patients with migraines. All treatment groups showed improvements as measured by headache ratings and medication use, relative to wait list controls. It is important to note that subjects with high scores on the Stanford Hypnotic Susceptibility Scale, Form A (Weitzenhoffer & Hilgard, 1959) showed meaningful decrements on outcome variables at the 1-year follow-up, across treatment conditions, when compared with those who scored low on this measure.

Several additional controlled studies on hypnosis with headaches have been published over the past decade with similar results. Melis, Rooimans, Spierings, and Hoogduin (1991) had 26 patients with chronic headaches undergo 4 weeks of baseline observation, and then randomly assigned them either to four weekly 1-hr sessions of hypnosis supplemented by home practice audiotape or to 4 weeks of no treatment (wait list). The hypnosis intervention was described as including the "flow off" technique (expressing and changing the headache as a visual image) as well as suggestions for moving the pain to other areas of the body. The hypnosis group reported significantly more improvement on number of headaches, headache hours, and headache days than the wait list control group did. Although the investigators used the Stanford Hypnotic Clinical Scale for Adults to describe their sample, they did not report on any association between suggestibility and outcome.

Spinhoven and his colleagues have published a number of randomized studies that indicate that hypnosis is essentially equivalent to autogenic training (in Spinhoven, Linssen, Van Dyck, & Zitman, 1992, autogenic training consisted of suggestions for hand heaviness, hand warming, and coolness of the forehead) in controlling tension headaches. Using 56 patients in a within-subjects, randomized design, they found that both hypnosis and autogenic training improved average headache pain intensity, psychological distress, and headache relief relative to a wait list control group. Hypnosis consisted of four sessions (over the course of 8 weeks) of suggestions for relaxation, imaginative inattention, and pain displacement and transformation. Similarly, ter Kuile et al. (1994) reported that in 146 subjects, hypnosis and autogenic training showed effects on headache duration and intensity over a wait list control but were no different from one another. Subjects who scored high on the Stanford Hypnotic Clinical Scale for Adults showed greater treatment effects posttreatment and at follow-up than did those who scored low, independent of treatment condition. The hypnosis treatment was similar to that used in the Spinhoven et al. study, but it included cognitive–behavioral interventions on maladaptive cognitive responses.

Zitman, Van Dyck, Spinhoven, and Linssen (1992) took 79 patients with headaches and first randomly assigned them to autogenic training or to "future-oriented" hypnosis (FI) that was not labeled as hypnosis. FI treatment largely involved having patients imagine themselves in a future situation in which pain reduction had been achieved. In the second phase, 6 months later, all patients who received either autogenic training or FI in the first phase were offered FI again, except that in this phase FI was "openly presented as a hypnotic technique" (p. 221). All three treatments appeared to be equally effective in reducing Headache Index scores. However, at 6-month follow-up, the FI group practicing what was explicitly labeled as hypnosis showed the greatest improvement on the Headache Index—and this improvement was statistically significantly greater than that reported by the attention control condition. There are at least two plausible explanations for the greater impact of the second hypnosis intervention. First, this higher efficacy may have been due to the fact that at the follow-up to the second phase, these subjects had received twice as much treatment (14 sessions total) as they had at the end of the first phase. Second, it is also possible that explicitly labeling the procedures as hypnosis might have been responsible for the treatment advantage.

The findings for the headache studies in aggregate are consistent with the conclusion of a review performed by Spinhoven (1988), that the effects of hypnotic treatments for headaches do not differ significantly from those of autogenic or relaxation training. K. A. Holroyd and Penzien (1990) reached the same conclusion in a more recent review. The only exception to this is Zitman et al.'s (1992) finding with FI, but this finding might reflect a dose effect (because subjects in this condition received more hypnosis than the subjects in the autogenic treatment condition) or an increased expectancy effect caused by an explicit labeling of the intervention as hypnosis.

It is notable that in those studies that included measures of suggestibility, patients showed more improvement with headache control if they scored high on tests of hypnotic suggestibility, independent of whether they received hypnosis, autogenic training or relaxation. Along these lines, the many similarities between hypnotic treatment and relaxation interventions, such as autogenic training, are worth noting. In fact, Edmonston (1991) has argued that hypnosis cannot be differentiated from, and in fact may be, a form of deep relaxation. On the other hand, relaxation and autogenic training both often include hypnotic-like suggestions for comfort, focused attention, and changes in perceptions, so perhaps these should be considered variants of hypnotic treatment. To complicate matters further, Spanos and Chaves (1989a, 1989b, 1989c) have long argued that positive responses to suggestions for pain control can be achieved without the induction of a hypnotic state. Studies on the hypnotic control of headache pain therefore raise two important questions: (a) What role does relaxation play in the effects of hypnotic analgesia (particularly given the role of tension in causing many forms of headaches)? and (b) What role do suggestions (i.e., hypnosis) play in the effects of relaxation training?

Chronic pain other than headache. Controlled trials of hypnosis for chronic pain conditions other than headache are few, but do provide some preliminary evidence that hypnosis is effective for reducing pain for a number of chronic pain conditions (see

Tables 3 and 4). We were able to identify four such studies. D. Spiegel and Bloom (1983) examined pain control and other variables in women with chronic cancer pain from breast carcinoma (as opposed to pain from cancer-related medical procedures discussed in the *Acute Pain* section). Fifty-four women were assigned to either a usual treatment control condition (n = 24) or to a group receiving usual treatment and weekly group therapy for up to 12 months (n = 30). The women in group therapy were, in turn, assigned to groups that either did or did not have brief (5–10 min) self-hypnosis as a part of their group therapy treatment (the nature of treatment was based on H. Spiegel & Spiegel, 1978). Both support groups showed improvement in pain control over usual treatment. However, women who received self-hypnosis showed an improvement above and beyond that of other interventions on reduced pain intensity.

One controlled study examined the effects of hypnosis among persons with refractory fibromyalgia (Haanen et al., 1991). Haanen and colleagues randomly assigned patients with this diagnosis to groups that received either eight 1-hr sessions of hypnotherapy (supplemented by a self-hypnosis home practice audiotape) over a 3-month period or 12 to 24 hr of physical therapy (massage and muscle relaxation training) for 12 weeks, with follow-up at 24 weeks. The investigators found larger improvements in the patients who received hypnosis than in the patients who received physical therapy on measures of muscle pain, fatigue, sleep disturbance, and overall assessment of outcome and distress scores. These differences were maintained through the follow-up assessment. Although this study is limited in that the control condition and the hypnosis condition were not equivalent in terms of patient contact and time, the findings are important because they provide one of the few tests of hypnosis in a chronic pain sample other than persons with headaches that used a randomized design.

Two controlled studies have been reported on hypnosis with chronic pain of mixed etiology. Melzack and Perry (1975) examined the effects of hypnosis and alpha biofeedback in 24 patients with a variety of chronic pain problems, including back pain (n = 10), peripheral nerve injury (n = 4), cancer (n = 3), arthritis (n = 2), amputation (n = 2), trauma (n = 2), and "head pain" (n = 1). Patients were randomly assigned to one of three groups; 12 received 6 to 12 sessions of hypnosis plus alpha training, 6 received hypnosis alone, and 6 received alpha training alone. Pain was assessed just before and just after each treatment session. The authors reported that alpha training had the smallest effect on pain, followed by hypnosis, which had a greater, but not statistically significant, effect on pain reduction. The combination of alpha training and hypnosis, however, had an impressive impact on pain reduction, as measured by scales from the McGill Pain Questionnaire (Melzack & Perry, 1975). Fifty-eight percent of the patients reported a reduction of pain of 33% or greater. The authors acknowledged that their study design could not rule out placebo effects as a possible explanation for the reductions in pain observed because there was not a placebo condition or even a no-treatment condition. Certainly, however, the findings indicate that the further study of the potential additive effects of hypnosis with other treatments for chronic pain is warranted.

Edelson and Fitzpatrick (1989) also looked at patients (N = 27) with mixed etiologies for pain, with back pain being the most frequent. Patients were randomly assigned to four 1-hr sessions of an attention control (supportive, nondirective discussions), a cognitive–behavioral, or a hypnosis group. The hypnosis group received the same information as the cognitive–behavioral group but after a standard hypnotic induction. The cognitive–behavioral group showed increases in walking and decreases in sitting relative to the control group and the hypnosis group, while the hypnosis group showed improvements in subjective ratings of pain only (McGill Pain Questionnaire total score) relative to the attention control condition.

Five additional investigations deserve mention even though they did not use random assignment to experimental (hypnosis) and control conditions. Using a multiple baseline design, Simon and Lewis (2000) reported that 28 patients with temporal mandibular disorder pain showed improved pain control at 6-month follow-up after receiving six sessions of hypnotic analgesia. This pain had previously been refractory to other treatments. Crasilneck (1995) used hypnosis with 12 patients who had what he described as intractable organic pain. His intervention involved multiple inductions within the same sessions followed by six specific suggestions for pain management, including pain displacement, age regression to a time period prior to the onset of pain, and a reexperiencing of the experience of being pain free, and glove anesthesia. He reported 80%–90% relief of pain at 1-year follow-up. M. Jensen, Barber, Williams-Avery, Flores, and Brown (2001) examined the effects of hypnosis with analgesia suggestions among 22 patients with spinal cord injury-related pain. They found that 86% of their sample reported a decrease in pain following a hypnotic induction and analgesia suggestions relative to prehypnosis pain levels. Dinges et al. (1997) used self-hypnosis as part of a cognitive–behavioral treatment program in an attempt to manage pain from sickle cell disease. Thirty-seven children, adolescents, and adults provided 4 months of baseline data before undergoing the combination of behavioral and self-hypnotic treatment. Findings indicated a substantial decrease in pain-related episodes following treatment. Finally, James, Large, and Beale (1989) evaluated self-hypnosis using a multiple baseline design for 5 patients with chronic pain and who were selected for high scores on hypnotic susceptibility tests. They found variable outcomes, with 2 of the patients reporting significant improvement, 2 reporting little change (although these 2 did find that self-hypnosis was effective on some occasions), and 1 reporting no apparent benefit.

Summary of chronic pain studies. The findings of chronic pain studies parallel, in some ways, those from acute etiologies. Compared with no-treatment, standard care, or attention conditions, hypnotic analgesia procedures result in significantly greater reductions in a variety of measures of pain. However, when hypnosis is compared with other treatments, in particular with other treatments that share many characteristics with hypnosis (e.g., suggestions for relaxation and competing sensations) such as autogenic and relaxation training, hypnosis is less often found to be superior to these alternative treatments. This finding is somewhat in contrast to the several acute pain studies demonstrating the superiority of hypnosis to other treatments. However, in none of these studies has hypnosis been shown to be less effective than any other treatment for reducing pain. Moreover, it is possible that hypnosis may be less time consuming and more efficient than either autogenic or relaxation training. At the very least, the question of relative efficiency of hypnosis, autogenic training, and relaxation training should be investigated in future studies.

Methodological Issues of Hypnotic Analgesia Research

Although the results of this review indicate that hypnotic analgesia results in decreased pain from a variety of acute and chronic pain conditions, several important methodological issues make firm conclusions regarding the efficacy of hypnotic analgesia difficult to make. For example, the numbers of patients in published controlled trials tend to be low, which limits the power to detect statistical differences between treatment conditions. Hypnotic interventions also vary widely from study to study. Moreover, although several studies referred to citations or scripts to describe their experimental intervention, only Lang et al. (2000) described a carefully detailed manualized procedure. There is clearly a need for more randomized clinical trials that include larger samples and standardized hypnotic procedures, particularly in the area of chronic pain (other than that caused by headaches). Three additional key methodological issues that deserve detailed discussion include suggestibility, nonspecific versus specific effects, and practice–dose effects.

Hypnotic Suggestibility

As discussed above, one of the most robust findings in the laboratory pain hypnosis literature has been the association between hypnotic pain reduction and hypnotic suggestibility as measured by hypnotizability scales (R. Freeman et al., 2000; E. R. Hilgard, 1969; E. R. Hilgard & Hilgard, 1975; E. R. Hilgard & Morgan, 1975; Knox et al., 1974; Miller et al., 1991). Moreover, Montgomery et al. (2000) found suggestibility to be an important variable in their meta-analysis of both experimental and clinical studies.

Patterson et al. (1997) have previously suggested that the relationship between suggestibility and pain control may not necessarily generalize well to clinical situations. For example, Gillett and Coe (1984) reported that they found no differences in response to hypnotic analgesia between low and high suggestibility patients undergoing painful dental procedures. In the current review, of the controlled studies we examined, seven assessed the association between suggestibility and outcome—four acute pain studies (R. M. Freeman et al., 1986; Harmon et al., 1990; Lang et al., 1996; Liossi & Hatira, 1999) and three chronic pain studies (Andreychuk & Skriver, 1975; Friedman & Taub, 1984; ter Kuile et al., 1994). Of these, all but one demonstrated a positive association between suggestibility and at least one outcome measure; Lang et al. (1996) was the only exception. In several studies, patients scoring high on tests of hypnotic suggestibility often showed as much benefit from other psychological treatments (autogenic training, relaxation, cognitive–behavioral) as they did from hypnosis (Andreychuk & Skriver, 1975; Friedman & Taub, 1984; Liossi & Hatira, 1999; ter Kuile et al., 1994). High suggestibility was also associated with long-term treatment effects in the one study that examined this (Friedman & Taub, 1984).

Thus, on the basis of the available studies, there does appear to be some association between clinical effect and suggestibility. Moreover, unlike many of the studies in the hypnotic analgesia literature of experimental pain, subjects in these studies were not specifically selected from the high and low ends of hypnotizability scales. Social–cognitive theorists have maintained that little can be concluded about the importance of suggestibility if medium susceptible subjects are not included in experimental designs (Kirsch & Lynn, 1995). The fact that the studies in the current review included subjects representing all ranges of suggestibility argues even more strongly for the potential importance of this variable in predicting analgesic treatment outcome in clinical populations.

Of course, the fact that an association exists between hypnotic suggestibility and treatment outcome does not necessarily mean that only persons with high screening scores should be offered hypnotic analgesia. Just because highly suggestible patients benefit more, on average, than those low on this variable does not mean that patients falling in the medium or low range would never benefit. In their discussion of this issue, Montgomery et al. (2000) showed that although highly suggestible people may obtain the most benefit, persons with medium scores can report pain relief from hypnotic analgesia, and even those with low suggestibility scores showed an effect size greater than zero (albeit the effect size for this group was very close to zero). Montgomery et al. concluded that 75% of the population could obtain "substantial" pain relief from hypnotic analgesia; given that the rates of highly suggestible people in the population is roughly 30% (E. R. Hilgard & Hilgard, 1975), this would certainly indicate that analgesic effects extend well beyond those scoring at the high end of the curve on this variable.

In addition, there is some evidence that people can increase their suggestibility with training and practice. For example, J. Holroyd (1996) has suggested that hypnotic analgesia can be improved through manualized training programs for patients. Similarly, Barabasz (1982) has demonstrated that restrictive environmental stimulation (REST) can increase both suggestibility scores and experimental pain tolerance (to shocks). Barabasz and Barabasz (1989) indeed demonstrated this finding among persons with chronic pain; subjects were able to increase their Stanford Hypnotic Susceptibility Scale scores and tolerance to ischemic pain following REST. It would seem that a primary benefit of research on suggestibility and response to analgesia is that it can be useful to identify patients that can respond readily and can also indicate those that might need additional training or support.

Nonspecific Versus Specific Effects

A second important issue concerning studies of clinical hypnotic analgesia is that of nonspecific effects. Frequently referred to in the literature as placebo effects, the term *nonspecific* better captures effects common to all treatments but not specific to the treatment being examined (Kazdin, 1979). Ideally, clinical trials not only determine that a treatment is effective relative to no treatment, or to a no-treatment waiting period, but also to a treatment condition designed to control for nonspecific effects. Designing such control conditions for hypnosis treatment is particularly challenging, however, because there are so many components to hypnotic interventions used in the clinical setting. For example, in many of the studies we reviewed, hypnosis included an induction, deepening, and suggestions for pain relief within the context of the induction. Studies in the laboratory have indicated that not all of these components are necessary for pain reduction and other perceptual phenomena (Chaves, 1993), although these findings have not been replicated in clinical pain populations. An ideal study would independently manipulate each of the components of what has traditionally been included in hypnotic treatments and compare these components to a "placebo" condition that controls for therapist time and patient expectancy but might not otherwise be expected to affect pain. A series of such studies would help determine the extent to which an induction, deepening suggestions, or analgesia suggestions are necessary or sufficient for pain reduction, and also help determine the extent to which hypnotic analgesia results in reductions of pain over and above the effects of expectancy and therapist attention.

Along the same lines, the question of whether an intervention is labeled as hypnosis has been brought to the fore in this review. Although all of the investigators clearly viewed the interventions tested in the studies reviewed as hypnosis, and it is likely that in most cases the interventions were presented as such to the study participants, it was often not specifically made clear that the patients studied were informed that they were undergoing hypnosis; this was particularly the case in studies with children. Moreover, in two of the studies, the investigators viewed their intervention as hypnosis, but specifically did not label it as such (Faymonville et al., 1997; Zitman et al., 1992). This brings up the important definitional issue of whether a patient who unknowingly undergoes an induction has received hypnosis, and whether such labeling influences the outcome of treatment. Ideally, future studies would include conditions in which the patient is told or not told the intervention is hypnosis, in order to disentangle the effects of this variable on treatment efficacy.

Although no clinical study on hypnotic analgesia published to date has systematically manipulated the label of the procedure tested (as *hypnosis* or not), some of the studies reviewed in this article did manipulate other components of the interventions, and so shed some preliminary light on the contributions of each to outcome. For example, several studies indicated that hypnotic pain control was significantly more effective than a condition in which patients received an equivalent amount of attention from the psychologist (Patterson et al., 1992; Patterson & Ptacek, 1997; Syrjala et al., 1992; Wakeman & Kaplan, 1978). In addition, a few studies included a control group in which the attention from the psychologist was labeled as hypnosis (Everett et al., 1993; Patterson & Ptacek, 1997; Patterson et al., 1989; Zitman et al., 1992), and most of these found the hypnotic intervention to be superior to the control intervention that had been labeled as hypnosis for patients. Several studies included control with relaxation and deep breathing (Davidson, 1962; Katz et al., 1987; Zeltzer & LeBaron, 1982) and the majority of studies on headache pain have compared hypnosis with treatment groups that have used autogenic training or progressive relaxation (see Table 3).

Not only is it important to seek to control for and test the relative contributions of the components of hypnosis but that studies determine the relative efficacy of various specific hypnotic suggestions. Tables 2 and 4, for example, list the many different hypnotic inductions and suggestions given in the studies reviewed in this article. Given the research that has demonstrated differential neurophysiological responding to different specific suggestions (e.g., Rainville et al., 1999), much more attention needs to be paid to the specific suggestions that are provided during treatment. It is very likely that some suggestions will be more effective for reducing pain experience than others. At a minimum, authors must provide clear descriptions of the specific suggestions made to the participants in any clinical trial. Ideally, these would be standardized and consistent across the patients within a trial. Better yet, investigators could systematically manipulate different suggestions within the same trial to determine which provide the greatest relief, decreases in global suffering, and improvements in function.

Practice and Dose Effects

A third issue that becomes apparent when examining the controlled trials of hypnotic analgesia for clinical pain concerns the marked variability in the amount of hypnotic treatment administered. Often, in the chronic pain studies for example, hypnotic treatment was provided in individual weekly sessions that lasted 45 min to 1.5 hr for 4 to 10 sessions over the course of 1 or 2 months. However, some patients received much less treatment at a time (e.g., 5–10 min of group hypnotic treatment at the end of a group therapy session; D. Spiegel & Bloom, 1983) or received treatment spread out over a longer period of time (e.g., sessions provided at intervals of 10–14 days; Anderson et al., 1975).

Only two studies with acute pain provided patients with audiotaped hypnosis instructions or suggestions to supplement those provided by the clinician, although both of these studies showed robust treatment effects (Harmon et al., 1990; Syrjala et al., 1992). However, many of the studies on chronic pain included audiotaped supplements and, although they all showed improvement over no treatment, effects were generally similar to those from autogenic or relaxation training studies (whose subjects also were often provided with audiotapes for practice; see Table 3). Unfortunately, none of the studies we reviewed included the presence or absence of an audiotape as an independent variable. Thus, at this time, we are not able to draw firm conclusions regarding the relative importance of home practice to treatment effects for either acute or chronic pain treatment.

Future research is needed to determine the extent to which there is a dose effect for hypnotic analgesia (e.g., by systematically varying the amount of hypnotic treatment received), as well as determine whether home practice improves the short- or long-term effects of hypnotic analgesia. At a minimum, controlled studies need to take these factors into account when designing experimental treatments and to ensure that they clearly indicate the number and length of hypnotic sessions administered, the extent to which subjects were required to practice outside of the sessions, and of great importance, whether the subjects complied with the practice recommendations.

The Puzzle of Chronic Pain

This review indicates positive analgesic effects for the use of hypnosis with both chronic and acute pain. However, studies with acute pain often demonstrated that hypnosis is superior to other psychological interventions for pain; such has not been the case with chronic pain. In carefully scrutinizing the hypnotic suggestions given for chronic pain in the studies reviewed (see Table 4), we discovered that, as a whole, clinical studies performed with patients with chronic pain often appear to provide hypnotic suggestions that fail to appreciate the multifaceted and complex nature of pain. Our contention is that hypnosis is often applied to chronic pain in a simplistic manner, and that effect sizes and treatment duration could be enhanced if clinicians and researchers used this treatment with a more comprehensive understanding of this problem (or at least reported this if it was indeed their practice). The following sections provide the rationale for this argument. In the remainder of this review we address some of the factors we believe may account for the inconsistent findings of hypnotic analgesia with chronic pain.

Pain Versus Suffering

A particularly vexing issue in applying hypnosis to chronic pain is that treatment must often address suffering rather than, or at least in addition to, pain (Fordyce, 1988) because chronic pain often persists in the absence of tissue damage (Loeser, 1982). There are at least five mechanisms that can result in suffering or pain behavior in the absence of nociception (tissue damage), and they are frequently present in patients with chronic pain. First, this group often has psychological disorders that, when treated, might alleviate the pain (Chibnall & Duckro, 1994; Geisser, Roth, Bachman, & Eckert, 1996; Romano & Turner, 1985). Second, patients with chronic pain often hold specific beliefs about their pain that are maladaptive, such as the beliefs that the source of their pain requires a biomedical solution, that pain is a signal of harm or physical damage, and that they are necessarily disabled by pain (M. P. Jensen, Turner, Romano, & Lawler, 1994); effective treatment involves modifying such thoughts (Turner & Romano, 2001). Third, somatization and somatosensory amplification are associated with chronic pain and a tendency to experience higher levels of pain (Barsky, Goodson, & Lane, 1988; Wilson et al., 1994). Fourth, operant or learning factors (social reinforcement in the form of unemployment compensation or attention from a solicitous spouse) often maintain pain behaviors in persons with chronic pain, well after a lesion is healed (Fordyce, 1976). Finally, chronic pain is thought to be maintained, at least in part, by deactivation, guarding and changes in body mechanics (Fordyce, 1976), and classic treatment involves systematic increases in strength and mobility, as well as multidisciplinary treatment with goals of returning patients to work, decreasing physician visits, lessening dependence on pain medication, and increasing functional activity (Turk & Okifuji, 1998).

Although appreciating such contributions to chronic pain may be apparent to theorists and practitioners in this area, studies on hypnotic analgesia of chronic pain problems make little or no mention of these factors. When chronic pain or suffering is primarily due to one or more of the factors discussed above, pain reduction may not be the primary goal of treatment. Pain treatment programs often have multiple indicators of treatment outcome, and pain reduction is often regarded to be less important than indicators of more functional activity (Turk & Okifuji, 1998). In fact, when hypnosis is used with some patients with chronic pain to reduce pain, the effect may be counterproductive. If a person with chronic pain is demonstrating illness conviction, he or she might regard hypnotic analgesia as a magical means to eliminate nociceptive input when the focus of treatment should be on any number of those factors discussed above. Yet, in almost every report or study discussed on the use of hypnosis with chronic pain, the primary role of hypnosis has been to decrease pain.

We believe that the impact of hypnosis on chronic pain might be strengthened if suggestions are geared toward reducing suffering or pain behaviors, or increasing activity and "well" behaviors, in addition to, or even in some cases rather than, suggestions for pain reduction. Chaves and Dworkin (1997) have pointed out that hypnosis has not been applied to chronic pain rehabilitation. In support of this conclusion is the fact that in all of the studies we reviewed there was no mention of providing suggestions for increasing activity for chronic pain or for fitting suggestions into the context of a larger treatment program (see Table 4). Rather, suggestions were almost exclusively geared toward relaxation, comfort, and analgesia. Hypnotic suggestions might be targeted toward increasing activity that is safely within the confines of the patient's limitations. Because patients with chronic pain are often depressed and perhaps grieving loss of activity, relationships, or employment, suggestions can also be targeted toward improvement of affective state (Yapko, 1992). Another potentially useful application of hypnosis might be to help the patients alter their model of the etiology of pain. One of the biggest challenges in treating chronic pain is to motivate patients to engage in treatment, and one novel application would be to combine it with recent models for engaging patients in the treatment process (M. P. Jensen, 1996; Kerns & Rosenberg, 2000).

Increasing Treatment Effect

Montgomery et al. (2000) concluded from their meta-analysis of experimental and clinical studies that most people can benefit from hypnotic analgesia. Perhaps of equal importance with respect to chronic pain are findings from Kirsch, Montgomery and Sapirstein (1995), who performed a meta-analysis of 18 studies in which cognitive–behavioral therapy was compared with the same therapy supplemented by hypnosis. The results of their analysis indicated a substantial effect size with the addition of hypnosis; the authors estimated that more than 70% of the patients benefited from adding hypnotherapy to the treatment. We believe a neglected question is whether hypnosis can increase the treatment effects of multidisciplinary treatment programs. For example, Kirsch et al. reported that when hypnosis is added to an obesity program, weight loss is maintained over longer treatment periods. An effective practitioner working with patients with obesity certainly knows that treatment for this problem is multidimensional, involving increasing activity, stimulus control, and self-monitoring (Levitt, 1993; Wadden & Bell, 1990). An obesity specialist would also see the folly of using hypnosis as an isolated intervention for eliminating appetite. Isolated attempts to reduce pain levels in some patients with chronic pain via hypnosis is analogous to attempting to reduce appetite in patients with obesity. Hypnosis adds to the effects of a comprehensive program for weight loss, and it seems reasonable to hypothesize that it would do the same for chronic pain.

This notion was apparent as early as 1975, when Melzack and Perry (1975) demonstrated the efficacy of hypnosis with chronic pain in a controlled study (though admittedly not one including a placebo condition). To reiterate, the investigators found neither biofeedback nor hypnosis to be effective in themselves; however, the combination of treatments resulted in significantly enhanced clinical effects. More studies with chronic pain should investigate the use of hypnosis for chronic pain in concert with other approaches.

Specifying Suggestions

Studies with pain induced in the laboratory suggest that the nature of the hypnotic suggestion is an influential variable in outcome. Perhaps the most salient example comes from the studies examining the impact of hypnotic analgesia on sensory versus affective pain. As discussed above, a number of researchers have speculated whether hypnosis has a greater effect on sensory versus affective components of pain (Price & Barber, 1987; Price et al., 1987), and Rainville et al.'s (1999) recent study indicated that the crucial variable was the nature of the hypnotic suggestion. Specifically, suggestions for sensory reductions of pain resulted in decreased activity in the somatosensory cortex, and suggestions for affective pain reduction led to decreased activity in the part of the brain that processes more emotional and suffering information. The one occasion where investigators in the Spinhoven laboratory (Zitman et al., 1992) found an advantage of hypnosis over autogenic training was when future oriented suggestions for pain control were made. Although yet to be tested in a controlled clinical trial, it follows that if a clinician desires that patients have pain control over the long term, then it is important to provide them with that suggestion specifically (J. Barber, 1998). Hypnotic suggestions for analgesia should also be targeted toward both sensory and affective dimensions of pain. Following the logic presented in the immediately preceding sections, if the goal of treatment is to increase activity, return to work or change an individual's model of pain, then it makes sense to tailor at least some of the hypnotic suggestions accordingly.

Analgesic Suggestions for Chronic Pain

In spite of our recommendations for targeting hypnotic suggestions for multiple aspects of chronic pain treatment, we certainly acknowledge that in many cases suggestions for analgesia with such patients would be appropriate. Certainly pain that has ongoing nociceptive input (e.g., cancer, spinal cord injury, arthritis, diabetic neuropathy) and fewer of the nonnociceptive factors maintaining it may be more responsive to hypnotic analgesia. In his prolific writing on clinical applications of hypnosis, Erickson (1980; Erickson & Rossi, 1981; Erickson, Rossi, & Rossi, 1976) reported a number of anecdotally effective suggestions for chronic pain, including (a) those for the direct abolition of pain, (b) amnesia, (c) analgesia, (d) anesthesia, (e) posthypnotic relief, (f) time distortion, (g) reinterpretation of the experience, (h) dissociation, and (i) displacement. It is interesting, then, that Erickson noted that suggestions for the direct abolition of pain or complete anesthesia seldom showed lasting results (Erickson et al., 1976). He often recommended instead that the patient's chronic pain be moved on a continuum to a less unpleasant level. As an example, Erickson (1980) suggested that a patient with a severe malignant pain would experience that sensation as an unpleasant itching mosquito bite.

Although not tested in any empirical studies, several writers have emphasized the need to provide suggestions for pain control to patients with chronic pain on several occasions over the course of time (J. Barber, 1996; Crasilneck, 1995). We earlier described J. Holroyd's (1996) point that hypnosis can be repeatedly practiced even by those low in suggestibility much like a form of meditation (see also Alden & Heap, 1998), and Barabasz's (1982; Barabasz & Barabasz, 1989) findings that both hypnotizability and pain tolerance can be increased with restricted environmental stimulation. Along the same lines, the prevailing clinical wisdom is that most patients receiving hypnosis for chronic pain should be taught self-hypnotic skills that generalize beyond the treatment setting. Few, if any, writers have suggested that chronic pain can be modified through a single session, and most of the studies we reviewed with this clinical problem used audiotapes to supplement clinical work. The fact that clinicians who are successful with chronic pain usually provide treatment over multiple sessions introduces the confounds inherent in psychotherapy. We simply cannot determine whether reported reductions in pain result from hypnotic suggestions, some artifacts of the therapeutic relationship, or (perhaps more likely) some combination of these factors. This is an area that is certainly in need of further exploration.

Another question that requires investigation concerns the relative efficacy of hypnotic analgesia for different types of pain problems. For example, it is reasonable to hypothesize that suffering that is maintained by social–financial disincentives may be less likely to respond to suggestions for analgesia. However, there are multiple forms of chronic pain, many of which are known to show varying responses to therapeutic modalities. The aforementioned headache studies suggest, for example, that headache pain responds equally well to hypnosis and autogenic training, but this seems to be the only definitive line of research for a specific pain etiology. Researchers need to determine the types of pain most responsive to hypnotic interventions (e.g., musculoskeletal, neuropathic, malignant or other causes of pain). Clinicians likely have their opinions concerning which types of pain they can treat effectively with hypnosis, but at this point, such conjectures remain as hypotheses to be tested.

Even if the goal of treatment is to increase physical activity, suggestions for pain relief might be of value. A patient who is skeptical about psychological treatment might be given suggestions for pain relief, with the hope that this would not only produce a short-term (and perhaps long-term) reduction in suffering and pain intensity but also increase rapport with the clinician and investment in treatment. This might pave the way for the often more difficult task of changing patients' beliefs about pain etiology and engaging them in the challenging exercises and lifestyle changes that are an integral component of many successful chronic pain treatments.

Summary and Conclusions

Pain is a health care issue that results in significant suffering and financial cost. The time has arrived to determine whether there is enough scientific evidence to justify the use of hypnosis as a viable treatment for pain. For the most part, the focus of most laboratory-based studies has been on examining the effects of hypnosis on perceived pain intensity. The results of these studies demonstrate consistent effects of hypnosis on pain reduction, and have contributed to the theoretical understanding of hypnotic analgesia. More recently, a number of neurophysiological studies have taken these findings to a new level of sophistication.

In this article we sought to provide a comprehensive review of the controlled trials of hypnosis for clinical pain. The findings from acute pain studies demonstrate consistent clinical effects with hypnotic analgesia that are superior to attention or standard care control conditions, and often superior to other viable pain treatments. Although earlier reviews did not provide support for the efficacy of hypnosis for chronic pain, these reviews were based on very few controlled clinical trials. In the past 2 decades, a greater number of controlled trials of hypnosis for chronic pain have been published. The findings from these studies show that hypnotic analgesia is consistently superior to no treatment but equivalent to relaxation and autogenic training for chronic pain conditions.

A number of important methodological issues surfaced in this review, the primary ones being the importance of measuring hypnotic suggestibility, controlling for nonspecific effects, and considering dose effects. Our findings suggest that acute and chronic pain represent disparate clinical issues for hypnotic analgesia; the treatment of chronic pain involves multidimensional assessment and treatment, and the clinician or hypnotist treating such problems should have an appreciation of the complexity of this problem. Although controlled clinical studies on hypnotic analgesia have substantial room for improvement, at this point the available evidence indicates that hypnosis is a viable intervention for both acute and chronic pain conditions.

References

Alden, P., & Heap, M. (1998). Hypnotic pain control. *International Journal of Clinical and Experimental Hypnosis, 46,* 62–76.

Anderson, J. A., Basker, M. A., & Dalton, R. (1975). Migraine and hypnotherapy. *International Journal of Clinical and Experimental Hypnosis, 23,* 48–58.

Andreychuk, T., & Skriver, C. (1975). Hypnosis and biofeedback in the treatment of migraine headache. *International Journal of Clinical and Experimental Hypnosis, 23,* 172–183.

Appel, P. R. (1992). The use of hypnosis in physical medicine and rehabilitation. *Psychiatric Medicine, 10,* 133–148.

Arendt-Nielsen, L., Zachariae, R., & Bjerring, P. (1990). Quantitative evaluation of hypnotically suggested hyperaesthesia and analgesia by painful laser stimulation. *Pain, 42,* 243–251.

Barabasz, A. F. (1982). Restricted environmental stimulation and the enhancement of hypnotizability: Pain, EEG alpha, skin conductance and temperature responses. *International Journal of Clinical and Experimental Hypnosis, 30,* 147–166.

Barabasz, A. F., & Barabasz, M. (1989). Effects of restricted environmental stimulation: Enhancement of hypnotizability for experimental and chronic pain control. *International Journal of Clinical and Experimental Hypnosis, 37,* 217–231.

Barabasz, A. F., & Lonsdale, C. (1983). Effects of hypnosis on P300 olfactory evoked potential amplitudes. *Journal of Abnormal Psychology, 92,* 520–523.

Barber, J. (1977). Rapid induction analgesia: A clinical report. *American Journal of Clinical Hypnosis, 19,* 138–147.

Barber, J. (1996). Hypnotic analgesia: Clinical considerations. In J. Barber (Ed.), *Hypnosis and suggestion in the treatment of pain* (pp. 85–118). New York: Norton.

Barber, J. (1998). The mysterious persistence of hypnotic analgesia. *International Journal of Clinical and Experimental Hypnosis, 46,* 28–43.

Barber, J., & Mayer, D. (1977) Evaluation of the efficacy and neural mechanism of a hypnotic analgesia procedure in experimental and clinical dental pain. *Pain, 4,* 41–48.

Barber, T. X., & Hahn, K. W. J. (1962). Physiological and subjective responses to pain-producing stimulation under hypnotically suggested and waking-imagined "analgesia." *Journal of Abnormal and Social Psychology, 65,* 411–415.

Barber, T. X., Spanos, N. P., & Chaves, J. F. (1974). *Hypnotism: Imagination and human potentialities.* Elmsford, NY: Pergamon Press.

Barsky, A. J., Goodson, D. K., & Lane, R. S. (1988). The amplification of somatic symptoms. *Psychosomatic Medicine, 50,* 510–519.

Bowers, K. S. (1990). Unconscious influences and hypnosis. In J. L. Singer (Ed.). *Repression and dissociation: Implications for personality theory, psychopathology, and health* (pp. 143–178). Chicago: University of Chicago Press.

Bowers, K. S. (1992). Imagination and dissociation in hypnotic responding. *International Journal of Clinical and Experimental Hypnosis, 40,* 253–275.

Bowers, K. S., & LeBaron, S. (1986). Hypnosis and hypnotizability: Implications for clinical intervention. *Hospital and Community Psychiatry, 37,* 457–467.

Bradley, L. A. (1996). Cognitive–behavioral therapy for chronic pain. In R. J. Gatchel & D. C. Turk (Eds.), *Psychological approaches to pain management: A practitioner's handbook* (pp. 131–147). New York: Guilford Press.

Braffman, W., & Kirsch, I. (1999). Imaginative suggestibility and hypnotizability: An empirical analysis. *Journal of Personality and Social Psychology, 77,* 578–587.

Campbell, D., & Stanley, J. (1963). Experimental and quasi-experimental designs for research on teaching. In N. Gage (Ed.), *Handbook of research on teaching* (pp. 171–246). Chicago: Rand McNally.

Chapman, C. R., Nakamura, Y., & Flores, L. Y. (1999). Chronic pain and consciousness: A constructivist perspective. In R. J. Gatchel & D. C. Turk (Eds.), *Psychosocial factors in pain: Critical perspectives* (pp. 35–55). New York: Guilford Press.

Chaves, J. F. (1986). Hypnosis in the management of phantom limb pain. In E. Dowd & J. Healy (Eds.), *Case studies in hypnotherapy* (pp. 198–209). New York: Guilford Press.

Chaves, J. F. (1989). Hypnotic control of clinical pain. In N. P. Spanos & J. F. Chaves (Eds.), *Hypnosis: The cognitive–behavioral perspective.* Buffalo, NY: Prometheus Books.

Chaves, J. F. (1993). Hypnosis in pain management. In J. W. Rhue, S. J. Lynn, & I. Kirsch (Eds.), *Handbook of clinical hypnosis.* Washington, DC: American Psychological Association.

Chaves, J. F. (1994). Recent advances in the application of hypnosis to pain management. *American Journal of Clinical Hypnosis, 37,* 117–129.

Chaves, J. F., & Barber, T. X. (1974). Acupuncture analgesia: A six factor theory. *Psychoenergetic Systems, 1,* 11–21.

Chaves, J. F., & Barber, T. X. (1976). Hypnotic procedures and surgery: A critical analysis with applications to acupuncture analgesia. *American Journal of Clinical Hypnosis, 18,* 217–236.

Chaves, J. F., & Brown, J. M. (1987). Spontaneous coping strategies for pain. *Journal of Behavioral Medicine, 10,* 263–276.

Chaves, J. F., & Dworkin, S. F. (1997). Hypnotic control of pain: Historical perspectives and future prospects. *International Journal of Clinical and Experimental Hypnosis, 45,* 356–376.

Chen, A. C. N., Chapman, C. R., & Harkins, S. W. (1979). Brain evoked potentials are functional correlates of induced pain in man. *Pain, 6,* 305–314.

Chibnall, J. T., & Duckro, P. N. (1994). Post-traumatic stress disorder in chronic post-traumatic headache patients. *Headache, 34,* 357–361.

Crasilneck, H. B. (1979). Hypnosis in the control of chronic low back pain. *American Journal of Clinical Hypnosis, 22,* 71–78.

Crasilneck, H. B. (1995). The use of the Crasilneck Bombardment Technique in problems of intractable organic pain. *American Journal of Clinical Hypnosis, 37,* 255–266.

Crasilneck, H. B., Stirman, J. A., & Wilson, B. J. (1955). Use of hypnosis in the management of patients with burns. *Journal of the American Medical Association, 158,* 103–106.

Crawford, H. J. (1990). Cognitive and psychophysiological correlates of hypnotic responsiveness and hypnosis. In M. L. Mass & D. Brown (Eds.), *Creative mastery in hypnosis and hypnoanalysis: A Festschrift for Erika Fromm* (pp. 47–54). Hillsdale, NJ: Erlbaum.

Crawford, H. J. (1994). Brain dynamics and hypnosis: Attentional and disattentional processes. *International Journal of Clinical and Experimental Hypnosis, 42,* 204–232.

Crawford, H. J., Knebel, T., Kaplan, L., Vendemia, J. M., Xie, M.,

Jamison, S., & Pribram, K. H. (1998). Hypnotic analgesia: 1. Somatosensory event-related potential changes to noxious stimuli and 2. Transfer learning to reduce chronic low back pain. *International Journal of Clinical and Experimental Hypnosis, 46,* 92–132.

Dane, J. R. (1996). Hypnosis for pain and neuromuscular rehabilitation with multiple sclerosis: Case summary, literature review, and analysis of outcomes. *International Journal of Clinical and Experimental Hypnosis, 44,* 208–231.

Danziger, N., Fournier, E., Bouhassira, D., Michaud, D., De Broucker, T., Santarcangelo, E., et al. (1998). Different strategies of modulation can be operative during hypnotic analgesia: A neurophysiological study. *Pain, 75,* 85–92.

Davidson, J. (1962). An assessment of the value of hypnosis in pregnancy and labor. *British Medical Journal, 2,* 951–952.

De Pascalis, V., Magurano, M. R., & Bellusci, A. (1999). Pain perception, somatosensory event-related potentials and skin conductance responses to painful stimuli in high, mid, and low hypnotizable subjects: Effects of differential pain reduction strategies. *Pain, 83,* 499–508.

De Pascalis, V., Magurano, M. R., Bellusci, A., & Chen, A. C. (2001). Somatosensory event-related potential and autonomic activity to varying pain reduction cognitive strategies in hypnosis. *Clinical Neurophysiology, 112,* 1475–1485.

De Pascalis, V., & Perrone, M. (1996). EEG asymmetry and heart rate during experience of hypnotic analgesia in high and low hypnotizables. *International Journal of Psychophysiology, 21,* 163–175.

Dinges, D. F., Whitehouse, W. G., Orne, E. C., Bloom, P. B., Carlin, M. M., Bauer, N. K., et al. (1997). Self-hypnosis training as an adjunctive treatment in the management of pain associated with sickle cell disease. *International Journal of Clinical and Experimental Hypnosis, 45,* 417–432.

Dingwall, E. J. (1967). *Abnormal hypnotic phenomena* (Vol. 1). London: Churchill.

Dixon, M., & Laurence, J. (1992). Two hundred years of hypnosis research: Questions resolved? Questions unanswered! In E. Fromm & M. R. Nash (Eds.), *Contemporary hypnosis research* (pp. 34–66). New York: Guilford Press.

Dynes, J. B. (1947). Objective method for distinguishing sleep from the hypnotic trance. *Neurological Psychiatry, 57,* 84–93.

Eastwood, J. D., Gaskovski, P., & Bowers, K. S. (1998). The folly of effort: Ironic effects in the mental control of pain. *International Journal of Clinical and Experimental Hypnosis, 46,* 77–91.

Edelson, J., & Fitzpatrick, J. L. (1989). A comparison of cognitive-behavioral and hypnotic treatments of chronic pain. *Journal of Clinical Psychology, 45,* 316–323.

Edmonston, W. E., Jr. (1991). Anesis. In S. J. Lynn & J. W. Rhue (Eds.), *Theories of hypnosis: Current models and perspectives* (pp. 197–237). New York: Guilford Press.

Erickson, M. (1980). *Innovative hypnotherapy* (Vol. 4). New York: Irvington.

Erickson, M., & Rossi, E. (1981). *Experiencing hypnosis: Therapeutic approaches to altered states.* New York: Irvington.

Erickson, M., Rossi, E., & Rossi, S. (1976). *Hypnotic realities: The induction of clinical hypnosis and forms of indirect suggestion.* New York. Irvington.

Esdaile, J. (1957). *Hypnosis in medicine and surgery.* New York: Julian Press.

Evans, F. J. (1989). Hypnosis and chronic pain. Two contrasting case studies. *Clinical Journal of Pain, 5,* 169–176.

Evans, M. B., & Paul, G. L. (1970). Effects of hypnotically suggested analgesia on physiological and subjective responses to cold stress. *Journal of Consulting and Clinical Psychology, 35,* 362–371.

Everett, J. J., Patterson, D. R., Burns, G. L., Montgomery, B. K., & Heimbach, D. M. (1993). Adjunctive interventions for burn pain control: Comparison of hypnosis and Ativan: The 1993 Clinical Research Award. *Journal of Burn Care and Rehabilitation, 14,* 676–683.

Ewin, D. M. (1983). Emergency room hypnosis for the burned patient. *American Journal of Clinical Hypnosis, 26,* 5–8.

Ewin, D. M. (1984). Hypnosis in surgery and anesthesia. In W. C. Wester II & A. H. Smith Jr. (Eds.), *Clinical hypnosis: A multidisciplinary approach.* Philadelphia: Lippincott.

Ewin, D. M. (1986). Emergency room hypnosis for the burned patient. *American Journal of Clinical Hypnosis, 29,* 7–12.

Faymonville, M. E., Mambourg, P. H., Joris, J., Vrijens, B., Fissette, J., Albert, A., & Lamy, M. (1997). Psychological approaches during conscious sedation. Hypnosis versus stress reducing strategies: A prospective randomized study. *Pain, 73,* 361–367.

Finer, B., & Graf, K. (1968). Circulatory changes accompanying hypnotic imagination of hyperalgesia and hypoalgésia in causalgic limbs. *Zeitschrift fur die Gesamte experimentelle Medizin einschliesslich experimentelle Chirurgie, 146,* 97–114.

Finer, B. L., & Nylen, B. O. (1961). Cardiac arrest in the treatment of burns, and report on hypnosis as a substitute for anesthesia. *Plastic and Reconstructive Surgery, 27,* 49–55.

Flowers, C. E., Littlejohn, T. W., & Wells, H. B. (1960). Pharmacologic and hypnoid analgesia: Effect upon labor and the infant response. *Obstetrics and Gynecology, 16,* 210–221.

Fordyce, W. E. (1976). *Behavioral methods for chronic pain and illness.* St. Louis: Mosby Year Book.

Fordyce, W. E. (1988). Pain and suffering. *American Psychologist, 43,* 276–283.

Freeman, R., Barabasz, A., Barabasz, M., & Warner, D. (2000). Hypnosis and distraction differ in their effects on cold pressor pain. *American Journal of Clinical Hypnosis, 43,* 137–148.

Freeman, R. M., Macaulay, A. J., Eve, L., Chamberlain, G. V., & Bhat, A. V. (1986). Randomised trial of self hypnosis for analgesia in labour. *British Medical Journal (Clinical Research Ed.), 292,* 657–658.

Friedman, H., & Taub, H. A. (1984). Brief psychological training procedures in migraine treatment. *American Journal of Clinical Hypnosis, 26,* 187–200.

Gainer, M. J. (1992). Hypnotherapy for reflex sympathetic dystrophy. *American Journal of Clinical Hypnosis, 34,* 227–232.

Gatchel, R. J., & Epker, J. (1999). Psychosocial predictors of chronic pain and response to treatment. In R. J. Gatchel & D. C. Turk (Eds.), *Psychosocial factors in pain: Clinical perspectives* (pp. 412–434). New York: Guilford Press.

Geisser, M. E., Roth, R. S., Bachman, J. E., & Eckert, T. A. (1996). The relationship between symptoms of post-traumatic stress disorder and pain, affective disturbance and disability among patients with accident and non-accident related pain. *Pain, 66,* 207–214.

Gilboa, D., Borenstein, A., Seidman, D., & Tsur, H. (1990). Burn patients' use of autohypnosis: Making a painful experience bearable. *Burns, 16,* 441–444.

Gillett, P. L., & Coe, W. C. (1984). The effects of rapid induction analgesia (RIA), hypnotic susceptibility and the severity of discomfort on reducing dental pain. *American Journal of Clinical Hypnosis, 27,* 81–90.

Goldstein, A., & Hilgard, E. R. (1975). Lack of influence of the morphine antagonist naloxone on hypnotic analgesia. *Proceedings of the National Academy of Sciences, 72,* 2041–2043.

Greene, R. J., & Reyher, J. (1972). Pain tolerance in hypnotic analgesic and imagination states. *Journal of Abnormal Psychology, 79,* 29–38.

Gruzelier, J., Allison, J., & Conway, A. (1988). A psychophysiological differentiation between hypnotic behaviour and simulation. *International Journal of Psychophysiology, 6,* 331–338.

Haanen, H. C., Hoenderdos, H. T., van Romunde, L. K., Hop, W. C., Mallee, C., Terwiel, J. P., & Hekster, G. B. (1991). Controlled trial of hypnotherapy in the treatment of refractory fibromyalgia. *Journal of Rheumatology, 18,* 72–75.

Halliday, A. M., & Mason, A. A. (1964). Cortical evoked potentials during hypnotic anaesthesia. *Electroencephalography and Clinical Neurophysiology, 16,* 312–314.

Hargadon, R., Bowers, K. S., & Woody, E. Z. (1995). Does counterpain imagery mediate hypnotic analgesia? *Journal of Abnormal Psychology, 104,* 508–516.

Harmon, T. M., Hynan, M. T., & Tyre, T. E. (1990). Improved obstetric outcomes using hypnotic analgesia and skill mastery combined with childbirth education. *Journal of Consulting and Clinical Psychology, 58,* 525–530.

Hartland, J. (1971). *Medical and dental hypnosis.* Baltimore: Williams & Wilkins.

Hernandez-Peon, R., Dittborn, J., Borlone, M., & Davidovich, A. (1960). Modifications of a forearm skin reflex during hypnotically induced anesthesia and hyperesthisia. *Acta Neurológica Latinoamericana, 6,* 32–42.

Hilgard, E. R. (1967). A quantitative study of pain and its reduction through hypnotic suggestion. *Proceedings of the National Academy of Sciences, 57,* 1581–1586.

Hilgard, E. R. (1969). Pain as a puzzle for psychology and physiology. *American Psychologist, 24,* 103–113.

Hilgard, E. R., & Hilgard, J. R. (1975). *Hypnosis in the relief of pain.* Los Altos, CA: Kaufmann.

Hilgard, E. R., & Morgan, A. H. (1975). Heart rate and blood pressure in the study of laboratory pain in man under normal conditions and as influenced by hypnosis. *Acta Neurobiologiae Experimentalis, 35,* 741–759.

Hilgard, J. R., & LeBaron, S. (1984). *Hypnotherapy of pain in children with cancer.* Los Altos, CA: Kaufman.

Hofbauer, R. K., Rainville, P., Duncan, G. H., & Bushnell, M. C. (1998). Cortical representation of the sensory dimension of pain. *Journal of Neurophysiology, 86,* 402–411.

Holroyd, J. (1996). Hypnosis treatment of clinical pain: Understanding why hypnosis is useful. *International Journal of Clinical and Experimental Hypnosis, 44,* 33–51.

Holroyd, K. A., & Penzien, D. B. (1990). Pharmacological versus non-pharmacological prophylaxis of recurrent migraine headache: A meta-analytic review of clinical trials. *Pain, 42,* 1–13.

Holzman, A. D., Turk, D. C., & Kerns, R. D. (1986). The cognitive–behavioral approach to the management of chronic pain. In A. D. Holzman & D. C. Turk (Eds.), *Pain management: A handbook of psychological treatment approaches* (pp. 31–50). New York: Pergamon Press.

Iserson, K. V. (1999). Hypnosis for pediatric fracture reduction. *Journal of Emergency Medicine, 17,* 53–66.

Jack, M. S. (1999). The use of hypnosis for a patient with chronic pain. *Contemporary Hypnosis, 16,* 231–237.

James, F. R., Large, R. G., & Beale, I. L. (1989). Self-hypnosis in chronic pain. A multiple baseline study of five highly hypnotisable subjects. *Clinical Journal of Pain, 5,* 161–168.

Jensen, M., & Barber, J. (2000). Hypnotic analgesia of spinal cord injury pain. *Australian Journal of Clinical and Experimental Hypnosis, 28,* 150–168.

Jensen, M., Barber, J., Williams-Avery, R., Flores, L., & Brown, M. (2001). The effect of hypnotic suggestion on spinal cord injury pain. *Journal of Back and Musculoskeletal Rehabilitation, 14,* 3–10.

Jensen, M. P. (1996). Enhancing motivation to change in pain treatment. In R. J. Gatchel & D. C. Turk (Eds.), *Psychological approaches to pain management: A practitioner's handbook* (pp. 78–111). New York: Guilford Press.

Jensen, M. P., Turner, J. A., Romano, J. M., & Lawler, B. K. (1994). Relationship of pain-specific beliefs to chronic pain adjustment. *Pain, 57,* 301–309.

Katz, E. R., Kellerman, J., & Ellenberg, L. (1987). Hypnosis in the reduction of acute pain and distress in children with cancer. *Journal of Pediatric Psychology, 12,* 379–394.

Kazdin, A. E. (1979). Nonspecific treatment factors in psychotherapy outcome research. *Journal of Consulting and Clinical Psychology, 47,* 846–851.

Kerns, R. D., & Rosenberg, R. (2000). Predicting responses to self-management treatments for chronic pain: Application of the pain stages of change model. *Pain, 84,* 49–55.

Kiernan, B., Dane, J., Phillips, L., & Price, D. (1995). Hypnotic analgesia reduces R-III nociceptive reflex: Further evidence concerning the multifactorial nature of hypnotic analgesia. *Pain, 60,* 39–47.

Kihlstrom, J. F. (1985). Hypnosis. *Annual Review of Psychology, 36,* 385–418.

Kihlstrom, J. F. (1992). Hypnosis: A sesquicentennial essay. *International Journal of Clinical and Experimental Hypnosis, 50,* 301–314.

Kirsch, I., & Lynn, S. J. (1995). The altered state of hypnosis. *American Psychologist, 50,* 846–858.

Kirsch, I., Montgomery, G., & Sapirstein, G. (1995). Hypnosis as an adjunct to cognitive–behavioral psychotherapy: A meta-analysis. *Journal of Consulting and Clinical Psychology, 63,* 214–220.

Knox, V. J., Gekoski, W. L., Shum, K., & McLaughlin, D. M. (1981). Analgesia for experimentally induced pain: Multiple sessions of acupuncture compared to hypnosis in high- and low-susceptible subjects. *Journal of Abnormal Psychology, 90,* 28–34.

Knox, V. J., Handfield-Jones, C. E., & Shum, K. (1979). Subject expectancy and the reduction of cold pressor pain with acupuncture and placebo acupuncture. *Psychosomatic Medicine, 41,* 477–486.

Knox, V. J., Morgan, A. H., & Hilgard, E. R. (1974). Pain and suffering in ischemia: The paradox of hypnotically suggested anesthesia as contradicted by reports from the "hidden observer." *Archives of General Psychiatry, 30,* 840–847.

Knox, V. J., & Shum, K. (1977). Reduction of cold-pressor pain with acupuncture analgesia in high- and low-hypnotic subjects. *Journal of Abnormal Psychology, 86,* 639–643.

Kroptov, E. A. (1997). Somatosensory. *International Journal of Psychophysiology, 27,* 1–8.

Kuttner, L. (1988). Favorite stories: A hypnotic pain-reduction technique for children in acute pain. *American Journal of Clinical Hypnosis, 30,* 289–295.

Lambert, S. (1996). The effects of hypnosis/guided imagery on the post-operative course of children. *Developmental and Behavioral Pediatrics, 17,* 307–310.

Lang, E. V., Benotsch, E. G., Fick, L. J., Lutgendorf, S., Berbaum, M. L., Berbaum, K. S., et al. (2000). Adjunctive non-pharmacological analgesia for invasive medical procedures: A randomised trial. *Lancet, 355,* 1486–1490.

Lang, E. V., Joyce, J. S., Spiegel, D., Hamilton, D., & Lee, K. K. (1996). Self-hypnotic relaxation during interventional radiological procedures: Effects on pain perception and intravenous drug use *International Journal of Clinical and Experimental Hypnosis, 44,* 106–119.

Lenox, J. R. (1970). Effect of hypnotic analgesia on verbal report and cardiovascular responses to ischemic pain. *Journal of Abnormal Psychology, 75,* 199–206.

Levitt, E. E. (1993). Hypnosis in the treatment of obesity. In J. W. Rhue, S. J. Lynn, & I. Kirsch (Eds.), *Handbook of clinical hypnosis* (pp. 533–553). Washington, DC: American Psychological Association.

Liossi, C., & Hatira, P. (1999). Clinical hypnosis versus cognitive behavioral training for pain management with pediatric cancer patients undergoing bone marrow aspirations *International Journal of Clinical and Experimental Hypnosis, 47,* 104–116.

Loeser, J. D. (1982). Concepts of pain. In M. Stanton-Hicks & R. Boas (Eds.), *Chronic low back pain* (pp. 145–148). New York: Raven.

Malone, M. D., & Strube, M. J. (1988). Meta-analysis of non-medical treatments for chronic pain. *Pain, 34,* 231–244.

Mauer, M. H., Burnett, K. F., Ouellette, E. A., Ironson, G. H., & Dandes, H. M. (1999). Medical hypnosis and orthopedic hand surgery: Pain perception, postoperative recovery, and therapeutic comfort. *International Journal of Clinical and Experimental Hypnosis, 47,* 144–161.

McGlashan, T. H., Evans, F. J., & Orne, M. T. (1969). The nature of hypnotic analgesia and placebo response to experimental pain. *Psychosomatic Medicine, 31,* 227–246.

Meier, W., Klucken, M., Soyka, D., & Bromm, B. (1993). Hypnotic hypo- and hyperalgesia: Divergent effects on pain ratings and pain-related cerebral potentials. *Pain, 53,* 175–181.

Melis, P. M., Rooimans, W., Spierings, E. L., & Hoogduin, C. A. (1991). Treatment of chronic tension-type headache with hypnotherapy: A single-blind time controlled study. *Headache, 31,* 686–689.

Melzack, R. (1990, February). The tragedy of needless pain. *Scientific American, 262,* 27–33.

Melzack, R., & Perry, C. (1975). Self-regulation of pain: The use of alpha-feedback and hypnotic training for the control of chronic pain. *Experimental Neurology, 46,* 452–469.

Melzack, R., & Wall, P. (1973). *The challenge of pain.* New York: Basic Books.

Meszaros, I., Banyai, E. I., & Greguss, A. C. (1980). Evoked potential, reflecting hypnotically altered state of consciousness. In G. Adam, I. Meszaros, & E. I. Banyai (Eds.), *Advances in physiological sciences: Vol. 17. Brain behavior* (pp. 467–475). Oxford, England: Pergamon.

Miller, M. F., Barabasz, A. F., & Barabasz, M. (1991). Effects of active alert and relaxation hypnotic inductions on cold pressor pain. *Journal of Abnormal Psychology, 100,* 223–226.

Montgomery, G. H., DuHamel, K. N., & Redd, W. H. (2000). A meta-analysis of hypnotically induced analgesia: How effective is hypnosis? *International Journal of Clinical and Experimental Hypnosis, 48,* 138–153.

Morgan, A. H., & Hilgard, J. R. (1978–1979a). The Stanford Hypnotic Clinical Scale for Adults. *American Journal of Clinical Hypnosis, 21*(2–3), 134–147.

Morgan, A. H., & Hilgard, J. R. (1978–1979b). The Stanford Hypnotic Clinical Scale for Children. *American Journal of Clinical Hypnosis, 21*(2–3), 148–169.

Moya, F., & James, L. S. (1960). Medical hypnosis for obstetrics. *Journal of the American Medical Association, 174,* 80–86.

Patterson, D. R. (2001). Is hypnotic pain control effortless or effortful? *Hypnos, 28,* 132–134.

Patterson, D. R., Adcock, R. J., & Bombardier, C. H. (1997). Factors predicting hypnotic analgesia in clinical burn pain. *International Journal of Clinical and Experimental Hypnosis, 45,* 377–395.

Patterson, D. R., Everett, J. J., Burns, G. L., & Marvin, J. A. (1992). Hypnosis for the treatment of burn pain. *Journal of Consulting and Clinical Psychology, 60,* 713–717.

Patterson, D. R., & Ptacek, J. T. (1997). Baseline pain as a moderator of hypnotic analgesia for burn injury treatment. *Journal of Consulting and Clinical Psychology, 65,* 60–67.

Patterson, D. R., Questad, K. A., & Boltwood, M. D. (1987). Hypnotherapy as a treatment for pain in patients with burns: Research and clinical considerations. *Journal of Burn Care and Rehabilitation, 8,* 263–268.

Patterson, D. R., Questad, K. A., & DeLateur, B. J. (1989). Hypnotherapy as an adjunct to pharmacologies for the treatment of pain from burn debridement. *American Journal of Clinical Hypnosis, 31,* 156–163.

Price, D. D., & Barber, J. (1987). An analysis of factors that contribute to the efficacy of hypnotic analgesia. *Journal of Abnormal Psychology, 96,* 46–51.

Price, D. D., & Barrell, J. J. (2000). Mechanisms of analgesia produced by hypnosis and placebo suggestions. In E. A. Mayer & C. B. Saper (Eds.), *Progress in brain research* (Vol. 122, pp. 255–271). New York: Elsevier Science.

Price, D. D., Harkins, S. W., & Baker, C. (1987). Sensory-affective relationships among different types of clinical and experimental pain. *Pain, 28,* 297–307.

Rainville, P., Carrier, B., Hofbauer, R. K., Bushnell, M. C., & Duncan, G. H. (1999). Dissociation of sensory and affective dimensions of pain using hypnotic modulation. *Pain, 82,* 159–171.

Rainville, P., Duncan, G. H., Price, D. D., Carrier, B., & Bushnell, M. C. (1997, August 15). Pain affect encoded in human anterior cingulate but not somatosensory cortex. *Science, 277,* 968–971.

Rausch, V. (1980). Cholecystectomy with self-hypnosis. *American Journal of Clinical Hypnosis, 22,* 124–129.

Romano, J. M., & Turner, J. A. (1985). Chronic pain and depression: Does the evidence support a relationship? *Psychological Bulletin, 97,* 18–34.

Sacerdote, P. (1978). Teaching self-hypnosis to patients with chronic pain. *Journal of Human Stress, 4,* 18–21.

Schlutter, L. C., Golden, C. J., & Blume, H. G. (1980). A comparison of treatments for prefrontal muscle contraction headache. *British Journal of Medical Psychology, 53,* 47–52.

Sharav, Y., & Tal, M. (1989). Masseter inhibitory periods and sensations evoked by electrical tooth-pulp stimulation in subjects under hypnotic anesthesia. *Brain Research, 479,* 247–254.

Shor, R. E. (1962). Physiological effects of painful stimulation during hypnotic analgesia under conditions designed to minimize anxiety. *International Journal of Clinical and Experimental Hypnosis, 10,* 183–202.

Siegel, E. F. (1979). Control of phantom limb pain by hypnosis. *American Journal of Clinical Hypnosis, 21,* 285–286.

Simon, E. P., & Lewis, D. M. (2000). Medical hypnosis for temporomandibular disorders: Treatment efficacy and medical utilization outcome. *Oral Surgery, Oral Medicine, Oral Pathology, Oral Radiology, and Endodontics, 90,* 54–63.

Smith, J. T., Barabasz, A., & Barabasz, M. (1996). Comparison of hypnosis and distraction in severely ill children undergoing painful medical procedures. *Journal of Counseling Psychology, 42,* 187–195.

Smith, S. J., & Balaban, A. B. (1983). A multidimensional approach to pain relief: Case report of a patient with systemic lupus erythematosus. *International Journal of Clinical and Experimental Hypnosis, 31,* 72–81.

Spanos, N. P. (1986). Hypnotic behavior: A social psychological interpretation of amnesia, analgesia and trance logic. *Behavioral and Brain Sciences, 9,* 449–467.

Spanos, N. P., & Chaves, J. F. (1989a). The cognitive–behavioral alternative in hypnosis research. In N. P. Spanos & J. F. Chaves (Eds.), *Hypnosis: The cognitive–behavioral perspective* (pp. 9–16). Buffalo, NY: Prometheus Books.

Spanos, N. P., & Chaves, J. F. (1989b). Future prospects for the cognitive–behavioral perspective. In N. P. Spanos & J. F. Chaves (Eds.), *Hypnosis: The cognitive–behavioral perspective* (pp. 437–446). Buffalo, NY: Prometheus Books.

Spanos, N. P., & Chaves, J. F. (1989c). Hypnotic analgesia, surgery and reports of nonvolitional pain reduction. *British Journal of Experimental and Clinical Hypnosis, 6,* 131–139.

Spanos, N. P., & Katsanis, J. (1989). Effects of instructional set on attributions of nonvolition during hypnotic and nonhypnotic analgesia. *Journal of Personality and Social Psychology, 56,* 182–188.

Spanos, N. P., Kennedy, S. K., & Gwynn, M. I. (1984). Moderating effects of contextual variables on the relationship between hypnotic susceptibility and suggested analgesia. *Journal of Abnormal Psychology, 93,* 285–294.

Spanos, N. P., Perlini, A. H., Patrick, L., Bell, S., & Gwynn, M. I. (1990). The role of compliance in hypnotic and nonhypnotic analgesia. *Journal of Research in Personality, 24,* 433–453.

Spiegel, D., Bierre, P., & Rootenberg, J. (1989). Hypnotic alteration of somatosensory perception. *American Journal of Psychiatry, 146,* 749–754.

Spiegel, D., & Bloom, J. R. (1983). Group therapy and hypnosis reduce metastatic breast carcinoma pain. *Psychosomatic Medicine, 45*, 333–339.

Spiegel, H., & Bridger, A. A. (1970). *Manual for Hypnotic Induction Profile: Eye-roll levitation method.* New York: Soni Medica.

Spiegel, H., & Spiegel, D. (1978). *Trance and treatment.* Washington, DC: American Psychiatric Press.

Spinhoven, P. (1988). Similarities and dissimilarities in hypnotic and nonhypnotic procedures for headache control: A review. *American Journal of Clinical Hypnosis, 30*, 183–194.

Spinhoven, P., Linssen, A. C., Van Dyck, R., & Zitman, F. G. (1992). Autogenic training and self-hypnosis in the control of tension headache. *General Hospital Psychiatry, 14*, 408–415.

Stern, J. A., Brown, M., Ulett, G. A., & Sletten, I. (1977). A comparison of hypnosis, acupuncture, morphine, valium, aspirin, and placebo in the management of experimentally induced pain. In W. E. Edmonston Jr. (Ed.), *Annals of the New York Academy of Sciences: Vol. 296. Conceptual and investigative approaches to hypnosis and hypnotic phenomena* (pp. 175–193). New York: New York Academy of Sciences.

Stowell, H. (1984). Event related brain potentials and human pain: A first objective overview. *International Journal of Psychophysiology, 1*, 137–151.

Sutcher, H. (1997). Hypnosis as adjunctive therapy for multiple sclerosis: A progress report. *American Journal of Clinical Hypnosis, 39*, 283–290.

Sutcliffe, J. P. (1961). "Credulous" and "skeptical" views of hypnotic phenomena: Experiments in esthesia, hallucination, and delusion. *Journal of Abnormal and Social Psychology, 62*, 189–200.

Syrjala, K. L., Cummings, C., & Donaldson, G. W. (1992). Hypnosis or cognitive behavioral training for the reduction of pain and nausea during cancer treatment: A controlled clinical trial. *Pain, 48*, 137–146.

Tan, S. (1982). Cognitive and cognitive–behavioural methods for pain control: A selective review. *Pain, 12*, 201–228.

ter Kuile, M. M., Spinhoven, P., Linssen, A. C., Zitman, F. G., Van Dyck, R., & Rooijmans, H. G. (1994). Autogenic training and cognitive self-hypnosis for the treatment of recurrent headaches in three different subject groups. *Pain, 58*, 331–340.

Turk, D. C., & Flor, H. (1999). Chronic pain: A biobehavioral perspective. In R. J. Gatchel & D. C. Turk (Eds.), *Psychosocial factors in pain: Critical perspectives* (pp. 18–34). New York: Guilford Press.

Turk, D. C., & Okifuji, A. (1998). Treatment of chronic pain patients: Clinical outcomes, cost-effectiveness, and cost-benefits of multidisciplinary pain centers. *Critical Reviews in Physical and Rehabilitation Medicine, 10*, 181–208.

Turner, J. A., & Chapman, C. R. (1982). Psychological interventions for chronic pain: A critical review. II. Operant conditioning, hypnosis, and cognitive–behavioral therapy. *Pain, 12*, 23–46.

Turner, J. A., & Romano, J. M. (2001). Cognitive–behavioral therapy for chronic pain. In J. D. Loeser, S. H. Butler, C. R Chapman, & D. C. Turk (Eds.). *Bonica's management of pain* (3rd ed., pp. 1751–1758). Philadelphia: Lippincott Williams & Wilkins.

Wadden, T. A., & Bell, S. T. (1990). Obesity. In A. S. Bellack, M. Hersen, & A. E. Kazdin (Eds.), *International handbook of behavior modification and therapy* (2nd ed., pp. 449–473). New York: Plenum Press.

Wakeman, J. R., & Kaplan, J. Z. (1978). An experimental study of hypnosis in painful burns. *American Journal of Clinical Hypnosis, 21*, 3–12.

Weinstein, E. J., & Au, P. K. (1991). Use of hypnosis before and during angioplasty. *American Journal of Clinical Hypnosis. 34*, 29–37.

Weitzenhoffer, A. M., & Hilgard, E. R. (1959). *Stanford Hypnotic Susceptibility Scale Forms A & B.* Palo Alto, CA: Consulting Psychologists Press.

West, L. J., Niell, K. C., & Hardy, J. D. (1952). Effects of hypnotic suggestion on pain perception and galvanic skin response. *American Medical Association Archives of Neurology and Psychiatry, 68*, 549–569.

Williams, D. A. (1999). Acute pain (with special emphasis on painful medical procedures). In R. J. Gatchel & D. C. Turk (Eds.), *Psychosocial factors in pain: Critical perspectives* (pp. 151–163). New York: Guilford Press.

Wilson, L., Dworkin, S. F., Whitney, C., & LeResche, L. (1994) Somatization and pain dispersion in chronic temporomandibular disorder pain. *Pain, 57*, 55–61.

Wright, B. R., & Drummond, P. D. (2000). Rapid induction analgesia for the alleviation of procedural pain during burn care. *Burns, 26*, 275–282.

Yapko, M. (1992). *Hypnosis and the treatment of depressions.* New York: Brunner/Mazel.

Zachariae, R., & Bjerring, P. (1994). Laser-induced pain-related brain potentials and sensory pain ratings in high and low hypnotizable subjects during hypnotic suggestions of relaxation, dissociated imagery, focused analgesia, and placebo. *International Journal of Clinical and Experimental Hypnosis, 42*, 56–80.

Zeltzer, L., & LeBaron, S. (1982). Hypnosis and nonhypnotic techniques for reduction of pain and anxiety during painful procedures in children and adolescents with cancer. *Journal of Pediatrics, 101*, 1032–1035.

Zitman, F. G., Van Dyck, R., Spinhoven, P., & Linssen, A. C. (1992). Hypnosis and autogenic training in the treatment of tension headaches: A two-phase constructive design study with follow-up. *Journal of Psychosomatic Research, 36*, 219–228.

Received April 26, 2001
Revision received July 31, 2002
Accepted November 12, 2002 ■

Part VIII
Professional and Legal Issues

[29]

Scientific Status of Refreshing Recollection by the Use of Hypnosis

Council on Scientific Affairs

• The Council finds that recollections obtained during hypnosis can involve confabulations and pseudomemories and not only fail to be more accurate, but actually appear to be less reliable than nonhypnotic recall. The use of hypnosis with witnesses and victims may have serious consequences for the legal process when testimony is based on material that is elicited from a witness who has been hypnotized for the purposes of refreshing recollection.

(*JAMA* 1985;253:1918-1923)

THE USE of hypnosis by appropriately trained physicians or psychologists has been recognized as a valid therapeutic modality by the American Medical Association since 1958.[1] No such consensus exists regarding the use of hypnosis as a means to refresh memory. There have been increasingly frequent attempts, however, to utilize hypnosis to aid witnesses and victims to remember forgotten details and to testify to these recollections. Similarly, confessions[2-4] have been obtained from hypnotized suspects, mitigating circumstances[5] (including exoneration[6,7]) have been elicited from defendants, and information[8] has been reported by plaintiffs who were hypnotized to overcome presumed amnesia.

Considerable controversy[9] has developed concerning the validity of using hypnosis in this manner. Some appellate courts have held that hypnotically refreshed memory may form the basis for testimony, and it is up to the judge or jury to consider the possible difficulties introduced by hypnosis in determining the weight of the evidence.[10,11] Other courts have held that no individual who has ever been hypnotized should be allowed to testify concerning a matter where memory has been "refreshed" during hypnosis.[12,13] Still others have ruled that specific guidelines on the way hypnosis is carried out must be followed to assess whether in any given instance testimony based upon hypnotically refreshed recollections is admissible.[14,15]

The charge of the Panel was to evaluate the scientific evidence concerning the effect of hypnosis on memory. (The Panel limited its deliberations to hetero-hypnosis [where both a hypnotist and a subject are involved]. Self-hypnosis or spontaneous hypnosis may occur. There is anecdotal evidence that memory may be affected by these other hypnotic states. However, there is no empirical evidence with which to evaluate such effects at this time.) Accordingly, the Panel did not deal with legal cases or with questions where no scientific data are available, but rather focused on the effects of hypnosis on memory reports under a variety of conditions. Since there is an appreciable amount of literature on this topic and a diversity of views within the Panel, the scientific literature on the following aspects of this question was carefully reviewed: (1) memory during hypnotic age regression, (2) hypnotic enhancement of rote memory, (3) hypnotic enhancement of recognition memory for meaningful and complex material, (4) hypnotic enhancement of recall memory for meaningful and complex material, (5) hypnotic enhancement of memory for analogue events, (6) clinical case and field reports, and (7) pertinent reviews of the literature.

Throughout its deliberations, the Panel recognized that the situation in the real world rarely allows a reliable assessment of the accuracy of recall since it is very difficult and sometimes impossible to be certain what really happened. Thus, useful data cannot be obtained in life situations unless a hypnotic memory report leads to clearly independent physical evidence.

Only in controlled studies is it known what the individual actually observed and is it possible to compare the accuracy of memory in the non-

This report was prepared by a panel of the Council on Scientific Affairs consisting of Martin T. Orne, MD, PhD, Chairman; A David Axelrad, MD; Bernard L. Diamond, MD; Melvin A. Gravitz, PhD; Abraham Heller, MD; Charles B. Mutter, MD; David Spiegel, MD; and Herbert Spiegel, MD. Rogers J. Smith, MD, served as liaison from the Council on Scientific Affairs. Matthew H. Erdelyi, PhD, John F. Kihlstrom, PhD, and Donald Rossi, PhD, participated as consultants to the Panel, and John M. Bradford, MBChB, DPM, participated as a resource person. Frederick J Evans, PhD (Society for Clinical and Experimental Hypnosis); Fred H. Frankel, MBChB, DPM (International Society of Hypnosis); and Harold J. Wain, PhD (American Society of Clinical Hypnosis), served as liaisons to the Panel from their respective societies. Janice Hutchinson, MD, was secretary to the Panel.

From the Council on Scientific Affairs, American Medical Association, Chicago

Resolution 5 (A-82), adopted unanimously by the House of Delegates on Dec 5, 1984, and referred by the Board of Trustees to the Council on Scientific Affairs, called upon the American Medical Association to "study the subject of refreshing recollection by the use of hypnosis of witnesses and victims of crime, and prepare a report on the present scientific status of this matter"

This report is not intended to be construed or to serve as a standard of medical care Standards of medical care are determined on the basis of all of the facts and circumstances involved in an individual case and are subject to change as scientific knowledge and technology advance and patterns of practice evolve This report reflects the views of scientific experts and reports in the scientific literature as of December 1984

Reprint requests to Council on Scientific Affairs, American Medical Association, 535 N Dearborn St, Chicago, IL 60610 (John C. Ballin, PhD).

hypnotic state and in hypnosis. Although these studies are relevant to the use of hypnosis for memory enhancement in uninvolved witnesses, it must be recognized that they may not reproduce the level of motivation and the intensity of feeling that can be aroused by some criminal acts.

THE NATURE OF HYPNOSIS

There is no single, generally accepted theory of hypnosis, nor is there consensus about a single definition. Despite some controversy on technical points among experts, most authorities agree that hypnosis requires at least superficial cooperation of the subject, the development of rapport, and the subject's focusing of attention. Typically, some form of induction procedure or "ceremony" is carried out that is believed by both doctor and patient to be effective in bringing about hypnosis, after which the subject becomes increasingly responsive to the explicit and implicit suggestions of the hypnotist (or someone designated by the hypnotist). During this process, the subject is invited to suspend critical judgment and to accept rather than to question the suggestions given.

When hypnosis has been established, it can be recognized by administering a series of different test suggestions of varying degrees of known difficulty, typically involving alterations of perception, motor control, or memory. The degree to which these suggestions are followed and experienced as real and involuntary indicates the extent to which hypnosis has taken place. Although different theorists account for the phenomena of hypnosis in different ways, there is consensus that these events occur, are real to the subject, and may be utilized clinically.

Modern research, both in the laboratory[16] and in the field[17,18] has documented that individuals differ in their ability to experience hypnosis and that this difference is a relatively stable trait, although even highly hypnotizable subjects can choose not to respond (or not to respond as well as they are able). Most but not all individuals are able to experience some degree of hypnosis.

Thus, hypnosis involves the focusing of attention; increased responsiveness to suggestions; suspension of disbelief with a lowering of critical judgment; potential for altering perception, motor control, or memory in response to suggestions; and the subjective experience of responding involuntarily.

SCIENTIFIC EVIDENCE CONCERNING HYPNOTICALLY REFRESHED MEMORY

Hypnosis has been used in an attempt to refresh memory in two major ways. The first derives from its use in psychotherapy and involves hypnotic age regression; the hypnotized individual is asked to relive an experience or emotion that may not be consciously recalled. The second involves suggesting to the hypnotized individual, directly or indirectly through the use of metaphors, that specific events or information be remembered; this approach is the one most often used with victims and witnesses when hypnosis is employed to refresh recall.

Memory During Hypnotic Age Regression

The use of hypnosis to reexperience affect associated with a traumatic event goes back well over a century. In hypnotic age regression, patients may behave in a manner that seems appropriate to the age at which the traumatic event appeared to have occurred. Their recollections are generally related to past traumatic events, and under hypnosis they may relive these events with intense affect. Characteristically, patients may describe a myriad of details (such as the expression on a parent's face or a spot on the carpet) that would not be accessible to someone who had not been present at the suggested time. Finally, patients often obtain relief of symptoms related to events relived during the session.

This phenomenon was sufficiently compelling to convince Freud initially that hypnotic recollections represented an accurate portrayal of past events. He eventually recognized,[19] however, that these remembrances reflected an emotional reality but were not necessarily historically accurate—rather, they were generally a combination of fantasies, desires, and fears as well as actual recollections of different periods of time.

Much of the more recent research on hypnotic age regression has sought to establish that the individual actually reexperienced past events and functioned both psychologically and physiologically at the age that he appeared to be reliving. Although this claim has not been supported by carefully controlled scientific studies,[20] there is still some controversy about this matter based on single case reports.[21]

The aspect of age regression that is directly relevant to the Panel's deliberations concerns the historical accuracy of the recalled material. In clinical practice, it is often difficult to verify independently even a few novel details that the patient reports in hypnosis (and one cannot assume, because one or another detail might have been correct, that other details that are not verified are also correct). Controlled laboratory studies that have attempted in various ways to verify the accuracy of recall in hypnotic age regression have not supported the claims of single case reports. It is the consensus of the Panel that hypnotic age regression is the subjective reliving of earlier experiences as though they were real—which does not necessarily replicate earlier events.

Hypnotically Suggested Increased Recall

A hypnotic procedure to refresh recall that is frequently used with victims and witnesses is the "television technique."[22] Prior to hypnosis, it is explained to the subject that everything a person sees, hears, or experiences is recorded in the subconscious and can be accurately accessed in hypnosis. Once hypnotized, the subject is told to imagine a television screen in his mind and that he will soon begin to see a documentary of the to-be-remembered event. As in a sporting event on television, he will be able to stop motion, go fast forward or backward, and "zoom in" in order to see any detail that might otherwise not be clear. Finally, it is explained that, while he may see himself in this documentary and accurately observe what happens, he need not experience any of the troublesome feelings or pain that may have occurred at the time, but rather will see in an objective manner the events that transpired.

The "television technique" is not merely presented to the subject as a metaphor, but rather represents a belief of how memory is organized and is the premise for assuming that hypnosis can actually refresh memory. The author and main proponent of this technique states: "The subconscious mind is alert and on duty 24 hours a day, seven days a week; it never sleeps."[22(p11)] "Because the perceptual apparatus works in a cybernetic fashion, much like a giant videotape recorder, the plethora of information perceived by the sensory system is recorded and stored in the brain at a subconscious level."[23(p40)] The assumption, however, that a process analogous to a multichannel videotape recorder inside the head records all sensory impressions and stores them in their pristine form indefinitely is not consistent with research findings or with current theories of memory.

Hypnotic Enhancement of Rote Memory

Any tape recorder theory of memory that asserts that hypnosis can access all memories would also have to assert that hypnosis enhances the recollection even of meaningless material learned by rote. After reviewing numerous studies, the Panel concluded that there is no scientific evidence that hypnosis increases the recall memory of nonsense syllables or other meaningless material.

Hypnotic Enhancement of Recognition Memory for Meaningful and Complex Material

Recognition memory involves providing information to the subject, who is asked to decide on the correctness of the information either by responding "yes" or "no" or by choosing among several alternatives. After reviewing the relevant scientific data, the Panel agreed that there is no evidence from research laboratory studies (of normal persons) that recognition memory can be enhanced by hypnosis. The experimental literature has not systematically addressed the question of whether these findings apply to individuals such as the perpetrators or victims of crime or significantly emotionally involved witnesses. However, one field study[24] has addressed this question, and its findings indicate that in a real-life situation there is also no increase in recognition memory with hypnotized witnesses or victims of crimes.

Hypnotic Enhancement of Recall Memory for Meaningful and Complex Material

Recall memory involves asking the individual to recollect freely some prior experience in response to minimal cues provided by the questioner. Recall memory for meaningful and complex material, as studied in the literature, uses pictures, poetry, and prose as stimuli. One classic study[25] shows apparent increased memory during hypnosis for poetry learned many years previously. Subjects were able to produce more of the poem during hypnosis than they were in the nonhypnotic state; however, when the remembered passages were compared with the original poem, it turned out that subjects improvised freely or confabulated in the style of the poet. Although to the observer their apparent increased hypnotic memory was compelling, it was found that hypnotized subjects produced more words overall, both correct and incorrect, by filling in gaps in memory with plausible phrases.

After reviewing the extensive literature, the Panel concluded that hypnosis can increase the number of meaningful items remembered but it also increases overall productivity; thus, hypnosis increases the number of both correct and incorrect statements. Because the amount of response productivity has not been adequately controlled in any study to date, it is not possible to determine whether hypnosis causes an increase in memory or whether hypnosis causes a relaxation of the response criterion (that is, a subject accepts a less rigorous standard for what he experiences as a "memory"), which would result in an increase in the number of responses produced. There are no techniques based on the individual's report that can discriminate reliably between a true and false memory report in any specific case.

Hypnotic Enhancement of Memory for Analogue Events

Analogue studies investigate the interaction of hypnosis and memory, employing stimulus materials and experimental procedures that attempt to resemble the real-world situations in which hypnosis is applied. Generalization from the laboratory to the real world depends on the degree to which the laboratory situation accurately represents the field situation.

Although some analogue studies have examined memory for material that is laden with affect, none of these reach the levels of trauma that may be encountered in the field. Furthermore, the motives of experimental subjects and the consequences to them of participation in the procedures differ from those of actual witnesses and victims. Thus, the available literature is more directly relevant to those cases in which preexisting psychopathology and traumatic reactions are not involved. In the studies reviewed, the literature indicates that hypnosis can lead to an increment in productivity, yielding increases in both accurate and false recollections. Although the Panel recognizes that there are many factors—including leading questions—that affect eyewitness testimony in the nonhypnotic state, subjects in hypnosis are more vulnerable to the biasing effects of leading questions. In some studies, hypnotizability appears to be the important variable; in others, the induction of hypnosis is the major factor; in still others, the determining factor is the interaction of hypnotizability and the induction of hypnosis.

The Panel concluded that the current literature does not support the use of hypnosis for casual or moderately involved witnesses. With respect to cases where there is a preexisting psychopathology and/or extreme emotional trauma, the current experimental literature is not definitive.

Clinical Case and Field Reports

In addition to laboratory research, there are clinical case reports that appear to demonstrate memory enhancement in hypnosis. The vast majority of these reports are anecdotal, and most fail to provide independent corroboration of the memories recovered in hypnosis or to establish that hypnosis was responsible for any effects observed. An extensive consecutive case series[26] has been reported from one police agency, but it includes only the subjective impressions of the police investigators concerning the emergence and validity of new information obtained. A more objective tally of results[24] from this same agency, in fact, offers no support for the view that hypnosis can effectively increase the production of accurate memory over what can be achieved by appropriate methods employed without hypnosis; however, the study did not provide evidence that hypnosis produced more distortion in memory.

Pertinent Reviews of the Literature

Published reviews of both experimental and field studies prepared independently of this Panel's deliberations support the conclusions described above. One review[27] finds no clear documentation in either the clinical or experimental literature that hypnosis can improve memory. Other reviewers, although persuaded by the clinical evidence that increases in accurate recollection can occur, agree that hypnosis can also lead to increases in false recollection and confabulation. This also occurs with victims or witnesses of crimes who suffer from traumatic amnesia or posttraumatic stress disorder.

EFFICACY OF HYPNOSIS TO REFRESH MEMORY

Review of the scientific literature indicates that when hypnosis is used to refresh recollection, one of the following outcomes occurs: (1) hypnosis produces recollections that are not substantially different from nonhypnotic recollections; (2) it yields recollections that are more inaccurate than nonhypnotic memory; or, most frequently, (3) it results in more information being reported, but these recollections contain both accurate and inaccurate details. When the third condition results, the individual is less likely to be able to discriminate between accurate and inaccurate recollections. There are no data to support a fourth alternative, namely, that hypnosis increases remembering of only accurate information.

Contrary to what is generally believed by the public, recollections obtained during hypnosis not only fail to be more accurate but actually appear to be generally less reliable than nonhypnotic recall. Furthermore, whereas in nonhypnotic memory reports there is usually a positive relationship between the accuracy of recollections and the confidence that the subject places in those recollections, both the hypnotic procedure and hypnotizability may serve to distort this relationship. The scientific literature indicates that hypnosis can increase inaccurate response to leading questions without a change in confidence,[28,29] or it can increase the subject's confidence in his memories without affecting accuracy,[30,11] or it can increase errors while also falsely increasing confidence.[11,12] In no study to date has there been an increase in accuracy associated with an appropriate increase in confidence in the veracity of recollections. Consequently, hypnosis may increase the appearance of certitude without a concurrent increase of veracity.

In the case of fugues (in which an individual forgets his identity), hypnosis can be an effective clinical procedure to help the person recover his identity. When used in this manner, hypnosis may serve to reinstate the individual's prior recollections. On the other hand, when an individual has a specific amnesia, particularly when it is associated with severe mental or physical trauma, recollections may or may not be obtained during hypnosis and, if obtained, they may or may not be accurate.[11,14] As with other hypnotically refreshed recollections, neither the hypnotist nor the subject can distinguish between actual memories and pseudomemories without subsequent independent verification.

As a therapeutic technique, hypnosis may be helpful in dealing with the emotional consequences of a traumatic event; that is, a recollection may have emotional validity even if it may not be historically accurate. Thus, it is not important for the therapist to concern himself with the veracity of what is remembered under hypnosis, but rather to help the patient integrate this material in an ego-syntonic way to deal with the traumatic events that are presumed to have occurred.

COMPLICATIONS OF HYPNOTICALLY REFRESHED MEMORY

The complications associated with using hypnosis to refresh memory involve both the effects on the hypnotized individual and the effects on others due to the material elicited during hypnosis.

Impact on the Hypnotized Person

When an individual is asked to undergo hypnosis for the public good, as in the case of witnesses or victims of crime, the authorities become responsible for ensuring that the procedure is carried out in a way that minimizes any possible negative consequences to the volunteer. Fortunately, the use of hypnosis is remarkably safe with individuals who do not have psychopathological problems or emotional concerns about the material to be discussed under hypnosis and who are not given ego-dystonic suggestions.

Witnesses and victims, however, are not selected for their mental health, and there may be psychodynamic reasons why they are unwilling or unable to recall the events in question. Although rare, there have been instances of individuals hypnotized for the purpose of aiding recall who became seriously disturbed during the session and continued to remain so for some time thereafter.[15] Under these circumstances, it is not sufficient to suggest that their discomfort will pass and to provide reassurance, since it is likely that the untoward response is due to strong affect stirred by an attempt to recall the events in question. For these reasons, the Panel believes that it is essential that hypnosis be conducted by a psychiatrist or a psychologist who is competent to help the witness or victim deal with overwhelming affect. This professional should have appropriate clinical training as well as special experience in the clinical and investigative use of hypnosis.

To accomplish these aims, it is the responsibility of a physician or psychologist using hypnosis for any reason first to carry out a clinical assessment of the subject's state of mind in order to evaluate his or her suitability for hypnosis. Special consideration needs to be given to individuals who appear to have posttraumatic stress disorders associated with complete or partial amnesias. The Panel feels that it is not appropriate merely to seek to breach the amnesia and elicit recall; the positive or negative consequences of such a procedure must be evaluated. In particular, it is important to help the subject integrate any new information elicited. A single session hardly ever can be considered appropriate treatment for traumatic amnesia or posttraumatic stress disorder. If such a diagnosis is considered, provisions for active follow-up need to be ensured.

Furthermore, in a therapeutic setting, the Panel is concerned that the patient, the clinician, and the integrity of the information obtained from hypnotized victims and witnesses be protected. This is best accomplished by obtaining adequate tape recordings of all sessions after the crime. Recordings should be obtained even in a therapeutic setting, with individuals who may be required to testify in court at some later date. Although, with the patient's permission, copies of these taped recordings may be made available to the authorities, it would be desirable for the therapist to maintain his own original recordings of the sessions.

Impact of Credible but Inaccurate Hypnotic Recall

Not only is there a question about the accuracy of a subject's recollection during hypnosis, but there is also the problem that hypnosis leads to an increased vulnerability to subtle cues and implicit suggestions that may distort recollections in specific ways, depending upon what is communicated to the subject. Both the expectations of the hypnotist and the prior beliefs of the subject may determine the content of confabulations or pseudomemories during hypnosis.[14-16] The manner in which a question is framed can influence the response and even produce a response when there is actually no memory.[17] To the extent that a suspicion may be transformed into a vivid pseudomemory in hypnosis, there may be serious consequences to the legal process when testimony is based on material that is elicited from a witness who has been hypnotized for the purposes of refreshing recollection about the incident in question.

The Panel believes that, in order to minimize a potential miscarriage of justice, it must be communicated clearly to the authorities that neither the subject nor the hypnotist can differentiate between accurate recollections and pseudomemories obtained through hypnosis without subsequent independent verification. If a case involving such a situation comes to trial, this caveat must be made clear.

USE OF HYPNOSIS WITH DEFENDANTS

Although such use is beyond the scope of the Panel's charge, it was felt appropriate to comment briefly on the use of hypnosis with defendants. In the Panel's view, there is no justification for the prosecution's use of hypnosis with a suspect.[2]

When defendants show clear evidence of amnesia, hypnosis may be requested by the defense. In occasional cases, hypnosis has yielded important information that was later corroborated by physical evidence.[18] Under these circumstances, it is essential to maintain the same procedural safeguards as would obtain with a witness or victim. Moreover, it is necessary to keep in mind that untrained individuals with no special knowledge of hypnosis are capable of simulating or faking hypnosis sufficiently well to deceive even experienced hypnotists. Furthermore, individuals in deep hypnosis are able to exert considerable control over their statements and may willfully lie. Consequently, the statements made by a defendant under hypnosis may be self-serving and purposively deceptive. The Panel concludes that a physician or psychologist who testifies about the use of hypnosis with a defendant has an obligation to emphasize the need for independent corroborative evidence and the questionable reliability of memories that have not been so corroborated.

SUMMARY AND RECOMMENDATIONS

The Panel has agreed that there is no evidence of increased recollection by means of hypnosis for recall memory of meaningless material or of recognition memory for any types of material. When hypnosis is used for recall of meaningful past events, there is often new information reported.[25,39] This may include accurate information as well as confabulations and pseudomemories. These pseudomemories may be the result of hypnosis transforming the subjects' prior beliefs into thoughts or fantasies that they come to accept as memories. Furthermore, since hypnotized subjects tend to be more suggestible, subjects become more vulnerable to incorporating any cues given during hypnosis into their recollections.

The Panel found no evidence to indicate that there is an increase of only accurate memory during hypnosis and recognized that there is no way for either the subject or the hypnotist to distinguish between those recollections that may be accurate and those that may be pseudomemories. External corroboration does not necessarily establish that the recollection of the hypnotic subject is independent of suggestion. It was concluded that hypnosis can be useful during the investigative process, when even a single correct recall may lead to important new evidence and where it matters relatively little if the hypnotized subject also produces many incorrect responses. This use of hypnosis is in stark contrast to its use with a witness who is to testify in court. There is controversy in the literature over whether hypnosis does, in fact, provide useful investigative information. Reports claiming success are anecdotal; a controlled study[24] did not support such claims. The value of such investigative use of hypnosis must be balanced against the potential testimonial incapacitation or restriction of evidence by the hypnotic subject as a trial witness.

Hypnosis can be effective in helping some individuals provide memory reports pertaining to events about which they are amnesic. Such recollections, however, may or may not be accurate, although they may be profoundly important in the psychotherapeutic treatment of the individual.

Based on the findings of the Panel, the Council on Scientific Affairs recommends the following:

- The use of hypnosis with witnesses and victims to enhance recall should be limited to the investigative process. Specific safeguards (detailed below) should be employed to protect the welfare of the subject and the public and to provide the kind of record that is essential to evaluate the additional material obtained during and after hypnosis.
- Prior to the induction of hypnosis in an investigative context, a psychological assessment of the subject's state of mind should be carried out and a detailed history of the individual's recollections obtained in a nonleading fashion. Statements such as "I can't remember anything" should not be accepted at face value but should lead to careful exploration of

whatever memory is available. Clinical, forensic, and experimental experience indicate that several nonhypnotic techniques may facilitate recall; for example, repeated recall efforts, even when the subject claims to remember nothing more, can enhance memory.[40] If, after repeated attempts to obtain recall, the decision is made to use hypnosis, it is essential to elicit the subject's expectations and fantasies about hypnosis and to deal with misconceptions. Before proceeding with hypnosis, informed consent should be obtained from the subject.

• Hypnosis should be conducted by a psychiatrist or psychologist, skilled in the clinical and investigative use of hypnosis, who is aware of the legal implications of the use of hypnosis for investigative purposes within the jurisdiction in which he or she practices. The clinician conducting the hypnosis session should take care to avoid leading or inadvertently cueing the subject. A complete taped and/or precise written record of the clinician's prior knowledge of the case must be made. Complete videotape recordings of the prehypnotic evaluation and history, the hypnotic session, and the posthypnotic interview showing both the subject and the hypnotist should be obtained.

• Ideally, only the subject and the psychiatrist/psychologist should be present when the subject is hypnotized. At times, exceptions may be necessary, such as allowing a law enforcement official who is not familiar with the details of the case to provide special expertise, such as a forensic expert or police artist, or such as permitting the parent of an anxious child to remain in the room. The need for the presence of additional individuals must be weighed carefully against the added risk of inadvertently cueing the hypnotized person.

• Although the specific form of hypnotic induction is relatively unimportant, some test suggestions of known difficulty should be given that provide information about the subject's ability to respond to hypnosis; standardized hypnotizability tests may also be used. Regardless of the specific procedure used to focus the subject's attention in hypnosis on the events to be remembered, the hypnotist should elicit at least one free narrative recall first and avoid any questions about specifics; instead, encouraging remarks without specific content (such as "go on," "continue," or "yes") should be used. After obtaining unpressured, free recall in hypnosis, it may be necessary to ask more specific (but nonleading) questions. Before asking such questions, it should be made clear to the subject that the response, "I don't know," is acceptable.

• The subject's response to the termination of hypnosis and the posthypnotic discussion about the experience of hypnosis are of major importance in assessing the subject's response to hypnosis. The videotape recording should include the complete posthypnotic discussion.

• Medical responsibility for the health and welfare of the subject cannot be abrogated by the investigative intent of a hypnotic session.

• Finally, the Panel recommends that the American Medical Association encourage continued research (1) to help clarify the effects of hypnosis on recall, (2) to enhance understanding of the kinds of functional amnesias that affect some victims and witnesses of crimes, and (3) to shed light on the nature of normal and pathological human memory.

References

1 American Medical Association. Medical use of hypnosis *JAMA* 1958,168:186-189.

2. *People v Leyra*, 302 NJ 353, 98 NE2d 553 (1951)

3. *People v Boyd*, Ind No. 81-C-6190 (Cir Ct Ill Feb 28, 1983).

4 *State v Forney*, No. 25A-83 (App Div NC Jan 19, 1983)

5 *People v Shelly*, Ind No 1340/73 (Sup Ct NY 1973).

6 *People v Ritchie*, No C-36932 (Sup Ct Cal April 7, 1977, unrep)

7. *State v Papp*, No 78-02-00229 (CP Summit Co, Ohio, Lorain Co No 16862 March 23, 1978, unrep), appealed, US Sup Ct No. 79-5091, *cert denied* Oct 1, 1979.

8 *Landry v Garrett Chevrolet Inc*, 430 So2d 1051 (La App 4th Cir), writs granted, 434 So2d 1103 (La 1983), 433 So2d 1105 (La 1983), 433 So2d 1139 (La App 4th Cir Feb 10, 1984), *writs denied* (not yet rep)

9 Diamond BL Inherent problems in the use of pretrial hypnosis on a prospective witness. *Calif Law Rev* 1980,68 313-349

10 *State v McQueen*, 295 NC 96, 244 SE2d 414 (1978)

11 *United States v Adams et al*, 581 F2d 193 (9th Cir 1978), *cert denied*, —US—, 99 S Ct 621 (1978)

12 *People v Shirley*, 31 Cal 3d 18, 641 P2d 775, 181 Cal Rptr 243 (1982)

13 *State v Collins*, 296 Md 670 (1983).

14 *State v Hurd*, 173 NJ Sup Ct 333, 414 A2d 291, *aff'd*, 86 NJ 525, 432 A2d 86 (1981)

15. *State v Beachum*, 97 NM 682, 643 P2d 246 (Ct App 1981)

16 Hilgard ER *Hypnotic Susceptibility*. New York, Harcourt Brace & World, 1965.

17 Frankel FH, Apfel RJ, Kelly SF, et al: The use of hypnotizability scales in the clinic: A review after six years. *Int J Clin Exp Hypn* 1979;27 63-73.

18. Spiegel H, Spiegel D: *Trance and Treatment: Clinical Uses of Hypnosis* New York, Basic Books Inc, 1978.

19. Freud S. *A Case of Hysteria, Three Essays on Sexuality, and Other Works*. London, Hogarth Press, 1953, p 274.

20. O'Connell DN, Shor RE, Orne MT. Hypnotic age regression. An empirical and methodological analysis. *J Abnorm Psychol* 1970,76(monogr 3) 1-32.

21. Spiegel H, Shor G, Fischman S An hypnotic ablation technique for the study of personality development. *Psychosom Med* 1945,7 272-278.

22. Reiser M· *Handbook of Investigative Hypnosis*. Los Angeles, LEHI Publishing Co, 1980

23 Reiser M Hypnosis as a tool in criminal investigation. *Police Chief* 1976,46 36,39-40

24. Sloane MC: *A Comparison of Hypnosis vs Waking State and Visual vs. Non-Visual Recall Instructions for Witness/Victim Memory Retrieval in Actual Major Crimes*, doctoral dissertation. Florida State University, Tallahassee, 1981.

25. Stalnaker JM, Riddle EE. The effect of hypnosis on long-delayed recall. *J Gen Psychol* 1932;6.429-440.

26 Reiser M, Nielson M. Investigative hypnosis. A developing specialty *Am J Clin Hypn* 1980,23:75-84.

27. Smith MC: Hypnotic memory enhancement of witnesses: Does it work? *Psychol Bull* 1983;94:387-407.

28 Putnam WH. Hypnosis and distortions in eyewitness memory *Int J Clin Exp Hypn* 1979, 27:437-448.

29 Zelig M, Beidleman WB: The investigative use of hypnosis: A word of caution *Int J Clin Exp Hypn* 1981,29 401-412

30 Sheehan PW, Tilden J Effects of suggestibility and hypnosis on accurate and distorted retrieval from memory *J Exp Psychol Learn Mem Cogn* 1983,9 283-293

31. Dywan J *Hypermnesia, Hypnosis and Memory Implications for Forensic Investigation*, doctoral dissertation University of Waterloo, Waterloo, Ontario, 1983.

32 Timm HW *A Theoretical and Empirical Examination of the Effects of Forensic Hypnosis on Eyewitness Recall* Presented at the Ninth International Congress of Hypnosis and Psychosomatic Medicine, Glasgow, Scotland, Aug 22-27, 1982

33 Udolf R *Handbook of Hypnosis for Professionals* New York, Van Nostrand Reinhold Co, 1980, p 213

34 Spiegel H Hypnosis and evidence Help or hindrance? *Ann NY Acad Sci* 1980,347 73-85

35 Kleinhauz M *Hypnosis in Criminal Investigation—Ethical and Practical Implications* Presented at the Ninth International Congress of Hypnosis and Psychosomatic Medicine, Glasgow, Scotland, Aug 22-27, 1982

36 Orne MT The use and misuse of hypnosis in court *Int J Clin Exp Hypn* 1979;27 311-341.

37 Mutter C *The Use of Hypnosis With Defendants*. Presented at the 26th Annual Meeting of the American Society of Clinical Hypnosis, Dallas, Nov 14-19, 1983

38 *State v Staggers*, No 74-243 (Cir Ct Fla April 23, 1974)

39 Dywan J, Bowers KS The use of hypnosis to enhance recall *Science* 1983,222 184-185

40 Erdelyi MH, Kleinbard J Has Ebbinghaus decayed with time? The growth of recall (hypermnesia) over days. *J Exp Psychol Hum Learn Mem* 1978;4 275-289

[30]

Recalling the Unrecallable: Should Hypnosis Be Used to Recover Memories in Psychotherapy?

Steven Jay Lynn, Timothy G. Lock, Bryan Myers, and David G. Payne[1]

Department of Psychology, Binghamton University, Binghamton, New York

Our observations have shown . . . that the memories which have become the determinants of hysterical phenomena persist for a long time with astonishing freshness and with the whole of their affective colouring . these experiences are completely absent from the patients' memory when they are in a normal psychical state, or are only present in highly summary form Not until they have been questioned under hypnosis do these memories emerge with the undiminished vividness of a recent event (Breuer & Freud, 1893–1895/1955, p. 9)

Recommended Reading

Brown, D., Scheflin, A.W., & Hammond, D.C. (1997). *Memory, trauma treatment, and the law.* New York: Norton.

Kirsch, I., & Lynn, S.J. (1995). The altered state of hypnosis: Changes in the theoretical landscape. *American Psychologist, 50,* 846–858.

Lynn, S.J., Martin, D., & Frauman, D.C. (1996). Does hypnosis pose special risks for negative effects? *International Journal of Clinical and Experimental Hypnosis, 44,* 7–19.

McConkey, K.M., & Sheehan, P.W. (1995). *Hypnosis, memory, and behavior in the forensic setting.* New York: Guilford Press.

Of course, not too long after this famous quote, Freud spurned hypnosis[2] in favor of other techniques such as free association, dream analysis, and interpretation But the idea that hypnosis is a royal road to unconscious or suppressed memories lingers to the present day. Survey research (cf. Lynn, Myers, & Malinoski, in press) indicates that between 20% and 34% of modern psychotherapists use hypnosis to help patients "recall the unrecallable" and to establish the historical "truth" or basis of current problems. Hypnosis would be valuable in such instances if it were a reliable technique for recovering accurate memories. However, in this review, we contend this is not the case.

It is worth noting at the outset that a review of the use of hypnosis in forensic situations (see Karlin & Orne, 1996; Scheflin, in press) is beyond the scope of this article, and that when hypnotic procedures are combined with behavioral and psychophysiological procedures, there is a proven benefit for interventions that are not focused on retrieving memories (Kirsch, Montgomery, & Sapirstein, 1995) The concerns and caveats we present here apply specifically to the use of hypnosis as a technique for unearthing historically accurate memories[3] in psychotherapy.

ACCURATE AND INACCURATE MEMORIES IN HYPNOSIS

On the basis of his review of 34 studies, Erdelyi (1994) concluded that hypnosis does not increase recognition of previously presented meaningful stimuli (e.g., poetry, meaningful pictures) or recognition or recall of nonmeaningful stimuli (e.g., nonsense syllables, word lists) Although Erdelyi noted that hypnosis increases recall of meaningful stimuli, it also increases false recollections. Indeed, when hypnotic and nonhypnotic conditions are compared and the sheer volume of responses is controlled, hypnotic recall is no more accurate than nonhypnotic recall (e.g., Erdelyi, 1994).

Support for Erdelyi's conclusions can be found in a meta-analysis reported by Steblay and Bothwell (1994) Their analysis summarized 24 studies, among which were studies that appeared after those included in Erdelyi's review. Steblay and Bothwell found no reliable differences in performance on structured tests of accurate recall[4] when subjects were hypnotized versus when they were not hypnotized. It is true that three studies in Steblay and Bothwell's analysis did report a superiority of recall in hypnotized subjects when recall was measured using unstructured free recall tests. However, in four more recent studies conducted in our laboratory (e.g., Abrams & Lynn, 1996), hypnotized subjects either fared no better or performed worse than nonhypnotized subjects on tests of accurate recall whether these tests were unstructured or structured. Furthermore, motivational instructions that urged subjects to "try your best on the recall test" yielded equivalent or superior recall compared with hypnosis.

Thus, the evidence does not seem to support the conclusion that hypnosis improves accurate recall. Whether hypnosis reduces inaccurate recall (e.g., distortions of presented stimuli, intrusions of nonpresented stimuli or events that never occurred) is a separate question. Recall errors are not uncommon. However, Steblay and Bothwell's (1994) analysis of six studies revealed that hypnotized participants, compared with nonhypnotized control subjects, produced more false memories in response to misleading questions or false information. Moreover, Steblay and Bothwell's analysis of five studies of recall revealed that hypnotized participants, compared with control subjects, generated more errors that were not prompted by misleading questions or the stimuli themselves. In short, hypnosis is not a reliable technique for augmenting accurate recall and generally results in a trade-off of errors for accurate remembrances.

Unwarranted Recall Confidence

Nonhypnotized persons are often overconfident about the accuracy of their memories (Spanos, 1996). However, hypnotized individuals are often (but not always) more confident about what they recall than nonhypnotized individuals, regardless of whether the information is accurate or not (Steblay & Bothwell, 1994). The magnitude of the overconfidence effect associated with hypnosis ranges from small to substantial, when present. An association between hypnotizability and confidence has also been documented, with highly hypnotizable participants particularly prone to what are called confident errors (i.e., being confident of inaccurate memories; Sheehan, 1988).

Hypnosis and Emotional Stimuli

It has been claimed that hypnosis may have particular utility as a memory recovery technique with traumatized persons because trauma blocks memory due to the state-dependent nature of memory. That is, retrieving a traumatic memory may depend on the congruence of the current context and mood with the context and mood at the time the event occurred, and hypnosis has the ability to reinstate those original conditions (Hammond et al., 1995, p. 15). This conclusion is not warranted or is questionable for the following reasons. First, although research has not compared hypnotic versus nonhypnotic recall in the presence of traumatic stimuli, studies with emotional and arousing yet not personally threatening stimuli (e.g., films of shop accidents and fatal stabbings, a mock "live" assassination, and a murder videotaped serendipitously) yield an unambiguous conclusion: Hypnosis does not improve recall of emotionally arousing events, and arousal level does not affect hypnotic recall (Lynn et al., in press). Second, controversy exists (Ofshe & Singer, 1994; Scheflin & Brown, 1996) regarding whether and to what degree emotional trauma can block memory for single, repeated, or prolonged events. And third, as Shobe and Kihlstrom note in this issue, hypnosis often involves relaxation suggestions that would not be expected to reinstate the traumatic context.

We agree that it is appropriate to question the generalizability of laboratory research to real traumatic situations, and to exhort researchers to devise creative designs that better approximate real-life situations. Nevertheless, the available evidence fails to support the contention that hypnosis has special promise for helping traumatized individuals regain lost memories.

Hypnotic Age Regression

In a review of more than 60 years of research on hypnotic age regression (a technique in which a subject is asked to respond to specific hypnotic suggestions to think, feel, or act like a child at a particular age), Nash (1987) found that the behaviors and experiences of age-regressed adults were often different from those of actual children. No matter how compelling such age-regression experiences appear to observers, they reflect participants' fantasies and beliefs and assumptions about childhood; they rarely, if ever, represent literal reinstatements of childhood experiences, behaviors, and feelings.

In one illustrative study (Nash, Drake, Wiley, Khalsa, & Lynn, 1986), subjects age-regressed to age 3 years reported the identity of their transitional objects (e.g., blankets, teddy bears). Parents of 14 hypnotized subjects and 10 role-playing control subjects were asked to verify this information. The results showed that hypnotized subjects were less accurate than control subjects in identifying the specific transitional objects they had used. Hypnotic subjects' hypnotic recollections, for example, matched their parents' reports only 21% of the time, whereas role-players' reports were corroborated by their parents 70% of the time. This research, like other studies reported in the age-regression literature (cf. Nash, 1987), indicates that age-regression experiences can be compelling yet inaccurate.

DETERMINANTS OF PSEUDOMEMORIES

In the studies we review in this section, the usual procedure was to provide participants with deliberately misleading suggestions during hypnosis or nonhypnotic control procedures and measure the extent to which the participants accepted the false information as true following hypnosis or the control procedure. When such information is accepted, it is referred to as a pseudomemory. Sometimes people with high hypnotizability scores report more pseudomemories than people with medium hypnotizability scores, but in general, both groups report more pseudomemories than people with low hypnotizability scores. The fact that people with medium and even low hypnotizability scores report pseudomemories indicates that the effect is not limited to a small and highly select segment of the population (Lynn & Nash, 1994; Orne, Whitehouse, Dinges, & Orne, 1996). Interestingly, highly hypnotizable subjects report more pseudomemories than other people in nonhypnotic as well as hypnotic conditions, implicating a general suggestibility factor in the genesis of pseudomemories (see Lynn et al, in press).

The rates at which pseudomemories are reported are influenced by the perceived verifiability and memorability of the to-be-remembered events. Rates for distinctive events (e.g., a telephone ringing in a classroom) that do not often occur in the real world are generally low (12% to 25%) in hypnotic contexts. However, when the events are impossible to verify (e.g., whether a person was awakened on a particular night by a noise), or are not particularly memorable (e.g., a door slamming in a hall the previous week), pseudomemory rates are much higher (45% to 80%; Lynn et al., in press).

Situational variables are influential determinants of pseudomemory reports. Pseudomemory rates decrease (but are by no means eliminated) when previously hypnotized subjects are offered a monetary reward for distinguishing between a false suggestion and an actual occurrence, when rapport with the experimenter is degraded, and when subjects are cross-examined (cf. Lynn et al., in press).

Several studies (see Lynn et al., in press) have compared pseudomemory rates of hypnotized subjects with pseudomemory rates of nonhypnotized imagining subjects or of role-playing subjects instructed to respond in terms of their understanding of how hypnotized subjects would respond in the experimental situation. Because these studies used very leading suggestions, it is not surprising that hypnotized and nonhypnotized persons responded comparably. This research indicates that false memories are by no means limited to hypnotic conditions and underscores the role of perceptions of the situation and situational cues in the formation of pseudomemories. However, this research does not mean that hypnotized persons are not genuinely confused or misled with respect to the false information they remember.

In another line of research, McConkey, Labelle, Bibb, and Bryant (1990) found that if testing took place immediately after hypnosis, approximately 50% of hypnotizable subjects reported a pseudomemory. However, when subjects were contacted by telephone at home 4 to 24 hr later by an experimenter who was not part of the earlier session, the rate decreased dramatically to 2.5%. Barnier and McConkey (1992) found that the pseudomemory rate declined from 60% (for a false suggestion that a thief depicted in a series of slides was wearing a scarf) to 10% when the experimental context shifted to imply that the experiment had ended.

By questioning subjects at their homes by telephone after the formal experiment was completed, and by implying that the experiment was terminated, these studies might have engendered subtle pressure on subjects to reverse their earlier pseudomemory reports. Hence, this program of research does not satisfactorily resolve the issue of whether pseudomemory reports reflect genuine memory alterations or merely alterations in reports in conformance with variations in the situational context.

Although McConkey's research indicates that pseudomemory reports are malleable, other research indicates this is not always the case For instance, Spanos and McLean (1986) showed that participants reversed their initial hypnotic pseudomemory reports when they were informed they could distinguish "real" and "false" memories if they accessed a "hidden observer" that could discriminate them. However, in three studies, we (see Lynn et al, in press) were unable to reverse pseudomemory reports by informing participants that they would be able to distinguish false and accurate memories. Hence, pseudomemory reports are not invariably sensitive to contextual manipulations and can be obdurate to modification.

The American Society of Clinical Hypnosis (ASCH) recently advanced guidelines (Hammond et al, 1995) intended to define principles of practice in the use of hypnosis for exploring, uncovering, and working through memories. The guidelines refer to the potentially contaminating effects (e.g., increase in volume of information reported and confidence that what is recalled is true) of suggestions and expectations that memory will increase during hypnosis (e.g., "You can and will recall everything") and say that such effects may be controlled considerably "when neutral expectations are created prior to hypnosis and during hypnotic induction and age regression" (p. 28).

The guidelines inspired a recent study of prehypnotic expectancies (Green, Lynn, & Malinoski, in press) comparing the pseudomemory rates of highly hypnotizable participants "warned" prior to hypnosis that hypnosis can lead to false memories with pseudomemory rates of highly hypnotizable participants who received no special instructions prior to hypnosis. During hypnosis, all subjects were given the suggestion that they had been awakened by a noise during a night of the previous week.[5] Prior to hypnosis, all of the participants indicated they had slept through the night

Participants who were warned were less likely to accept the suggestion during hypnosis: 38% of the warned participants did so, versus 75% of the unwarned participants. Hence, warnings reduced participants' suggestibility during hypnosis. However, an analysis of those persons who accepted the suggestion during hypnosis showed that the warning had no effect on their posthypnotic pseudomemories: Among this group, 75% of those persons who had been warned and 58% of those who had not been warned stated immediately after hypnosis that the noise had occurred in reality (i.e., reported a pseudomemory). After extensive questioning, during a final confidential assessment, 58% of the warned participants who had accepted the noise suggestion during hypnosis reported the pseudomemory, compared with 50% of the unwarned participants. Furthermore, warned participants were just as confident in their false memories as were unwarned participants.

In summary, when participants are warned about the deleterious effects of hypnosis on memory, suggestibility is reduced, but the risk of pseudomemories is by no means eliminated. Future research should evaluate the possibility that this risk will be further reduced when the full ASCH guidelines (e.g., avoiding leading questions and attempting to establish neutral expectations about the effects of hypnosis on memory prior to, during, and after hypnosis) are followed.

CONCLUSIONS

If clinicians were concerned only about accurate information, then hypnosis might be a useful memory recovery technique insofar as it can lower the threshold for reporting both accurate and inaccurate memories. To be sure, hypnosis does not always produce memory errors. Kluft (in press), for example, has reported that he was able to corroborate a number of hypnotically evoked memories of sexual abuse reported by patients in his clinical practice diagnosed with dissociative identity disorder (formerly known as multiple personality disorder). In most instances, however, it is not only impractical or inappropriate, but impossible to corroborate memories of patients in psychotherapy. Because clinicians and clients are not, as a rule, able to differentiate accurate and inaccurate memories, the yield of accurate memories must be weighed against the risk of memory errors associated with the hypnotic context. As Steblay and Bothwell (1994) concluded, "Hypnosis is not necessarily a source of accurate information; at worst it may be a source of inaccurate information provided with confident testimony" (p. 649).

Such concerns raise the question of whether hypnosis should be demonized and banished from the arena of psychotherapies. We contend that to do so would be a serious mistake that would deprive clinicians of a valuable technique that can be used successfully in many contexts outside that of memory recovery, including the treatment of persons who remember traumatic experiences without the use of any special techniques.

The literature on memory recovery and hypnosis is complex, and future research may change our assessment. For instance, if the available evidence indicated that safeguards can eliminate memory errors while preserving a recall advantage for hypnosis, we would acknowledge that hypnosis may have a useful role in improving recall. However, this has not, as yet, been demonstrated.

Nor has it been shown that the memory recovery component of psychotherapies contributes to their efficacy to begin with. Indeed, many nonhypnotic procedures geared toward memory recovery are inherently suggestive in nature (i.e., there is "something" to be recalled that will improve present functioning), and may well carry a pseudomemory risk equal to or greater than that of hypnosis. The attempt to recover suppressed memories is complex and risky business whether hypnosis is used or not. Certainly each clinician must ultimately weigh the costs versus the benefits of any psychotherapeutic technique. In our view, however, the data indicate that the answer to the question of whether hypnosis should be used to recover historically accurate memories in psychotherapy is "no."

Acknowledgments—We would like to thank the following individuals for their helpful comments on earlier versions of this manuscript: Maggie Bruck, Etzel Cardena, Joseph Green, Albrecht Inhoff, John Kihlstrom, Irving Kirsch, Michael Langone, Stephen Lisman, Elizabeth Loftus, Peter Malinoski, Lisa Marmelstein, Ralph Miller, Michael Nash, Alan Scheflin, Peter Sheehan, and Jane Stafford

Notes

1 Address correspondence to Steven Jay Lynn, Psychology Department, Binghamton University, Binghamton, NY 13902-6000.

2. The term hypnosis refers to a social situation in which a person designated as a hypnotist attempts to influence the experiences and behaviors of a subject or patient The suggestions administered in the hypnotic situation typically call for changes in sensation, perception, affect, cognition, and control over behavior or psychophysiological processes (e.g., heart rate). Hypnotizability, or hypnotic responsiveness, refers to observed or reported responsivity to suggestions following a hypnotic induction Participants range on a continuum of hypnotizability according to how many suggestions they accept, or pass. People who pass 3 or fewer suggestions out of 12 have a score that is conventionally considered low (about 15%–20% of the population), those who pass 4 to 8 suggestions have scores considered medium (about 60%–70% of the population), and those who pass 9 to 12 suggestions are regarded as highly hypnotizable (about 15%–20% of the population).

3 Of course, it could be, and has been, argued that memories retrieved during hypnosis, or any psychotherapeutic technique for that matter, need not be "historically accurate" to have therapeutic value. We acknowledge that all memories produced in psychotherapy and other contexts are not necessarily accurate, that memory is not an unbiased and permanent record of events as they unfolded in the past, and that it is possible that behavioral change in psychotherapy may come about regardless of the historical truth of memories. However, we agree with Spence (1994) and with Kihlstrom (in press) that, as a rule, "narrative truth is no substitute for historical truth" (Kihlstrom, p. 38), and that when clients place stock in false narratives, they may be diverted from confronting and resolving important issues in therapy.

4. In structured recall tests, subjects are required to respond to specific questions about the to-be-recalled material. Such tests can be contrasted with unstructured recall tests, in which subjects are not cued or questioned about the specific content of the information to be recalled (e.g., "Write down everything you can remember").

5. It is important to emphasize that because this study did not evaluate the full ASCH guidelines, generalization to the complete set of procedures mandated by ASCH may be hazardous

References

Abrams, L, & Lynn, S J (1996) *The independent and interactive effects of hypnosis and mnemonic aids on delayed eyewitness recall* Unpublished manuscript, Ohio University, Athens

Barnier, A J, & McConkey, K M (1992) Reports of real and false memories The relevance of hypnosis, hypnotizability, and the context of memory test *Journal of Abnormal Psychology, 101,* 521–527

Breuer, J, & Freud, S (1955) Studies on hysteria In J Strachey (Ed), *The standard edition of the complete psychological works of Sigmund Freud* (Vol 2) London· Hogarth Press (Original work published 1893–1895)

Erdelyi, M (1994) Hypnotic hypermnesia The empty set of hypermnesia *International Journal of Clinical and Experimental Hypnosis, 42,* 379–390

Green, J P, Lynn, S J, & Malinoski, P (in press) Hypnotic pseudomemories The effects of warnings and hidden observer instructions *Applied Cognitive Psychology*

Hammond, D C, Garver, R B, Mutter, C B, Crasilneck, H B, Frischholz, E, Gravitz, M A, Hibler, N S., Olson, J., Scheflin, A, Spiegel, H, & Wester, W (1995) *Clinical hypnosis and memory Guidelines for clinicians and for forensic hypnosis* Des Plaines, IL American Society of Clinical Hypnosis Press

Karlin, R A, & Orne, M T (1996) Commentary on Borawick v Shay. Hypnosis, social influence, incestuous child abuse, and satanic ritual abuse The iatrogenic creation of horrific memories for the remote past *Cultic Studies Journal, 13,* 42–95

Kihlstrom, J (in press) Exhumed memory In S J Lynn & K M McConkey (Eds), *Truth in memory* New York Guilford Press

Kirsch, I, Montgomery, G, & Sapirstein, G (1995) Hypnosis as an adjunct to cognitive behavioral psychotherapy A meta-analysis *Journal of Consulting and Clinical Psychology, 63,* 214–220

Kluft, R P (in press) Reflections on the traumatic memories of dissociative identity disorder patients In S J Lynn & K M McConkey (Eds), *Truth in memory* New York Guilford Press

Lynn, S J, Myers, B., & Malinoski, P (in press) Hypnosis, pseudomemories, and clinical guidelines A sociocognitive perspective In J D Read & D S Lindsay (Eds), *Recollections of trauma Scientific studies and clinical practice* New York. Plenum Press

Lynn, S J, & Nash, M R (1994) Truth in memory Ramifications for psychotherapy and hypnotherapy *American Journal of Clinical Hypnosis, 36,* 194–208

McConkey, K M, Labelle, L, Bibb, B C, & Bryant, R A (1990) Hypnosis and suggested pseudomemory The relevance of test context *Australian Journal of Psychology, 42,* 197–206

Nash, M R (1987) What, if anything, is age regressed about hypnotic age regression? A review of the empirical literature *Psychological Bulletin, 102,* 42–52

Nash, M R, Drake, M, Wiley, R, Khalsa, S, & Lynn, S J (1986) The accuracy of recall of hypnotically age regressed subjects *Journal of Abnormal Psychology, 95,* 298–300

Ofshe, R J, & Singer, M T (1994) Recovered-memory therapy and robust repression Influence and pseudomemories *International Journal of Clinical and Experimental Hypnosis, 42,* 391–410

Orne, E C, Whitehouse, W G, Dinges, D F, & Orne, M T (1996) Memory liabilities associated with hypnosis Does low hypnotizability confer immunity? *International Journal of Clinical and Experimental Hypnosis, 44,* 354–369

Scheflin, A W (in press) False memories and buridan's ass A response to Karlin & Orne "Hypnosis, social influence, incestuous child abuse, and satanic ritual abuse The iatrogenic creation of horrific memories for the remote past" *Cultic Studies Journal*

Scheflin, A W, & Brown, D (1996) Repressed memory or dissociative amnesia What the science says *Journal of Psychiatry and Law, 24,* 143–188

Sheehan, P (1988) Confidence, memory, and hypnosis In H Pettinati (Ed), *Hypnosis and memory* (pp 96–127) New York Guilford Press

Spanos, N P (1996) *Multiple identities and false memories* Washington, DC American Psychological Association

Spanos, N P, & McLean, J (1986) Hypnotically created pseudomemories Memory distortions or reporting biases? *British Journal of Experimental and Clinical Hypnosis, 3,* 155–159

Spence, D P (1994) *The rhetorical voice of psychoanalysis Displacement of evidence by theory* Cambridge, MA Harvard University Press

Steblay, N M, & Bothwell, R K (1994) Evidence for hypnotically refreshed testimony The view from the laboratory *Law and Human Behavior, 18,* 635–651

[31]

THE ALLEGED DANGERS OF STAGE HYPNOSIS

Michael Heap

Centre for Psychotherapeutic Studies, University of Sheffield, Sheffield, UK

Introduction

From time to time, the safety of hypnosis and its possible misuse are subjected to attention in the learned literature and the mass media. In the UK in the 1990s, there was a surge of interest in stage hypnosis shows, probably owing to the activities of Paul McKenna, who gave popular televised performances. Owing to some legal claims of physical injury, including the tragic death of one participant (Heap, 1995), the possible hazards of stage hypnosis occupied much media attention, and numerous allegations of psychological injury were publicized. These included three lawsuits in which the present author was engaged for the defence. One of these is examined in detail in this issue (Heap, 2000). Another lawsuit, brought against McKenna, is the subject of a separate paper by Graham Wagstaff, one of the expert witnesses for the defendant (Wagstaff, 2000). In this paper I shall examine other cases and attempt to lay some ground rules for investigating claims made against stage hypnotists.

The law on stage hypnosis in the UK

In the UK, organizers of stage hypnosis shows in places of public entertainment must apply for a licence from the local council. This is enshrined in the 1952 Hypnotism Act. The act arose from some concerns about the safety of stage hypnosis. In 1948, a woman made allegations of negligence and assault against a stage hypnotist during one of his performances (*Raines-Bath* vs *Slater*). The plaintiff was initially awarded damages for negligence but the verdict was quashed on appeal (see Waxman, 1988).

Since then, there have been a number of published accounts by writers in the UK and abroad, in which it is claimed that psychological distress, and sometimes physical injury, were caused to a participant or even a member of the audience by the actions of a stage hypnotist (Erickson, 1962; Waxman, 1978, 1981, 1988, 1989; Kleinhauz, Drefuss, Beran, Goldberg and Axikri, 1979; Kleinhauz and Beran, 1981, 1984; Misra, 1985; MacHovec, 1986, 1988; Echterling and Emmerling, 1987; Crawford, Kitner-Triolo, Clarke and Olesko, 1992).

In the late 1980s, the UK Home Office drew up guidelines for the conduct of stage hypnosis to be attached to licences, with a view to protecting the participants (Home Office, 1989).

Recent allegations of harm by stage hypnotists

In more recent years, several cases have been the subject of private legal action. In 1995, a young man sued a stage hypnotist when he injured himself while running away from an imaginary army of giant mice. He claimed to have a phobia of mice. His case was unsuccessful. At about the same time, a woman successfully sued

Glasgow's Pavilion Theatre after breaking her leg when she fell off the stage during a stage hypnosis show.

In 1993, a healthy young woman, Sharron Tabarn, died during the night after taking part in stage hypnosis. The verdict of the inquest was death by natural causes. I have presented an analysis of this case elsewhere (Heap, 1995). The mother of the deceased understandably felt that stage hypnosis was a necessary factor in accounting for her daughter's death. She and others mounted a campaign to have stage hypnosis prohibited. She was also granted leave to appeal against the coroner's verdict on her daughter's death, and her lawyers presented a mass of documents to the royal courts. However, the judge considered that hypnosis was probably not implicated in her death and the original verdict was upheld.

Following the publicity stimulated by this campaign, other people came forward with accounts about how they too had been harmed by participating in stage hypnosis shows. As a result, at least four civil cases were brought against stage hypnotists by alleged victims. The author has examined documents relating to all of these, and has provided expert witness testimony in three. One of these has been discontinued without any settlement, one is ongoing, and I have provided an account of the third in this issue (Heap, 2000). The fourth is *Gates* vs *McKenna* (Wagstaff, 2000).

While these four cases were in progress, the UK Home Office set up a panel of experts to study evidence concerning the alleged dangers of stage hypnosis. The members of this group were psychologists and psychiatrists who had no particular expertise in hypnosis and therefore no prejudices either way. The report and recommendations of this panel were announced in October 1995 (Home Office, 1995). The panel concluded that stage hypnosis does not pose a significant mental health risk that would warrant its prohibition. After consulting a wide range of people the panel brought out a revised set of model conditions (Home Office, 1996).

Analysis of cases

It is clear from the documents that I have inspected in the above four cases that, in each instance, the plaintiff's side made a number of popular assumptions that are unwarranted or ill-supported from a study of the available scientific evidence concerning hypnosis.

Assumption 1: The stage hypnotist places the participants in a deep trance

In all of these cases the statements of claim by the plaintiff's side alleged that the stage hypnotist places the participants in a deep state of trance. For example, in one case it was asserted that hypnosis 'involves the interference with the conscious will of the subject(s)' and 'they are induced to perform acts that would be embarrassing and/or distasteful to them if fully conscious'.

It is not difficult to understand why such assumptions are made. Typically, the participants in a stage hypnosis show respond immediately and vividly to the suggestions given, as though they are indeed under the complete control of the hypnotist. Some of the stunts seem to call for quite unusual imagined experiences – as, for example, when a young man is told that he has fallen in love with a broomstick, or when all participants are told that someone in the audience has stolen their 'belly buttons' and they must find out who it is. At other times, when they are not required to be active, participants may seem to have entered some kind of stuporous state as they sit slumped in their chairs. Sometimes an individual who is noted for his or her calm and reticent demeanour seems to undergo a personality change once he or she is up on stage and has been 'induced'.

There is every reason to believe that people will behave exactly like 'genuine' stage hypnosis participants if they are given enough incentive, such as money. However, the participants do not usually receive any material reward for their efforts. Nevertheless, some onlookers will simply interpret participants' activities as indicating that they are 'just acting'. Others, however, believe that they would behave in the way they do only if they were in some special mental state. This difference in interpretation is also evident among the participants themselves: some ascribe their outlandish behaviour to the fact that they were merely cooperating with the hypnotist; others have no ready and obvious explanation of why they responded in the manner they did – hence the explanation that the hypnotist puts them into a 'trance' and they are thus somehow under his or her power. Indeed, the fact that the stage hypnotist usually carries out a 'trance-inducing' ceremony at the beginning of the act and a 'trance-terminating' ritual at the end, serves to confirm this explanation. Moreover, because their behaviours and experiences are apparently so immediate and dramatic, people are inclined to believe that participants in stage hypnosis must be in especially deep trances or must be very deeply hypnotized.

Despite this, the evidence from the hypnosis literature indicates that under equivalent contextual demands and expectations, and possessing the same cognitive skills, commitment and involvement, 'non-hypnotized' participants are indistinguishable from participants who have been ceremonially 'put into a trance' (Barber, Spanos and Chaves, 1974; Kirsch, 1991).

This is actually implied in manuals of stage hypnosis (Meeker and Barber, 1971), and some stage hypnotists dispense with the 'trance-inducing' rituals altogether yet conduct their act in the same way. Prominent among these is the American illusionist and stage hypnotist George Kresge, *aka* 'The Amazing Kreskin' (Baker, 1990). Kresge specifically instructs his participants, whom he does not test for suggestibility, to remain awake and not 'go into a trance'. Similarly, in the UK, the magician Martin S. Taylor (Hoggart and Hutchinson, 1995) holds stage hypnosis shows without using hypnosis, sometimes in order to circumvent local prohibitions. Indeed, some *magicians* use stage hypnosis stunts, again without any attempt to 'induce hypnosis' – for example, the suggestion that the participants are unable to rise from their chair or that they are receiving an electric shock from their chair or from each other.

One can therefore state with confidence that the salient determining factors in the behaviour and experiences of the participants at a stage hypnosis show are their own skills, attributes and commitment to the task, the definite expectations concerning how they should respond, the effect of audience pressure, the stage hypnotist's demands, and the effects of being among a group of participants (see also Meeker and Barber, 1971).

One manifestation of these factors is the difference in the quality of the responses of stage participants and that of patients undergoing hypnosis treatment. For example, a patient responding to the suggestion of imagining being a child again will generally remain relatively unchanged in his or her demeanour, although occasionally he or she may speak in a soft voice, more child-like than usual; stage participants, on the other hand, fidget, giggle, jump off their chairs and run around, fight with one another, and so on. When told that they are riding a horse (perhaps in order to recreate feelings associated with their favourite pastime) patients may again show little change in their behaviour except perhaps for slight rhythmical movements of the body; contrariwise, stage participants respond wildly, jumping up and down in their chairs, slapping their thighs, and so on. When given suggestions that they are feeling tired and sleepy, relatively little outward change is noted in the responses of patients, whereas stage participants slump in their chairs, drape themselves over one another, and even slide to the floor as though in a stupor. These differences in behaviour do not arise because the stage participants are 'in a deeper trance' or are 'more deeply hypnotized' than their counterparts in the clinic; in all three of the foregoing scenarios, patients in the clinic, despite minimal overt change, may report having profound and vivid experiences of the imagined or suggested effects. Clearly, the differences arise because the demands on the stage participants are that they must be immediately responsive and give a highly visible and flamboyant performance for the entertainment of the audience. Such is decidedly not the case in the clinic.

Nevertheless, we may speculate that defining the situation as 'hypnotic' has the following implications:

1. It may provide participants with a more potent excuse or justification for behaving in a disinhibited manner.
2. It will affect the way the participants explain their experiences and behaviour. For example, as was stated earlier, many participants will attribute their behaviour and experiences to their having been 'in a trance'.
3. Some participants may be more likely to assume that they are less able to resist the entertainer's instructions if they identify themselves as being 'hypnotized'.
4. The attribution 'hypnotized' as opposed to 'acting' or 'imagining' may itself have adverse consequences for some participants; this will be discussed in due course.

Assumption 2: Participants in a stage hypnosis show are extremely high in suggestibility or hypnotic susceptibility

Most stage hypnotists initially select their participants by their response to a simple suggestibility test, often the 'hand-clasp' suggestion, whereby members of the audience are told that they are unable to separate their interlocked fingers. These participants may then be put through a traditional trance-inducing ceremony, although some entertainers use a dramatic-looking 'rapid induction' method whereby eye-fixation on the hypnotist's hand is followed by the participant's falling backwards on to the stage floor with the hypnotist's assistance. Non-responders and uncooperative participants may then be deselected. Sometimes the number of participants is sufficiently large to allow further selection of the more entertaining members of the group, as the performance proceeds.

These preliminaries would not reliably select those who, in research papers, are identified by extensive psychometric tests as being of high hypnotic susceptibility; nor is it necessary to the performance that they do so. A person may prove to be a good subject for stage hypnosis for several reasons that are not related to hypnotic susceptibility. The ability to act in an improvised and hilarious manner is obviously one. It follows from these considerations, and those discussed under the previous heading, that one can make no reliable assumptions about people's hypnotic susceptibility by virtue of their participating in a stage hypnosis show, other than that they are more likely to be more susceptible than average. Evidence on the measured susceptibility of participants for stage hypnosis bears this out (Crawford, Kitner-Triolo, Clarke and Olesko, 1992).

Assumption 3: If the stage hypnotist does not cancel a suggestion properly then a participant may be compelled to respond to the suggestion on leaving the place of entertainment

Examples of such cases, given by Waxman (1978, 1988), are a man who continued the search for his navel and consulted a policeman, and a woman who squawked like a chicken every time she heard a whistle. A more recent case, reported in a tabloid newspaper (*The People*, 19 February 1995), concerned a man who filed a lost-property notice after he had been told that his brain had gone missing. The last-mentioned case may be dismissed as a stunt, but by what criteria? In this issue of *Contemporary Hypnosis* (Heap, 2000), I describe the case of a man who claimed to have experienced an overwhelming desire to have sexual intercourse with his furniture and domestic appliances following a stage hypnosis show. Two consultant psychiatrists and the man's general medical practitioner supported this claim on the basis that he was acting on a post-hypnotic suggestion.

Modern laboratory research, clinical experience and current theoretical understanding of hypnosis and suggestion indicate that a subject's response to a post-hypnotic suggestion is constrained in the following ways:

1. The suggested response must be within the subject's repertoire of abilities.
2. The response must be acceptable to the subject and compatible with the context in which it is given. For example, it is unlikely that the suggestion that the subject 'squawk like a chicken' would elicit that response in the clinical setting.
3. Although the suggestion may be experienced by the subject as having a compulsive quality, it involves cognitive effort on the subject's part (Barnier and McConkey, 1998) and may be overridden by the subject's own volition if such is demanded by the situation.
4. The influence of the suggestion is easily overridden by existing competing habits.
5. The subject's impulse to respond to the suggestion usually dissipates with time.
6. The influence of the suggestion is determined by the explicit and implicit demands of the context; when those demands are perceived as no longer operative, the subject stops responding. For example, in experiments on highly susceptible subjects, the response to post-hypnotic suggestion ceases when the experiment seems to have been temporarily suspended or when the subjects perceive themselves as no longer obliged to behave in the manner required by the experimenter; or even, although not always, when they are no longer under his or her surveillance (Fisher, 1954; Spanos, Menary, Brett, Cross and Ahmed, 1987).

Hence, the assertion that participants for stage hypnosis are endangered by the possibility of uncancelled suggestions is made on weak grounds. Of particular salience is the fact that when the stage hypnosis show has ended, important influences such as the context and the reason for acting on the suggestion are removed. This is not the case, say, after a session of clinical hypnosis, when the requirement is for the suggested response (for example, recalling a nauseous experience when putting a cigarette to one's lips) to persist in the person's everyday life; likewise in the case of a scientific experiment on the effect of post-hypnotic suggestions on the subject's everyday behaviour.

I shall later emphasize that any claim of injury following stage hypnosis should be framed according to established diagnostic criteria in medicine and psychiatry.

Perhaps, for example, a genuine instance of adverse and inappropriate perseveration of hypnotic responding could be explained in terms of obsessive-compulsive tendencies on the person's part. Such a person may feel compelled to continue responding because he or she believes that for some reason the requirement to respond is still operative (for example, 'the suggestion was not properly removed') and that *not* to respond would be (in the manner of obsessional thinking) problematical in some way.

Assumption 4: The stage hypnotist may not take a participant fully out of the hypnotic trance when the performance is over

This allegation was also made by the two psychiatrists and general practitioner involved in the case I describe in Heap (2000). Indeed, the initial diagnosis offered by the plaintiff's psychiatrist was that in the weeks after the stage hypnosis show, he had been in a 'trance-like, semi-hypnotic waking state'. Examples from the literature include that described by Kleinhauz and Beran (1981). This was a teenager who was admitted to hospital after participating in a stage hypnosis show. She had fallen into a deep stupor and could not be roused. Neurological and other medical investigations were negative, whereupon a number of psychiatric diagnoses were made without reference to her experience of stage hypnosis. She was in this condition for six days, at which point she was then seen by the main author of the paper, whose opinion was that she was in a pathological post-hypnotic state. The patient responded well to psychotherapy but after some months she was readmitted to hospital, once more in a deep stupor. No stage hypnosis was involved this time and the therapists therefore concluded that the girl was engaging in manipulation; her state of entrancement was now self-induced in order to control and punish her therapist for what she saw as his rejection of her, and was an attempt to regain his special attention.

In another, very anecdotal case described by Kleinhauz and Beran (1984), a male student had symptoms of acute psychosis, including bizarre behaviour, withdrawal, apathy, passivity and 'megalomania'. He had been previously hypnotized by a friend to help him prepare for an examination. The authors state, 'It is possible to conclude that his symptomatology had been entirely a product of a continuing hypnotic state' (1984: 287).

There is an obvious problem here of how one diagnoses a condition that has a limitless range of presenting symptoms, as revealed by the above examples. It is also clear from the discussion of assumption 1 that the notion that a person may remain wholly or partially in some special 'state of hypnotic trance' has little support in the scientific literature.

One interpretation of this assumption that may have some rational basis is to adopt a 'weak' definition of the notion of 'trance' – namely, a normal state of focused attention and detachment from ongoing reality (Heap, 1996). From this perspective we can say that a person who has 'not been adequately alerted from trance' is someone who may still be preoccupied with the thoughts, images, memories and feelings that he or she has been experiencing during hypnosis. On occasion, this may be hazardous (for example, if he or she has to drive home through busy traffic), but it is continuous with everyday experience and is normally transient and self-terminating. It may be that some individuals who have strong dissociative tendencies are more inclined to these after-effects. As well as this, where hypnosis has been used as a relaxation procedure, as with similar methods, individuals may feel groggy or drowsy on alerting, and may need some time to recover. However, this is not a special kind of drowsiness or grogginess that is uniquely hypnotic and thus in some way especially dangerous or pathological.

None of this supports the contention that participants in stage hypnosis are at risk by the hypnotist's 'not releasing them from their trance', in the same way that a witch or wizard may not release a victim from a magic spell. The hypnotist's task is to inform the subject that the hypnotic session is now over (or the subject may make that decision for himself or herself) and it is time to orient himself or herself to the immediate present.

Some ground rules for assessing claims

Even without reference to actual claims of harm, it is not difficult to understand how, from a rational and scientifically informed consideration of the subject, stage hypnosis could, in certain circumstances, cause distress. Participants usually experience hypnosis as intense and unusual, and the term 'hypnosis' has 'spooky' and 'mind-controlling' connotations. Some people, especially those of an anxious nature, may regret participating, as they may believe that they were under the complete control of the hypnotist. The context of stage hypnosis may make it difficult for some participants to decline to respond or to disengage completely if they wish. A stage hypnotist may suggest an experience that a participant may usually find distressing – for example, engaging in an activity about which he or she has a phobia, or, in the case of a female participant, that she has lost one of her breasts and must find out who has it.

However, when assessing claims, it is important to acknowledge an essential fact, one which has emerged over the past 100 years of scientific inquiry – namely, that hypnosis is not a pathological state, and, where adverse reactions are evoked, these are not the result of any unique psychopathological features because of the person's experience of hypnosis.

It is necessary, therefore, that any claim of psychological injury due to stage hypnosis should be investigated on its own merits according to the following criteria:

1. The exact nature of the plaintiff's disorder should be described and defined according to established diagnostic criteria in medicine and psychiatry.
2. It should be made clear in terms of current knowledge of psychology and psychiatry how the complainant's alleged symptoms have been caused by the stage hypnotist's actions.
3. The possible role of hypnosis should be described with reference to current learned and scientific knowledge concerning the nature of hypnosis.

The case of *Gates* vs *McKenna*

This case, in which the plaintiff alleged that he had a schizophrenic illness after participating in a stage hypnosis show, is described more fully by Wagstaff in this issue (Wagstaff, 2000). In view of what has been stated earlier, it is worth mentioning that initially the plaintiff's psychiatrist offered a fairly orthodox, though highly tenuous, explanation of the possible causal connection between the plaintiff's experience of stage hypnosis and his subsequent mental illness. He contended that as schizophrenia is known to be precipitated by 'life events or environmental stressors', the plaintiff developed a schizophrenic illness because stage hypnosis is 'an environmental event or stressor'. The term 'life event' as used here, however, seems to have acquired an extraordinary elasticity, and it is revealing that the same psychiatrist, in a report on another alleged victim of stage hypnosis, this time with a diagnosis of major depression, stated that depression may be precipitated by 'life events', the 'life event' in this case again being stage hypnosis.

It is not too difficult, therefore, to understand how the plaintiff's legal representatives were attracted to the idea that the state of mind into which their client was allegedly placed could be expressed in terms of neurophysiological changes, and that these changes, at least according to one line of theorizing, also underlie the condition that he allegedly had following the defendant's actions. Neither, however, it is difficult to acknowledge the great weakness of this stance.

It is instructive to compare this claim with an example of the persistence of psychological disturbance following neurological insult, namely post-concussional state. It is established beyond doubt that a blow or sudden jolt to the head may have neurological effects described as 'concussion', and that these may be corroborated by physical examination of the patient at the time. There is good evidence that even a year later some effects (headache, lack of concentration, irritability, and so on) may persist (Blakely and Harrington, 1993; Wright and Telford, 1996). Extensive neurological and neuropsychological examination and brain scanning may raise the suspicion of residual organic impairment. Yet in any individual personal injury claim, it may still be difficult to make a convincing case of post-concussional syndrome, and the defence may readily find expert witnesses to challenge this diagnosis (Bohnen and Jolles, 1992).

One great weakness of the plaintiff's case was that it was speculated, largely on a theoretical basis, that the verbal communications of the defendant triggered clinically significant changes in the plaintiff's neurophysiological functioning. Again, on theoretical grounds, the plaintiff's psychiatric symptoms were linked to these putative neurophysiological changes. Yet no results of any neurological examination, brain scan or neurological assessment were offered by the plaintiff's side.

In this case the plaintiff's problem was schizophrenia, yet, prior to this case no authoritative writer was seriously arguing that 'hypnosis causes schizophrenia'. Neither was there any good evidence that hypnosis or stage hypnosis could precipitate the mental deterioration that Gates reportedly displayed in the days and months following his experience.

These considerations raise the question of how one may demonstrate negligence in such a case and whether the defendant could reasonably have foreseen and forestalled the harm that was alleged to have transpired through his actions. For obvious reasons, the UK Home Office model conditions on stage hypnosis (Home Office, 1996) do not require that the entertainer conduct a mental state examination on his or her participants. He or she is advised to inform the audience that participants should be of 'normal physical and mental health'. However, the plaintiff's side in this case asserted that he had no history of psychiatric problems nor was there anything to suggest that he was at risk of developing a mental illness.

Notwithstanding this, anyone reading accounts of *Gates* vs *McKenna* (Wagstaff, 2000) will ponder the following: whether or not this question applies to this particular case, is it advisable for a person with a psychotic predisposition to take part in stage hypnosis? Intuitively, from the earlier discussion of the possible hazards of stage hypnosis, one is likely to feel that this is not the sort of activity in which someone with psychotic tendencies should engage.

Conclusions

People who use hypnosis in therapy, or who investigate hypnosis from a scientific standpoint, can feel no particular obligations to stage hypnotists. I, for one, am convinced that when hypnosis is used for the purposes of entertainment it gives the public a completely misguided impression of what it actually is and how it may be used therapeutically. However, we must hold steadfast to a rational and scientific understanding of the subject, one that is consistent with mainstream psychology, the neurosciences and their related disciplines. This requires an attitude of impartiality and objectivity when one is asked to assess claims of harm against untrained 'hypnotherapists' or stage hypnotists. In this paper I have attempted to set some ground rules for this kind of work, which have these considerations in mind.

References

Baker RA (1990) They Call it Hypnosis. Buffalo, NY: Prometheus.

Barber TX, Spanos NP, Chaves JF (1974) Hypnosis, Imagination and Human Potentialities. New York: Pergamon.

Barnier AJ, McConkey KM (1998) Posthypnotic responding: Knowing when to stop helps keep it going. International Journal of Clinical and Experimental Hypnosis 46: 204–19.

Blakely TA, Harrington DE (1993) Mild head injury is not always mild: Implications for damage litigation. Medicine, Science and Law 33: 231–42.

Bohnen N, Jolles J (1992) Neurobehavioral aspects of postconcussive symptoms after mild head injury. Journal of Nervous and Mental Diseases 180: 683–92.

Crawford HJ, Kitner-Triolo M, Clarke SW, Olesko B (1992) Transient positive and negative experiences accompanying stage hypnosis. Journal of Abnormal Psychology 101: 663–7.

Echterling LG, Emmerling DA (1987) Impact of stage hypnosis. American Journal of Clinical Hypnosis 29: 149–54.

Erickson MH (1962) Stage hypnosis back syndrome. American Journal of Clinical Hypnosis 3: 141–2.

Fisher S (1954) The role of expectancy in the performance of posthypnotic behaviour. Journal of Abnormal Psychology 49: 503–7.

Heap M (1995) A case of death following stage hypnosis: analysis and implications. Contemporary Hypnosis 12: 99–110.

Heap M (1996) The nature of hypnosis. The Psychologist 9: 498–501.

Heap M (2000) A legal case of a man complaining of an extraordinary sexual disorder following stage hypnosis. Contemporary Hypnosis 17: 143–9.

Hoggart S, Hutchinson M (1995) Bizarre Beliefs. London: Richard Cohen.

Home Office (1989) Model conditions to be attached to public entertainments licenses. Annex to Home Office Circular No 42/1989.

Home Office (1995) Report of the Expert Panel Appointed to Consider the Effects of Participation in Performances of Stage Hypnosis.

Home Office (1996) Model conditions to be attached to licences for the performance of stage hypnotism. Annex to Home Office Circular No 39/1996.

Kirsch I (1991) The social learning theory of hypnosis. In SJ Lynn, JW Rhue (eds) Theories of Hypnosis: Current Models and Perspective. New York: Guilford Press, pp. 439–65.

Kleinhauz M, Beran B (1981) Misuses of hypnosis: A medical emergency. International Journal of Clinical and Experimental Hypnosis 29: 148–61.

Kleinhauz M, Beran B (1984) Misuse of hypnosis: A factor in psychopathology. American Journal of Clinical Hypnosis 26: 148–61.

Kleinhauz M, Drefuss DA, Beran B, Goldberg T, Axikri D (1979) Some after-effects of stage hypnosis: A case study of psychopathological manifestations. International Journal of Clinical and Experimental Hypnosis 27: 7–19.

MacHovec FJ (1986) Hypnosis Complications. Springfield, IL: Charles C. Thomas.
MacHovec FJ (1988) Hypnosis complications: Risk factors and prevention. American Journal of Clinical Hypnosis 31: 40–9.
Meeker WB, Barber TX (1971) Toward an explanation of stage hypnosis. Journal of Abnormal Psychology 77: 61–70.
Misra P (1985) Hazards of stage hypnosis. Paper presented at the 10th International Congress of Hypnosis and Psychosomatic Medicine, Toronto, 10–16 August.
Spanos NP, Menary E, Brett PJ, Cross W, Ahmed Q (1987) Failure of hypnotic responding to occur outside the experimental setting. Journal of Abnormal Psychology 96: 52–7.
Wagstaff GF (2000) Can hypnosis cause madness? Contemporary Hypnosis 17(3): 97–111.
Waxman D (1978) Misuse of hypnosis. British Medical Journal ii: 571.
Waxman D (1981) Hypnosis: A Guide for Patients and Practitioners. London: George Allen and Unwin.
Waxman D (1988) The problems of stage hypnotism. In M Heap (ed.) Hypnosis: Current Clinical, Experimental and Forensic Practices. London: Croom Helm, pp. 426–33.
Waxman D (1989) Hartland's Medical and Dental Hypnosis. London: Ballière Tindall.
Wright JC, Telford R (1996) Postconcussive symptoms and psychological distress. Clinical Rehabilitation 10: 334–6.

Address for correspondence:
Dr Michael Heap, BSc, MSc, PhD
Centre for Psychotherapeutic Studies,
University of Sheffield,
10 Claremont Crescent,
Sheffield S10 2TA.
Email: m.heap@sheffield.ac.uk

[32]

Immediate and Persisting Effects of Misleading Questions and Hypnosis on Memory Reports

Alan Scoboria
University of Connecticut

Giuliana Mazzoni
Seton Hall University

Irving Kirsch
University of Connecticut

Leonard S. Milling
University of Hartford

Immediate and persisting effects of misleading questions and hypnosis on memory reports were assessed. After listening to a story, 52 highly suggestible students and 59 low and medium suggestible students were asked misleading or neutral questions in or out of hypnosis. All participants were then asked neutral questions without hypnosis. Both hypnosis and misleading questions significantly increased memory errors, and misleading questions produced significantly more errors than did hypnosis. The 2 effects were additive, so that misleading questions in hypnosis produced the greatest number of errors. There were no significant interactions with level of hypnotic suggestibility. Implications of these findings for the per se exclusion of posthypnotic testimony are discussed.

Hypnosis has received considerable attention in recent years as a method of enhancing eyewitness memory reports. Although some studies have suggested that hypnosis may have a small effect on improving memory accuracy, the effect is unreliable and has been linked to factors that are not specific to hypnosis (Erdelyi, 1994). Most of the studies in this area indicate that hypnotic procedures do not increase the accuracy of memory. Instead, it results in increased error rates and enhanced confidence in the accuracy of both true and false retrieved details (for reviews, see Erdelyi, 1994; Kebbell & Wagstaff, 1998; Orne, Whitehouse, Dinges, & Orne, 1996).

The negative effects of hypnosis on posthypnotic memory reports have led to a per se exclusion of posthypnotic testimony by witnesses in a number of states. Under this rule, any testimony occurring during or after a hypnotic procedure is inadmissible in court, and the only testimony a previously hypnotized witness can provide consists of statements recorded before the hypnotic procedure. A per se exclusion is presently applied to hypnotically refreshed testimony in approximately two thirds of the states. However, because of the Sixth Amendment to the U.S. constitution, which guarantees various rights to an accused person in a criminal trial, defendants who have been hypnotized for memory enhancement are permitted to testify (Scheflin, Spiegel, & Spiegel, 1999).

Hypnosis is only one of a number of suggestive procedures that can negatively impact the accuracy of memory reports (see Mazzoni, in press, for a review of procedures that result in memory distortions). For example, similar distortions can be obtained through the use of misleading questions (reviewed in Loftus, 1979). Leading questions involve material that inherently suggests a desired or correct answer to the subject. For example, the question "Did the woman have one or two children?" implies that the woman has children and that one of the options provided is correct. When the suggested material is inaccurate, the leading question is in fact a misleading question. A number of studies have demonstrated that variations in questions as small as a single word can affect an individual's response (Loftus & Zanni, 1975).

Although both hypnosis and misleading questions appear to have negative effects on the accuracy of memory reports, their status in court is quite different. Leading questions can be objected to in the courtroom, but witnesses are not barred from testifying on matters about which they have previously been asked leading questions. This difference between the legal status of hypnosis and that of leading questions reveals an implicit assumption that the effects of prior exposure to hypnosis are more pernicious than those of prior exposure to leading questions. However, there appear to be no empirical data addressing this issue. One purpose of the present study is to provide a comparison of the effects of hypnosis and misleading questions on memory reports. Per se exclusion of testimony from witnesses who have been hypnotized, but not of testimony from witnesses who have been asked leading questions, would be supported empirically only if the effects of hypnosis were more pernicious than those of misleading questions.

A second purpose of this study is to investigate the effects of hypnosis and hypnotic suggestibility on the immediate and persisting effects of misleading questions. The questions are: Does

---

Alan Scoboria and Irving Kirsch, Department of Psychology, University of Connecticut; Giuliana Mazzoni, Department of Psychology, Seton Hall University; Leonard S. Milling, Department of Psychology, University of Hartford.

The data described herein were collected by Alan Scoboria as partial fulfillment of requirements for a master's degree in clinical psychology at the University of Connecticut. We thank Gregory Bivens, Jason Gerchewski, Chris Giulietti, Michelle Malarney, Laura Martinelli, and Mark Relyea for their assistance in data collection and analysis. We thank David Kenny for his advice on statistical analyses.

Correspondence concerning this article should be addressed to Giuliana Mazzoni, Department of Psychology, Seton Hall University, South Orange, New Jersey 07079. E-mail: mazzongi@shu.edu

hypnosis potentiate the negative effects of misleading questions? Does hypnotic suggestibility moderate the effect of misleading questions? Is there an interaction between these two variables, such that hypnosis potentiates the effects of misleading questions only to the extent that participants are hypnotically suggestible? Do these effects persist when misleading questions are replaced by neutral questions asked outside of hypnosis?

Previous studies have produced mixed results. The induction of hypnosis potentiated the leading question effect in two studies (Putnam, 1979; Zelig & Beidleman, 1981), but failed to affect responses to misleading questions in three others (Linton & Sheehan, 1994; Sheehan, Garnett, & Robertson, 1993; Sheehan & Linton, 1993). Compared with people low in hypnotic suggestibility, highly suggestible participants yielded to more misleading questions in three studies (Linton & Sheehan, 1994; Sheehan et al., 1993; Sheehan & Linton, 1993), but not in a fourth (Register & Kihlstrom, 1988). Interactions between hypnotic suggestibility and the effects of hypnosis on responses to misleading questions have not been reported in any study.

The Register and Kihlstrom (1988) study was the only one of these studies that assessed the persisting effects of misleading questions, but it did not assess the effects of inducing hypnosis. Persisting effects were also assessed by Sheehan, Grigg, and McCann (1984). They reported that highly suggestible participants who had been hypnotized and asked misleading questions subsequently made more errors to neutral questions than did low suggestible participants. However, the low suggestible participants in the Sheehan et al. (1984) study were simulators who had been asked to pretend to be hypnotized.

The effects of misleading questions can best be assessed by comparing responses to misleading questions with responses to neutral questions. Thus, a definitive answer to the question of whether hypnosis increases the effects of misleading questions would require comparisons of responses to the same number of misleading and neutral questions with and without hypnosis. This has not been assessed in previous studies. Also, most studies select for high and low levels of suggestibility, thus ignoring the majority of people who are moderately responsive to suggestion. Furthermore, no previous study evaluating the combined effects of hypnosis and misleading questions has provided a baseline measurement of natural memory errors made because of normal processes such as forgetting. The accurate assessment of the individual and combined effects of misleading questions and hypnosis on memory requires a no-treatment control group to which the other groups may be compared. In the present experiments, this is provided by including a group of participants who are asked neutral questions outside of hypnosis.

The experiment reported here assesses the independent and combined effects of hypnosis and misleading questions on memory accuracy in a stratified sample of high, moderate, and low suggestible individuals. These effects were assessed twice. For the first assessment, half the participants were hypnotized and the other half were not. Within each of these conditions, half were given misleading questions and the other half were given neutral questions. During the second assessment, none of the participants were hypnotized and all were asked neutral forms of the questions. This corresponds to the common situation in which a person is asked neutral questions outside of hypnosis, after previously having been asked misleading questions about the same material, either in or out of hypnosis.

Method

Participants

Participants were 111 undergraduate students (64 women, 37 men, ages 18–21) at the University of Connecticut, selected from 1,000 students who had been screened for hypnotic suggestibility on the Carleton University Responsiveness to Suggestibility Scale (CURSS; Spanos, Radtke, Hodgins, Bertrand, & Stam, 1981) in groups of 1 to 50 participants. Participants received course credit for their involvement. To enhance the likelihood of finding a hypnotic effect if there was one, highs were overrepresented in the sample. Thus, 52 highly suggestible participants (scores of 5–7 on the CURSS) and 59 medium (scores of 3–4) and low (scores of 0–2) suggestible participants were included in the study. Because of experimenter error, exact scores on the CURSS were not retained. Instead, the following scores were used to indicate suggestibility: high = 3, medium = 2, low = 1. Data were collected over two semesters. The experiment was conducted with high suggestible participants in one semester and low and medium suggestible participants in the other.

Measures

Hypnotic suggestibility. Hypnotic suggestibility was measured by using behavioral scores on the CURSS. The CURSS consists of a hypnotic induction and seven test suggestions. Self-reported behavioral scores on the CURSS are obtained by having participants complete a questionnaire on which they indicate whether they had made the behavioral response called for by the suggestion (0 = no; 1 = yes). Behavioral responsiveness to suggestion is assessed as the sum of these ratings. A test–retest reliability coefficient of .67 has been reported (Spanos, Radtke, Hodgins, Bertrand, Stam, & Dubreuil, 1983, p. 560). Construct validity is indicated by a correlation of .62 between CURSS and the Harvard Group Scale of Hypnotic Susceptibility, Form A, and a correlation of .65 between the CURSS and the Stanford Hypnotic Susceptibility Scale: Form C (Spanos, Radtke, Hodgins, Bertrand, Stam, & Moretti, 1983). We used the Comey and Kirsch (1999) modification of the CURSS suggestions. In this version of the CURSS, instructions and cues for goal-directed fantasies are replaced by additional repetitions of the suggestion. This modification of the CURSS results in a more normal distribution of response scores. Comey and Kirsch reported internal consistency coefficients (Cronbach's alphas) of .63 for behavioral scores on this version of the CURSS (p. 71).

Recall. We constructed a new measure of recall to assess the effects of hypnosis and misleading questions on memory reports. Our measure of recall was derived from Register and Kihlstrom's (1988) modification of the Gudjonsson Suggestibility Scale (GSS; Gudjonsson, 1984). The GSS assesses individual differences in susceptibility to suggestive questioning and the tendency to change answers as a result of social pressure. A narrative is read to participants, who are then asked to report what they can recall about the story. Following a 40-min distraction period, participants are again asked what they can recall. They are then asked a series of 20 questions, 15 of which contain misleading information (i.e., information that is not contained in the story or that contradicts information contained in the story). Participants then receive negative feedback; they are informed that a number of responses were incorrect and that they therefore will be asked the questions a second time. Responses are scored for yield (acceptance of the misinformation in the misleading questions) and shift (changes in responses at the second questioning).

Register and Kihlstrom (1988) modified the GSS for use with an American sample. Their modification contains a slightly different story and questions. More important for the purpose of this study, it contains two sets of questions. The first set of questions consists of 18 misleading questions and 6 neutral questions. The second set consists of 24 neutral questions, containing no leading characteristics. For each misleading question in the first set, there is a corresponding neutral question in the second. For example, the misleading question "Did the woman have one or two children?" in Set 1 was replaced by the neutral question "Did the woman have any children?" in Set 2. We modified two of the neutral questions from the Register and Kihlstrom version. "Describe the complexions of the assailants" was changed to "Of what race or races were the assailants?" "Describe the woman's husband's attitude during the police interview" was modified to read "What was the woman's husband's attitude, if any, during the police interview?" to eliminate what was decided to be a leading question.

The GSS was designed as a measure of individual differences in interrogative suggestibility, which is the tendency to yield to social pressure and misleading information during interrogations. Our study did not concern interrogative suggestibility. Instead, its purpose was to assess the effects of hypnosis and misleading questions on the accuracy of memory reports. This was assessed by categorizing participants' responses to misleading and nonleading questions as *correct, incorrect,* or *don't know* (DK; when the participant stated that he or she did not know the answer to a question). Although the questions used to elicit these reports were derived from a modified version of the GSS, the primary measures of the dependent variables of this study are not contained in that scale. Answers to questions were tape recorded, transcribed, and then categorized independently by two raters. Yield (reporting answers consistent with the misinformation in the misleading question) was also scored (as in the GSS), but only for participants in the misleading question groups. Note that yield constitutes a subset of error responses.

Responses to misleading and neutral questions were scored one point each. Half points were scored when answers provided both correct and incorrect information (e.g., "Of what race or races were the assailants?"; response: "Asian and White"; correct response "1 was Asian, the others were not known"; response scored as half correct, half error). Interrater reliability was calculated with Pearson correlations on the scores for each category. For Trial 1, these coefficients were .97 for correct responses, .98 for DK responses, .95 for errors, and .99 for yield. For Trial 2, the correlations were .82 for correct responses, .95 for DK responses, and .98 for errors, and .96 for yield. Disagreements were resolved through discussion.

Procedure

The experiment was designed as a 2 × 2 factorial, involving misleading or neutral questions administered in or out of hypnosis. Thus, the four cells were misleading questions in hypnosis (L + H), misleading questions without hypnosis (L), neutral questions in hypnosis (H), and the control condition (C) consisting of neutral questions without hypnosis. Six undergraduate experimenters, who were unaware of the variables being studied, administered experimental procedures. Participants who had been prescreened on the CURSS were contacted by telephone and invited to take part in an individual 90-min memory experiment. Participants randomized to hypnotic conditions were informed that their participation would involve their being hypnotized and that this presented no danger to them whatsoever. No rationale for the use of hypnosis was provided. Participants in nonhypnotic conditions were not aware of the use of hypnosis in the study.

After the signing of informed consent, participants were played the taped narrative. They were then asked to recall all that they could about the narrative. This was followed by a 40-min distraction period, in which participants completed forms that were unrelated to the study. These were the quality of relationships inventory (Pierce, Sarason, & Sarason, 1991), the State Self-Esteem Scale (Heatherton & Polivy, 1991), and the Positive Affect/Negative Affect Scale (Watson, Clark, & Tellegen, 1988). Participants were then asked to recall as much as possible about the narrative. At this point, half the participants were hypnotized by means of an audiotaped hypnotic induction, and the remaining participants continued to complete the distraction task. Hypnotized participants received the following audiotaped suggestion for memory enhancement:

> Now please keep your eyes closed and continue to relax. In a moment, you will be asked a series of questions about the story you have heard. You will be able to answer these questions while remaining deeply relaxed and hypnotized. You will find it very easy to focus your attention and concentration on the story that you have heard. The answers to the questions will come easily and effortlessly to mind, in your mind's eye, and you will have no trouble remembering the information and answering the questions. An interesting thing about hypnosis and memory is that the more details you recall, the easier you will find it to recall even more. Although you are still deeply hypnotized, you will be able to open your eyes when you are asked to do so, to speak, and to follow the instructions of the experimenter.

Half the participants were then asked the set of misleading questions, and the other half were asked the set of neutral questions. This first trial provided an assessment of the immediate effects of hypnosis and misleading questions. Hypnotized participants were then brought out of hypnosis. Following a 10-min distracter period, all participants were asked the set of neutral questions. This second trial provided an assessment of the persisting effects of the prior use of hypnosis and misleading questions. When participants provided unclear or multiple answers, the research assistant prompted participants to clarify their responses.

Results

Means and standard deviations of correct responses, DK responses, and errors on Trials 1 and 2 are reported in Table 1. Also included in Table 1 are means and standard deviations for accuracy rates, scored as correct responses as a proportion of the sum of correct and incorrect responses. These data were analyzed with a regression analyses using Type I sums of squares,[1] in which the main effects for hypnosis, misleading questions, and hypnotic suggestibility were entered one at a time, followed by the interaction terms. This was supplemented by analyses of covariance, with hypnotic suggestibility as the covariate. Both analyses yielded the same pattern of results for hypnosis, misleading questions, and the interaction of these two factors. Therefore, we present only the data from the regression, which also provides tests of the interactions with suggestibility. The results of these analyses are presented in Table 2. Significance was found only for main effects of hypnosis and misleading questions. Effect sizes (*d*) were calculated as the standardized mean difference between the conditions being compared.

Analyses of correct responses revealed a significant immediate effect of hypnosis. Examination of Table 1 indicates that while they were hypnotized, participants in hypnotic conditions remembered more correct information than did participants in the nonhypnotic conditions ($d = 0.42$). However, this effect did not persist after hypnosis had been terminated ($d = 0.28$). Analyses of DK responses revealed significant immediate and persisting main effects of hypnosis compared with no-hypnosis (Trial 1, $d = 0.96$; Trial 2, $d = 0.65$) and misleading questions compared with neutral

[1] This is also known as a hierarchical decomposition of the sum-of-squares. Each term is adjusted for only the terms that precede it in the model. However, the error variance for each term is given from the last equation with all the terms in it.

Table 1
Means and Standard Deviations for Correct Responses, Don't Know (DK) Responses, and Errors

	Condition							
	M + H		M		H		C	
Variable	*M*	*SD*	*M*	*SD*	*M*	*SD*	*M*	*SD*
Trial 1								
Correct	15.32	2.73	14.09	3.47	15.21	2.90	13.86	3.27
DK	1.00	1.33	3.89	3.86	4.61	2.77	6.79	2.71
Errors	7.57	2.95	5.91	3.17	3.93	2.55	3.07	1.70
Accuracy	0.67	0.13	0.70	0.14	0.79	0.12	0.82	0.11
Trial 2								
Correct	14.39	2.56	13.52	2.73	14.67	2.58	14.00	3.18
DK	2.68	1.54	4.82	3.15	5.32	3.25	6.89	3.67
Errors	6.89	2.06	5.59	2.53	3.89	2.77	3.04	2.03
Accuracy	0.66	0.11	0.70	0.11	0.78	0.13	0.82	0.12

Note. M + H = misleading questions and hypnosis; M = misleading questions; H = hypnosis; C = control.

questions (Trial 1, $d = 1.23$; Trial 2, $d = 0.82$). Participants in both hypnotic and misleading questions conditions made fewer DK responses than those in nonhypnotic and neutral question conditions. Analyses of errors revealed significant immediate and persisting main effects of hypnosis compared with no hypnosis (Trial 1, $d = 0.49$; Trial 2, $d = 0.46$) and misleading questions compared with neutral questions (Trial 1, $d = 1.25$; Trial 2, $d = 1.18$). Both independent variables led to increased error rates. Analyses of accuracy rates revealed significant and persisting main effects of misleading questions (Trial 1, $d = 1.92$; Trial 2, $d = 2.04$). Compared with neutral questions, misleading questions resulted in significantly lower accuracy rates for questions to which participants provided an answer. None of the interactions were significant.

There are two questions of interest that are not directly assessed in the regression analyses. These are: Do the effects of hypnosis and misleading questions differ in magnitude, and Are the combined effects of misleading questions and hypnosis greater than their individual effects? Because interactions with suggestibility did not approach significance, we used the following three sets of post hoc *t* tests to answer these questions: (a) hypnosis alone versus misleading questions alone, (b) hypnosis and misleading questions combined versus misleading questions alone, and (c) hypnosis and misleading questions combined versus hypnosis

Table 2
Regression Analyses of Correct Responses, Don't Know (DK) Responses, Errors, and Accuracy on Misleading Questions, Hypnosis, and Suggestibility

	Correct		DK		Errors		Accuracy	
Variable	F^a	η^2	F^a	η^2	F^a	η^2	F^a	η^2
Trial 1								
Hypnosis (H)	4.70*	.04	22.73**	.18	6.33*	.06	1.69	.02
Leading questions (M)	0.08	.00	36.75**	.26	40.20**	.28	25.37**	.20
Suggestibility (S)	0.03	.00	0.67	.01	0.12	.00	0.01	.00
H × M	0.01	.00	0.45	.00	0.63	.01	0.04	.00
H × S	1.07	.01	0.76	.01	0.08	.00	0.41	.00
M × S	0.02	.00	0.54	.00	0.18	.00	0.01	.00
H × M × S	0.09	.00	0.02	.00	0.07	.00	0.01	.00
Trial 2								
Hypnosis (H)	2.10	.02	10.39**	.09	5.90*	.05	2.45	.02
Leading questions (M)	0.52	.01	16.54**	.14	37.53**	.27	30.48**	.23
Suggestibility (S)	0.00	.00	0.32	.00	0.52	.01	0.44	.01
H × M	0.03	.00	0.24	.00	0.25	.00	0.91	.00
H × S	0.48	.01	0.01	.00	0.16	.00	0.64	.00
M × S	1.23	.01	0.14	.00	1.00	.01	0.38	.01
H × M × S	0.01	.00	0.18	.00	0.17	.00	0.72	.00

[a] $df = (1, 103)$.
$^*p < .05$. $^{**}p < .01$.

alone. These analyses were performed on errors and DK responses. Correct responses were not analyzed because the overall analysis failed to reveal an effect of misleading questions, and accuracy was not analyzed because the overall analysis failed to reveal an effect of hypnosis.

The first comparison revealed significant differences in errors between hypnosis-only group and misleading-questions-only group, immediate, $t(55) = 2.55$, $p < .05$, $d = 0.69$; persistent, $t(55) = 2.37$, $p < .05$, $d = 0.64$. Thus, although significant increases in errors were produced by both hypnosis and misleading questions, the misleading questions produced significantly more errors than hypnosis. No differences were found for DK responses.

The second comparison revealed significant differences in errors and DK responses between participants who were asked misleading questions during hypnosis and those who were asked misleading questions without being hypnotized, immediate errors, $t(53) = 2.01$, $p < .05$, $d = 0.54$; persistent errors, $t(53) = 2.10$, $p < .05$, $d = 0.57$; immediate DK responses, $t(53) = 3.74$, $p < .01$, $d = 1.11$; persistent DK responses $t(53) = 3.21$, $p < .01$, $d = 0.91$. More errors and fewer DK responses were made when participants were asked misleading questions in hypnosis than when asked misleading questions without hypnosis.

The third comparison revealed significant immediate and persisting differences in both errors and DK responses between people who were asked misleading questions in hypnosis and those who were asked neutral questions in hypnosis, immediate errors, $t(54) = 4.94$, $p < .01$, $d = 1.32$; persistent errors, $t(54) = 4.60$, $p < .01$, $d = 1.24$; immediate DK responses, $t(54) = 6.22$, $p < .01$, $d = 1.76$; persistent DK responses, $t(54) = 3.88$, $p < .01$, $d = 1.10$. The two procedures combined resulted in significantly more errors and fewer DK responses than either procedure alone.

Finally, we analyzed the effect of hypnosis on yields to the information contained in misleading questions among participants who had been assigned to the misleading question condition. Mean number of yields to misleading questions on Trials 1 and 2 as a function of whether participants had been hypnotized is reported in Table 3. These data were analyzed by a regression analyses by using Type I sums of squares, in which hypnosis was entered first, followed by hypnotic suggestibility and the interaction between hypnosis and suggestibility. The results of these analyses are presented in Table 4. They indicate that hypnosis significantly enhanced the tendency to yield to misleading questions ($d = 0.59$), but this effect was no longer significant when the misleading questions were replaced by neutral questions ($d = 0.41$). Neither the main effects of hypnotic suggestibility nor the interactions of hypnosis with hypnotic suggestibility approached significance.

Table 3
Immediate and Persisting Yields to Misleading Questions as a Function of Hypnosis

Trial	Condition: Hypnosis *M*	Hypnosis *SD*	No hypnosis *M*	No hypnosis *SD*
1	7.04	2.91	5.22	3.25
2	4.54	2.27	3.70	1.84

Table 4
Regression Analyses of Yields on Hypnosis and Hypnotic Suggestibility

Variable	F^a	η^2
Trial 1		
Hypnosis (H)	4.62*	.08
Suggestibility (S)	0.36	.01
H × S	0.08	.00
Trial 2		
Hypnosis (H)	2.13	.04
Suggestibility (S)	0.01	.00
H × S	0.11	.00

[a] $df = (1, 51)$.
* $p < .05$.

Discussion

This study assessed the separate and combined effects of misleading questions and hypnosis on responses to a series of objective questions about a tape-recorded narrative. The experimental manipulations provide an analogue of situations that occur in the legal context. Witnesses in legal cases are examined before testifying in court, and there is no control over the degree to which leading questions are used in these pretrial interrogations. Leading questions are sometimes asked during court proceedings as well. In this case, an objection may be raised, and the question might be rephrased. Nevertheless, prior exposure to a leading question may affect subsequent responses. Similarly, concerns about the effect of hypnosis on a witness's testimony relate to the prior use of hypnosis, as hypnosis is never induced while a witness is on the stand. As in court testimony, in this study the final memory reports were obtained after hypnosis had been terminated and after misleading questions had been replaced by neutral questions.

In this study, both hypnosis and misleading questions led participants to produce incorrect responses, rather than say they did not know the answer to a question. Misleading questions produced significantly more memory errors than did hypnosis, and the two effects were additive, so that the combination of misleading questions and hypnosis produced significantly more errors than either manipulation alone. Also, misleading questions produced a significant decrease in accuracy.

Consistent with the results of two prior studies (Putnam, 1979; Zelig & Beidleman, 1981), but inconsistent with three others (Linton & Sheehan, 1994; Sheehan et al., 1993; Sheehan & Linton, 1993), we found that hypnosis potentiated the tendency to yield to misleading questions. As in Sheehan et al. (1984), the negative effects of hypnosis on memory persisted after hypnosis had been terminated. Like Register and Kihlstrom (1988), but unlike data reported by Sheehan and his colleagues (Linton & Sheehan, 1994; Sheehan et al., 1993; Sheehan & Linton, 1993), yields to misleading questions were not significantly associated with hypnotic suggestibility.

Because misleading questions produced more errors than hypnosis, our data provide little support for a per se exclusion of posthypnotic testimony in the absence of a similar exclusion of testimony that has been obtained after witnesses have been exposed to leading questions. Either of two options would be consistent with the data observed in this study: (a) that the per se exclusion rule be extended to witnesses who have been asked leading questions or (b) that the per se exclusion of posthypnotic testimony be dropped.

It is important to stress, however, that the results of this study do not provide any support for the use of hypnosis to enhance memory. Although there was a significant increase in correct responding during hypnosis, it did not persist when participants were asked questions outside of hypnosis. Furthermore, it was accompanied by a similar increase in memory errors, which did persist after participants had been brought out of hypnosis. Nevertheless, our data argue against singling out hypnosis as a particularly pernicious procedure. Hypnosis produced significantly fewer errors than misleading questions. These data are inconsistent with a per se exclusion of testimony from witnesses who have been questioned under hypnosis, but not from witnesses who have previously been asked leading questions.

The Dissociation Between Hypnosis and Misleading Questions

The results of this study also suggest that two different mechanisms are responsible for the increase in memory errors observed in hypnosis and after being asked misleading questions. The decrease in DK responses produced by hypnosis was accompanied by almost identical increases in both correct and incorrect responses. Specifically, there was a mean of 1.30 more correct responses and 1.28 more errors in the hypnotic condition than in the nonhypnotic condition. In contrast, the decrease in DK responses produced by misleading questions was accompanied by an equivalent increase in errors. For example, on Trial 1, there was an average of 3.28 fewer DK responses and 3.26 more errors in the misleading questions condition than in the neutral question condition. Thus, participants exposed to misleading questions evidenced a shift from reporting not knowing the answer to particular questions about a past experience to reporting inaccurate information, whereas participants exposed to hypnosis shifted from reporting not knowing to reporting both accurate and inaccurate information.

This dissociation between the effects of hypnosis and the effects of misleading questions suggests that those effects may be due to different mechanisms. The key to the dissociation is the presence or absence of misleading cues. It is commonly believed that hypnosis enhances memory, and this belief may lead to a criterion shift in which the level of certainty required for a person to produce a response is lowered, such that participants are more likely to report information about which they are relatively uncertain (see Koriat & Goldsmith, 1996). However, if they are not provided with misleading cues, some of the answers produced by the criterion shift are likely to be accurate, whereas others will be inaccurate. Thus, there is an increase in production of responses (i.e., the significant decrease in DK responses in our data) that is not accompanied by a significant increase in accuracy.

In contrast, misleading questions provide inaccurate cues about how to answer the questions. For example, the misleading question "Did the woman have one or two children?" incorrectly implies that the woman had children, when, in fact, this information was not present in the story that participants heard. These misleading cues produce an increase in errors and also a decrease in accuracy. In future studies, it would be useful to analyze the effects of hypnosis and misleading questions on memory using signal detection analyses, which is precluded in the present study by the use of recall rather than recognition data and by the presence of three response categories, resulting in an inability to hold the number of correct and incorrect responses used to calculate hit rates and false alarms to constant output levels (see Klatzky & Erdelyi, 1985). It would also be useful to examine the separate and combined effects of hypnosis and misleading questions on participants' confidence in their responses, as this has been reported to be affected by hypnosis (Erdelyi, 1994; Kebbell & Wagstaff, 1998; Orne et al., 1996).

Immediate and Persisting Effects of Misleading Questions

Almost all of the errors made on Trial 1 by participants subjected to misleading questions were yields to the misinformation contained in the question. When interpreted in conjunction with the mean error and DK responses in the two groups asked only neutral questions, these data indicate that misleading questions produced two shifts in response. The first is a shift from not knowing the answer to providing an incorrect answer, which can be deduced from the significantly smaller number of DK responses in the misleading questions conditions than in the neutral questions conditions. The second shift in response is from one incorrect answer to another. This can be deduced from the fact that participants not asked misleading questions produced errors that were inconsistent with the information contained in the misleading questions (which they were not asked), whereas almost all of the errors made by participants in the misleading questions condition were influenced by the misinformation contained in the misleading questions. Thus, besides producing additional errors, yields to misleading questions replaced the errors that would have been made without the misleading cues.

On Trial 2, when the misleading questions were replaced by neutral questions, the effect of misleading questions on yield scores was no longer significant. Nevertheless, misleading questions continued to increase errors in memory reports. Thus, when misleading questions were replaced by neutral questions, participants continued to err in their responses, but the errors were less likely to contain the specific misinformation contained in the misleading question. The following typical example of how this occurred is instructive. One of the misleading questions was "Was the woman's purse brown?" (In fact, the color of the purse had not been mentioned in the story.) At Time 1, 15 students yielded to this misleading question by answering "yes," and only 3 students provided a different incorrect answer. On Trial 2, this misleading question was replaced with the neutral question, "What color was the woman's bag?" Only 3 of the participants who had previously been asked the misleading question responded with the answer "brown." However, 12 students in this condition responded erroneously by providing a different color. It is possible that by the second trial, the participants had forgotten some of the specific misinformation contained in the misleading questions, but retained a sense of knowing the answer (perhaps remembering that they had given an answer to it on the previous trial), which they then supplied incorrectly. Alternatively, not recalling the color, but feeling that they ought to, participants may have simply generated a color. In either case, these data suggest that yields may underestimate the deleterious effects of misleading questions, when scored after the misleading question has been replaced by a neutral question. Misleading questions may enhance the likelihood of error even when the misleading information is not accessible, thereby decreasing accuracy.

Conclusions

Both hypnosis and misleading questions produce deleterious effects on memory reports. These effects persist after hypnosis is terminated and misleading questions are replaced by neutral questions. Misleading questions produce significantly more errors than hypnosis, and the two effects are additive, such that misleading questions asked during hypnosis elicit significantly more errors than either procedure alone.

Hypnosis produces a shift from DK responses to both accurate and inaccurate responses, which is consistent with the hypothesis that its effects are due to a criterion shift. Misleading questions produce a shift from DK responses to errors, almost all of which are yields to the misleading information contained in the questions. The result is a significant decrease in accuracy. Thus, hypnosis and misleading questions appear to produce deleterious effects by different mechanisms.

When misleading questions are replaced by neutral questions, the prior exposure to misleading questions continues to produce errors in responding, but the errors are less likely to contain the misleading information provided in the misleading questions. In this circumstance, yields are likely to be an underestimate of the deleterious effects of misleading questions, because most of the errors produced by the prior exposure to the misleading cues would no longer be scored as yields.

In summary, our data indicate that the effects of prior exposure to misleading questions are more pernicious than those of prior exposure to hypnosis. These data challenge the logic behind a per se exclusion of testimony from witnesses who have previously been hypnotized, but no per se exclusion of testimony from witnesses who have previously been asked misleading questions.

References

Comey, G., & Kirsch, I. (1999). Intentional and spontaneous imagery in hypnosis: The phenomenology of hypnotic responding. *International Journal of Clinical and Experimental Hypnosis, 47,* 65–85.

Erdelyi, M. H. (1994). Hypnotic hypermnesia: The empty set of hypermnesia. *International Journal of Clinical and Experimental Hypnosis, 42,* 379–390.

Gudjonsson, G. (1984). A new scale of interrogative suggestibility. *Personality and Individual Differences, 7,* 195–199.

Heatherton, T. F., & Polivy, J. (1991). Development and validation of a scale for measuring state self-esteem. *Journal of Personality and Social Psychology, 60,* 895–910.

Kebbell, M. R., & Wagstaff, G. F. (1998). Hypnotic interviewing: The best way to interview eyewitnesses? *Behavioral Sciences and the Law, 16,* 115–129.

Klatzky, R. L., & Erdelyi, M. H. (1985). The response criterion problem in tests of hypnosis and memory. *The International Journal of Clinical and Experimental Hypnosis, 33,* 246–257.

Koriat, A., & Goldsmith, M. (1996). Monitoring and control processes in the strategic regulation of memory accuracy. *Psychological Review, 103,* 490–517.

Linton, C. P., & Sheehan, P. W. (1994). The relationship between interrogative suggestibility and susceptibility to hypnosis. *Australian Journal of Clinical and Experimental Hypnosis, 22,* 53–64.

Loftus, E. F. (1979). *Eyewitness testimony.* Cambridge, MA: Harvard University Press.

Loftus, E. F., & Zanni, G. (1975). Eyewitness testimony: The influence of the wording of a question. *Bulletin of the Psychonomic Society, 5,* 86–88.

Mazzoni, G. (in press). False memories. *European Psychologist.*

Orne, E. C., Whitehouse, W. G., Dinges, D. F., & Orne, M. T. (1996). Memory liabilities associated with hypnosis: Does low hypnotizability confer immunity? *International Journal of Clinical and Experimental Hypnosis, 44,* 354–369.

Pierce, G. R., Sarason, I. G., & Sarason, B. R. (1991). General and relationship-based perceptions of social support: Are two constructs better than one? *Journal of Personality and Social Psychology, 50,* 845–855.

Putnam, W. H. (1979). Hypnosis and distortions in eyewitness memory. *International Journal of Clinical and Experimental Hypnosis, 27,* 437–448.

Register, P. A., & Kihlstrom, J. F. (1988). Hypnosis and interrogative suggestibility. *Personality and Individual Differences, 9,* 549–558.

Scheflin, A. W., Spiegel, H., & Spiegel, D. (1999). Forensic uses of hypnosis. In A. K. Hess & I. B. Weiner (Eds.), *The handbook of forensic psychology* (2nd ed., pp. 474–498). New York: Wiley.

Sheehan, P. W., Garnett, M. S., & Robertson, R. (1993). The effects of cue level, hypnotizability and state instruction on responses to leading questions. *International Journal of Clinical and Experimental Hypnosis, 41,* 287–304.

Sheehan, P. W., Grigg, L., & McCann, T. (1984). Memory distortion following exposure to false information in hypnosis. *Journal of Abnormal Psychology, 93,* 259–265.

Sheehan, P. W., & Linton, C. P. (1993). Parameters influencing response to leading questions. *Australian Journal of Clinical and Experimental Hypnosis, 21,* 1–14.

Spanos, N. P., Radtke, H. L., Hodgins, D. C., Bertrand, L. D., & Stam, H. J. (1981). *The Carleton University Responsiveness to Suggestion Scale.* Unpublished manuscript, Carleton University, Ottawa, Canada.

Spanos, N. P., Radtke, H. L., Hodgins, D. C., Bertrand, L. D., Stam, H. J., & Dubreuil, D. L. (1983). The Carleton University Responsiveness to Suggestion Scale: Stability, reliability, and relationships with expectancy and "hypnotic experiences." *Psychological Reports, 53,* 555–563.

Spanos, N. P., Radtke, H. L., Hodgins, D. C., Bertrand, L. D., Stam, H. J., & Moretti, P. (1983). The Carleton University Responsiveness to Suggestion Scale: Relationship with other measures of hypnotic susceptibility, expectancies, and absorption. *Psychological Reports, 53,* 723–734.

Watson, D., Clark, L., & Tellegen, A. (1988). Development and validation of brief measures of positive and negative affect: The PANAS Scales. *Journal of Personality and Social Psychology, 54,* 1063–1070.

Zelig, M., & Beidleman, W. B. (1981). The investigative use of hypnosis: A word of caution. *International Journal of Clinical and Experimental Hypnosis, 29,* 401–412.

Received February 19, 2001
Revision received November 8, 2001
Accepted November 9, 2001 ■

Name Index

For Product Safety Concerns and Information please contact our EU representative GPSR@taylorandfrancis.com Taylor & Francis Verlag GmbH, Kaufingerstraße 24, 80331 München, Germany

Printed and bound by CPI Group (UK) Ltd, Croydon, CR0 4YY
11/06/2025
01899267-0001